Communications in Computer and Information Science 2830

Rationale
The CCIS series is devoted to the publication of proceedings of computer science conferences. Its aim is to efficiently disseminate original research results in informatics in printed and electronic form. While the focus is on publication of peer-reviewed full papers presenting mature work, inclusion of reviewed short papers reporting on work in progress is welcome, too. Besides globally relevant meetings with internationally representative program committees guaranteeing a strict peer-reviewing and paper selection process, conferences run by societies or of high regional or national relevance are also considered for publication.

Topics
The topical scope of CCIS spans the entire spectrum of informatics ranging from foundational topics in the theory of computing to information and communications science and technology and a broad variety of interdisciplinary application fields.

Information for Volume Editors and Authors
Publication in CCIS is free of charge. No royalties are paid, however, we offer registered conference participants temporary free access to the online version of the conference proceedings on SpringerLink (http://link.springer.com) by means of an http referrer from the conference website and/or a number of complimentary printed copies, as specified in the official acceptance email of the event.

CCIS proceedings can be published in time for distribution at conferences or as post-proceedings, and delivered in the form of printed books and/or electronically as USBs and/or e-content licenses for accessing proceedings at SpringerLink. Furthermore, CCIS proceedings are included in the CCIS electronic book series hosted in the SpringerLink digital library at http://link.springer.com/bookseries/7899. Conferences publishing in CCIS are allowed to use our online conference service (Meteor) for managing the whole proceedings lifecycle (from submission and reviewing to preparing for publication) free of charge.

Publication process
The language of publication is exclusively English. Authors publishing in CCIS have to sign the Springer CCIS copyright transfer form, however, they are free to use their material published in CCIS for substantially changed, more elaborate subsequent publications elsewhere. For the preparation of the camera-ready papers/files, authors have to strictly adhere to the Springer CCIS Authors' Instructions and are strongly encouraged to use the CCIS LaTeX style files or templates.

Abstracting/Indexing
CCIS is abstracted/indexed in DBLP, Google Scholar, EI-Compendex, Mathematical Reviews, SCImago, Scopus. CCIS volumes are also submitted for the inclusion in ISI Proceedings.

How to start
To start the evaluation of your proposal for inclusion in the CCIS series, please send an e-mail to ccis@springer.com

Pierangela Bruno · Francesco Calimeri ·
Francesco Cauteruccio · Mauro Dragoni ·
Fabio Stella · Giorgio Terracina
Editors

Artificial Intelligence for Healthcare, and Hybrid Models for Coupling Deductive and Inductive Reasoning

First International Joint Conference, HC@AIxIA+HYDRA 2025
Bologna, Italy, October 25–26, 2025
Proceedings

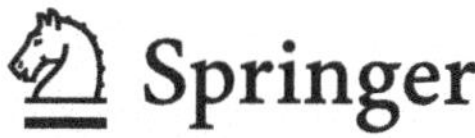
Springer

Editors
Pierangela Bruno
University of Calabria
Rende, Italy

Francesco Calimeri
University of Calabria
Rende, Italy

Francesco Cauteruccio
University of Salerno
Fisciano, Italy

Mauro Dragoni
Fondazione Bruno Kessler
Povo, Trento, Italy

Fabio Stella
Università degli Studi di Milano-Bicocca
Milan, Italy

Giorgio Terracina
University of Calabria
Rende, Italy

ISSN 1865-0929 ISSN 1865-0937 (electronic)
Communications in Computer and Information Science
ISBN 978-3-032-16707-1 ISBN 978-3-032-16708-8 (eBook)
https://doi.org/10.1007/978-3-032-16708-8

This Springer imprint is published by the registered company Springer Nature Switzerland AG
The registered company address is: Gewerbestrasse 11, 6330 Cham, Switzerland

Preface

This volume contains a collection of revised selected papers presented at the 4th International Joint Workshop of Artificial Intelligence for Healthcare (HC@AIxIA) and Hybrid Models for Coupling Deductive and Inductive Reasoning (HYDRA), held in Bologna, Italy, during October 25–26, 2025 and co-located with the 28th European Conference on Artificial Intelligence (ECAI). HC@AIxIA+HYDRA 2025 was jointly organized by the University of Calabria, University of Milano-Bicocca, Fondazione Bruno Kessler, and University of Salerno.

In a rapidly evolving world where AI is increasingly embedded in critical sectors, integrating advanced reasoning methods into practical applications not only enhances technological capabilities but also addresses pressing societal challenges, making this integration both useful and profoundly interesting. The joint HYDRA and HC@AIxIA workshop provides a unique platform for exploring the intersection of foundational AI research and practical applications across multiple domains. It also brings together the research themes of hybrid deductive-inductive reasoning in artificial intelligence (HYDRA) and the application of AI in healthcare (HC@AIxIA). By exploring the synergies between advanced reasoning methods and their application across diverse domains, including but not limited to healthcare, the workshop aims to foster interdisciplinary collaboration and innovation.

The workshop welcomed original research contributions, summaries of recent work, and work-in-progress studies on frameworks, applications, and methodologies for combining deductive and inductive approaches. It invites a wide multidisciplinary spectrum of researchers, industrialists, entrepreneurs, and healthcare practitioners: submissions were welcomed from a range of stakeholders, including computer scientists, health informaticians, and emergency medicine experts; public health experts, epidemiologists, clinicians, etc.; national and international public health agencies; epidemic intelligence systems providers; NGOs and agencies; industry and startups. Collaborations across disciplines bridged the gap between theory and practice and fostered actionable AI-driven solutions across diverse domains.

The content of this volume is related to the following subjects:

- Hybrid inductive-deductive approaches to AI
- Integration of logic programming paradigms (e.g., ASP, CSP) in inductive scenarios
- New methods for combining deductive and inductive systems
- Knowledge representation and reasoning to enhance inductive processes
- Evaluation of Hybrid Reasoning Methods
- Ethical and social implications of hybrid AI systems
- Knowledge representation and formal reasoning in healthcare
- Probabilistic graphical models and causal networks for clinical decision-making
- Personalized medicine and computer-interpretable clinical guidelines
- Ethical and legal considerations in medical AI
- Machine learning methods, data mining, and statistical methods for clinical decision support

- Learning, representation, and reasoning with time
- Methods for diagnosis, treatment selection, treatment planning, and prognosis
- Monitoring patients in healthcare
- Ontologies and medical vocabularies
- Support for natural language generation/understanding in connection with electronic patient records
- Deductive and inductive systems in eHealth scenarios
- Tools for supporting authoring, execution, and maintenance of clinical protocols and guidelines
- Tools for building and deployment of clinical decision-support systems.

The HC@AIxIA+HYDRA 2025 conference gathered 61 submissions from authors from 20 different countries. From these, 40 high-quality papers were accepted and presented during the workshop. All submissions underwent a rigorous double-blind peer-review process with 4 reviews per submission. The current volume contains 40 papers which were selected by the Program Committee for the Springer post-proceedings.

All the papers selected for the post-proceedings volume are given in the form presented by the authors. These papers are of interest to everyone working in the field of artificial intelligence, data science, and healthcare.

We thank all the authors for their interest in HC@AIxIA+HYDRA 2025, the members of the Program Committee for their contributions, and the reviewers for their peer-reviewing efforts.

November 2025

Pierangela Bruno
Francesco Calimeri
Francesco Cauteruccio
Mauro Dragoni
Fabio Stella
Giorgio Terracina

Organization

Workshop Chairs

Pierangela Bruno	University of Calabria, Italy
Francesco Calimeri	University of Calabria, Italy
Francesco Cauteruccio	University of Salerno, Italy
Mauro Dragoni	Fondazione Bruno Kessler, Italy
Fabio Stella	Università degli Studi di Milano - Bicocca, Italy
Giorgio Terracina	University of Calabria, Italy

Program Committee

Mario Alviano	University of Calabria, Italy
Alessia Amelio	University G. d'Annunzio Chieti–Pescara, Italy
Luca Anselma	Università di Torino, Italy
Gianluca Apriceno	Fondazione Bruno Kessler, Italy
Simone Bartucci	Università della Calabria, Italy
Riccardo Bellazzi	University of Pavia, Italy
Francesco Bellocchio	Fresenius Medical Care, Italy
Paola Berchialla	University of Turin, Italy
Alice Bernasconi	Fondazione IRCCS Istituto Nazionale dei Tumori, Italy
Alessio Bottrighi	University of Eastern Piedmont, Italy
Andreas Brännström	Umeå University, Sweden
Andrea Brunello	University of Udine, Italy
Luciano Caroprese	University "G. d'Annunzio" of Chieti-Pescara, Italy
Paola Cavalcante	Fondazione IRCCS Istituto Neurologico Carlo Besta, Italy
Davide Chicco	Università di Milano-Bicocca, Italy
Stefano Cirillo	University of Salerno, Italy
Marco Colussi	University of Milan, Italy
Richard Comploi-Taupe	Siemens, Austria
Anthony Constantinou	Queen Mary University of London, UK
Erica Coppolillo	University of Calabria, Italy
Stefania Costantini	University of L'Aquila, Italy
Alessandro Dal Palù	University of Parma, Italy

Edoardo De Rose	University of Calabria, Italy
Luigi Di Biasi	University of Salerno, Italy
Carmine Dodaro	University of Calabria, Italy
Jonas Ehrhardt	Helmut Schmidt University, Germany
Esra Erdem	Sabanci University, TR
Grazia Ferrara	University of Salerno, Italy
Zini Floriano	Free University of Bozen-Bolzano, Italy
Francesca Gasparini	Università Milano-Bicocca, Italy
Daniele Germano	Sapienza University of Rome, Italy
René Heesch	Helmut Schmidt University, Germany
Giovambattista Ianni	Università della Calabria, Italy
Antonio Ielo	Università della Calabria, Italy
Alberto Lavelli	Fondazione Bruno Kessler, Italy
Fabrizio Lo Scudo	University of Calabria, Italy
Peter Lucas	Radboud University Nijmegen, Netherlands
Marco Maratea	University of Calabria, Italy
Cinzia Marte	University of Calabria, Italy
Giuseppe Mazzotta	University of Calabria, Italy
Giovanni Melissari	DLVSystem, Italy
Lucia Migliorelli	Università Politecnica Delle Marche, Italy
Sara Moccia	Università degli Studi "G. d'Annunzio" Chieti – Pescara, Italy
Sara Montagna	Università degli Studi di Urbino Carlo Bo, Italy
Stefania Montani	Università del Piemonte Orientale, Italy
Brais Muñiz Castro	University of Coruña, Spain
Giovanna Nicora	Università degli Studi di Pavia, Italy
Rafael Peñaloza	University of Milano-Bicocca, Italy
Pierpaolo Pierpaolo	University of Glasgow, UK
Luigi Portinale	Università del Piemonte Orientale, Italy
Alessandro Quarta	University of Calabria, Italy
Daniele Radicioni	University of Turin, Italy
Marta Ranzini	Humanitas Research Hospital, Italy
Fabio Rinaldi	IDSIA USI-SUPSI, Switzerland
Niccolò Rocchi	University of Milano-Bicocca, Italy
Luca Romeo	University of Macerata, Italy
Lucia Sacchi	University of Pavia, Italy
Nicola Saccomanno	University of Udine, Italy
Leonardo Sanna	Fondazione Bruno Kessler - FBK, Italy
Marco Scutari	IDSIA, Switzerland
Alberto Signoroni	University of Brescia, Italy
Christel Sirocchi	Friedrich-Alexander-Universität Erlangen-Nürnberg, Germany

Contents

Rehabilitation & Human-Robot Interaction

Differentially Private Fine-Tuning of Self-Supervised Learning Models for Human Activity Recognition on Wearables 3
Oktay Ozan Güner, Sergio Consoli, Vicenç Gómez, and Mario Ceresa

Using Multi-modal Generative Models for Creating Speech Therapy Material 21
Mihir Mulye, Stefan Conrad, and Stefan Knecht

AI for Diagnosis & Medical Imaging

MultiH-EU: An AI-Driven Decision Support System for Multi-disease Diagnosis 37
Diogen Babuc and Teodor-Florin Fortiş

RAG-Enhanced LLMs for Interactive Explainability in Clinical Decision Support Systems 50
Lorenzo Mannocci, Francesca Naretto, Lucia Passaro, and Anna Monreale

KaiMed: A Hybrid Multi-Agent AI Platform for Clinical Reasoning and Cross-Specialty Discovery 64
Francesco Barbato, Filippo Sorichetti, Emanuele Ielo, and Lorenzo Megliola

Comparing Different Positional Encodings for the Interpretation of Medical Images 78
Andrea Santomauro, Giorgio Leonardi, and Luigi Portinale

Short Communications

Designing a Multimodal Dataset for AI-Based Prognosis in STEMI 93
Simone Bartucci, Edoardo De Rose, Alessandro Quarta, Rossella Quarta, Alessia Donata Camarda, Alberto Polimeni, and Francesco Calimeri

Automatic Explainable Progress Prediction of Wet Age-Related Macular Degeneration 99
Riccardo Fidanza, Daniele Meli, and Emilia Maggio

Explaining Medical Time Series Classification Through Boundary-Aware Feature Analysis 105
Christel Sirocchi and Damiano Verda

A Logic-Based Framework for Inferring Medical Events (Extended Abstract) 120
Yvon K. Awuklu, Meghyn Bienvenu, Katsumi Inoue, Vianney Jouhet, and Fleur Mougin

When ‘Scarce’ Becomes ‘*Too* Scarce’: The Rare Diseases Drama 126
Alice Bernasconi, Federico Pirola, Alessio Zanga, and Antonio Balordi

Application of Nonlinear Autoregressive Neural Network for Prediction of HIV Infections in Poland 132
Marek Landowski and Anna Landowska

SEDformer: Path Signatures and Transformers to Predict Newborns Movement Symmetry 138
Philippe Rambaud, Arpad Rimmel, Imen Trabelsi, Justine Zini, Alexandra Wodecki, Emmanuelle Motte Signoret, François Jouen, Joanna Tomasik, and Jean Bergounioux

LLM-Assisted Conformance Checking for Medical Processes 152
Giorgio Leonardi, Stefania Montani, and Manuel Striani

Temporal Data Modeling and Analysis

LUME-DBN: Full Bayesian Learning of DBNs from Incomplete Data in Intensive Care 167
Federico Pirola, Fabio Stella, and Marco Grzegorczyk

Using Temporal Features to Improve Accuracy in Multivariate Pattern Analysis (MVPA) of M/EEG Data 182
Fatemeh Barazesh Morgani, Erin Goddard, and Gustavo Batista

Relevance-Aware Thresholding in Online Conformal Prediction for Time Series 196
Théo Dupuy, Binbin Xu, Stéphane Perrey, Jacky Montmain, and Abdelhak Imoussaten

Hidden Rhythms: an Embedding Framework for Downstream Tasks Validated on ECG Data ... 218
Simone Bartucci, Edoardo De Rose, Francesca Filice, Francesco Calimeri, and Simona Perri

Generating Patient Cohorts from Electronic Health Records Using Two-Step Retrieval-Augmented Text-to-SQL Generation ... 231
Angelo Ziletti and Leonardo D'Ambrosi

Which Metadata Matters? Evaluating Predictive Features for Environmental Time Series ... 243
Ann-Kathrin Dörr, Tina Schmidt, Jens Schoth, Ivana Kraiselburd, and Folker Meyer

Causal Modeling and Data Reasoning

An Automatic Alignment Strategy for Medical Ontologies: the MedPix 2.0 Case Study ... 257
Luigi Colucci Cante, Mariangela Graziano, Irene Siragusa, Beniamino Di Martino, and Roberto Pirrone

Learning a Causal Model for Intracranial Pressure in Patients with Traumatic Brain Injury ... 270
Alessio Zanga, Francesca Graziano, Giuseppe Citerio, Paola Rebora, Stefania Galiberti, Shubhayu Bhattacharyay, David K. Menon, Ewout W. Steyerberg, and Fabio Stella

Survival Hidden Markov Model ... 283
Alessandro Bregoli, Francesco Bellocchio, Luca Neri, and Fabio Stella

An Approach Leveraging Deep Learning and Stream Reasoning for Dynamic Task Assignments Balancing Productivity and Well Being ... 296
Luca Laboccetta, Francesco Calimeri, Davide Iacopino, Salvatore Iiritano, Marta Maria, Simona Perri, Massimiliano Ruffolo, and Giorgio Terracina

Machine Learning and Statistical Insights Into Hospital Stay Durations: The Italian Healthcare Administrative Data Case ... 308
Marina Andrić and Mauro Dragoni

Patient management

Depth Sensor Based AI-Services for Nursing Homes ... 323
Rinu Elizabeth Paul, Lucas Deichsel, and Tanja Schultz

A Hybrid Inductive-Deductive Approach for Resource-Efficient Suicide Risk Detection in Counseling Conversations 336
Ron Franco, Avi Segal, and Kobi Gal

Triage Discrimination: Myth or Reality? 352
Justin Armanini and Fabio Stella

Neuro-symbolic and Multi-modal Learning

Expert-Guided POMDP Learning for Data-Efficient Modeling in Healthcare 369
Marco Locatelli, Arjen Hommersom, Roberto Clemens Cerioli, Daniela Besozzi, and Fabio Stella

A Hybrid Evolutionary Fuzzy Neural Approach for Maternal Health Risk Prediction 384
Gianluca Apriceno, Marina Segala, Giovanni Valer, Nicola Muraro, Vincenzo Netti, Paulo Vitor de Campos Souza, and Mauro Dragoni

Multi-view Multi-instance Learning for Health Recovery Monitoring in Older Adults 398
Veselka Boeva, Alexander J. O. Ojutkangas, and Shahrooz Abghari

An LBBD Approach for Solving the Chemotherapy Treatment Scheduling Problem 412
Simone Caruso, Carmine Dodaro, Marco Maratea, Cinzia Marte, and Marco Mochi

Large Language Models in Healthcare

Automated Machine Learning to Enhance Knowledge Retrieval in Retrieval-Augmented Generation Pipelines 429
Matteo Magnini, Gianluca Aguzzi, Leonardo Sanna, Simone Magnolini, Patrizio Bellan, Mauro Dragoni, and Sara Montagna

Exploring Large Language Models as Digital Health Coaches: A Role-Play Approach to Brief Action Planning 441
Marco Bolpagni, Leonardo Sanna, Simone De Carli, Silvia Gabrielli, and Mauro Dragoni

Assessing Temporal Reasoning of Large Language Models on Structured Temporal Clinical Data 453
Gianluca Apriceno, Tania Bailoni, and Mauro Dragoni

Unified Peripartum Database with Natural-Language-to-SQL Capabilities at Udine University Hospital: Design and Prototype 467
Doriana Armenise, Ginevra Battello, Andrea Brunello, Lorenza Driul, Angelo Montanari, Elisa Rizzante, Nicola Saccomanno, Andrea Salvador, Serena Xodo, and Silvia Zermano

Are We Ready for Multi-agent Systems to Deliver Structured Mental Health Support? Lessons from Adapting Self-Help+ Intervention 481
Leonardo Sanna, Marco Bolpagni, Valentina Fietta, Simone De Carli, Mattia Franzin, Giorgia Gavioli, Lorenzo Gios, Susanna Pardini, Anna Elena Nicoletti, Silvia Rizzi, Silvia Gabrielli, and Mauro Dragoni

Healthcare applications

Query Carefully: Detecting the Unanswerables in Text-to-SQL Tasks 497
Jasmin Saxer, Isabella Maria Aigner, Luise Linzmeier, Andreas Weiler, and Kurt Stockinger

Multi-agent Dynamic Resource Allocation: A Reinforcement Learning Approach 510
Stefania Costantini, Giovanni De Gasperisù, Pasquale De Meo, Francesco Gullo, and Alessandro Provetti

Author Index 523

Rehabilitation & Human-Robot Interaction

Differentially Private Fine-Tuning of Self-Supervised Learning Models for Human Activity Recognition on Wearables

Oktay Ozan Güner[1(✉)], Sergio Consoli[2], Vicenç Gómez[1], and Mario Ceresa[2]

[1] Universitat Pompeu Fabra, Barcelona, Spain
oktayozan.guner01@estudiant.upf.edu, vicen.gomez@upf.edu
[2] European Commission, Joint Research Centre (DG JRC), Ispra, Italy
sergio.consoli@ec.europa.eu, mario.ceresa@ec.europa.eu

Abstract. The surge in wearable technology for health has advanced personalized Human Activity Recognition (HAR), yet introduces privacy concerns under EU regulations such as the GDPR, the AI Act and the European Health Data Space (EHDS). This paper examines fine-tuning approaches for self-supervised models on wearable data, using Differentially Private Stochastic Gradient Descent (DP-SGD) to balance privacy and utility. Using the PAMAP2 dataset and the HarNet10 model, we compare classifier head and full model fine-tuning. Our results show that tuning only the classifier head (4.83% of parameters) preserves higher accuracy and F1-scores while significantly reducing vulnerability to membership inference attacks compared to non-private baselines. This strategy provides a lightweight and regulation-compliant framework for privacy-preserving HAR on wearables.

Keywords: Wearable Technology · Human Activity Recognition · Differential Privacy · Fine-Tuning · Privacy-Utility Trade-off

1 Introduction

The advancement of wearable technologies fundamentally transforms personal health monitoring [27]. As wearables spread among increasingly larger populations, they offer substantial benefits, including tracking physical activity, heart rate, and sleep patterns. This enables AI-driven applications to provide personalized fitness recommendations, monitor health metrics and even warn users of injury risks by leveraging personalized models [19]. However, the collection of sensitive data at scale introduces significant security and privacy concerns.

Deep learning techniques [13,17,34], such as CNN/LSTM variants, have become the dominant approach for sensor-based human activity recognition (HAR) to learn spatio-temporal features directly from raw data and generally

P. Bruno et al. (Eds.): HC_AIxIA_HYDRA 2025, CCIS 2830, pp. 3–20, 2026.
https://doi.org/10.1007/978-3-032-16708-8_1

outperforming classical machine learning methods [20]. Architectural improvements have further enhanced feature extraction and, in some cases, computational efficiency through mechanisms such as attention and modality transfer [2,12]. More recently, self-supervised learning (SSL) has allowed researchers to pre-train foundation models for wearables, alleviating the scarcity of labeled data. These models can then be adapted to downstream tasks with minimal supervision, showing strong domain and modality transfer [11,33]. Although vision-based privacy-preserving methods using low-resolution imagery exist for HAR tasks [25,29], their deployment remains challenging, while sensor-based systems that replace sensitive features with non-sensitive ones provide empirical privacy against user re-identification [14].

Despite these advances, most studies lack the formal privacy guarantees. Within the European Union (EU), privacy concerns are addressed by a stringent regulatory landscape. The General Data Protection Regulation (GDPR)[1] sets strict rules for processing personal data. In addition, the AI Act[2] categorizes AI use cases into high, medium, and low risk, aiming to mitigate risks associated with AI technologies. The European Health Data Space (EHDS)[3] seeks to create a unified framework that empowers individuals with greater control over their health information for primary and secondary use, enhancing transparency and trust in data handling practices. To comply with these regulations, researchers have turned to privacy-preserving techniques such as Federated Learning (FL) [9], which offers a promising approach by training models on decentralized data sources. However, even when FL is applied, there remains a risk that sensitive data can be partially or fully reconstructed from the shared model updates through model-inversion attacks. Thus, malicious third parties could extract sensitive information from the data [3]. To mitigate such sensitive information leaks, Differential Privacy (DP) [1,7,10] is recommended as an additional layer of protection [3]. DP injects calibrated noise into the data or gradients during training, which obscures the contribution of any single data point and thus lowers the risk of reconstruction. However, this protection introduces a trade-off, as the noise required for privacy can significantly reduce model performance and computational efficiency [3]. Exploring various options and scenarios to find an acceptable privacy-utility trade-off is crucial, yet it remains a significant challenge. This allows stakeholders to make informed decisions based on their specific privacy requirements and utility goals.

This paper explores the impact of fine-tuning strategies on the privacy-utility trade-off for HAR on wearable devices, to address the gap between state-of-the-art models and individuals' privacy guarantees. We show that updating only a small fraction of a self-supervised foundation model (HarNet10) [33] with Dif-

[1] European Union Regulation, EU 2016/679 (General Data Protection Regulation): https://eur-lex.europa.eu/eli/reg/2016/679/oj/eng.

[2] European Union Regulation, EU 2024/1689 (Artificial Intelligence Act): https://eur-lex.europa.eu/eli/reg/2024/1689/oj/eng.

[3] European Union Regulation, EU 2025/327 (European Health Data Space): https://eur-lex.europa.eu/eli/reg/2025/327/oj/eng.

ferentially Private Stochastic Gradient Descent (DP-SGD) [1,4,26] can provide strong privacy guarantees while maintaining high model utility.

Our study is guided by the following research questions:

RQ1: What is the utility loss of applying gradient perturbation to different fine-tuning strategies?
RQ2: Does the theoretical privacy guarantee of gradient perturbation align with empirical privacy against membership inference attacks in a real-life scenario?
RQ3: Which fine-tuning strategy offers a better balance between privacy and model utility for the HAR task?

Two sequential experiments are designed[4], as described below, to address the research questions:

1. **Privacy–Utility Trade-Off (Experiment 1):** comparison of two fine-tuning strategies through a comprehensive analysis of their utility loss under identical DP settings.
2. **Empirical Resilience (Experiment 2):** simulation of a membership inference attack to evaluate whether the theoretical privacy guarantee of the best fine-tuning strategy translates into practical resilience when compared to its non-private baseline.

The rest of the paper is structured as follows. In Sect. 2, we describe the dataset and the preprocessing steps. Section 3 details the differentially private fine-tuning strategies, while Sect. 4 presents our experimental setup and evaluation protocol. Section 5 discusses the empirical findings, emphasizing the privacy–utility trade-offs revealed by our experiments. Finally, Sect. 6 summarizes our main results and limitations, offering suggestions for future research.

2 Datasets and Preprocessing

We used the PAMAP2 Physical Activity Monitoring dataset [23], publicly available in the UCI Machine Learning Repository. It contains wearable sensor data from nine subjects (eight male, one female) who performed 18 physical activities recorded by three inertial measurement units (IMUs) placed on key body parts[5]. Each subject followed a protocol of 12 core and six optional activities, yielding more than 10 h of data per participant [24].

To ensure a balanced and comparable benchmark for the fine-tuning strategies, we restricted the analysis to the eight most widely performed of the 12 core activities: lying, ironing, sitting, vacuum cleaning, walking, standing, ascending stairs, and descending stairs. Only subject 109 was excluded, as it did not perform all eight activities. We retained only the well-calibrated 16g accelerometer

[4] https://github.com/oozanguner/dpsgd-finetuning-harnet.

[5] The dataset comprises synthetic data and does not involve real patient or citizen data. It is designed for research purposes only and does not reflect actual individual activities or personal information.

axes from the hand-worn IMU, consistent with the modality used in pre-training the foundation model (HarNet10), and discarded the 6g channel. After time-ordering and imputing missing data via linear interpolation, the signals were downsampled from 100 Hz to 30 Hz and segmented into 10-second windows with 50% overlap. Windows dominated by transient activities (activity ID 0) for more than half their duration were discarded. The remaining were assigned a single activity label based on the activity class that appears most often within each window.

This preprocessing yielded a total of 2,887 samples across all subjects. The dataset was well balanced, with each subject contributing between 345 and 379 samples, providing a reliable basis for the fine-tuning experiments.

3 Methods

3.1 Pre-trained Model and Fine-Tuning Strategies

In this study, we adopted the open-source HarNet10 foundation model, which is based on an 18-layer ResNet-V2 architecture with one-dimensional convolutions treated as a common feature extractor [33]. The model was pre-trained using multi-task SSL on the UK-Biobank dataset, which contains over 700k person-days of unlabeled data from wrist-worn accelerometers [33]. The SSL tasks that shared the same feature extractor, including Arrow of Time, Permutation and Time Warping, yielded a 1024-dimensional feature vector [33]. For downstream applications, the architecture was designed to have an additional fully-connected layer with 512 units placed between the feature extractor and the final classification layer [33]. We investigated two fine-tuning strategies on the PAMAP2 dataset: (i) classifier head fine-tuning, freezing the feature extractor layers and updating only the final classifier layers (4.83% of parameters), and (ii) full model fine-tuning, in which all 10 million parameters of the model were updated [33].

3.2 Differential Privacy via Gradient Perturbation (DP-SGD)

Differential Privacy [1,8] provides a rigorous framework to ensure that the outcome of an algorithm does not substantially change when any single individual's data is added or removed. The privacy guarantee is controlled by two parameters: ε, the privacy budget, and δ, the probability that the guarantee may fail.

Formally, a randomized algorithm $\mathcal{M} : \mathcal{D} \rightarrow \mathcal{R}$ with domain $\mathcal{D}$ and range $\mathcal{R}$ is said to be (ε, δ)-differentially private if

$$\Pr[\mathcal{M}(d) \in S] \leq e^{\varepsilon} \Pr[\mathcal{M}(d') \in S] + \delta, \tag{1}$$

for all datasets $d, d' \in \mathcal{D}$ differing in at most one record and for all measurable subsets $S \subseteq \mathcal{R}$, where ε is the privacy budget and δ the failure probability, with $\varepsilon \geq 0$ and $0 \leq \delta \leq 1$ [1].

To enforce this guarantee during optimization, Differentially Private Stochastic Gradient Descent (DP-SGD) [1] clips the ℓ_2-norm of each per-sample gradient to a fixed bound and adds calibrated Gaussian noise to the aggregated gradient. The update rule for the model parameters θ at step t is:

$$\theta_{t+1} = \theta_t - \eta_t \tilde{g}_t, \qquad \tilde{g}_t = \frac{1}{L}\left(\sum_{i \in L_t} \bar{g}_t(x_i) + \mathcal{N}(0, \sigma^2 C^2 I)\right), \tag{2}$$

where $\bar{g}_t(x_i)$ is the clipped gradient of sample x_i, L the batch size, L_t the mini-batch at step t, C the clipping bound, σ the noise scale, and η_t the learning rate.

We used Opacus [32] to implement DP-SGD through vectorized operations, which enabled efficient computation. Because this procedure repeats over many steps, the privacy budget ε accumulates over training epochs, resulting in a privacy guarantee (ε, δ) [1]. Opacus also validates DP compatibility and disallows batch-dependent layers that would break per-sample gradients [32]. Therefore, HarNet10's BatchNorm layers were replaced with GroupNorm [30] to remain batch-independent. Instead of normalizing over the batch dimension, GroupNorm divides each sample channel into groups and normalizes within each group independently of other samples in a batch. Thus, by avoiding the mixing of information across samples, it demonstrates stable and often superior performance with small batch sizes while yielding comparable results with typical batch sizes like 32, 16, compared to BatchNorm [30]. To assess the sensitivity of the privacy budget (ε) to the noise scale (σ), we fixed the clipping bound at $C = 1$ and fine-tuned the model with $\sigma \in \{1, 5, 10\}$. The default privacy accountant (PRVAccountant) in Opacus was used to track the cumulative privacy budget (ε) over training steps [32], with a fixed failure probability $\delta = 10^{-5}$ [1]. This setup enabled us to quantify the trade-off between noise level and model utility at each training step.

4 Experimental Design and Settings

Concerning the model fine-tuning setup, we used a batch size of 32 and an initial learning rate of 10^{-3}, combined with adaptive scheduling. We then minimized cross-entropy loss using the AdamW optimizer (weight decay=0.01) to provide effective regularization and prevent overfitting. To help prevent overfitting, we also applied an early stopping criterion based on the validation loss, with a patience of 10 epochs, and set a maximum of 20 training epochs as an upper bound rather than using a fixed number of epochs. Furthermore, ReduceLROnPlateau was employed as a learning rate scheduler that reduces the learning rate by a factor of 0.1 when the validation loss stopped improving for 3 consecutive epochs.

In Experiment 1, we fine-tuned the foundation model with both fine-tuning strategies using the DP parameters (σ, C, and δ) to identify the best strategy for subsequent experiments. In Experiment 2, only the winning strategy and its non-private counterpart were fine-tuned as target models to assess resilience against an adversary. Their non-private baselines were also trained to enable utility loss comparison. In the following we describe the two sequential experiments that we have carried out to evaluate privacy-utility trade-off when adapting the self-supervised foundation model to a sensor-based HAR task.

4.1 Experiment 1: Privacy-Utility Assessment

We adopted two nested, subject-wise stratified group K-fold schemes to split the subjects into training, validation, and test sets while ensuring a balanced distribution of activity labels [6,33]. This setup was chosen to avoid data leakage across subjects. Before training, all samples were standardized to zero mean and unit variance on the training set of each inner fold, and the resulting scaler was applied unchanged to the corresponding validation and test sets. In the outer loop ($K = 4$), two subjects were withheld for testing in each fold, while in the inner loop ($K = 3$), the best epoch was selected using two validation subjects from the remaining six. We computed test accuracy and macro-F1 [18] for both fine-tuning strategies and their non-private counterparts, and then calculated utility loss from these metrics to quantify the degradation of each strategy relative to its non-private baseline. To test whether the strategies differed significantly, we applied a two-tailed paired t-test [16] to the differences in performance metrics (accuracy and macro-F1) measured on the test sets of the outer loop. For each metric, we assessed the normality of the paired differences using the Shapiro-Wilk test [22]. If normality was confirmed, we used the paired t-test, otherwise the Wilcoxon signed-rank test ($\alpha = 0.05$) [16]. We also reported Cohen's d [28] to assess the practical importance of the results. This analysis determined which fine-tuning strategy was carried forward to Experiment 2 to evaluate its resilience against a real-life adversary.

4.2 Experiment 2: Empirical Privacy via Membership Inference Attack

Following the procedure of Rahman et al. [21], we attacked the selected DP strategy from Experiment 1 and its non-private counterpart, using them as target models (Fig. 1). A hold-two-subject-out cross-validation scheme was applied, excluding Subjects 102 and 103 from fine-tuning. The remaining subjects were trained using three-fold cross-validation to select the best-performing model, which was then tested on Subjects 102 and 103. All samples from the training subjects were labeled as members, and those from the test subjects as non-members, serving as the ground-truth membership labels.

To train an effective adversary, we first built five non-private shadow models with the same architecture and hyperparameters as the target models, using data only from the held-out subjects in a subject-wise split (Subject 102 for shadow training, Subject 103 for shadow validation). These shadow models were trained on samples not seen by the target models. We then trained an attack model to predict whether a data point was a member or non-member. We used the XGBClassifier algorithm [5] for its effectiveness in handling noisy data, typical of membership inference tasks, and its computational efficiency [31]. The attack

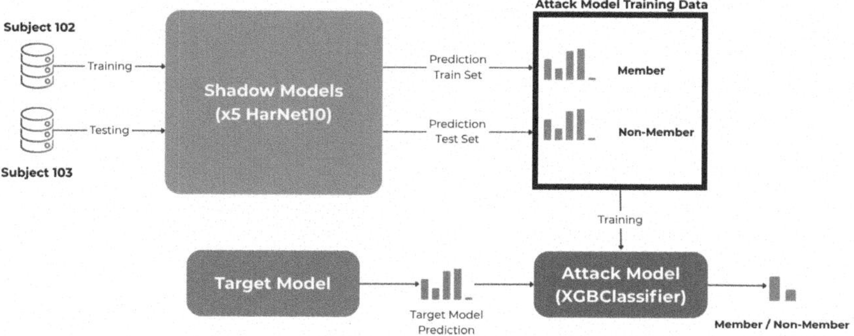

Fig. 1. Membership inference pipeline: five shadow models with the HarNet10 architecture produce probability vectors labeled Member/Non-Member to train an XGBClassifier attacker, which then predicts membership from the target model's probabilities.

model was trained on the probability vectors (eight activities) produced by the shadow models for their member and non-member sets. It was configured with a learning rate of 10^{-1}, 200 boosting rounds, a maximum tree depth of 6, and early stopping after 10 rounds. Finally, we evaluated attack success on the target models using ROC-AUC [15], computed from the true positive rate (TPR) versus the false positive rate (FPR) across thresholds. An AUC of 0.5 indicates random guessing (high resilience), while 1.0 indicates high vulnerability. This evaluation assessed whether the theoretical privacy guarantee from Experiment 1 translated into practical resilience against a real-life adversary.

5 Results and Discussion

5.1 Privacy-Utility Trade-Off

Figure 2 shows the results for Experiment 1 regarding test accuracy (top) and macro-F1 score (bottom). Horizontal lines denote the non-private fine-tuned models, used as baselines to compute the utility loss under DP-SGD for the two strategies (classifier head vs. full model). These baselines generalized well, with less than 2% gaps between test and validation scores. Specifically, the classifier head strategy achieved $73.5 \pm 1.69\%$ test accuracy and $70.99 \pm 2.32\%$ test macro-F1, while the full model yielded $71.56 \pm 6.67\%$ and $71.04 \pm 6.43\%$, respectively.

For a noise level of $\sigma = 1$, freezing the feature extractor layers (classifier head strategy) preserved more utility than full model fine-tuning. The classifier head achieved $62.33 \pm 5.56\%$ accuracy and $58.18 \pm 6.04\%$ macro-F1, outperforming the full model's $56.88 \pm 6.56\%$ and $45.04 \pm 7.08\%$. As the noise increased, accuracies converged (at $\sigma = 10$: 33.24 vs. 33.49%), but macro-F1 remained higher for the classifier head ($27.37 \pm 3.93\%$ vs. $22.60 \pm 5.09\%$). Table 1 in Appendix A reports detailed results, including mean $\pm$ standard deviation scores from the nested cross-validation (subject-wise), the average epoch of best validation performance, and the final privacy budget (ε) for each experiment.

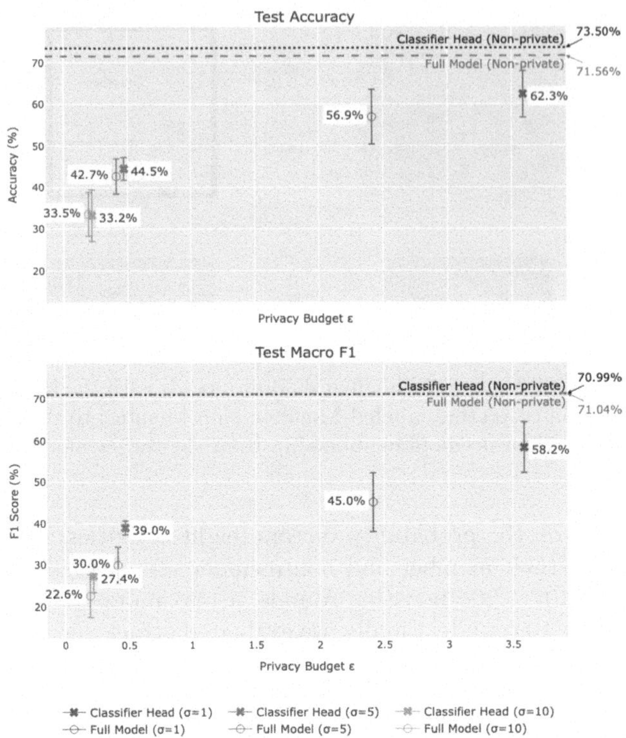

Fig. 2. Test accuracy (top) and macro-F1 score (bottom) with respect to the privacy budget values (ε) for classifier head and full model fine-tuning strategies. Horizontal lines indicate non-private baselines.

The classifier head experiments consumed larger privacy budgets (ε) than the full model variants at the same noise scales (σ), as confirmed by the privacy accountant, because training continued longer before early stopping. For example, at $\sigma = 1$ the classifier head consumed $\varepsilon \approx 3.59$, corresponding to 15.19% utility loss in accuracy, whereas the full model consumed $\varepsilon \approx 2.42$, with 20.51% utility loss (full figures are available in Tables 2–3 in Appendix B). The classifier head incurred less utility loss in both accuracy and macro-F1. The differences were particularly pronounced in macro-F1, with $\sim$ 18.0% utility loss for the classifier head at $\varepsilon \approx 3.59$ versus $\sim$ 36.6% for the full model at $\varepsilon \approx 2.42$.

To validate our findings, we performed the statistical analysis described in Sect. 4.1. At the lowest noise scale ($\sigma = 1$), where utility losses were minimal for both strategies, the paired differences across outer folds ($K = 4$) followed a normal distribution (Shapiro–Wilk test; $p = 0.826$ for accuracy, $p = 0.956$ for macro-F1). The two-tailed paired t-test showed that the classifier head strategy significantly outperformed the full model (62.33% vs. 56.88% for accuracy; 58.18% vs. 45.04% for macro-F1), with $p = 0.019$ for accuracy and $p = 0.004$ for macro-F1. Effect sizes (Cohen's d) were also very large ($d = 2.30$ for accuracy;

$d = 3.95$ for macro-F1). While these results justify advancing the classifier head strategy to Experiment 2, they also clarify its trade-off: although the classifier head is less privacy-efficient than full model fine-tuning (consuming a larger ε per unit of σ), it is more utility-efficient for a given level of privacy protection in our setting, addressing **RQ1**. Our findings also indicate that the classifier head strategy better preserves the task-relevant information learned during pre-training from the noise injected by DP-SGD.

5.2 Empirical Privacy via Membership Inference Attack

Figures 3 and 4 show the accuracy profiles during optimization for the non-private and DP target models, respectively. The non-private target model reached 96.39% mean training accuracy, 74.21% mean validation accuracy, and 72.54% test accuracy. The DP target model reached 73.06% mean training accuracy, 64.43% mean validation accuracy, and 59.22% test accuracy, corresponding to 18.36% utility loss and a final privacy budget of $\varepsilon \approx 4.12$. Detailed epoch-wise training and validation accuracies are reported in Tables 4–5 in Appendix C.

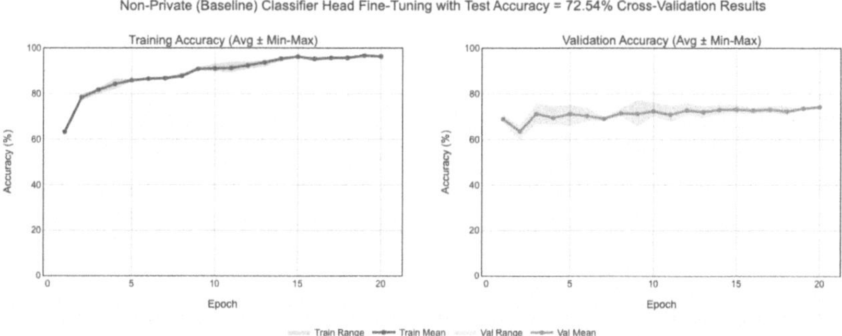

Fig. 3. Training and validation accuracy curves for the non-private target model using classifier head fine-tuning.

In terms of activity prediction, the non-private target model performed well on dynamic activities with repetitive arm motions, such as vacuum cleaning (92.8% recall), walking (86.2%), and ironing (85.1%). Errors mainly arose among activities with similar motion patterns, such as walking, ascending and descending stairs, ironing, and vacuum cleaning, as well as among static postures like lying, sitting, and standing. The DP target model showed lower recalls across classes (e.g., walking 86.2% $\rightarrow$ 74.8%; standing 62.0% $\rightarrow$ 43.5%), and confusion between walking and ascending stairs increased. For instance, 18.7% of walking samples were misclassified as ascending stairs by the DP target model, compared to 11.4% by its non-private counterpart. This suggests that the injected noise disproportionately affects activities that are already difficult to distinguish.

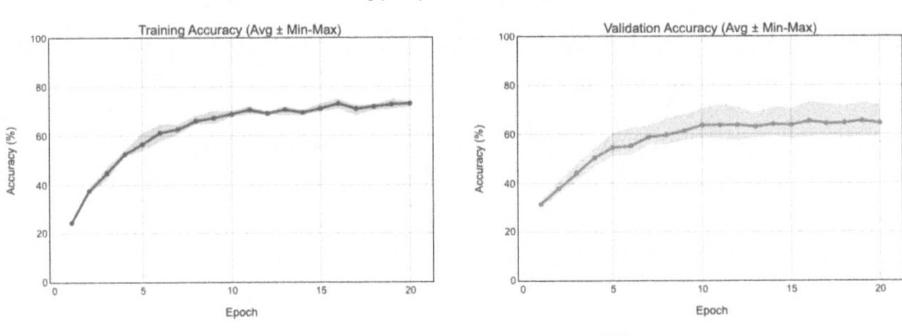

Fig. 4. Training and validation accuracy curves for the DP target model (σ=1) using classifier head fine-tuning.

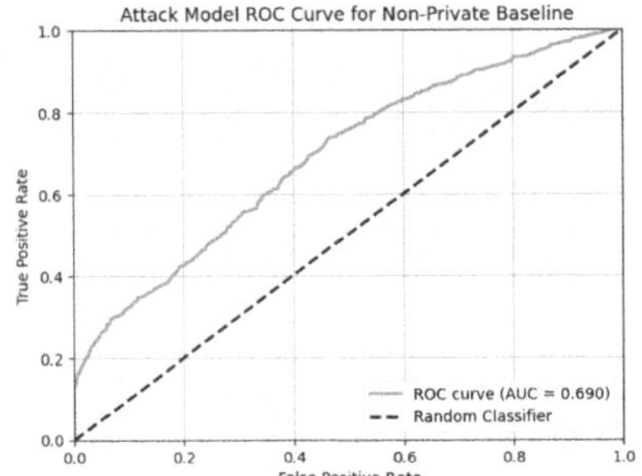

(a) ROC curve for the membership inference attack against the non-private target model.

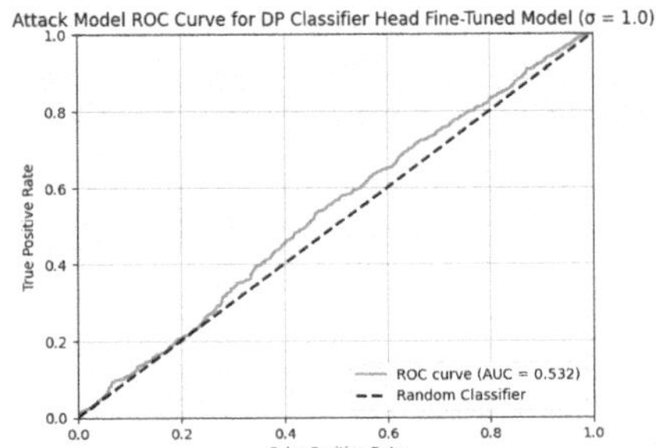

(b) ROC curve for the membership inference attack against the DP target model ($\sigma = 1.0$).

Fig. 5. ROC curves for the membership inference attack: (a) non-private target model; (b) DP target model ($\sigma = 1.0$).

Detailed confusion matrices of both models across all activities are provided in Fig. 6 in Appendix D.

Five non-private shadow models were trained to mimic the behavior of the target models and generate data for training the attack model. They achieved training accuracies ranging from 92.02% to 96.64% and test accuracies from 62.64% to 67.24% on the held-out subject (see Table 6, Appendix E). This performance pattern, consistent with the non-private target model, reflects a clear generalization gap between training and validation accuracy, which is important for ensuring the reliability of the attack setup. The attack model trained on the outputs of these shadow models reached 79.1% test accuracy with an AUC of 0.869, confirming its ability to distinguish between member and non-member outputs. When examining the resilience of the target models against the adversary, the attack model reached an AUC of 0.690 on the non-private target model, indicating clear vulnerability. In contrast, the DP target model

($\sigma = 1$) achieved an AUC of 0.532, close to random guessing, as shown in Fig. 5. Together with $\varepsilon = 4.12$, these results demonstrate that the theoretical privacy guarantee translates into practical resilience when the classifier head strategy is used, addressing **RQ2**. Furthermore, in relation to **RQ3**, the findings confirm that DP classifier head fine-tuning offers a better balance between privacy and utility than full model fine-tuning, as supported by the empirical privacy evaluation.

6 Conclusions

This paper explores the impact of fine-tuning strategies on the privacy-utility trade-off of the foundation model HarNet10 for human activity recognition (HAR). Our findings underscore the potential for privacy-enhancing techniques to be integrated into AI systems without compromising their utility. By freezing feature extractor layers, we effectively preserve task-relevant information, which is essential for accurate downstream tasks. Notably, the differentially private (DP) classifier head strategy showcased a significant reduction in the success of membership inference attacks, achieving near-random levels compared to non-private models. This approach, which fine-tunes only 4.83% of model parameters, illustrates a viable path toward creating AI solutions that are both privacy-preserving and effective, fostering trust in wearable data analysis. From a policy perspective, these results provide a foundation for developing guidance that promote the responsible use of AI in sensitive domains. However, our study comes with some limitations. First, we used a single dataset (PAMAP2) with only limited demographic variability and the experiments focused on one model (HarNet10) with fixed hyperparameters, employing only gradient perturbation (DP-SGD) with a Gaussian mechanism. Additionally, our privacy evaluation was limited to membership inference attacks. Future work will address these gaps by conducting broader privacy audits, assessing resilience against diverse attacks, and exploring other state-of-the-art HAR models to further optimize the privacy-utility balance. This ongoing research is crucial for informing policy decisions and advancing the development of trustworthy AI systems.

Appendix

A Comparison of the Fine-Tuning Strategies

B Privacy-Utility Trade-Off

C Performance of the Target Models

Table 1. Comparison of the test and validation scores under both fine-tuning strategies and different noise scales (σ).

Experiment	Fine-Tune Strategy	Test Acc (%)	Test F1 (%)	Val Acc (%)	Val F1 (%)	Best Val Epoch	Privacy Budget (ε)
Non-private baseline	Classifier Head	**73,5 ± 1,69**	70,98 ± 2,32	74,92 ± 2,49	72,83 ± 2,95	14,58 ± 4,88	-
Non-private baseline	Full Model	71,56 ± 6,67	**71,04 ± 6,43**	**75,17 ± 5,45**	**73,56 ± 5,49**	11 ± 4,87	-
Gradient Perturbation ($\sigma = 1.0$)	Classifier Head	62,33 ± 5,56	58,18 ± 6,04	61,78 ± 3,92	57,48 ± 3,80	15,5 ± 4,8	3,58 ± 0,62
Gradient Perturbation ($\sigma = 1.0$)	Full Model	56,88 ± 6,56	45,04 ± 7,08	60,37 ± 9,15	48,81 ± 9,30	6,75 ± 2,71	2,41 ± 0,44
Gradient Perturbation ($\sigma = 5.0$)	Classifier Head	44,53 ± 2,73	38,99 ± 1,65	44,68 ± 5,13	39,69 ± 3,93	19,08 ± 1,22	0,47 ± 0,01
Gradient Perturbation ($\sigma = 5.0$)	Full Model	42,7 ± 4,23	29,26 ± 4,42	43,89 ± 3,61	31,26 ± 3,57	15,08 ± 4,34	0,41 ± 0,06
Gradient Perturbation ($\sigma = 10.0$)	Full Model	33,49 ± 5,28	22,60 ± 5,09	33,81 ± 7,68	23,04 ± 7,04	15,58 ± 3,77	0,19 ± 0,02
Gradient Perturbation ($\sigma = 10.0$)	Classifier Head	33,24 ± 6,21	27,37 ± 3,93	32,52 ± 7,02	27,46 ± 6,37	19,25 ± 0,97	0,22 ± 0

Table 2. Comparison of utility loss in the test set under different noise scales, in the classifier head fine-tuning strategy. The table quantifies the privacy-utility trade-off by showing the degradation in test accuracy and F1-score relative to the non-private baseline for increasing levels of noise (σ).

Experiment	Fine-Tune Strategy	Metric	Score (%)	Utility Loss (%)	Privacy Budget (ε)
Non-private baseline	Classifier Head	Acc F1	73,50 70,99	- -	-
Gradient Perturbation ($\sigma = 1.0$)	Classifier Head	AccF1	62,33 58,18	**15,19** **18,04**	3,59
Gradient Perturbation ($\sigma = 5.0$)	Classifier Head	AccF1	44,54 39,00	39,41 45,06	0,47
Gradient Perturbation ($\sigma = 10.0$)	Classifier Head	AccF1	33,25 27,38	54,77 61,43	0,23

Table 3. Comparison of utility loss in the test set under different noise scales, in the full model fine-tuning strategy. The table quantifies the privacy-utility trade-off for the full model approach, showing the degradation in test accuracy and F1-score relative to its non-private baseline for increasing levels of noise (σ).

Experiment	Fine-Tune Strategy	Metric	Score (%)	Utility Loss(%)	Privacy Budget (ε)
Non-private baseline	Full Model	Acc F1	71,56 71,04	- -	-
Gradient Perturbation ($\sigma = 1.0$)	Full Model	AccF1	56,88 45,04	**20,51 36,59**	2,42
Gradient Perturbation ($\sigma = 5.0$)	Full Model	AccF1	42,71 29,97	40,32 57,82	0,41
Gradient Perturbation ($\sigma = 10.0$)	Full Model	AccF1	33,49 22,60	53,20 68,19	0,20

Table 4. Non-Private Classifier Head Fine-Tuned Target Model Training and Validation Accuracy over Epochs. The table shows the mean and standard deviation of the model's accuracy on the training and validation sets for each of the 20 training epochs.

Epoch	Training Accuracy	Validation Accuracy
1	63.21 ± 1.27	68.98 ± 1.84
2	78.39 ± 1.4	63.53 ± 3.41
3	81.65 ± 1.41	71.23 ± 4.54
4	84.25 ± 2.47	69.46 ± 4.62
5	85.87 ± 0.6	71.03 ± 4.71
6	86.52 ± 0.42	70.28 ± 3.13
7	86.8 ± 0.56	69.06 ± 0.76
8	87.87 ± 1.16	71.44 ± 2.06
9	90.88 ± 0.74	71.14 ± 5.83
10	91.06 ± 1.96	72.32 ± 3.59
11	91.27 ± 2.6	70.83 ± 3.76
12	92.5 ± 1.64	72.77 ± 2.88
13	93.71 ± 1.63	71.97 ± 2.63
14	95.39 ± 0.72	73.04 ± 2.24
15	96.33 ± 0.39	73.13 ± 1.94
16	95.36 ± 0.88	72.75 ± 1.53
17	95.8 ± 0.29	73.09 ± 1.68
18	95.8 ± 0.41	72.3 ± 2.08
19	96.84 ± 1.18	73.58 ± 0.52
20	96.39 ± 0.34	74.21 ± 1.22

Per-class Recall for Non-Private Baseline (σ=0)

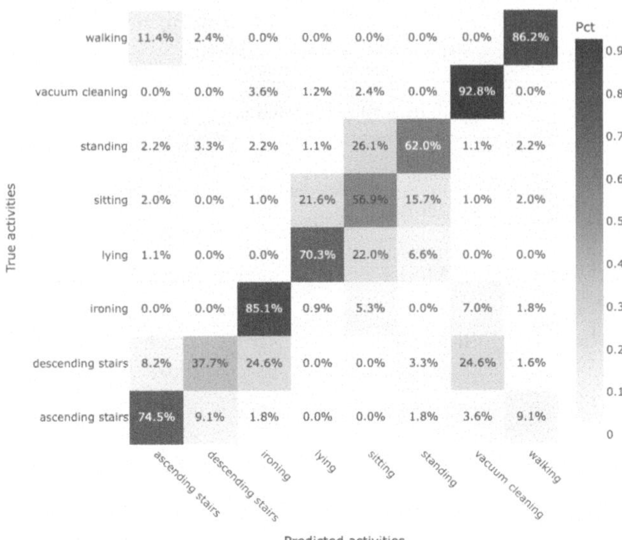

(a) Per-class recall confusion matrix for the non-private target model on the test set.

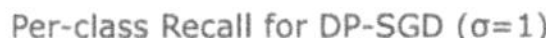

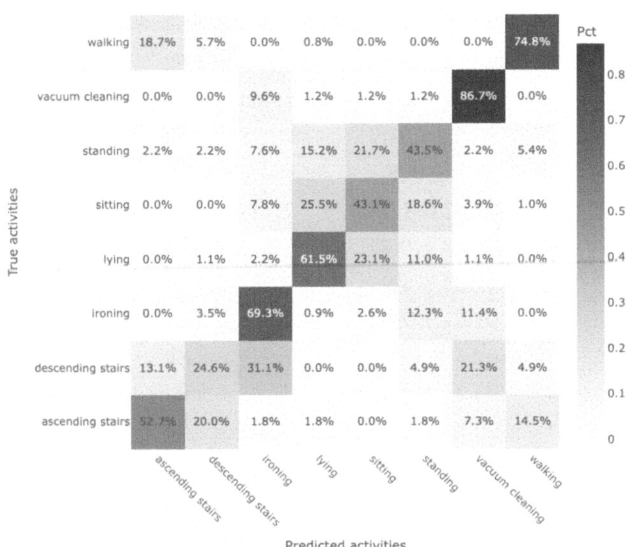

(b) Per-class recall confusion matrix for the DP target model ($\sigma = 1$) on the test set.

Fig. 6. Per-class recall confusion matrices on the test set: (a) non-private target model; (b) DP target model ($\sigma = 1$).

Table 5. DP Classifier Head Fine-Tuned Target Model (σ=1) Training, Validation Accuracy, and Epsilon over Epochs. The table shows the progression of the mean and standard deviation for the model's training accuracy, validation accuracy, and the cumulative privacy budget (ε) for each of the 20 training epochs.

Epoch	Training Accuracy	Validation Accuracy	$\mathcal{E}$
1	24.29 ± 0.25	31.28 ± 1.65	1.22 ± 0.01
2	37.46 ± 1.06	37.68 ± 3.1	1.52 ± 0.01
3	44.83 ± 2.69	44.14 ± 3.61	1.76 ± 0.01
4	52.33 ± 1.58	50.28 ± 3.93	1.97 ± 0.02
5	56.41 ± 4.1	54.41 ± 5.41	2.16 ± 0.02
6	61.2 ± 3.68	55.12 ± 6.72	2.33 ± 0.02
7	62.53 ± 2.08	58.67 ± 4.29	2.5 ± 0.02
8	65.99 ± 2.01	59.6 ± 6.14	2.65 ± 0.02
9	67.19 ± 2.88	61.26 ± 6.15	2.8 ± 0.02
10	68.79 ± 1.35	63.59 ± 6.29	2.94 ± 0.02
11	70.49 ± 1.75	63.59 ± 7.71	3.07 ± 0.02
12	69.1 ± 0.59	63.7 ± 6.97	3.2 ± 0.02
13	70.59 ± 2.02	63.08 ± 5.39	3.33 ± 0.02
14	69.41 ± 1.07	64.01 ± 6.46	3.45 ± 0.03
15	71.05 ± 1.83	63.69 ± 6.42	3.57 ± 0.03
16	73.05 ± 2.19	65.27 ± 7.47	3.69 ± 0.03
17	70.93 ± 2.3	64.28 ± 7.33	3.8 ± 0.03
18	71.82 ± 1.44	64.53 ± 6.62	3.91 ± 0.03
19	72.7 ± 2.14	65.37 ± 7.36	4.02 ± 0.03
20	73.06 ± 1.24	64.43 ± 6.76	4.12 ± 0.03

D Per-Class Performances of the Target Models

E Performance of the Shadow Models

References

1. Abadi, M., Chu, A., Goodfellow, I., McMahan, H.B., Mironov, I., Talwar, K., et al.: Deep learning with differential privacy. In: Proceedings of the ACM SIGSAC Conference on Computer and Communications Security, pp. 308–318 (2016)
2. Agac, S., Durmaz Incel, O.: On the use of a convolutional block attention module in deep learning-based human activity recognition with motion sensors. Diagnostics **13**(11), 1861 (2023)

Table 6. Performance metrics for the five non-private Shadow Models.

Shadow Models	Best Train Accuracy (%)	Best Validation Accuracy (%)	Test **Accuracy (%)**
1	96,64	90,00	65,23
2	94,12	83,33	67,24
3	92,02	90,00	62,64
4	95,38	93,33	66,95
5	93,70	86,67	65,80

3. Bacco, M., Kanellopoulos, S., Di Leo, M., Kotsev, A., Friis-Christensen, A.: Technology safeguards for the re-use of confidential data. JRC Technical Report JRC141298, European Commission, DG JRC, Ispra, Italy (2025)
4. Bassily, R., Smith, A., Thakurta, A.: Private empirical risk minimization: Efficient algorithms and tight error bounds. In: 2014 IEEE 55th Annual Symposium on Foundations of Computer Science. pp. 464–473 (2014)
5. Chen, T., Guestrin, C.: XGBoost: a scalable tree boosting system. In: Proceedings of the 22nd ACM SIGKDD International Conference on Knowledge Discovery and Data Mining, pp. 785–794 (2016)
6. Dehghani, A., Glatard, T., Shihab, E.: Subject cross validation in human activity recognition. ArXiv **abs/1904.02666** (2019)
7. Dwork, C., Roth, A.: The algorithmic foundations of differential privacy. Found. Trends Theor. Comput. Sci. **9**(3–4), 211–407 (2014)
8. Hurtado Ramírez, D., Porras Díaz, L., Rahimian, S., Auñón García, J.M., Irigoyen Peña, B., Al-Khazraji, Y., et al.: Technological enablers for privacy preserving data sharing and analysis. JRC Technical Report JRC134350, European Commission, DG JRC, Luxembourg, Luxembourg (2023)
9. Kairouz, P., McMahan, H.B., Avent, B., Bellet, A., Bennis, M., Bhagoji, A.N., et al.: Advances and open problems in federated learning. Foundations and Trends in Machine Learning **14**(1–2), 1–210 (2021)
10. Kang, Y., Liu, Y., Niu, B., Tong, X.Y., Zhang, L., Wang, W.: Input perturbation: a new paradigm between central and local differential privacy. ArXiv:abs/2002.08570 (2020)
11. Lei, Y., Cao, Y., Wang, W., Dong, Y., Yin, C., Cao, W., et al.: Watchguardian: Enabling user-defined personalized just-in-time intervention on smartwatch. ArXiv:abs/2502.05783 (2025)
12. Liao, T., Zhao, J., Liu, Y., Ivanov, K., Xiong, J., Yan, Y.: Deep transfer learning with graph neural network for sensor-based human activity recognition. In: 2022 IEEE International Conference on Bioinformatics and Biomedicine (BIBM), pp. 2445–2452. IEEE (2022)
13. Mahmud, S., Tanjid Hasan Tonmoy, M., Kumar Bhaumik, K., Mahbubur Rahman, A., Ashraful Amin, M., Shoyaib, M., et al.: Human activity recognition from wearable sensor data using self-attention. In: 24th European Conference on Artificial Intelligence, pp. 1332–1339. IOS Press (2020)
14. Malekzadeh, M., Clegg, R.G., Cavallaro, A., Haddadi, H.: Privacy and utility preserving sensor-data transformations. Pervasive Mob. Comput. **63**, 101132 (2020)
15. Mireshghallah, F., Goyal, K., Uniyal, A., Berg-Kirkpatrick, T., Shokri, R.: Quantifying privacy risks of masked language models using membership inference attacks.

In: Proceedings of the 2022 Conference on Empirical Methods in Natural Language Processing, pp. 8332–8347. Association for Computational Linguistics (2022)
16. Najmi, A., Sadasivam, B., Ray, A.: How to choose and interpret a statistical test? An update for budding researchers. J. Family Med. Primary Care **10**, 2763–2767 (2021)
17. Oluwalade, B., Neela, S., Wawira, J., Adejumo, T., Purkayastha, S.: Human activity recognition using deep learning models on smartphones and smartwatches sensor data. In: Proceedings of the 14th International Joint Conference on Biomedical Engineering Systems and Technologies. vol. 5, pp. 645–650 (2021)
18. Opitz, J.: A closer look at classification evaluation metrics and a critical reflection of common evaluation practice. Trans. ACL **12**, 820–836 (2024)
19. Piwek, L., Ellis, D.A., Andrews, S., Joinson, A.: The rise of consumer health wearables: promises and barriers. PLoS Med. **13**(2), e1001953 (2016)
20. Preatoni, E., Nodari, S., Lopomo, N.F.: Supervised machine learning applied to wearable sensor data can accurately classify functional fitness exercises within a continuous workout. Front. Bioeng. Biotechnol. **8**, 664 (2020)
21. Rahman, M., Rahman, T., Laganière, R., Mohammed, N.: Membership inference attack against differentially private deep learning model. Trans. Data Privacy **11**(1), 61–79 (2018)
22. Razali, N.M., Wah, Y.B.: Power comparisons of shapiro-wilk, kolmogorov-smirnov, lilliefors and anderson-darling tests. J. Stat. Model. Anal. **2**, 21–33 (2011)
23. Reiss, A.: PAMAP2 Physical Activity Monitoring. UCI Machine Learning Repository (2012). https://doi.org/10.24432/C5NW2H
24. Reiss, A., Stricker, D.: Introducing a new benchmarked dataset for activity monitoring. In: 2012 16th International Symposium on Wearable Computers, pp. 108–109 (2012)
25. Ryoo, M.S., Rothrock, B., Fleming, C., Yang, H.J.: Privacy-preserving human activity recognition from extreme low resolution. In: Proceedings of the 31st AAAI Conference on Artificial Intelligence. vol. 31, pp. 4255–4262 (2017)
26. Song, S., Chaudhuri, K., Sarwate, A.D.: Stochastic gradient descent with differentially private updates. In: 2013 IEEE Global Conference on Signal and Information Processing, pp. 245–248 (2013)
27. Statista: Global wearable device shipments from 2021 to 2028, by product category (in millions). Statista (2024). https://www.statista.com/statistics/1265326/wearables-worldwide-shipments-quarterly-by-product-category/. Accessed 5 July 2025
28. Sullivan, G.M., Feinn, R.S.: Using effect size-or why the p value is not enough. J. Grad. Med. Educ. **4**(3), 279–282 (2012)
29. Wang, Y., Cheng, Z., Yi, X., Kong, Y., Wang, X., Xu, X., et al.: Modeling the trade-off of privacy preservation and activity recognition on low-resolution images. In: Proceedings of the 2023 CHI Conference on Human Factors in Computing Systems, pp. 1–15. No. 589 (2023)
30. Wu, Y., He, K.: Group normalization. In: Ferrari, V., Hebert, M., Sminchisescu, C., Weiss, Y. (eds.) ECCV 2018. LNCS, vol. 11217, pp. 3–19. Springer, Cham (2018). https://doi.org/10.1007/978-3-030-01261-8_1
31. Xia, F., Liu, Y., Jin, B., Yu, Z., Cai, X., Li, H., et al.: Leveraging multiple adversarial perturbation distances for enhanced membership inference attack in federated learning. Symmetry **16**(12), 1677 (2024)
32. Yousefpour, A., Shilov, I., Sablayrolles, A., Testuggine, D., Prasad, K., Malek, M., et al.: Opacus: User-friendly differential privacy library in pytorch. In: NeurIPS 2021 Workshop Privacy in Machine Learning (2021)

33. Yuan, H., Chan, S., Creagh, A.P., Tong, C., Acquah, A., Clifton, D.A., et al.: Self-supervised learning for human activity recognition using 700,000 person-days of wearable data. NPJ Digital Med. **7**(1), 91 (2024)
34. Zhang, S., Li, Y., Zhang, S., Shahabi, F., Xia, S., Deng, Y., et al.: Deep learning in human activity recognition with wearable sensors: a review on advances. Sensors **22**(4), 1476 (2022)

Using Multi-modal Generative Models for Creating Speech Therapy Material

Mihir Mulye(✉), Stefan Conrad, and Stefan Knecht

Heinrich-Heine-University, Düsseldorf, Germany
{mihir.mulye,stefan.conrad,stefan.knecht}@uni-duesseldorf.de

Abstract. The process of collecting rehabilitation material for speech disorders can be resource intensive, consume a lot of time and effort, and can also constrain the possibilities of customization. Improvements in multimodal generative Machine Learning can help accelerate and enhance the efficiency of this process. In this paper, we explore the use of such models to create rehabilitation material for aphasia. We propose a novel pipeline that uses existing rehabilitation concepts to generate not only therapy tasks using Large Language Models (LLMs), and images using Text-to-Image (T2I) models but also generate prompts for creating images and the therapy tasks themselves. We observe that combinations of Qwen (LLM) with both Stable Diffusion Turbo and Flux (both T2Is) tend to generate images with higher T2I evaluation metrics. In addition, we also investigate using Large Language and Vision Assistant (LLaVa) as a visual question answering tool to supplement LLM generated answers. Our experiments indicate that the answers generated by LLaVa have a higher alignment with Qwen (average alignment of 0.751 and 0.782 for inputs from SDXL+Qwen and Flux+Qwen, respectively) compared to Llama (average alignment of 0.721 and 0.740 for inputs from SDXL+Llama and Flux+Llama, respectively).

Keywords: Generative Machine Learning · Aphasia Rehabilitation

1 Introduction

Speech disorders such as *Aphasia* affect a person's ability to properly use language to communicate with others. Rehabilitation is possible but requires extensive time and effort from therapists and patients. Therapy tasks such as *naming*, *repetition*, *comprehension*, among others, have to be customized to help patients practice different speech modalities. These tasks aim to improve language aspects by requiring patients to identify an object from an image, describe an image, or match the image corresponding to an audio prompt. It can be inferred from the task description that images play a crucial role in rehabilitation [2]. Currently, therapists and caregivers have to spend a significant amount of resources, namely time, effort, and money on image acquisition, definitions of pertinent questions-answers based on those images, and designing appropriate therapy exercises.

P. Bruno et al. (Eds.): HC_AIxIA_HYDRA 2025, CCIS 2830, pp. 21–34, 2026.
https://doi.org/10.1007/978-3-032-16708-8_2

Applying advances in multimodal generative Machine Learning (ML) to these routine tasks can allow the redirection of valuable resources to provide care and assistance to patients effectively.

In this work, we focus particularly on aphasia, a speech disorder primarily caused by stroke or brain injury. Our contributions in this paper are: (1) proposing a novel approach that uses multimodal generative machine learning models (such as Large Language Models (LLM) and Text-to-Image (T2I) models) to generate prompts, images, and pairs of question-answers solely from a list of aphasia therapy concepts, (2) first known application of the Large Language and Vision Assistant (LLaVa) to answer LLM generated questions based on the T2I generated images for the purpose of aphasia rehabilitation, (3) quantifying the quality of artificially generated images using the T2I evaluation metrics, and (4) to collate the generated material so that it can be used as a baseline dataset for aphasia therapy. The code along with the implementation details for this paper is available on GitHub[1].

2 Related Work

In this section, we provide an overview of the existing research.

Aphasia Rehabilitation Material Generation Using T2I: Research works [7,8] explore the possibility of using Text-to-Image (T2I) models to generate image rehabilitation material for aphasia. They use input prompts designed by Speech Language Pathologists (SLPs) that are based on existing aphasia rehabilitation material. [8] performs a qualitative analysis of the generated images without defining the evaluation criteria. This evaluation is prone to subjectivity and is therefore not reproducible. [7] calculates automated T2I evaluation metrics and performs a quantitative evaluation. However, these works use human designed input prompts that require time to design, introduce variations, and do not eliminate the cost in terms of therapists investing their time and effort. Additionally, these works only generate images for therapy tasks.

T2I Evaluation Metrics: Inception Score [9] assesses whether artificial images (i) look similar to a specific object (*image quality*) and (ii) correspond to a variety of objects (*image diversity*). It is mathematically defined as the Kullback-Leibler divergence between (1) marginal distribution for all generated images and (2) class probability distribution computed by a pretrained InceptionNet. CLIPScore [3] measures the cosine similarity between the Contrastive Language Image Pretraining (CLIP) embeddings of the input text and the generated image. Text-to-Image Faithfulness evaluation with Question Answering (TIFA) [4] proposes using a Question Answering (QA) model, Language Model (LM), and a

[1] https://github.com/mihirm05/multimodal_models_for_speech_rehab_material_generation.

Visual Question Answering (VQA) model to evaluate the alignment of a generated image with the input text prompt. The LM produces pairs of question and answers (which are later filtered using the QA) from the input text prompt. The prompt is used to generate images using the T2I to be evaluated. These generated images along with the filtered questions are used as inputs for the VQAs to compute TIFA. It is calculated by comparing the VQA responses with the answers generated by the combination of LM and QA.

Multimodal Models: Large Language and Vision Assistant (LLaVa) [5] is a multimodal model that combines vision encoders with LLMs to understand the image-text modality. The model takes image and text prompts as input and produces natural language output. It can be used for solving diverse sets of tasks such as image captioning, visual question answering, scene understanding, to name a few. There exists also a suite of commercial multimodal models such as GPT-4 [1], Gemini [10] among others that are not open source.

3 Methodology

In this section, we discuss the implementation details of our experiments. We use Kaggle's T4 GPUs for the computations. Figure 1 shows our proposed approach to generate rehabilitation material for aphasia from a list of existing therapy concepts. The following discussions describe our approach.

Input Concept List: In this context, concepts are singular words that describe nouns, verbs, or abstract ideas such as emotions, time of day, events, among others. Examples of concepts include verbs such as *singing*, *meeting*, nouns such as *duck*, *bus* and human feelings such as *fear*, *happy* among others. These concepts focus on improving various language aspects including vocabulary development, scene comprehension, and sentence formulation. The concepts considered in this work are taken from aphasia therapy[2]. In doing so, we ensure that the material generated by our approach is relevant to therapy. We start with a total of 548 concepts.

Prompt Generation: Our contribution is to use the concepts to generate prompts using Qwen [11] and Llama[3] (see Fig. 1). For each concept, we generate one prompt per LLM. To do so, we employ *in-context learning*. In-Context Learning is a method that enables LLMs to perform new tasks without the need for retraining or fine-tuning. This is achieved by providing a few examples of the said tasks within the input prompt itself. The user can specify the input and output that is expected for the new category of tasks, and the LLM adapts its inference accordingly. We use the following prompt as input for *in-context*

[2] https://www.aphasiatherapyonline.com/wordlists.

[3] https://huggingface.co/meta-llama/Llama-3.2-3B-Instruct.

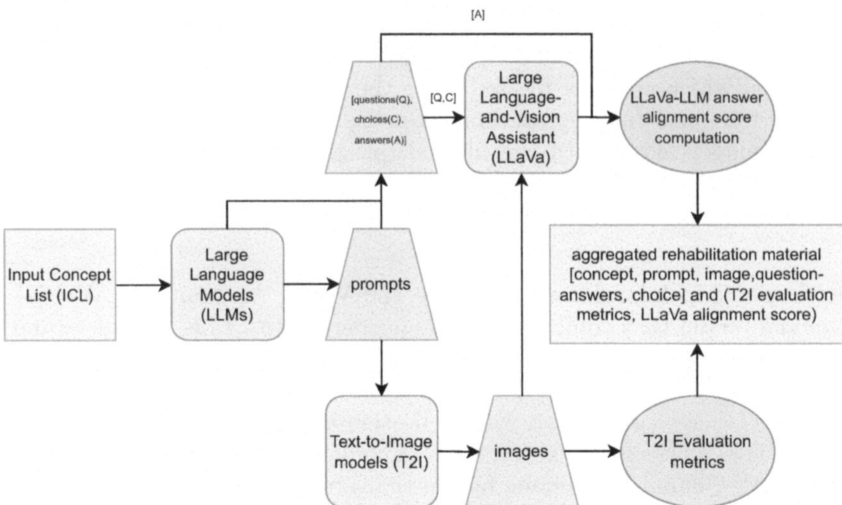

Fig. 1. Depiction of the proposed approach to generate aphasia rehabilitation material. Using just the *Input Concept List*, this pipeline creates prompts, images, question-answer pairs, and potential choices for the question which the therapists can use in designing rehabilitation tasks. We use *in-context learning* to generate prompts and the question-answers (and their corresponding choices). The details of *in-context learning* have been discussed in the text. Additionally, we compute the T2I evaluation metrics for generated images and the alignment score between the answers generated by LLM and LLaVa. In the figure, rectangles denote the pipeline inputs and the outputs, rounded rectangle denote the generative models, trapezoids show the generated material, and the ellipses indicate the evaluation metrics.

learning for prompt generation. Note that we have used a total of 10 examples for *in-context learning* but have provided only 3 examples in the text below for conciseness.

"You are a helpful assistant that generates OUTPUT from a given INPUT as shown in the examples. Do not add any extra explanation or commentary.
INPUT: football
OUTPUT: a realistic picture of football on a field, bright sunny day
INPUT: ambulance
OUTPUT: an action shot of ambulance weaving through the traffic with lights and sirens on
INPUT: cup
OUTPUT: a blue cup kept on the table, uniform lighting"

We use the same prompt as input for Qwen and Llama. The concepts are provided as the INPUT, whereas the desired generated prompt style is provided as the OUTPUT. The LLM then generates outputs in this format for new inputs. We manually verify if the generated prompts contain the input concepts and observe that from the initial 548 concepts, Qwen generates 449 prompts and Llama generates 408 prompts successfully. The failure to generate prompts for some concepts could be attributed to (i) the input concept being overly abstract, (ii) inherent limitations of the LLM, or (iii) suboptimal LLM parameter configurations (temperature, token window length), among others. However, a detailed analysis must be conducted to determine the exact cause and this is outside the scope of the current work. Next, we identify a total of 375 concepts for which both Qwen and Llama are able to generate prompts. We use the prompts corresponding to these concepts for further processing.

Question-Answer and Choice Generation: Using the filtered prompts generated in the previous step, we create four pairs of question-answer per prompt. We also create potential choices, one among which is the correct answer to the question. These choices can be used in case the therapy task needs to be in the form of a multiple choice question. As in prompt generation, we use *in-context learning* with Qwen and Llama to generate pairs of question-answer and the choices. The following prompt is designed as an input for *in-context learning.* Note that the same prompt is used as input for Qwen and Llama. We provided a total of 10 examples for the *in-context learning*, however, only 1 example is presented here to maintain conciseness.

"You reword text into a series of FOUR questions. Each question must be supported exactly in the text provided. The best answer is always from the text. Ask meaningful questions.
[USER]
PROMPT: a golden wheat field at sunset
[ASSISTANT]
PROMPT: a golden wheat field at sunset
QUESTION 1: What type of landscape is depicted?
CHOICES: [forest] [field] [desert] [mountain]
ANSWER: [field]
QUESTION 2: What time of day is shown in the image?
CHOICES: [morning] [noon] [sunset] [night]
ANSWER: [sunset]
QUESTION 3: What color is the field described as?
CHOICES: [green] [brown] [golden] [silver]
ANSWER: [golden]
QUESTION 4: Is there any water visible in the image?
CHOICES: [no] [yes]
ANSWER: [no] "

Additionally, as with prompt generation, we ensure that the generated question-answers adhere to the contents of the corresponding prompt and the image. This is necessary as LLMs are prone to hallucinations.

Image Generation: Using the LLM generated prompts, we create images using Flux[4][5] and SDXL Turbo[6]. With the rapidly advancing field of generative machine learning, it is natural to restrict the selection of models for our exploratory analysis. We select T2I models that are free to use and are not computationally intensive. The size of the generated images is 512×512×3. For each concept, we have two prompts, four generated images, and eight pairs of questions and answers.

Visual Question Answering with LLaVa: This is an exploratory analysis to verify whether multimodal models can be reliably used to answer image-based therapy questions and serve as a quality evaluation tool. We hypothesize that the answers generated by LLMs can be supplemented by using LLaVa as a visual question-answering assistant. This can potentially reduce the reliance on manual annotation of the LLM generated answers (that we conducted in the previous step) and could also accelerate the therapy material creation process. The input to the LLaVa are the questions and choices (generated by LLM), and images (generated by T2Is). LLaVa's output is the answer to the input questions based on the input images and choices. The prompt for LLaVa is provided below where the *<image>* indicates the placeholder for the input image during the inference step, q indicates the input question, and c indicates the input choice list for potential answers.

"<image> Answer the multiple-choice question based on the image.
Question: q
Choices: c
Respond with ONLY the correct answer."

Image Quality Evaluation: To quantify the quality of the generated images, we calculate the Inception Score (IS), CLIPScore, and TIFA. We compute four different versions of CLIPScore that use variations of the CLIP model, namely: *base16*, *base32*, *large14*, and *large14-336*. Similarly, for TIFA, we compute three variations that include different visual question answering modules namely, *git-base*, *git-large*, and *vilt*. Computing variations of the CLIPScore and TIFA provides a holistic evaluation of the generated images. For TIFA, we use the questions generated by Qwen and Llama, and generated images from the T2I models as input to the visual question answer module. It should be noted that this differs from the original implementation of TIFA, in which the questions are generated using the GPT-3 model. The theoretical ranges of the evaluation metrics are as follows: IS $\in$ [1, # of classes for which InceptionNet is trained], CLIPScore $\in$ [0, 100], and TIFA $\in$ [0, 1]. For all metrics, a higher value indicates better image quality.

[4] https://github.com/black-forest-labs/flux.
[5] https://www.kaggle.com/code/crischir/testing-flux1-flux-1-dev.
[6] https://huggingface.co/stabilityai/sdxl-turbo.

Visual Question Answering Quality Evaluation: To evaluate the performance of LLaVa, we first manually verify the alignment of the question-answer pairs (generated using LLMs) with the input prompt that was used to create the pairs. The manual verification is essential to eliminate potential errors introduced during generation. We use these verified LLM answers to evaluate the quality of the LLaVa output. For each image, we compare the LLaVa answers (to the corresponding questions) with our annotations (manually verified LLM answers) and obtain a value $\in [0, 1]$. A value of 0 indicates that LLaVa answered all the questions incorrectly, whereas 1 indicates that LLaVa answered all the questions correctly. We compute this for all the images and obtain an *alignment score* distribution. Next, we compute the mean (μ), the standard deviation (σ), and the coefficient of variation (cv) of this distribution. Naturally, a high μ and a low σ would indicate higher confidence in the LLaVa output.

For our implementation, the design choices in the experiments are based on the following considerations: generative multimodal models are (i) open source, (ii) free to use, and (iii) not compute intensive.

4 Results

In this section, we discuss the results of our experiments and analyze them. We describe the convention that we use in the following text. We refer to the images generated using a T2I model (say T) that takes input prompts generated using an LLM (say L) as T_L. For example, we refer to the images generated by $SDXL\_Turbo$ (T) using input prompts created using $Qwen$ (L), as $SDXL\_Qwen$.

The evaluation metrics in Table 1 are represented as $\mu \pm \sigma$ (cv) where μ, σ, and cv indicate the mean, the standard deviation, and the coefficient of variation of the metric distribution, respectively. The coefficient of variation is the ratio of the standard deviation to the mean and provides information on the degree of dispersion of the data around the mean value. A higher cv indicates greater variability in the distribution. Ideally, a T2I model should have high μ, and low σ and cv, as it indicates the model's capability of consistently generating good quality images. When analyzing cv, we operate under the assumption that the μ of the distributions are positive, not close to zero, and that the distributions are of comparable type. This means that the nature of the distributions being compared should not differ significantly.

Inception Score (IS): From Table 1, we observe that SDXL-Llama and Flux-Llama have the highest and lowest mean, respectively. Furthermore, Flux-Qwen and SDXL-Qwen have the lowest and highest cv, respectively. Notably, the μ of Flux-Qwen and SDXL-Llama do not differ significantly, and on further examination, we observe that the cv of Flux-Qwen is significantly less than that of SDXL-Llama. This indicates that Flux-Qwen is consistently capable of generating images that are almost as good as SDXL-Llama.

CLIPScore: We compute four variants of CLIPScore namely *base16*, *base32*, *large14*, and *large14-336*. From the values in Table 1, we observe that **(a)base16:**

Table 1. T2I evaluation metric scores shown as $\mu \pm \sigma$ (cv) of prompt-image pairs for the T2I models. **Row 1:** Inception Score, **Rows 2-5:** CLIP Score variants, and **Rows 6-8:** TIFA variants.

Metric	SDXL-Qwen	Flux-Qwen	SDXL-Llama	Flux-Llama
IS	15.361±1.989(0.129)	15.829±1.256(0.079)	**15.981±1.929(0.121)**	15.105±1.579(0.104)
base16	**32.498±2.437(0.074)**	32.290±2.574(0.079)	31.914±2.378(0.074)	31.874±2.608(0.081)
base32	32.266±2.488(0.077)	**32.330±2.605(0.080)**	31.994±2.589(0.080)	32.232±2.635(0.081)
large14	**27.218±2.672(0.098)**	27.064±2.897(0.107)	26.792±2.709(0.101)	26.664±2.923(0.109)
large14-336	**27.896±2.761(0.098)**	27.706±2.852(0.102)	27.496±2.627(0.095)	27.309±2.887(0.105)
git-base	0.564±0.269(0.478)	**0.577±0.253(0.439)**	0.574±0.255(0.444)	0.572±0.255(0.446)
git-large	0.589±0.258(0.439)	0.590±0.258(0.437)	0.579±0.251(0.434)	**0.593±0.244(0.411)**
vilt	0.295±0.230(0.782)	**0.295±0.229(0.777)**	0.288±0.227(0.787)	0.291±0.225(0.772)

SDXL-Qwen performs the best for this variation, as it has the highest μ and the lowest cv among all compared T2I models. In contrast, Flux-Llama performs the worst, as it has the lowest μ and highest cv of all models. **(b)base32:** For this variant, Flux-Qwen has the highest μ, while SDXL-Llama has the lowest μ. The cv values for both are the same, indicating a similar spread in the metric distribution relative to their respective means. **(c)large14:** SDXL-Qwen has the highest and lowest μ and cv, respectively, indicating consistent good quality images. In contrast, Flux-Llama has the lowest μ and highest cv, respectively, that translates to a wide metric distribution and inconsistent image quality. **(d)large14-336:** Flux-Llama has the lowest and highest μ and cv, respectively, for this metric, whereas SDXL-Qwen has the highest and the second lowest μ and cv, respectively.

TIFA: We compute three variants of TIFA based on the visual question answering model used namely, *git-base*, *git-large*, and *vilt*. We observe that **(a)git-base:** Flux-Qwen has the highest and lowest μ and cv, respectively, among all models. In addition, SDXL-Qwen performs the worst with the lowest and highest μ and cv, respectively. **(b)git-large:** Flux-Llama performs the best for this variant. In contrast, SDXL-Llama has the lowest μ and the third highest cv. **(c)vilt:** For this variant, both SDXL-Qwen and Flux-Qwen generate similar metric values. Both models perform better than the rest. SDXL-Llama performs the worst of all the compared models.

From the analysis of the T2I evaluation metrics, we note that the combination of $SDXL\_Qwen$ tends to generate images of better quality followed by $FLUX\_Qwen$. The metric distributions for CLIPScore and TIFA are provided in Figs. 2 and 3. It should be noted that automated metrics should be used with considerations. The IS and CLIPScore depend on the quality of the encoder used. This might affect the evaluation of images that contain classes that the encoder has not been trained on. For TIFA, the performance of the LM and the VQA determine the accuracy of the resulting metric. Hence, it is suggested to

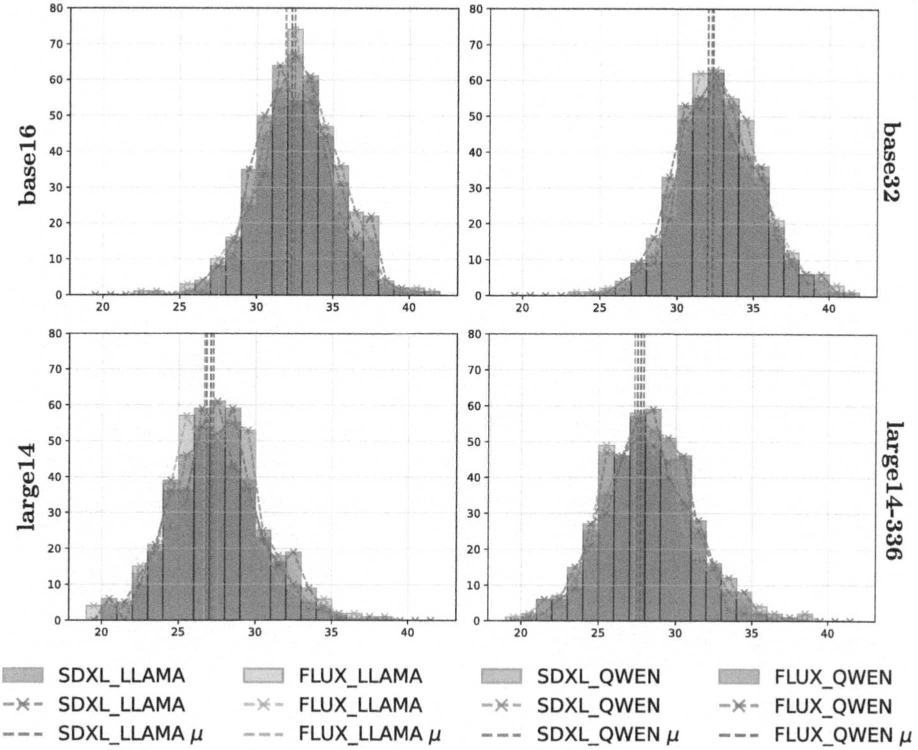

Fig. 2. Histograms of CLIPScore variants across different T2I models. The dashed vertical line indicates the mean score per T2I model. In each histogram, the x-axis indicates the metric score and the y-axis indicates the counts.

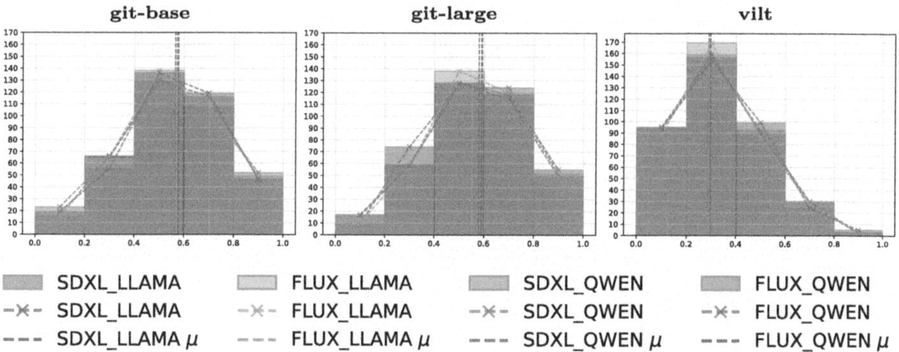

Fig. 3. Histograms of TIFA variants across different T2I models. The dashed vertical line indicates the mean score per T2I model. In each histogram, the x-axis indicates the metric score and the y-axis indicates the counts.

Table 2. Alignment scores for output of LLaVa with the answers generated by the LLMs. The score is presented as $\mu \pm \sigma$ (cv) for all the generated images. The histogram and the scatter plot for the distribution has been provided in Fig. 5 in the Appendix.

Metric	SDXL Qwen	SDXL Llama	Flux Qwen	Flux Llama
alignment score	0.751±0.222(0.290)	0.721±0.228(0.316)	**0.782±0.214(0.274)**	0.740±0.219(296)

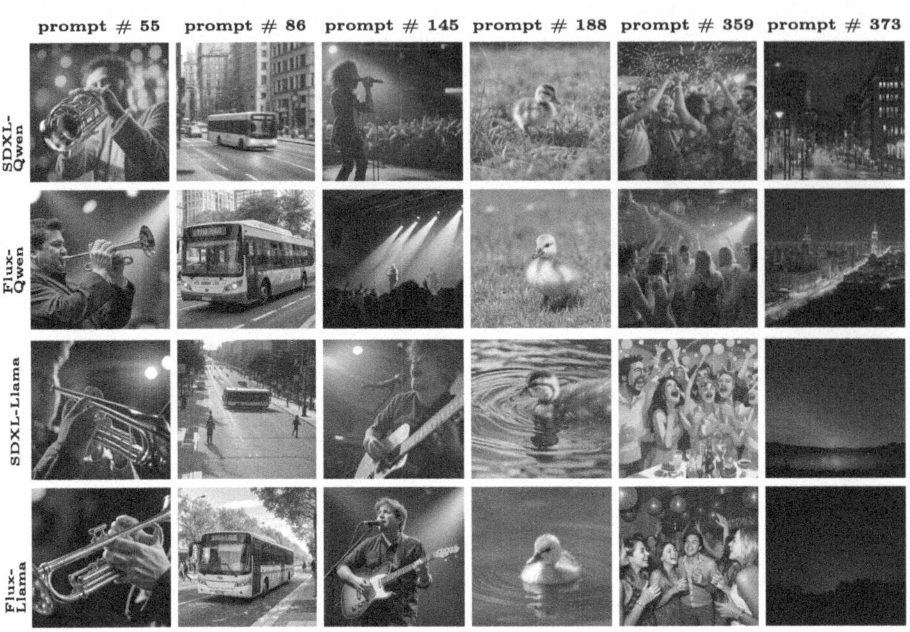

Fig. 4. Examples of generated images. The prompts follow this template: {*concept, Qwen generated prompt, Llama generated prompt*}. **#55:** {trumpet, [a musician playing a trumpet live, vibrant background], [a shiny trumpet held by a musician, brightly lit]}, **#86:** {bus, [a city bus driving down the street, busy urban environment], [a bus driving down the road, people walking on the sidewalk]}, **#145:** {sing, [a singer performing on stage, audience present], [a person singing with a guitar, action shot]}, **#188:** {duckling, [a cute duckling waddling happily in a grassy field], [a cute duckling swimming in the water, brightly lit]}, **#359:** {party, [a vibrant photo of people dancing and drinking at a festive party], [a lively party scene with people laughing and having fun]}, **#373:** {night, [a cityscape at night with illuminated buildings and streetlights], [a dark and quiet night scene with stars in the sky]}.

employ these automated metrics in conjunction with the knowledge of SLPs to establish the usability of generated images for rehabilitation.

LLaVa Alignment Score: This metric, as previously explained, computes the alignment of the LLaVa answers with the LLM generated answers. The objective of computing this metric score is to explore the potential of using LLaVa as a tool to supplement LLM generated answers. If the answers produced by LLaVa by using images (generated by T2I) and questions (generated by LLM) align with the answers (generated by LLM), it can serve as an auxiliary source of ground truth annotation, reducing manual efforts needed to verify the LLM generated answers. From Table 2, we observe that for LLaVa performs poorly when the questions are generated by Llama. On the other hand, when answering questions generated by Qwen, LLaVa tends to have a higher μ and a lower cv, indicating a better alignment. In this work, we manually verified the answers generated by LLM before computing the alignment score. The initial hypothesis that LLaVa can be used as a supplementary tool to validate LLM generated answers has shown potential and warrants further investigation.

The generated images are presented in Fig. 4 along with the corresponding input prompts. We find that the T2I models are able to generate images for *nouns* such as *duck* and *bus*. Also, these models are able to generate scenes such as *night*. However, for *verbs* such as *singing* and *partying*, the models tend to introduce abnormalities in the generated output. It is noteworthy that, since this is a rapidly evolving research domain, upcoming models might be able to address the shortcomings of the models that have been used in this work.

5 Conclusions and Future Work

In this research, we proposed an end-to-end pipeline using multimodal generative models to create aphasia training material that therapists can use to rehabilitate patients. We create prompts from a concept list; images and question-answer pairs from the generated prompts. We evaluate the T2I evaluation metrics and find that combinations of $SDXL\_Qwen$ and $FLUX\_Qwen$ tend to generate better images. We also conduct a preliminary investigation of using LLaVa as a supplementary tool to validate LLM generated answers. We find that LLaVa performs well in answering the Qwen generated questions (as compared to Llama generated questions). We conclude that the initial experiments with LLaVa have shown potential and the results justify further research.

As we discussed previously, expert evaluation of the generated rehabilitation material will be crucial to determine its practical usability. A potential solution could be to have the generated material evaluated by a pool of SLPs and the mean agreement score in conjunction with the automated metrics can be used to decide whether a particular generated data point should be included in the therapy or not. Additionally, patient feedback could also be used to improve the quality of the generated material. Another interesting research could be integrating the proposed pipeline in this work with rehabilitation frameworks such as [6]. LLMs can potentially also be used to design customized therapy tasks that are suited to individual patients. The research in this work can be extended and customized to other speech disorders.

A Appendix

Figure 5 shows the alignment score distribution for following: (i)$SDXL\_Llama$, (ii)$FLUX\_Llama$, (iii)$SDXL\_Qwen$, and (iv)$FLUX\_Qwen$

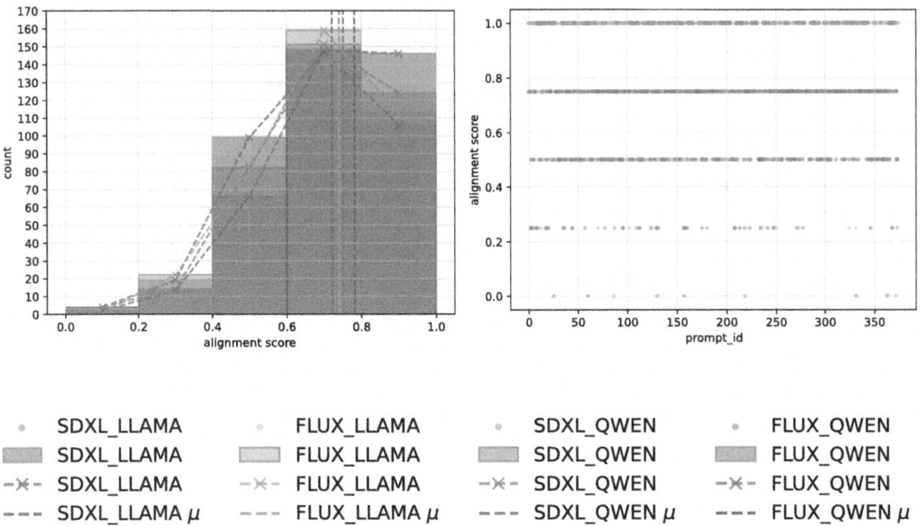

Fig. 5. Histogram (left) and Scatter plot (right) for the alignment score of LLaVa output to the answers generated by LLMs.

We provide only one example of the rehabilitation material generated in Table 3 for conciseness. Additional information on rehabilitation material and the relevant model configurations can be found at this link[7]. We observe a tendency for the LLaVa answers, especially for combinations where the input questions are provided by Llama, to be incorrect and result in a lower alignment score. This can also be inferred from the values in Table 2 where the combinations with Llama perform worse compared to the combinations with Qwen as LLM.

[7] https://github.com/mihirm05/multimodal_models_for_speech_rehab_material_generation.

Table 3. Rehabilitation material generated using multimodal machine learning models for the concept *night*. The concept is used as input to the LLMs to generate prompts (which are in turn used to generate images), pairs of question answers corresponding to the prompt, and potential choices. As an exploratory analysis, we use these generated questions and the images as input to LLaVa and obtain answers. This is to investigate if such multimodal models can be used as a helping tool to supplement LLM generated answers.

Concept	LLM generated [Prompt(P), Question(Q), Choice(C), Answer(A)]	LLaVa answers
night	**Qwen:** **P:** a cityscape at night with illuminated buildings and streetlights **Q1:** What setting is the scene described? **C:** [morning] [afternoon] [evening] [night] **A:** [night] **Q2:** What elements are illuminated? **C:** [trees] [buildings] [lanterns] [streetlights] **A:** [buildings, streetlights] **Q3:** What time of day is it? **C:** [dawn] [midday] [dusk] [night] **A:** [night] **Q4:** Are there any natural elements illuminated? **C:** [yes] [no] **A:** [no] **Llama:** **P:** a dark and quiet night scene with stars in the sky **Q1:** What is the overall atmosphere of the scene? **C:**[busy] [noisy] [peaceful] [stormy] **A:** [peaceful] **Q2:** What is visible in the scene? **C:** [trees] [mountains] [stars] [moon] **A:** [stars] **Q3:** Is the scene described as active or passive? **C:** [active] [passive] [busy] [quiet] **A:** [quiet] **Q4:** What is the time of day implied by the description? **C:** [day] [dawn] [night] [dusk] **A:** [night]	**SDXL-Qwen:** [Evening, Streetlights, Dusk, Yes] **FLUX-Qwen:** [Night, Buildings, Night, Yes] **SDXL-Llama:** [Peaceful, Stars, Passive, Night] **FLUX-Llama:** [Peaceful, Stars, Passive, Night]

References

1. Achiam, J., et al.: Gpt-4 technical report. arXiv preprint arXiv:2303.08774 (2023)
2. Brown, J., Thiessen, A.: Using images with individuals with aphasia: Current research and clinical trends. Am. J. Speech Lang. Pathol. **27**(1S), 504–515 (2018)
3. Hessel, J., Holtzman, A., Forbes, M., Bras, R.L., Choi, Y.: Clipscore: A reference-free evaluation metric for image captioning. arXiv preprint arXiv:2104.08718 (2021)
4. Hu, Y., et al.: Tifa: accurate and interpretable text-to-image faithfulness evaluation with question answering. In: Proceedings of the IEEE/CVF International Conference on Computer Vision, pp. 20406–20417 (2023)
5. Liu, H., Li, C., Wu, Q., Lee, Y.J.: Visual instruction tuning. Adv. Neural. Inf. Process. Syst. **36**, 34892–34916 (2023)
6. Mulye, M., Conrad, S., Knecht, S.: Proof of clinical feasibility of natural language learning with machines. In: Proceedings of the 35th GI-Workshop Grundlagen von Datenbanken (GvDB 2024). vol. 3710. CEUR-WS.org (2024)

7. Mulye, M., Conrad, S., Knecht, S.: Exploring applicability of text-to-image models for generating aphasia rehabilitation material. In: International Conference on AI in Healthcare, pp. 324–338. Springer (2025)
8. Pierce, J.E.: Ai-generated images for speech pathology–an exploratory application to aphasia assessment and intervention materials. Am. J. Speech Lang. Pathol. **33**(1), 443–451 (2024)
9. Salimans, T., Goodfellow, I., Zaremba, W., Cheung, V., Radford, A., Chen, X.: Improved techniques for training GANs. In: Advances in Neural Information Processing Systems, vol. 29 (2016)
10. Team, G., et al.: Gemini: a family of highly capable multimodal models. arXiv preprint arXiv:2312.11805 (2023)
11. Team, Q.: Qwen2.5: A party of foundation models (September 2024). https://qwenlm.github.io/blog/qwen2.5/

AI for Diagnosis & Medical Imaging

MultiH-EU: An AI-Driven Decision Support System for Multi-disease Diagnosis

Diogen Babuc(✉) and Teodor-Florin Fortiş

Computer Science Department, West University of Timişoara, V. Pârvan blvd., no. 4, 300223 Timişoara, Timiş, Romania
{diogen.babuc,florin.fortis}@uvt.ro

Abstract. Recent advancements in artificial intelligence (AI) have substantially impacted healthcare, particularly in disease diagnosis and prediction. This paper introduces an AI-driven decision support system (DSS) designed for multi-disease diagnosis. The DSS leverages custom deep learning architectures: convolutional neural networks, vision transformers, and hybrid models to perform precise and efficient medical image classification and predictive analytics. Image preprocessing is enhanced through masked and variational autoencoders. To enhance model performance and adaptability, the system employs neural architecture search methods guided by stochastic principles. The proposed DSS addresses significant challenges in deploying AI in healthcare, including cross-domain generalization and secure integration within medical settings. Federated learning techniques are incorporated to enable decentralized model training across multiple medical institutions. This integrated DSS showcases the transformative potential of AI in healthcare.

Keywords: multi-disease diagnosis · federated learning · neural architecture search · medical image processing · neural architectures

1 Introduction

The integration of artificial intelligence (AI) into healthcare enabled substantial advances in clinical diagnostics, risk prediction, and decision support [16]. Deep learning techniques, particularly convolutional neural networks (CNN) and vision transformers (ViT), have proven to be highly effective in the analysis of complex medical images. These innovations can be impactful in oncology, neurology, and ophthalmology, where early and precise detection is vital.

However, the clinical deployment of AI systems remains hindered by several key challenges. These include the need for robust generalization across diverse patient populations and data types, secure and ethical handling of sensitive medical data, and adaptability to decentralized healthcare infrastructures [17]. Furthermore, the capacity to perform multi-disease diagnosis, rather than targeting a single pathology, remains underexplored in real-world applications.

P. Bruno et al. (Eds.): HC_AIxIA_HYDRA 2025, CCIS 2830, pp. 37–49, 2026.
https://doi.org/10.1007/978-3-032-16708-8_3

This paper introduces `MultiH-EU`, an AI-driven decision support system (DSS) tailored for multi-disease diagnosis and clinical risk prediction. `MultiH-EU` leverages state-of-the-art deep learning approaches because it includes specialized CNN, ViT, and hybrid models, to provide high-precision classification across several diseases: colorectal and cervical cancer, Alzheimer's disease, diabetic retinopathy, and skin lesions. It also incorporates advanced image preprocessing to improve input quality and model robustness.

To further enhance performance and adaptability, the DSS applies neural architecture search (NAS) driven by stochastic optimization principles, enabling automated tuning of network parameters. In addition, federated learning ensures decentralized model training across medical institutions without compromising patient privacy [29].

The main contributions of this research can be summarized in the following major objectives:

1. Design and development of a modular AI-based DSS capable of diagnosing multiple diseases using diverse custom deep learning architectures across varied imaging and clinical datasets.
2. Implementation of secure and privacy-preserving AI training mechanisms to enable decentralized deployment in real-world healthcare environments.
3. Optimization of preprocessing and model performance through stochastic neural architecture search and innovative image enhancement techniques.

Together, these objectives position `MultiH-EU` as a comprehensive and clinically applicable AI platform, addressing the technical and ethical challenges of AI integration in healthcare.

2 Background Information and Related Works

This section outlines the foundational technologies and methodologies that underpin the `MultiH-EU` system. It highlights state-of-the-art advancements in federated learning, secure AI deployment, and neural architecture search, which collectively enable scalable, privacy-preserving, and high-performance multi-disease diagnosis [27].

2.1 Federated Learning and Secure AI Deployment in Clinical Environments

Federated Learning (FL) is a decentralized paradigm in which multiple clients (hospitals, diagnostic labs, or regional clinics) collaboratively train machine learning models without transferring raw patient data to a central server [18]. Instead, each participant trains a local model using its dataset and shares only hidden updates (gradients or model weights) with a central aggregator. This approach ensures compliance with privacy regulations such as GDPR and aligns with ethical standards in AI for healthcare. This subsection demonstrates how

FL is not only a privacy-preserving solution but also a scalable, maintainable component of real-world AI deployment in medicine [20].

In the MultiH-EU system, FL is a core component of the training pipeline, enabling geographically distributed institutions to contribute to model development while preserving full ownership of their data. Frameworks such as Metis-FL [5], Flower [9], Fed-BioMed [22], and SubstraFL [26] are employed to facilitate this process, supporting various deep learning architectures, including CNN, ViT, and hybrid models.

Colorectal polyp detection (Bionnica [7]). Colonoscopy data for colorectal polyps vary significantly across hospitals due to differences in imaging devices, labeling protocols, and staining. Bionnica, a custom CNN-based architecture, is trained using FL to aggregate insights from these heterogeneous sources without centralizing patient images.

Cervical cancer screening (BFIS [3] and BOVNet [8]). Screening centers in different regions often exhibit domain shifts in cytology image distributions due to varying staining protocols and imaging equipment. Federated training allows BFIS and BOVNet to generalize better by learning from distributed cytopathology datasets without centralizing sensitive images.

Alzheimer's detection (EDoViT-Alz [4], DAS-Alz [2]). Brain scan data from memory clinics or research institutes is particularly privacy-sensitive. FL enables collaborative modeling across neurology centers to improve detection accuracy while maintaining strict data governance.

Diabetic retinopathy (EI-ViT-Net [10]). FL is applied across multiple ophthalmology clinics, ensuring diverse patient coverage and improving generalization. This avoids the biases introduced by single-site data while protecting patient confidentiality.

Skin lesion classification (EDF+DVFS [6]). FL supports resource-constrained deployments (mobile dermatology units) that use on-device learning for skin lesion classification. Training models across distributed dermatological imaging centers improves classification robustness in diverse populations, while task scheduling is evaluated by energy consumption and CPU and GPU degradation.

2.2 Neural Architecture Search for Adaptive Model Optimization

The design of high-performing neural networks for medical image analysis is a complex task, often requiring extensive experimentation and domain expertise. Manual architecture engineering is time-consuming and prone to suboptimal configurations.

NAS addresses this challenge by automating the discovery of optimal model architectures based on defined performance objectives, such as classification accuracy, model size, and inference latency. In the MultiH-EU system, NAS plays a central role in tailoring model configurations for task-specific requirements, ensuring adaptability, scalability, and efficiency.

The NAS approach adopted in this work is guided by stochastic optimization principles, enabling efficient exploration of large architectural design spaces.

Randomized sampling, reinforcement learning, or evolutionary algorithms are employed to generate and evaluate candidate architectures dynamically [28].

NAS enables such specialization by adapting architectural parameters like depth, width, kernel sizes, and attention mechanisms to fit the specific needs of each dataset and task. Beyond accuracy, the NAS strategy employed in `MultiH-EU` also accounts for hardware-aware constraints to support real-world deployment. These include minimizing latency and maximizing energy efficiency for edge devices.

3 Methodology

The proposed system, `MultiH-EU`, is a modular, AI-driven DSS designed for secure, scalable, and high-accuracy multi-disease diagnosis. The methodology encompasses a layered approach involving disease-specific model design, distributed training, data security, and deployment optimization, as depicted in Fig. 1. It integrates advanced deep learning architectures, federated learning protocols, and preprocessing pipelines with a focus on real-world clinical applicability.

3.1 System Architecture Overview

Effective preprocessing of medical images is a critical component in AI-based diagnosis, directly influencing the performance and generalization of deep learning models. In `MultiH-EU`, disease-specific preprocessing pipelines are adopted to enhance feature extraction, improve robustness to noise, and handle domain variability. The system leverages advanced techniques such as masked autoencoders, variational autoencoders, CycleGAN [12], and zero-shot noise-to-noise (ZS-N2N) denoising [29], adapted to the unique characteristics of each disease type.

The Fig. 1 presents a comprehensive overview of the `MultiH-EU` methodology, depicting the full pipeline from data intake to deployment readiness. It begins with five core medical domains—colorectal polyps, retinopathy, cervical cells, skin lesions, and Alzheimer's—each contributing domain-specific datasets into the system. These data sources feed into a unified preprocessing and enhancement stage, to improve input quality. After preprocessing, the data is passed to the local model training phase, where disease-specific neural networks are trained within individual institutions using their private data. The outputs from these distributed models are then securely transmitted to a central node in the federated aggregation and security layer, which manages encoding updates and ensures compliance through mechanisms such as Latin Djokovic encoding [1]. Following aggregation, NAS is used to refine model designs, optimizing for performance and deployment constraints. The figure emphasizes the system's privacy-preserving design and its adaptability across multiple medical domains.

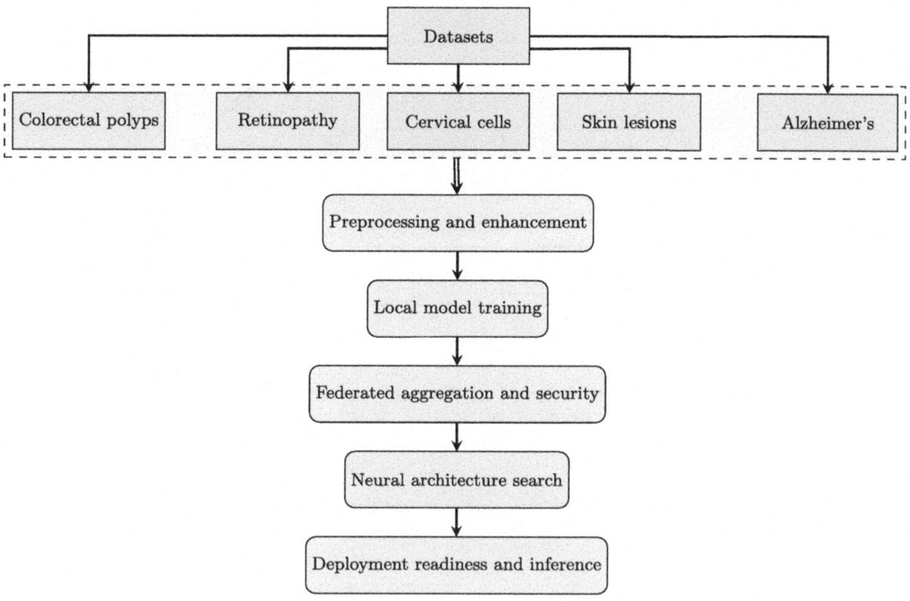

Fig. 1. Overview of the `MultiH-EU` logistics. Integrating data sources, preprocessing, federated training, NAS optimization, and multi-platform deployment.

The Fig. 2 illustrates the `MultiH-EU` methodology as a modular pipeline structured by medical use case. Each disease domain—colorectal polyps, cervical cancer, Alzheimer's disease, diabetic retinopathy, and skin lesions—is represented as an independent processing stream. For each case, relevant medical data is first preprocessed and then fed into a disease-specific AI model. These models are trained using federated learning frameworks appropriate for the data and institutional setup, including also a CI/CD-enabled hosted solution. Each framework supports privacy-preserving collaboration between clinical sites without sharing raw data. All model outputs from these distributed training environments are then directed into a unified aggregation and evaluation module. This final component is responsible for combining model updates, calculating performance metrics and ensuring consistent evaluation across all use cases. The figure emphasizes the system's modular design, secure learning strategy, and consistent evaluation approach across diverse medical domains.

Disease-specific AI modules. At the core of the system are disease-specific AI modules, each engineered for a targeted pathology: colorectal polyps, cervical cancer, Alzheimer's disease, diabetic retinopathy, and skin lesions, as Fig. 2 suggests. These modules are built using deep learning architectures tailored to each diagnostic domain, including convolutional neural networks, vision transformers, and hybrid models. The models are trained on domain-specific datasets, with custom preprocessing pipelines that reflect the unique visual and structural features of each disease.

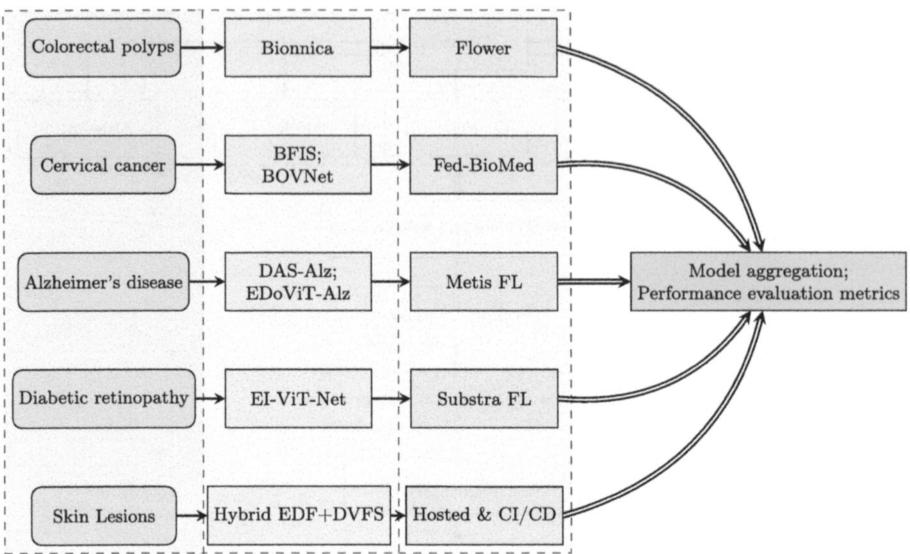

Fig. 2. `MultiH-EU` methodology per use case, integrating preprocessing, disease-specific AI models, federated learning frameworks, and evaluation metrics.

Federated learning engine. To ensure privacy-preserving collaboration across clinical partners, the system incorporates a federated learning engine built upon frameworks such as Metis-FL, Flower, Fed-BioMed, and SubstraFL. In this configuration, medical institutions train local models on private datasets without exposing raw data, and only encrypted model updates are shared with a central aggregator. This setup preserves data confidentiality while enabling the global model to benefit from a diverse range of patient populations and imaging conditions. The federated learning layer is fully integrated with the `MultiH-EU` training loop, enabling seamless synchronization and performance aggregation across nodes.

Hybrid coupling with clinical knowledge. To ensure real-world applicability, the inductive models are complemented by interfaces to deductive, rule-based components. These modules encode clinical constraints such as safety thresholds, triage protocols, or mandatory follow-up actions. They act as supervisory layers on top of the neural predictions. For instance, in screening scenarios, a positive classification may be cross-checked with domain-specific rules (lesion size or cytology grade thresholds) before generating a final recommendation.

Preprocessing and enhancement layer. Before inference or training, raw input data undergoes disease-specific enhancement in the preprocessing layer. Techniques such as masked autoencoders (for reconstructing masked image patches), variational autoencoders (for latent encoding of cellular features), CycleGANs (for domain adaptation between imaging styles), and zero-shot noise-to-noise denoising (for cleaning without clean target data) are applied to boost data quality. These preprocessing methods ensure that models receive standardized, information-rich input.

Model optimization layer. Once initial models are trained, the architecture is fine-tuned using a NAS process guided by stochastic optimization. NAS is applied to discover optimal model configurations—including depth, width, kernel size, and attention structure—for each pathology and dataset. The search process dynamically balances trade-offs between accuracy, inference time, and memory usage. This ensures the final model is not only high-performing but also adaptable to varying hardware constraints and use-case demands.

3.2 Training Workflow

The training pipeline in `MultiH-EU` is structured into five key phases: image preprocessing, local training, federated aggregation, neural architecture adaptation, and deployment. Each phase is tightly integrated with the others to support high model performance, cross-domain generalization, and secure training across distributed environments.

In the preprocessing phase, raw medical images are transformed into high-quality, standardized inputs suited for neural model consumption. Techniques vary by disease and imaging modality:

- **Noise reduction** via ZS-N2N denoising (see Eq. (1)). Given a noisy input image x, the model D_θ (parameterized denoiser) learns to predict a clean signal by minimizing:

$$\mathcal{L}_{\text{N2N}}(\theta) = \mathbb{E}_{x \sim \mathcal{X}} \left[\|D_\theta(x) - x'\|_2^2 \right] \tag{1}$$

  where x' is another independently sampled noisy version of x from the distribution $\mathcal{X}$, and $\|\cdot\|_2^2$ denotes the squared L2 norm.
- **Feature compression** using autoencoders (see Eq. (2)). The encoder E maps the input x to a latent representation z, and the decoder G reconstructs the image as $\hat{x}$:

$$z = E(x), \quad \hat{x} = G(z) \tag{2}$$

  with reconstruction loss (Eq. (3)) defined by:

$$\mathcal{L}_{\text{AE}} = \|x - \hat{x}\|_2^2 \tag{3}$$

  where $\hat{x}$ is the decoded approximation of the original input.
- **Domain adaptation** using CycleGAN (see Eq. (4)). The generators G and F translate between source and target image domains, and are optimized with the cycle consistency loss:

$$\mathcal{L}_{\text{cyc}}(G, F) = \mathbb{E}_{x \sim A}[\|F(G(x)) - x\|_1] + \mathbb{E}_{y \sim B}[\|G(F(y)) - y\|_1] \tag{4}$$

  where A and B represent distinct domains (e.g., different hospitals or devices), and $\|\cdot\|_1$ is the L1 norm.

3.3 Selected Datasets

To rigorously evaluate the performance, robustness, and generalizability of the MultiH-EU system, we conduct experiments on a combination of public benchmark datasets and proprietary clinical image repositories. The datasets are selected to reflect real-world variability in imaging modalities, acquisition conditions, and pathological diversity across the five targeted disease domains. Each dataset undergoes domain-specific preprocessing and is integrated into the federated learning and architecture optimization pipelines of MultiH-EU.

Colorectal polyps are evaluated using a combination of endoscopic video frames and histopathological slides sourced from public datasets such as Kvasir-SEG [14], CVC-ClinicDB [24], and proprietary clinical archives. These datasets include both hyperplastic and adenomatous polyps, which are critical for early colorectal cancer screening. The Bionnica CNN and MAE-enhanced preprocessing pipeline are applied to extract edge- and texture-sensitive features. For cervical cancer screening, the system uses datasets such as Herlev Pap Smear, SIPaKMeD, and internal cytology lab slides [21]. The data consists of high-resolution cellular images labeled with squamous intraepithelial lesion grades. VAEs and ZS-N2N denoising are employed to manage noise and inter-laboratory variation. MRI scans (T1-weighted) for Alzheimer's diagnosis are obtained from the Alzheimer's Disease Neuroimaging Initiative (ADNI) and supplemented with hospital-acquired imaging [13]. Preprocessing includes grayscale normalization and anatomical alignment. Attention-based ViT and CNN models (EDoViT-Alz and DAS-Alz) are used to highlight regions associated with neurodegeneration. Diabetic retinopathy analysis leverages fundus image datasets such as APTOS [11], EyePACS [23], and local ophthalmology center data. These datasets cover all DR severity levels (No DR, Mild, Moderate, Severe, and Proliferative). Domain variability is addressed through CycleGAN-based style adaptation and N2N denoising. The system uses dermoscopic datasets such as ISIC 2018 [15], HAM10000 [25], and institutional dermatology scans for skin lesion analysis. These include a diverse range of skin conditions, from benign nevi to malignant melanomas. The hybrid CNN-transformer models (BOVNet, Renesansa) and CycleGAN-based augmentation are used to account for variations in skin tone, lighting, and lesion forms [19].

4 Results and Discussion

This section evaluates the performance of the MultiH-EU system across five major disease domains. The evaluation focused on three main metrics—accuracy, area under the ROC curve (AUC), and F1-score—to assess classification quality and robustness. Models were tested using real-world benchmark and clinical datasets, each paired with preprocessing pipelines and optimized architectures via NAS.

The results confirm that domain-specific preprocessing and architecture tuning via NAS significantly enhance model performance. For example, Alzheimer's detection using EDoViT-Alz and DAS-Alz benefited from attention-driven ViTs,

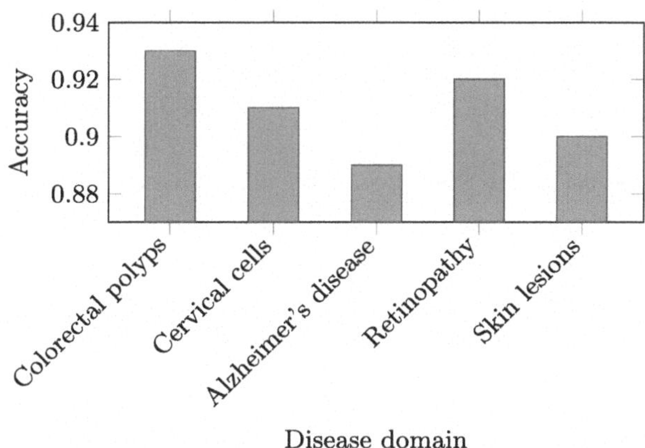

Fig. 3. Mean model accuracy for all disease categories in the `MultiH-EU` environment.

which increased focus on hippocampal and cortical regions. However, this domain showed slightly lower metrics compared to others due to higher intra-class variance and limited labeled data in some stages of progression (MCI). Skin lesion classification maintained strong performance despite the added challenge of deployment on resource-constrained devices. EDF+DVFS was optimized through latency-aware NAS and edge deployment scheduling, maintaining a balance between efficiency and performance. Across all domains, federated learning led to improved generalization compared to centralized baselines. Variability between hospitals (staining differences in cervical samples or different retinal fundus cameras) was effectively addressed by training across distributed data sources.

Figure 3 illustrates a bar chart of model accuracy per disease alongside a boxplot showing distribution across metrics. While colorectal polyps and retinopathy consistently outperform others, the variance in F1-scores highlights task-specific challenges. Alzheimer's results show the largest spread, reflecting sensitivity to image quality and clinical labels.

The statistical evaluation of the `MultiH-EU` system across five medical domains (Table 1a)—colorectal polyps, cervical cancer, Alzheimer's disease, diabetic retinopathy, and skin lesions—demonstrates consistently strong model performance based on five key indicators: accuracy, AUC, F1-score, precision, and sensitivity. Colorectal polyp detection achieved the highest overall accuracy at 0.93, along with an AUC of 0.95 and an F1-score of 0.92, reflecting excellent classification balance and strong discriminative ability. Cervical cancer and retinopathy models both showed robust performance, with F1-scores of 0.90 and 0.91 respectively, suggesting high reliability even under moderate domain shift.

The Alzheimer's model, while slightly lower in accuracy (0.89) and F1 (0.88), achieved a sensitivity of 0.90, which is critical in medical contexts where false negatives (missed diagnoses) carry high risk. Similarly, the skin lesion classifier maintained balanced precision (0.88) and sensitivity (0.90), underscoring its

Table 1. Comprehensive performance analysis of the diagnostic model across different disease types and ablation scenarios.

(a) Statistical performance indicators for each disease type.

Disease	Acc.	AUC	F1	Prec.	Sens.
Col. polyps	0.93	0.95	0.92	0.91	0.93
Cerv. cancer	0.91	0.92	0.90	0.89	0.91
Alzheimer's	0.89	0.90	0.88	0.86	0.90
Retinopathy	0.92	0.93	0.91	0.90	0.92
Skin lesions	0.90	0.91	0.89	0.88	0.90

(b) Ablation study: average accuracy across all domains.

Configuration	Avg. acc.
Full `MultiH-EU` (baseline)	0.91
w/o NAS	0.87
w/o Federated learning	0.88
w/o Denoising	0.89

suitability for deployment in real-time, mobile dermatological screening. Overall, the use of AUC as a complementary metric is crucial, especially in imbalanced datasets.

To assess the individual impact of architectural components, we conducted ablation experiments by incrementally disabling key system elements: FL, NAS, and denoising. As shown in Table 1b, each removal results in a measurable drop in performance across all diseases. The largest degradation occurred when NAS was disabled, underscoring its role in architecture optimization. These results highlight the synergistic value of combining preprocessing, decentralized learning, and architecture optimization in a unified pipeline. To validate robustness, we performed leave-one-site-out experiments across distributed clinical datasets. In each round, one institution's data was withheld from training and used only for testing. Table 2a shows the F1-scores across five runs. Despite institutional variability in imaging hardware and labeling protocols, the models retained strong predictive performance, validating the federated architecture's adaptability. Table 2b reports inference time and compressed model size for each disease domain on an Intel Core i7, 12th generation, with Iris X Graphics, using PyTorch.

Post-NAS and deployment optimizations successfully reduced inference latency below 30 ms for all models, which may be suitable for clinical and mobile use cases. Clinicians examined the regions highlighted by the system, labeling each as either concordant or discordant with established expert diagnostic markers (in a Google Forms example, when specifying the feedback). Cohen's Kappa index was employed to statistically quantify the level of inter-rater agreement between the clinicians' assessments and the system's highlighted regions. Subsequently, the proportion of correctly aligned regions was computed for each case.

To assess the contribution of federated learning, we compared three training paradigms: (1) centralized training using pooled datasets, (2) federated learning with global model aggregation, and (3) specific local training per institution. Table 3 shows that federated learning matches centralized performance (baseline) while outperforming isolated local models, all without compromising data privacy. This validates federated learning as a practical middle-ground solution,

Table 2. Benchmarking diagnostic model performance for generalizability and practical efficiency.

(a) Cross-institution generalization (Leave-One-Out).

Held-out site	**F1-score**
Hospital A (Cervical)	0.88
Hospital B (Retina)	0.89
Clinic C (Polyp)	0.90
Neuro Ctr D (Alzheimer)	0.85
SkinLab E (Skin)	0.87
Avg.	0.88

(b) Inference time and model size (edge-optimized).

Model	**Lat. (ms)**	**Size (MB)**
Bionnica	22.1	18.5
BFIS	19.8	16.3
EDoViT-Alz	28.5	21.0
EI-ViT-Net	24.3	20.4
EDF+DVFS	20.5	19.1

Table 3. Comparative effectiveness (F1-score), efficiency, and NAS search performance of training strategies across different models.

Model	Baseline	Federated	Local	NAS time (hrs)	Acc. (%)	Lat. (%)
Bionnica	0.92	0.91	0.86	36	+4.2	−16.5
BFIS	0.90	0.90	0.85	28	+3.7	−18.2
EDoViT-Alz	0.89	0.88	0.84	48	+4.5	−15.1
EI-ViT-Net	0.91	0.91	0.87	32	+3.9	−14.8
EDF+DVFS	0.89	0.89	0.83	30	+4.0	−17.0
Average	0.902	0.898	0.85	34.8	**+4.1**	**−16.3**

delivering strong performance with regulatory compliance and minimal compromise on generalization. In addition to standard metrics, we assessed 95% confidence intervals, expected calibration error, and Brier score for selected domains, highlighting model reliability.

5 Conclusions

This paper presented `MultiH-EU` configuration, a modular AI-driven decision support system designed for accurate, secure, and scalable multi-disease diagnosis and risk prediction. Through the integration of domain-specific deep learning models, advanced preprocessing techniques, federated learning frameworks, and neural architecture search, `MultiH-EU` delivers reliable classification performance across five clinically significant disease domains: colorectal polyps, cervical cancer, Alzheimer's disease, diabetic retinopathy, and skin lesions.

Empirical evaluations are applied, highlighting the effectiveness of model specialization and NAS-guided optimization. The federated learning engine proved crucial in preserving patient data privacy while enabling collaborative model training across distributed healthcare institutions. In addition, improvements such as zero-shot noise-to-noise denoising, CycleGAN-based adaptation, and lightweight deployment pipelines further contribute to the system's robustness and real-world applicability. The architecture's flexibility supports deployment across heterogeneous platforms, ensuring both diagnostic efficiency and accessibility.

Future work will explore the integration of multimodal clinical data, such as electronic health records and genomic sequences, to improve diagnostic scope.

Acknowledgments. This research was partially supported by the project "Romanian Hub for Artificial Intelligence - HRIA", in the program PCIDIF/709/PCIDIF_P4/OP1/RSO1.6/PCIDIF_A12 - Action 4.1 - MySMIS 351416.

References

1. Babuc, D.: An authentic algorithm for ciphering and deciphering called Latin Djokovic. arXiv preprint arXiv:2403.01463 (2024)
2. Babuc, D., Babuc, G.: Das-Alz: Alzheimer's disease classification using downscaled MRI scans and a reinforced convolutional neural network. In: 2024 IEEE 24th International Conference on Bioinformatics and Bioengineering (BIBE), pp. 1–7. IEEE (2024)
3. Babuc, D., Fortiş, A.E.: A customizable intelligent system for cervical cytology image classifications. In: International Conference on Complex, Intelligent, and Software Intensive Systems, pp. 82–93. Springer, Cham (2024)
4. Babuc, D., Fortiş, A.E.: Edovit-Alz: Alzheimer's disease identification with vision transformer using extremely downscaled MRI data. In: International Conference on P2P, Parallel, Grid, Cloud and Internet Computing, pp. 109–120. Springer, Cham (2024)
5. Babuc, D., Fortiş, T.F.: Federated learning platforms for privacy-preserving histopathological image classification. In: International Conference on Advanced Information Networking and Applications, pp. 317–328. Springer, Cham (2025)
6. Babuc, D., Fortiş, T.F.: Hybrid task scheduling for optimized neural network inference on skin lesions in resource-constrained systems. In: Proceedings of the 5th Workshop on Machine Learning and Systems, pp. 269–275 (2025)
7. Babuc, D., Ivaşcu, T., Ardelean, M., Onchiş, D.: Bionnica: a deep neural network architecture for colorectal polyps' premalignancy risk evaluation. medRxiv, pp. 2024–06 (2024)
8. Babuc, D., Onchis, D.: Bovnet: Cervical cells classifications using a custom-based neural network with autoencoders
9. Beutel, D.J., et al.: Flower: a friendly federated learning research framework. arXiv preprint arXiv:2007.14390 (2020)
10. Farcaş, A., Lobonţ, A., Babuc, D., Ivaşcu, T., Ştefănigă, S.A.: EI-vit-net: a vision transformer approach for diabetic retinopathy's decision support pipeline. In: 2024 IEEE 24th International Conference on Bioinformatics and Bioengineering (BIBE), pp. 1–6. IEEE (2024)
11. Gangwar, A.K., Ravi, V.: Diabetic retinopathy detection using transfer learning and deep learning. In: Evolution in Computational Intelligence: Frontiers in Intelligent Computing: Theory and Applications (FICTA 2020), vol. 1, pp. 679–689. Springer, Cham (2021)

12. Gidijala, K., Sagenela, V.K.: The conception of fundus multi-disease dataset (FMDD) using multi-spectral generative adversarial networks. Eng. Technol. Appl. Sci. Res. **15**(2), 21539–21544 (2025)
13. Hinrichs, C., et al.: Spatially augmented LPboosting for ad classification with evaluations on the ADNI dataset. Neuroimage **48**(1), 138–149 (2009)
14. Jha, D., et al.: Kvasir-seg: a segmented polyp dataset. In: International Conference on Multimedia Modeling, pp. 451–462. Springer, Cham (2019)
15. Kassem, M.A., Hosny, K.M., Fouad, M.M.: Skin lesions classification into eight classes for ISIC 2019 using deep convolutional neural network and transfer learning. IEEE Access **8**, 114822–114832 (2020)
16. Koski, E., Murphy, J.: AI in healthcare. In: Nurses and Midwives in the Digital Age, pp. 295–299. IOS Press (2021)
17. Kothinti, R.R.: Artificial intelligence in disease prediction: transforming early diagnosis and preventive healthcare (2024)
18. Lee, G.H., Shin, S.Y.: Federated learning on clinical benchmark data: performance assessment. J. Med. Internet Res. **22**(10), e20891 (2020)
19. Ma, S., Huang, J.: Combining multiple markers for classification using ROC. Biometrics **63**(3), 751–757 (2007)
20. Mohammad Amini, M., Jesus, M., Fanaei Sheikholeslami, D., Alves, P., Hassanzadeh Benam, A., Hariri, F.: Artificial intelligence ethics and challenges in healthcare applications: a comprehensive review in the context of the European GDPR mandate. Mach. Learn. Knowl. Extraction **5**(3), 1023–1035 (2023)
21. Ram, E., Stihl, E.: Impact of cell type selection on binary classification of cervical cancer using convolutional neural networks: a compatibility analysis of herlev and sipakmed (2023)
22. Silva, S., Altmann, A., Gutman, B., Lorenzi, M.: Fed-BioMed: a general open-source frontend framework for federated learning in healthcare. In: Albarqouni, S., et al. (eds.) DART/DCL -2020. LNCS, vol. 12444, pp. 201–210. Springer, Cham (2020). https://doi.org/10.1007/978-3-030-60548-3_20
23. Tariq, M., Palade, V., Ma, Y.: Transfer learning based classification of diabetic retinopathy on the kaggle eyepacs dataset. In: International Conference on Medical Imaging and Computer-Aided Diagnosis, pp. 89–99. Springer, Cham (2022)
24. TS, C., Jagadale, B.N.: Comparative analysis of u-net and deeplab for automatic polyp segmentation in colonoscopic frames using CVC-clinicdb dataset (2023)
25. Tschandl, P., Rosendahl, C., Kittler, H.: The ham10000 dataset, a large collection of multi-source dermatoscopic images of common pigmented skin lesions. Sci. Data **5**(1), 1–9 (2018)
26. Wu, C.Y., Gupta, P., Mohapatra, S.: Case studies and recommendations for designing federated learning models for digital healthcare systems. In: Federated Learning for Digital Healthcare Systems, pp. 301–323. Elsevier (2024)
27. Xie, S., Yu, Z., Lv, Z.: Multi-disease prediction based on deep learning: a survey. Comput. Model. Eng. Sci. **128**(2), 489–522 (2021)
28. Xie, S., Zheng, H., Liu, C., Lin, L.: SNAS: stochastic neural architecture search. arXiv preprint arXiv:1812.09926 (2018)
29. Zhaoyang, S., et al.: Exploring zero-shot learning for multi-disease diagnosis using vision transformers with tongue and facial imaging. Available at SSRN 4987853

RAG-Enhanced LLMs for Interactive Explainability in Clinical Decision Support Systems

Lorenzo Mannocci(✉), Francesca Naretto, Lucia Passaro, and Anna Monreale

University of Pisa, Pisa, Italy
lorenzo.mannocci@di.unipi.it,
{francesca.naretto,lucia.passaro,anna.monreale}@unipi.it

Abstract. Artificial Intelligence (AI) is increasingly embedded in high-risks decision-making systems across domains such as healthcare, finance, and the judicial system. As reliance on predictive models grows, so does the demand for Explainable AI (XAI) to ensure transparency, trust, and interpretability. However, existing XAI approaches often fail to present explanations in a format accessible to domain experts, limiting their practical utility. Large Language Models (LLMs) have recently emerged as a bridge between complex models and end-users, offering natural language explanations. Yet, their use introduces new risks, including hallucinated outputs and lack of source traceability. To address these challenges, we propose a Clinical Decision Support System (CDSS) that not only combines standard predictive models with XAI techniques but also incorporates a Retrieval-Augmented Generation module as an interactive enhancer. This module grounds explanations in verified medical knowledge, reformulates technical outputs into a human-like format, and enables users—such as clinicians—to actively query the system. By fostering an interactive, human-in-the-loop environment, our approach empowers domain experts to explore model decisions, contextualize explanations, and build trust in AI-assisted diagnostics. The study concludes with preliminary experiments validating the proposed methodology.

Keywords: explainable AI · human computer interaction · retrieval-augmented generation · large language models · clinical decision support system

1 Introduction

Artificial Intelligence (AI) has rapidly evolved to become a crucial component in decision-making systems across various fields, including healthcare [42], finance [7], law enforcement [38], and the judicial system [34]. The increasing reliance on predictive models in these domains necessitates the development of

P. Bruno et al. (Eds.): HC_AIxIA_HYDRA 2025, CCIS 2830, pp. 50–63, 2026.
https://doi.org/10.1007/978-3-032-16708-8_4

methods to explain their outputs, a requirement that has led to the emergence of Explainable Artificial Intelligence (XAI) [16,20]. XAI aims to make AI models more interpretable, transparent, and trustworthy, ensuring that domain experts and end-users can understand and assess the rationale behind automated decisions [10,31]. The need for trust and transparency in AI decision-making has also been recognized at the regulatory level. The European Union's AI Act [37], one of the first comprehensive legal frameworks for AI, emphasizes the importance of explainability, particularly for high-risk AI applications. The AI Act mandates that AI systems used in critical sectors provide clear, understandable, and verifiable explanations to ensure accountability and fairness. This regulatory push further underscores the necessity of effective XAI techniques that can meet both ethical and legal standards while supporting domain experts in making informed decisions.

Many high-risk applications depend on predictive models that significantly impact human lives. In healthcare, AI-driven diagnostic systems assist doctors in detecting diseases, recommending treatments, and predicting patient outcomes [42]. In the judicial system, predictive models inform parole decisions and risk assessments [34]. Despite their effectiveness, these models often operate as black boxes, making it difficult for domain experts to verify their outputs and detect potential biases. Without proper interpretability, decision-makers may struggle to trust AI-driven recommendations, leading to ethical, legal, and social concerns. Indeed, these explanations might be difficult to interpret, particularly for professionals outside the field of computer science, such as doctors, lawyers, or policymakers. The challenge lies in presenting these explanations in a way that aligns with the expertise and expectations of the end-users [9]. For example, rule-based explainability methods may generate decision rules with numerical thresholds that do not align with conventional domain knowledge. In medical applications, an AI model might define a risk threshold for blood pressure or glucose levels that deviates from commonly accepted medical guidelines, creating confusion among clinicians. Without proper contextualization, such outputs can diminish trust in the AI system rather than enhancing its credibility. Moreover, existing XAI methods often fail to present explanations in a format that is intuitive and easily digestible for domain experts. This limitation has led to the integration of Large Language Models (LLMs) as interfaces for explainability, offering a more natural and human-like explanations for AI predictions [3].

LLMs have been increasingly employed as mediators between complex AI models and domain experts, translating complex mathematical justifications into human-like explanations. By reformatting and simplifying the outputs of XAI techniques, LLMs can substantially enhance the interpretability of AI-driven decisions [3]. In a healthcare setting, for instance, an LLM can transform a technical explanation of a machine learning model's prediction into a structured summary that aligns with a physician's diagnostic workflow [23,30]. More recently, LLMs have been leveraged not only to translate explanations into natural language but also to enrich them with contextual information drawn from their pretrained knowledge [36]. However, this approach introduces an additional layer of complexity and potential risk. LLMs are known to occasionally produce inaccurate or misleading outputs, a phenomenon referred to as hallucinations [24]. Furthermore, these models typically do not provide access to the underlying sources that support their responses, limiting transparency and traceability [27].

One promising approach to mitigating LLM hallucinations in XAI is the use of Retrieval-Augmented Generation (RAG) [26]. RAG enhances LLM-generated explanations by grounding them in an external, domain-specific knowledge base. Instead of relying solely on the LLM's pre-trained knowledge, RAG retrieves relevant information from a curated database to provide more accurate and reliable explanations. In the context of XAI, RAG can address two critical challenges. First, it reduces the risk of hallucinations by ensuring that explanations are based on verified sources rather than probabilistic text generation. Second, it allows for the integration of domain-specific knowledge, ensuring that explanations adhere to established medical, legal, or financial guidelines. By leveraging RAG, AI-generated explanations can be aligned more closely with experts' expectations, thereby increasing trust and usability in real-world applications.

In this work, we present, to the best of our knowledge, the first Clinical Decision Support System (CDSS) that integrates standard predictive models with XAI techniques and RAG-enhanced explanations. The proposed system consists of three key components:

1. *Predictive Model*: A standard classifier, such as a neural network or a random forest, that generates predictions based on patient data;
2. *Explainer*: An explanation method that provides insights into the model's decision-making process through feature importance-based explanations (e.g., LIME [39] and SHAP [28]), decision rules (e.g., LORE [19]) or exemplars and counter-exemplars [18];
3. *RAG-Based enhancer module*: A module built on RAG that enhances explanations by grounding them in reliable medical knowledge, mitigating hallucinations, and transforming traditional explanations into more human-readable, context-aware formats. It also serves as an interactive tool, allowing end users to ask specific questions and explore the patient's clinical profile in relation to the model's predictions and explanations.

By combining standard classifiers with RAG-based explanations grounded in verified medical sources, our system enhances the trustworthiness and domain relevance of AI-driven medical decisions. This approach addresses key limitations of conventional XAI by providing interpretable, reliable insights tailored to healthcare professionals. The study concludes with *preliminary experiments* validating the proposed methodology.

2 Related Works

AI is transforming modern society, largely due to the rise of complex Machine Learning (ML) models with strong predictive capabilities. However, these models—such as deep neural networks and ensemble methods—are often considered black boxes due to their lack of transparency [20,31]. This opacity makes it difficult to identify biases in training data or explain decisions, which is especially concerning in high-stakes domains like healthcare, finance, and criminal justice. As Rudin argues [40], the lack of interpretability hinders trust, accountability, and real-world deployment of AI systems in regulated settings. At the same time, Large Language Models (LLMs) have opened new possibilities for generating intuitive, accessible explanations. Their ability to bridge technical and non-technical understanding supports the development of more human-centric, fair, and transparent AI systems.

We focus next on two key areas: post-hoc explanations, which analyze model behavior after predictions are made, and human-centered explanations, which adapt to user needs to improve interpretability.

2.1 Post-hoc Explanations

In the context of post-hoc explanation methods for black-box models applied to tabular data, both local and global approaches have been extensively studied and benchmarked [5]. Local explanation methods aim to interpret individual predictions by approximating the model's behavior in the vicinity of a specific instance. One of the most widely known techniques in this category is LIME, which builds a simple surrogate model—usually linear—on a locally perturbed dataset to estimate the contribution of each feature [39]. Although popular, LIME suffers from instability due to its random neighborhood generation strategy. A more theoretically grounded alternative is SHAP, which relies on Shapley values from cooperative game theory to assign each feature an importance score based on its marginal contribution across all possible feature combinations [28]. SHAP ensures consistency and local accuracy, making it a robust choice for feature attribution. Another relevant method is LORE, which employs genetic algorithms to generate a neighborhood and extracts interpretable decision rules, offering both factual and counterfactual explanations [19]. Other approaches provide local explanations which are based on exemplars or better counter-exemplars, which enable a counterfactual reasoning that in some sense produce suggestions to users on what is possible to change for obtaining a different decision from the machine learning model [18].

On the other hand, global explanation methods focus on understanding the model's logic over the entire input space. RuleFit combines decision rules extracted from tree ensembles with linear models to produce sparse, interpretable explanations of model behavior. Building upon this idea, SkopeRules uses ensemble techniques to extract a set of high-precision rules that summarize the model's decision boundaries [14]. More recently, Setzu et al. [41] proposed GLocalX, which aggregates local explanations to form a coherent global understanding of the model, effectively bridging the gap between local interpretability and global insight. These methods, differing in their assumptions and strategies, collectively contribute to the growing toolbox of post-hoc XAI techniques tailored for tabular data.

2.2 Human-Centered Explanations

Both post-hoc and intrinsic XAI methods have advanced model interpretability, yet a key challenge remains: ensuring explanations are truly comprehensible to end users. Human-centered XAI addresses this by aligning explanations with user needs through participatory design methods such as interviews and user studies [2,11,12]. This approach emphasizes contextualized explanations that integrate seamlessly into user workflows and are validated through real-world testing [25,45].

Recent work explores how LLMs can enhance explanation quality by generating adaptive, narrative-style outputs that combine predictions with counterfactuals [23,29]. For example, x-[plAIn] [30] uses a customized LLM to generate concise, audience-specific summaries of XAI methods. Narrative explanations are also being explored across data types, including tabular data [6,48], graphs [17,35], and images [44].

Initially framed as a data-to-text task, LLM-generated narratives have evolved to incorporate broader knowledge, adding context and reasoning beyond simple summaries [29]. A recent pilot study found users preferred such narratives over SHAP plots across several metrics [48]. This approach aligns with the concept of *self-explanations*, where models articulate reasoning to aid understanding [22]. However, it also introduces risks like adversarial helpfulness, where convincing but incorrect explanations may mislead users [1]. RAG helps mitigate this by grounding outputs in trusted sources, improving factual accuracy and transparency [15]. Similarly, Park et al. [36] combine LLMs with knowledge graphs to generate structured, domain-specific explanations that are both clinically accurate and contextually rich.

3 Method

In light of the growing need for human-centered explanations and the impressive capabilities of LLMs to generate human-like responses, challenges arise, particularly when LLMs produce convincing yet incorrect answers or exhibit hallucinations. These issues can compromise the reliability of explanations and erode user trust. To address these concerns, we propose leveraging RAG, a system that combines the generative power of LLMs with the reliability of external, grounded, and reliable sources. By integrating RAG, we ensure that the explanations are not only contextually rich and human-readable but also rooted in verifiable information, thereby enhancing both accuracy and transparency in the model's outputs. Figure 1 illustrates the approach proposed in this work, which combines traditional classifiers, such as black-box models, with standard explainers like LIME or SHAP, alongside an enhancement module based on RAG. The final output of this integrated method is then processed by a selector. In the following sections, we provide a detailed description of each step in the method.

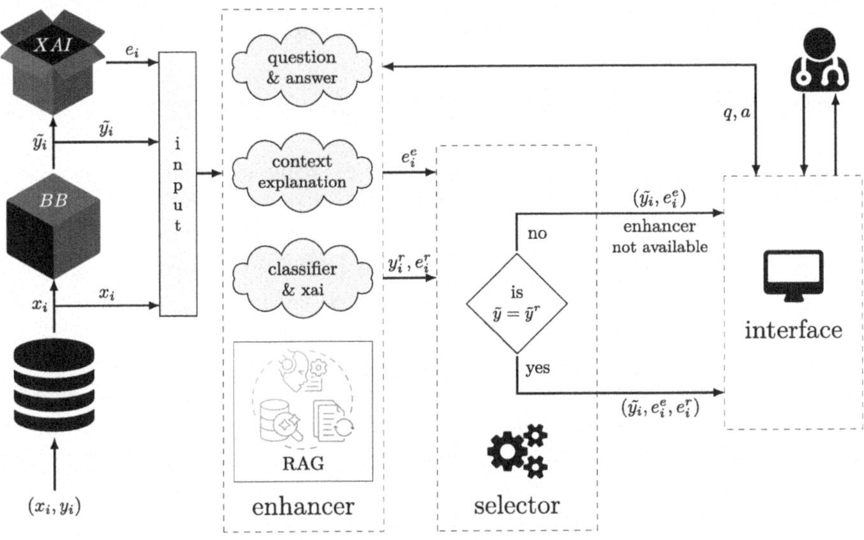

Fig. 1. Pipeline of the proposed Clinical Decision Support System (CDSS), integrating a predictive model, an explainer, a RAG-based enhancer that enriches and contextualizes explanations using external medical knowledge, and a selector module that governs information delivery based on confidence and consistency.

3.1 Black-Box Model and Explainer

A classification task is formally defined as follows. Given a dataset $D = \{(x_i, y_i)\}_{i=1}^n$, where $X = \{x_1, x_2, \ldots, x_n\}$ represents the input feature vectors, with $x_i \in \mathbb{R}^d$ for each i, and d being the dimensionality of the input space, and $Y = \{y_1, y_2, \ldots, y_n\}$ is the corresponding target vector, where each $y_i \in \{1, 2, \ldots, C\}$ represents a class label for the i-th data point. The goal is to learn a mapping $f : X \to \tilde{Y}$, where $\tilde{Y}$ is the predicted class label set. The model used to perform the classification is a black-box classifier BB, such that the predicted output $\tilde{y}_i = BB(x_i)$ is generated for each input x_i. This predicted label $\tilde{y}_i$ is then compared with the true label y_i for evaluation of the model's performance.

A local explainer is defined as a function that takes as input a specific instance x_i and its predicted label $\tilde{y}_i$, and outputs an explanation e_i. This explanation can take various forms, such as feature importance, decision rules, exemplars, etc. Formally, a local explainer can be defined as function $\phi : (X, \tilde{Y}) \to E$, where E is the explanation set. An explanation $e_i \in E$ aims to provide insight into the reasoning of the black-box classifier BB for the prediction $\tilde{y}_i$ of the specific instance x_i.

3.2 Enhancer

The enhancer module, based on RAG, is designed to support three distinct tasks: *context explanation*, *classifier and XAI*, and *question & answer*. Each component in the pipeline operates independently and could, in principle, be implemented using LLM instead of a RAG-based approach. However, rather than relying solely on the LLM's pre-trained knowledge, RAG retrieves relevant information from a curated medical database to generate more accurate, contextualized, and reliable explanations.

In the following we described in detail the three potential enhancer's tasks:

Context Explanation. This task enriches an existing explanation by converting the explanation into a human-like format and integrating context from the RAG's specialized corpus. This task takes as input the feature vector x_i, the prediction $\tilde{y}_i$ made by the classifier, and the initial explanation e_i generated by the local explainer, and provides an enhanced explanation e_i^e, by exploiting the RAG system. It can be formally defined as a function $C : (X, \tilde{Y}, E) \rightarrow \mathcal{E}$, where $\mathcal{E} = \{e_1^e, \ldots, e_n^e\}$ is the *enhanced explanation* set. In particular the RAG system enriches the explanation e_i by incorporating contextual knowledge from the corpus and transforming it into a more human-comprehensible format. The resulting output, e_i^e, is an enriched, human-like explanation that offers a clearer, more detailed understanding of the model's decision-making process, grounded in both the prediction and the context of the input data;

Classifier and XAI. In this task, the RAG serves as both a classifier and an explanation generator. Formally, the task can be defined as: $R : X \rightarrow (Y^r, E^r)$, where the RAG is provided with the input feature vector x_i and performs a classification along with an explanation supporting the prediction. The output consists of the predicted label y_i^r and an explanation e_i^r.

Question and Answer. This task is the most flexible method for interacting with the system, allowing users to request interactive explanations. It is performed at the end of the pipeline, once the user has received the initial results from the entire decision support system. In this task, a question q is provided as input along with the entire system's information. The output a is the answer to the question, which may take various forms depending on the nature of q. This task allows the user to query the system for additional information coming from the specialized corpus of the RAG, clarification, or deeper insights into the model's predictions and explanations, providing an interactive and dynamic way to explore and understand the decision-making process of the AI model.

3.3 Selector

The final component of the proposed method is the *selector*, serves as a filtering and governance layer for the information presented to the user. It receives as input the black-box model's prediction $\tilde{y}_i$, the enhanced explanation e_i^e, the enhancer's prediction y_i^r, and the enhancer's explanation e_i^r. The primary function of the selector is to implement the decision making strategy based on the input information, ensuring that the system refrains from presenting information when confidence is insufficient or conflicting. For example, a simple but effective implementation of the selector may involve outputting the enhancer's explanation e_i^r only if the black-box classifier's prediction $\tilde{y}_i$ matches the enhancer's prediction y_i^r. This strategy prioritizes trust in the black-box classifier, thereby mitigating the risk of misleading or hallucinated outputs that might arise from the RAG-based enhancer. Although this represents a minimal implementation, the design space for selector strategies is broad and can be extended to incorporate more sophisticated techniques for confidence estimation, consistency checking, and risk-aware decision-making, ultimately improving the reliability and robustness of the entire AI pipeline.

4 Experiments and Results

In this section, we show some preliminary results of a specific instantiation of our methodology.

4.1 Dataset and Experimental Setting

We evaluate our proposed method using the Pima Indians Diabetes Database [43], a publicly available dataset[1] originally provided by the National Institute of Diabetes and Digestive and Kidney Diseases. The goal is to diagnostically predict the presence of diabetes in a patient based on a set of clinical attributes. Prior to training, the dataset is standardized using a standard scaler, and we applied random oversampling to balance the class distribution by increasing the number of instances in the minority class, i.e., patients diagnosed with diabetes. As black-box model, we employed a Random Forest classifier trained on an 80/20 train-test split, using a grid search and 3-fold cross-validation to optimize the hyperparameters. For local explanations, we use LIME [39], which provides feature importance scores for each prediction. The enhancer module builds on the MedRAG framework[2], introduced by [46], leveraging the StatPearls corpus for clinical decision support and the MedCPT retriever tailored for biomedical content. The LLM used for generation is Mixtral[3]. Finally, the selector filters the enhancer's output, returning the RAG-based explanation e_i^r only when the enhancer's prediction y_i^r matches the black-box prediction $\tilde{y}_i$, ensuring that explanations are only provided when there is consistency across models.

The *Classifier & XAI* task receives as input the patient's DESCRIPTION, represented by the feature vector x_i. The *Context explanation* task extends this input by including the black-box PREDICTION $\tilde{y}_i$ and the corresponding EXPLANATION e_i provided by the explainer (LIME in this case). Lastly, the *Question & answer* task builds upon the inputs of the *Context explanation* task by incorporating a user-defined QUESTION q, which MedRAG must answer based on the available information. In Appendix A, we provide an example of input and output of the enhancer. Figure 3 illustrates the prompt templates employed by the enhancer module to query MedRAG, based on the specific tasks defined in Sect. 3. Instead, Fig. 4 shows an example instance from the PIMA dataset, for

---

[1] https://www.kaggle.com/datasets/uciml/pima-indians-diabetes-database (accessed: 19/07/2025).

[2] https://github.com/Teddy-XiongGZ/MedRAG (accessed: 19/07/2025).

[3] https://huggingface.co/mistralai/Mixtral-8x7B-Instruct-v0.1 (accessed: 19/07/2025).

Table 1. Classification performance comparison on test set between Random Forest and MedRAG.

model	diabetes	precision	recall	f1-score	accuracy	agreement
Random Forest	no	0.82	0.79	0.80	0.75	0.82
	yes	0.64	0.69	0.66		
MedRag	no	0.77	0.80	0.78	0.71	
	yes	0.60	0.56	0.58		

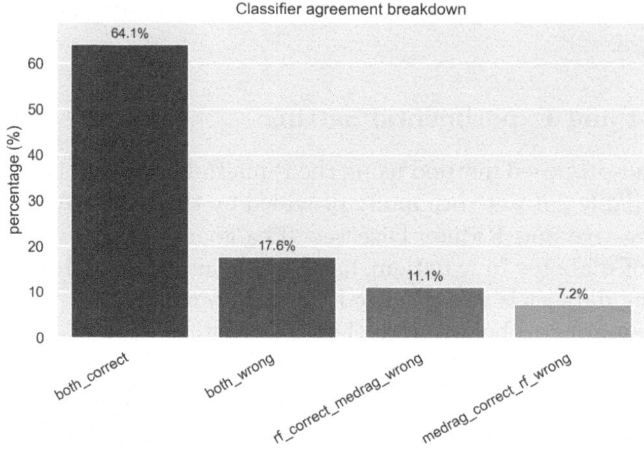

Fig. 2. Bar plot showing the agreement counts in the prediction task comparing Random Forest and MedRAG models.

which the selector's strategy is satisfied. In the table on the top left, we display the patient features along with the classifier's prediction $\tilde{y}_i$ and the enhanced prediction y_i^r generated by the RAG system. The top right section shows the feature importance values calculated using LIME, while the bottom section illustrates the output of the enhancer module based on the RAG system. It can be observed that the explanation provided by the RAG system is consistent with the one generated by LIME. Additionally, the RAG-based explanation includes references to the relevant documents in the corpus that support the explanation, thereby enabling the validation of the RAG's output.

4.2 Preliminary Results

In this work, we present a preliminary evaluation of the proposed methodology to highlight the importance of integrating both a predictive model and the RAG module within the same system. To this end, we compare the predictive performance of the Random Forest (RF) classifier and the MedRAG model on the Pima Indians Diabetes dataset. The results are reported in Table 1. Given the imbalanced nature of the dataset, with 65% of the records indicating no diabetes, the f1-score serves as the primary evaluation metric, alongside the recall for the "yes" class. This focus is driven by the importance of identifying as many diabetic cases as possible, even at the cost of some false positives. In this context, the Random Forest model outperforms MedRAG, particularly in the detection of diabetes cases, where it achieves an f1-score of 0.66 compared to MedRAG's 0.58. Furthermore, 82% of the time, both models agree on the prediction, which is the condition required for the selector to output the enhancer's explanation e^r. Figure 2 further breaks down this agreement, showing that the majority of instances where the models agree, they are correct. The second most frequent combination is when both models agree and are wrong. Notably, when the models disagree, the Random Forest model is more often correct than MedRAG, highlighting the greater reliability of the former in making accurate predictions.

5 Discussion and Conclusions

Our results show that the traditional Random Forest model outperformed the RAG-based system, supporting its continued use in our CDSS. Nonetheless, the strong agreement between the two models suggests that RAG-generated explanations can complement traditional ones, enhancing interpretability and user trust.

These *preliminary findings*, though promising, are limited by the small dataset, largely due to the computational cost of RAG. Expanding experiments to other clinical datasets and black-box models will help validate the system's generalizability. Future work should also explore: *i)* the impact to use a LLM tailored to medical domain instead of a generalist LLM, and *ii)* how factors like model confidence and explanation alignment affect the CDSS's reliability.

Privacy remains a major concern, particularly when integrating LLMs and RAG in healthcare [32,33]. Explanations often require access to sensitive clinical data, and using closed-source LLMs risks violating patient confidentiality and regulations like GDPR [8,47]. Addressing these challenges will require privacy-preserving techniques such as local inference, federated learning [13,21], and unlearning methods [4].

In summary, we propose a hybrid XAI approach that combines traditional models with generative enhancers to support interpretable, human-aligned AI in clinical contexts. While further validation is needed, this work takes a step toward more transparent and responsible decision support systems.

Acknowledgments. This research was partially supported by: The European Commission under the NextGeneration EU programme – National Recovery and Resilience Plan (PNRR), under agreements: PNRR - M4C2 - Investimento 1.3, Partenariato Esteso PE00000013 - "FAIR - Future Artificial Intelligence Research" - Spoke 1 "Human-centered AI", and SoBigData.it – "Strengthening the Italian RI for Social Mining and Big Data Analytics" – Prot. IR0000013 – Avviso n. 3264 del 28/12/2021. The European Union's Horizon Europe research and innovation programme for the project FINDHR (g.a. No. 101070212), and under the Excellent Science European Research Council (ERC) programme for the XAI project (g.a. No. 834756), and the HORIZON Europe projects TANGO - Grant Agreement n. 101120763 Views and opinions expressed are those of the author(s) only and do not necessarily reflect those of the European Union. Neither the European Union nor the granting authority can be held responsible for them.

A Input and Output Prompt for RAG

Input (classifier & xai)

You are a helpful medical expert. Your task is to classify a patient as having diabetes or not based on the provided medical data and using the relevant documents.

Based on the following information: {DESCRIPTION}, does the patient have diabetes?

Please provide a detailed explanation of the reasoning in "step_by_step_thinking" and a clear binary classification in "classification" where '1' indicates "Diabetes" and "0" indicates 'No Diabetes'. In addition, include a section with the feature importance ranking and another section with the specific rules that influenced the classification based on each feature. In these two sections, add only relevant exploited features for the decision. Organize your output in JSON format as Dict"step_by_step_thinking": Str(explanation), "classification": Int(0 or 1), "feature_importance_ranking": List[Str], "rules_applied": Dict[Str, Str]. Your responses will be used for research purposes only, so please provide a definite and clear answer.

Input (context explanation)

You are an AI assistant helping interpret the output of a machine learning model that predicts whether a patient has diabetes.

Based on the following information: {DESCRIPTION}. The machine learning model predicted: {PREDICTION}. According to LIME, the most influential features for this prediction were: {EXPLANATION}.

Use this information and any relevant medical background knowledge to generate a well-rounded, contextualized explanation.
The explanation should describe why the model made its prediction, referencing the most influential features and their values.
The explanation should be written in plain language suitable for a non-technical medical professional, and should include any relevant caveats or uncertainty if appropriate.

Input (question & answer)

You are an AI assistant helping interpret the output of a machine learning model that predicts whether a patient has diabetes. You receive a question from the doctor and you must give an answer.

Based on the following information: {DESCRIPTION}. The machine learning model predicted: {PREDICTION}. According to LIME, the most influential features for this prediction were: {EXPLANATION}. The doctor asked the following question: {QUESTION}.

Use this information and any relevant medical background knowledge to provide a clear, informative answer to the doctor's question. The answer should be written in plain language suitable for a non-technical medical professional, and should include any relevant caveats or uncertainty if appropriate.

context/background input information output indicator

Fig. 3. The prompt templates for the three tasks supported by the enhancer module are defined as follows. The *Classifier & XAI* task receives as input the patient's DESCRIPTION, represented by the feature vector x_i. The *Context explanation* task extends this input by including the black-box PREDICTION $\tilde{y}$ and the corresponding EXPLANATION e provided by the explainer (LIME in this case). Lastly, the *Question & answer* task builds upon the inputs of the *Context explanation* task by incorporating a user-defined QUESTION q, which MedRag must answer based on the available information.

Output (classifier & xai)

"step_by_step_thinking": "To classify whether a patient has diabetes or not, we need to compare the given patient's features with the diagnostic criteria for diabetes. The documents provided do not give specific criteria for diagnosing diabetes, but they do provide information about what to consider when diagnosing diabetes. The relevant documents for this task are Document [2] (Title: Prediabetes – Introduction), Document [5] (Title: Diabetes Mellitus Screening – Definition/Introduction), Document [6] (Title: Diabetes Mellitus Screening – Definition/Introduction – Type 2 Diabetes), and Document [8] (Title: Mean – Definition/Introduction). Based on the given patient's features, we can compare them to the diagnostic criteria for diabetes and prediabetes. The patient's age, pregnancies, blood pressure, skin thickness, insulin, BMI, and diabetes pedigree function are all relevant features to consider. The normal blood glucose level is between 70 mg/dL to 99 mg/dL. In patients with prediabetes, blood glucose levels are elevated between 110 mg/dL to 125 mg/dL. The patient's glucose level is 187.0, which is higher than the diagnostic criteria for prediabetes. Therefore, based on this single feature, we can classify the patient as having diabetes."

"classification": 1

"feature_importance_ranking": ["Glucose"]

"rules_applied": {"Glucose": "Glucose > 125 mg/dL (Diabetes)"}

Fig. 4. An example instance from the PIMA dataset is presented. In the table on the top left, we display the patient features along with the classifier's prediction $\tilde{y_i}$ and the enhanced prediction y_i^r generated by the RAG model. The top right section shows the feature importance values calculated using LIME, while the bottom section illustrates the output of the Enhancer module based on the RAG model.

References

1. Ajwani, R., Javaji, S.R., Rudzicz, F., Zhu, Z.: LLM-generated black-box explanations can be adversarially helpful. arXiv preprint arXiv:2405.06800 (2024)
2. Amershi, S., et al.: Guidelines for human-AI interaction. In: Conference on Human Factors in Computing Systems CHI, pp. 1–13 (2019)
3. Bilal, A., Ebert, D., Lin, B.: LLMs for explainable AI: a comprehensive survey. arXiv preprint arXiv:2504.00125 (2025)
4. Blanco-Justicia, A., et al.: Digital forgetting in large language models: a survey of unlearning methods. Artif. Intell. Rev. **58**(3), 90 (2025)
5. Bodria, F., Giannotti, F., Guidotti, R., Naretto, F., Pedreschi, D., Rinzivillo, S.: Benchmarking and survey of explanation methods for black box models. Data Min. Knowl. Disc. **37**(5), 1719–1778 (2023)
6. Burton, J., Al Moubayed, N., Enshaei, A.: Natural language explanations for machine learning classification decisions. In: International Joint Conference on Neural Networks IJCNN, pp. 1–9. IEEE (2023)
7. Cao, L.: AI in finance: challenges, techniques, and opportunities. ACM Comput. Surv. **55**(3), 1–38 (2022)
8. Chadwick, R., Blundell, S., Prendergast, E.: Assessments of the privacy compliance in commercial large language models (2024)
9. Conati, C., Barral, O., Putnam, V., Rieger, L.: Toward personalized XAI: a case study in intelligent tutoring systems. Artif. Intell. **298**, 103503 (2021)
10. Doshi-Velez, F., Kim, B.: Towards a rigorous science of interpretable machine learning. arXiv preprint arXiv:1702.08608 (2017)

11. Ehsan, U., Riedl, M.O.: Human-centered explainable AI: towards a reflective sociotechnical approach. In: Late Breaking Papers: Multimodality and Intelligence - HCI International Conference, pp. 449–466. Springer, Cham (2020)
12. Eiband, M., Schneider, H., Bilandzic, M., Fazekas-Con, J., Haug, M., Hussmann, H.: Bringing transparency design into practice. In: International Conference on Intelligent User Interfaces IUI, pp. 211–223 (2018)
13. Fontana, M., Naretto, F., Monreale, A.: A new approach for cross-silo federated learning and its privacy risks. In: IEEE International Conference on Privacy, Security and Trust (PST), pp. 1–10 (2021)
14. Friedman, J., Popescu, B.: Predictive learning via rule ensembles. Ann. Appl. Stat. **2** (2008)
15. Garigliotti, D.: Explaining LLM-based question answering via the self-interpretations of a model. In: Advances in Interpretable Machine Learning and Artificial Intelligence, co-located with ECML-PKDD (2024)
16. Giannotti, F., Naretto, F., Bodria, F.: Explainable for trustworthy AI. In: Human-Centered Artificial Intelligence: Advanced Lectures, pp. 175–195. Springer, Cham (2023)
17. Giorgi, F., Campagnano, C., Silvestri, F., Tolomei, G.: Natural language counterfactual explanations for graphs using large language models. arXiv preprint arXiv:2410.09295 (2024)
18. Guidotti, R.: Counterfactual explanations and how to find them: literature review and benchmarking. Data Min. Knowl. Discov. **38**(5), 2770–2824 (2024)
19. Guidotti, R., et al.: Stable and actionable explanations of black-box models through factual and counterfactual rules. Data Min. Knowl. Discov. **38**(5), 2825–2862 (2024)
20. Guidotti, R., Monreale, A., Ruggieri, S., Turini, F., Giannotti, F., Pedreschi, D.: A survey of methods for explaining black box models. ACM Comput. Surv. **51**(5), 1–42 (2018)
21. Haffar, R., Naretto, F., Sánchez, D., Monreale, A., Domingo-Ferrer, J.: GLOR-FLEX: local to global rule-based explanations for federated learning. In: International Conference on Fuzzy Systems FUZZ-IEEE, pp. 1–9. IEEE (2024)
22. Huang, S., Mamidanna, S., Jangam, S., Zhou, Y., Gilpin, L.H.: Can large language models explain themselves? A study of LLM-generated self-explanations. arXiv preprint arXiv:2310.11207 (2023)
23. Ichmoukhamedov, T., Hinns, J., Martens, D.: How good is my story? Towards quantitative metrics for evaluating -generated XAI narratives. arXiv preprint arXiv:2412.10220 (2024)
24. Ji, Z., et al.: Survey of hallucination in natural language generation. ACM Comput. Surv. **55**(12), 1–38 (2023)
25. Jiang, T., Sun, Z., Fu, S., Lv, Y.: Human-AI interaction research agenda: a user-centered perspective. Data Inf. Manage. **8**(4), 100078 (2024)
26. Lewis, P., et al.: Retrieval-augmented generation for knowledge-intensive NLP tasks. In: Advances in Neural Information Processing Systems NeurIPS, vol. 33, pp. 9459–9474 (2020)
27. Li, D., et al.: A survey of large language models attribution. arXiv preprint arXiv:2311.03731 (2023)
28. Lundberg, S.M., Lee, S.I.: A unified approach to interpreting model predictions. In: Advances in Neural Information Processing Systems NeurIPS, vol. 30 (2017)
29. Martens, D., Hinns, J., Dams, C., Vergouwen, M., Evgeniou, T.: Tell me a story! narrative-driven XAI with large language models. Decis. Support Syst. 114402 (2025)

30. Mavrepis, P., Makridis, G., Fatouros, G., Koukos, V., Separdani, M.M., Kyriazis, D.: XAI for all: can large language models simplify explainable AI? arXiv preprint arXiv:2401.13110 (2024)
31. Miller, T.: Explanation in artificial intelligence: insights from the social sciences. Artif. Intell. **267**, 1–38 (2019)
32. Naretto, F., Monreale, A., Giannotti, F.: Evaluating the privacy exposure of interpretable global explainers. In: International Conference on Cognitive Machine Intelligence CogMI, pp. 13–19. IEEE (2022)
33. Naretto, F., Pellungrini, R., Monreale, A., Nardini, F.M., Musolesi, M.: Predicting and explaining privacy risk exposure in mobility data. In: International Conference on Discovery Science, pp. 403–418. Springer, Cham (2020)
34. Nowotko, P.M.: AI in judicial application of law and the right to a court. Procedia Comput. Sci. **192**, 2220–2228 (2021)
35. Pan, B., Xiong, Z., Wu, G., Zhang, Z., Zhang, Y., Zhao, L.: Tagexplainer: narrating graph explanations for text-attributed graph learning models. arXiv preprint arXiv:2410.15268 (2024)
36. Park, C., Lee, H., Lee, S., Jeong, O.: Synergistic joint model of knowledge graph and LLM for enhancing XAI-based clinical decision support systems. Mathematics **13**(6), 949 (2025)
37. Parliament, E., Council: Artificial intelligence act (2024). https://eur-lex.europa.eu/eli/reg/2024/1689/oj/eng. Accessed 16 Apr 2025
38. Raaijmakers, S.: Artificial intelligence for law enforcement: challenges and opportunities. IEEE Secur. Priv. **17**(5), 74–77 (2019)
39. Ribeiro, M.T., Singh, S., Guestrin, C.: "Why should I trust you?" Explaining the predictions of any classifier. In: ACM International Conference on Knowledge Discovery and Data Mining SIGKDD, pp. 1135–1144 (2016)
40. Rudin, C.: Stop explaining black box machine learning models for high stakes decisions and use interpretable models instead. Nat. Mach. Intell. **1**(5), 206–215 (2019)
41. Setzu, M., Guidotti, R., Monreale, A., Turini, F., Pedreschi, D., Giannotti, F.: Glocalx-from local to global explanations of black box AI models. Artif. Intell. **294**, 103457 (2021)
42. Shaheen, M.Y.: Applications of artificial intelligence (AI) in healthcare: a review. ScienceOpen Preprints (2021)
43. Smith, J.W., Everhart, J.E., Dickson, W.C., Knowler, W.C., Johannes, R.S.: Using the ADAP learning algorithm to forecast the onset of diabetes mellitus. In: Annual Symposium on Computer Application in Medical Care, p. 261 (1988)
44. Wojciechowski, A., Lango, M., Dusek, O.: Faithful and plausible natural language explanations for image classification: a pipeline approach. arXiv preprint arXiv:2407.20899 (2024)
45. Wolf, C.T.: Explainability scenarios: towards scenario-based XAI design. In: International Conference on Intelligent User Interfaces IUI, pp. 252–257 (2019)
46. Xiong, G., Jin, Q., Lu, Z., Zhang, A.: Benchmarking retrieval-augmented generation for medicine. In: Findings of the Association for Computational Linguistics, ACL 2024 (2024)
47. Yao, Y., Duan, J., Xu, K., Cai, Y., Sun, Z., Zhang, Y.: A survey on large language model (LLM) security and privacy: the good, the bad, and the ugly. High-Confidence Comput. 100211 (2024)
48. Zytek, A., Pidò, S., Veeramachaneni, K.: LLMs for XAI: future directions for explaining explanations. arXiv preprint arXiv:2405.06064 (2024)

KaiMed: A Hybrid Multi-Agent AI Platform for Clinical Reasoning and Cross-Specialty Discovery

Francesco Barbato[1(✉)], Filippo Sorichetti[3,7], Emanuele Ielo[6], and Lorenzo Megliola[2,4,5]

[1] Naples, Italy
francescobarbatoingaero@gmail.com
[2] KaiMed, Varese, Italy
[3] Scuola Universitaria Superiore IUSS, Pavia, Italy
[4] HFARM College, Roncade, Italy
[5] University of Chichester, Chichester, UK
[6] Rome, Italy
[7] Università degli Studi di Pavia, Pavia, Italy

Abstract. KaiMed is a modular AI platform designed to support adaptive clinical reasoning in complex decision-making scenarios. Unlike traditional Clinical Decision Support Systems (CDSS)—which are often static, narrow in scope, and specialty-specific—KaiMed integrates symbolic and sub-symbolic approaches into a unified architecture to enable scalable, explainable, and cross-specialty medical reasoning.

The platform combines: (1) a clinically grounded knowledge graph derived from curated trials and peer-reviewed literature; (2) a semantic retrieval engine using vector embeddings to access unstructured scientific content; and (3) a multi-agent reasoning layer that coordinates specialized agents responsible for diagnosis, treatment, validation, and referral.

Each agent operates within a transparent workflow supervised by a central agent, dynamically interacting with both the knowledge graph and the semantic index to enable hybrid, context-aware reasoning that mirrors expert decision-making.

The system is evaluated in the domain of Inflammatory Bowel Disease (IBD), showing high scores in clarity, relevance, and perceived usefulness. Its performance across structured metrics (QAMAI, TDS, ACCS) surpasses direct LLM baselines, highlighting the benefits of agent coordination and knowledge-aware reasoning. Structured source attribution is implemented and being refined for improved traceability.

KaiMed is actively being extended to new domains—including urology and chronic rhinosinusitis—leveraging shared ontologies and a unified architecture to support cross-domain discovery.

Rather than replacing clinical expertise, KaiMed amplifies it—bridging fragmented knowledge, surfacing hidden connections, and supporting modular, transparent decision-making across medical specialties.

F. Barbato and E. Ielo—Independent Researcher, Contributor to the KaiMed Initiative (non-institutional affiliation).

P. Bruno et al. (Eds.): HC_AIxIA_HYDRA 2025, CCIS 2830, pp. 64–77, 2026.
https://doi.org/10.1007/978-3-032-16708-8_5

Keywords: AI for Clinical Reasoning · Explainable AI in Healthcare · Multi-Agent Reasoning · Medical Knowledge Graphs · Hybrid AI Architectures

1 Introduction

The accelerating growth of biomedical data has created unprecedented opportunities for clinical insight—but also exacerbated problems of knowledge fragmentation, cognitive overload, and a lack of integration across medical specialties. It is estimated that more than 80% of healthcare data is **unstructured and underutilized** [7], while diagnostic errors contribute to up to 10% of patient deaths and affect a significant portion of hospital adverse events [1,4].

Contemporary Clinical Decision Support Systems (CDSS) have addressed specific tasks, such as drug interaction checks or guideline reminders, but often remain **narrow in scope**, **static in logic**, and limited to **single-specialty use** [5]. Moreover, they are rarely designed to incorporate real-time scientific evidence, to handle ambiguous or incomplete information, or to support the **iterative reasoning** that defines expert clinical practice.

To address these limitations, we present *KaiMed*: a modular AI platform for **adaptive clinical reasoning**, designed to assist healthcare professionals in complex decision-making scenarios. Unlike recent frameworks such as MedAgent or MedKG-LLM, KaiMed emphasizes agent-level accountability and cross-specialty scalability, offering a unified workflow that combines symbolic and sub-symbolic reasoning.

- **structured knowledge graphs**, constructed from peer-reviewed clinical trials and publications,
- **semantic search** over recent scientific literature using vector-based retrieval,
- and a **multi-agent orchestration layer** enabling explainable and specialized medical reasoning.

The platform can be accessed through natural language and supports both **exploratory insight** and **case-specific consultation**. It is built to operate across multiple medical domains while maintaining **traceability**, **interoperability**, and **clinical alignment**.

This paper focuses on the application of KaiMed to a single representative use case—**Inflammatory Bowel Disease (IBD)**—to illustrate its architecture and evaluation methodology. However, the system is **domain-agnostic** by design, and structured to support **cross-specialty discovery**, **translational research**, and **multi-context deployment**.

Contributions of this work

This paper introduces the core technical innovations behind *KaiMed*, including:

1. A **hybrid reasoning system** integrating symbolic (knowledge graph) and sub-symbolic (semantic vector) representations.

2. A **multi-agent architecture**, with coordinated clinical agents mapped to real-world medical functions.
3. A methodology for constructing a **clinically grounded knowledge graph**, enriched through semantic normalization.
4. A **clinical evaluation framework** based on accuracy, disagreement, complexity, and quality assessment metrics.

Recent work confirms the growing impact of hybrid and agent-based architectures in clinical AI. Frameworks such as **MedAgent** [6] and **MedKG-LLM** [8] illustrate the benefits of combining agents with knowledge graphs, while benchmark initiatives like **MultiMedQA** [9] highlight the need for robust, multi-dimensional evaluation—further validating the direction pursued by KaiMed.

Ultimately, *KaiMed* aims to show that AI can support not only clinical answers, but **clinical thinking**—bridging evidence and expertise through **transparency**, **modularity**, and **medical reasoning**.

2 Related Work

Clinical decision-making has long been supported by rule-based **Clinical Decision Support Systems (CDSS)**, which offer alerts, guidelines, and risk stratifications. While effective in narrow contexts, traditional CDSS often lack flexibility, adaptability, and integration with unstructured or evolving evidence [5]. These limitations have motivated the development of more dynamic, AI-based systems capable of contextual reasoning.

Recent efforts have explored the use of **Medical Knowledge Graphs (KGs)** to structure domain knowledge and facilitate interpretable inference. Projects such as [3,8] demonstrate that graph-based models improve explainability and enable complex querying across diseases, drugs, and clinical entities. However, standalone KGs are limited in their capacity to generalize across ambiguous or novel inputs without substantial domain engineering.

To address this, **retrieval-augmented generation (RAG)** techniques have emerged, combining LLMs with semantic search over scientific corpora [2]. This hybrid approach allows systems to ground responses in up-to-date, context-relevant literature. Applied to healthcare, RAG pipelines have shown promise in tasks such as medical Q&A, patient summarization, and evidence retrieval [9].

More recently, the introduction of **multi-agent architectures** has opened a new direction in clinical AI. Inspired by human medical teams, systems like **MedAgent** [6] coordinate multiple specialized agents (e.g., diagnostician, researcher, triage) under a supervisory controller to tackle complex problems. These systems benefit from modularity and role clarity but are still emerging in terms of clinical integration and scalability.

KaiMed builds upon these approaches with a unified framework explicitly designed for transparency and cross-specialty reasoning.

3 System Architecture

This section details the modular architecture of *KaiMed*, organized into a **Data Layer and an Agentic Layer**, and explains how these components interact in clinical reasoning. As shown in Fig. 1, the architecture is organized into two primary layers:

- **The Data Layer**, which ingests, stores, and processes structured and unstructured clinical knowledge; and
- **The Agentic Layer**, which manages the reasoning process through a team of specialized agents and human-in-the-loop interaction.

These layers are connected via a shared pipeline that enables **hybrid reasoning**, combining evidence from curated medical literature, semantic embeddings, and domain-specific ontologies with explainable, role-driven agent workflows.

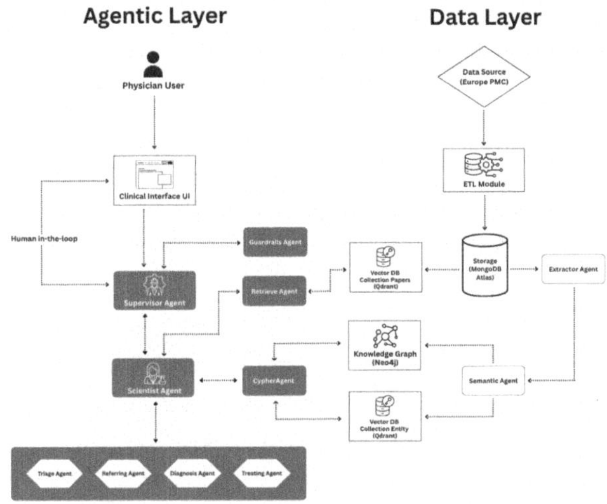

Fig. 1. KaiMed Platform Architecture.

3.1 Knowledge Graph Layer

At the heart of the Data Layer is a **medical knowledge graph (KG)**, encoding clinically relevant relationships extracted from peer-reviewed literature, particularly clinical trials. A custom ETL pipeline retrieves, filters, and parses articles from trusted sources (e.g., Europe PMC). Textual data is processed via medical ontologies and LLM-based agents to extract structured triples (e.g., *Disease – Treated With – Drug*).

The graph is stored in Neo4j, with typed nodes (e.g., *Disease, Drug, Symptom, Test*) and semantically rich relationships (e.g., *Treated With, Has Complication, Diagnoses*) enriched with attributes like treatment line or clinical severity.

Although this paper presents a use case in **Inflammatory Bowel Disease (IBD)**, the graph model supports multi-specialty separation through a graph property, allowing both isolated and cross-domain reasoning in future applications.

This module is part of the Data Layer shown in Fig. 1.

3.2 Vector Retrieval Layer

To complement the symbolic graph, *KaiMed* includes a **semantic search engine** built on **Qdrant**, a high-performance vector database. Thousands of medical articles are embedded using a transformer-based sentence encoder and indexed to allow **retrieval-augmented generation (RAG)**.

Agents can submit natural language queries that are converted into embedding vectors and compared against the corpus using cosine similarity. This enables real-time access to evolving medical evidence and contextual matching beyond exact term overlap—especially useful in ambiguous scenarios not covered by the structured KG.

Each document in Qdrant includes metadata fields (e.g., *title, abstract, source, domain*) and can be filtered by specialty or publication type, aligning results with the knowledge graph's scope and provenance.

This component complements the knowledge graph within the Data Layer (see Fig. 1).

3.3 Multi-agent Control Layer

KaiMed's reasoning logic is implemented in the Agentic Layer through a **multi-agent architecture**, orchestrated by a central **Supervisor Agent**. This agent routes clinical requests to role-specific agents, each designed to emulate a medical function.

Agents operate asynchronously within a shared state graph implemented via **LangGraph**, enabling dynamic task routing and intermediate memory. Each agent may interact with the KG, the Vector DB, or both—depending on the reasoning needs of the task.

This modular orchestration mirrors interdisciplinary clinical practice and enables **transparent, explainable AI behaviors**—each agent's contribution is observable, traceable, and independently verifiable.

KaiMed's architecture brings together **structured medical knowledge**, **semantic evidence retrieval**, and **agent-based reasoning** into a single pipeline- designed to scale across domains while maintaining **explainability**, **adaptability**, and **traceability** in real-world clinical environments.

4 Knowledge Graph Construction

The *KaiMed* knowledge graph (KG) is built to represent clinically relevant relationships extracted from peer-reviewed medical literature, particularly clinical trials. It serves as a central symbolic substrate for reasoning over diseases, treatments, symptoms, diagnostics, and outcomes.

4.1 Data Sources and ETL Pipeline

The initial corpus is constructed from authoritative sources, primarily Europe PMC, focusing on **clinical trials** and **review articles** published within the last decade. Documents are selected using disease-specific queries (e.g., *"Inflammatory Bowel Disease"*) and filtered by publication type and quality (excluding preprints and non-peer-reviewed content).

A custom **ETL pipeline** ingests these documents into a structured format with metadata like title, abstract, publication date, type. These records are stored in **MongoDB** for preprocessing before KG extraction.

4.2 Extraction and Semantic Normalization

To convert unstructured content into graph data, *KaiMed* employs two sequential LLM-based components:

- The **Extractor Agent** analyzes the text and outputs clinical triples in the form (subject, relation, object), enriched with entity types and attributes (e.g., *"Inflammatory Bowel Disease"* Treated With *"Infliximab"*, Curative).
- The Semantic Agent normalizes entities by resolving synonyms, abbreviations, and variants through ontologies, alias mapping, and vector similarity. Each concept is assigned a unique identifier, with redundant forms merged into a single descriptive node.

4.3 Graph Model and Ontology

The graph is implemented in **Neo4j**, with typed nodes (e.g., *Disease, Drug, Test, Symptom*) and directed, attribute-rich edges (e.g., *Treated With, Diagnoses, Has Risk Factor*). The ontology is designed to be **general and extensible**, enabling future domains to reuse or specialize core concepts.

Each node and relationship is tagged with a graph property to allow for **domain-level separation** (e.g., `"graph": "ibd"`), which enables scoped queries and supports cross-domain expansion while maintaining a **single-instance deployment**.

4.4 Clinical Integration

Graph nodes are linked to **real patient instances** extracted from clinical trials, creating patient-centric subgraphs. This enables agents to reason not only over abstract clinical knowledge but also over concrete patterns observed in actual patients, reflecting real-world variability in case presentations and outcomes.

The KG can be queried directly by agents via Cypher, either to:

- retrieve specific relationships (e.g., treatments for a condition),
- validate hypotheses (e.g., known comorbidities),
- or explore surrounding evidence via graph traversal.

5 Multi-agent Workflow

KaiMed uses a multi-agent framework to decompose clinical reasoning into specialized sub-tasks, each handled by a distinct agent. These agents are coordinated by a central **Supervisor Agent**, which routes input, state, and intermediate results based on the clinical context.

The multi-agent workflow is implemented using **LangGraph**, a stateful orchestration layer that enables dynamic execution paths and memory between components. Each agent receives a shared state object, can invoke tools (e.g., KG queries, literature search), and returns enriched outputs to be passed downstream.

5.1 Agent Roles and Functions

Table 1. Roles and functions of agents in the KaiMed workflow

Agent	Function
Supervisor Agent	Central orchestrator; analyzes user input and delegates to appropriate agents.
Triage Agent	Collects and structures patient information; ensures completeness of clinical data.
Diagnosis Agent	Suggests primary and differential diagnoses based on evidence.
Treating Agent	Recommends therapeutic strategies, considering guidelines and trial evidence.
Scientist Agent	Conducts external literature reviews using semantic search (Qdrant).
Referring Agent	Determines whether a specialist referral is clinically indicated.
Guardrails Agent	Prevents non-medical or inappropriate system usage.

Each agent is implemented as an independent language model function, guided by a prompt template, tools, and logic boundaries. Agents can reason autonomously, but always within the structured flow enforced by the supervisor (Table 1).

5.2 Integration with Knowledge Modules

Agents interact with both data sources:

- **Knowledge Graph (Neo4j)**: queried via Cypher through a dedicated KG interface agent. Enables retrieval of structured clinical relationships (e.g., *IBD* → Treated With → *Infliximab*).
- **Semantic Vector DB (Qdrant)**: accessed via similarity search API, supporting retrieval-augmented generation. Useful for rapidly identifying relevant studies, reviews, or outcome data.

This hybrid integration allows agents to blend formal medical knowledge with recent unstructured evidence, simulating the information-seeking behavior of human clinicians.

5.3 Example Clinical Use Case

Input:

"Male, 32 years old, history of Crohn's disease. Persistent abdominal pain, weight loss, CRP (C-Reactive Protein) > 20, loose stools for 6 weeks. No current biologic treatment."

Workflow:

1. Triage Agent structures the clinical case and flags severity indicators (chronic inflammation, weight loss, duration).
2. Diagnosis Agent confirms flare-up of Crohn's disease; considers possible complications (e.g., strictures).
3. Treating Agent queries the KG to identify first-line and escalation therapies. Suggests biologics (e.g., infliximab) and dietary modification.
4. Scientist Agent performs literature retrieval to validate efficacy and safety of the proposed biologic for this profile.
5. Referring Agent recommends gastroenterology consultation for colonoscopy and potential biologic initiation.

Outcome:

KaiMed returns a structured report summarizing the suggested diagnosis, recommended treatment, evidence links, and reasoning path—supporting clinician decision-making while retaining transparency.

6 Evaluation Framework

To assess the clinical performance of *KaiMed*, we implemented a structured evaluation framework combining quantitative metrics, expert-grounded scores, and comparative baselines. Although the evaluation focuses on Inflammatory Bowel Disease (IBD), the methodology is domain-agnostic.

Each case is evaluated across multiple dimensions:

6.1 Evaluation Metrics

Table 2. Evaluation metrics and scales.

Metric	Description	Scale
ACCS	Amsterdam Clinical Challenge Scale. Measures the inherent clinical complexity of the case.	1–5
TDS	Total Disagreement Score. Measures divergence between AI diagnosis and ground truth.	0–3
QAMAI	Quality Assessment of Machine-Generated Information. Evaluates six domains: Accuracy, Clarity, Relevance, Completeness, Source Citation, Perceived Usefulness.	1–5 per domain

All evaluations are conducted using LLM-assisted scoring and expert-reviewed ground truths. For benchmarking purposes, direct model outputs (GPT-4o-mini) are compared with *KaiMed* agent responses. GPT-4o-mini was selected as baseline due to its wide availability and general-purpose capabilities; future work will include comparisons with specialized medical LLMs (Table 2).

6.2 Clinical Sample Case Evaluation

Prompt:

A 50-year-old woman with a severe ulcerative colitis flare, high fever, tachycardia, and abdominal distension. She has not responded to IV corticosteroids after 72 h.

Expected Ground Truth:

Initiate urgent surgical management – she likely has toxic megacolon. Involve colorectal surgery team immediately.

KaiMed Agent Output (Excerpt):

"...This presentation is consistent with toxic megacolon. The patient has failed medical management and shows signs of systemic instability (fever, tachycardia). Surgical consultation is urgently indicated for potential colectomy. Continue supportive care and initiate preoperative planning..."

The case received an **ACCS score of 5/5**, indicating high clinical complexity, and a **TDS of 1.5/3**, reflecting moderate disagreement with expert ground truth. In terms of informational quality, **KaiMed's output scored 5.0 across all QAMAI domains—Accuracy**, Clarity, Relevance, Completeness, and Usefulness—with a Source Citation score of 3.4.

This individual case illustrates the system's ability to identify urgent clinical trajectories with high precision. Broader performance trends across a larger cohort are discussed next.

6.3 QAMAI and Baseline Comparison

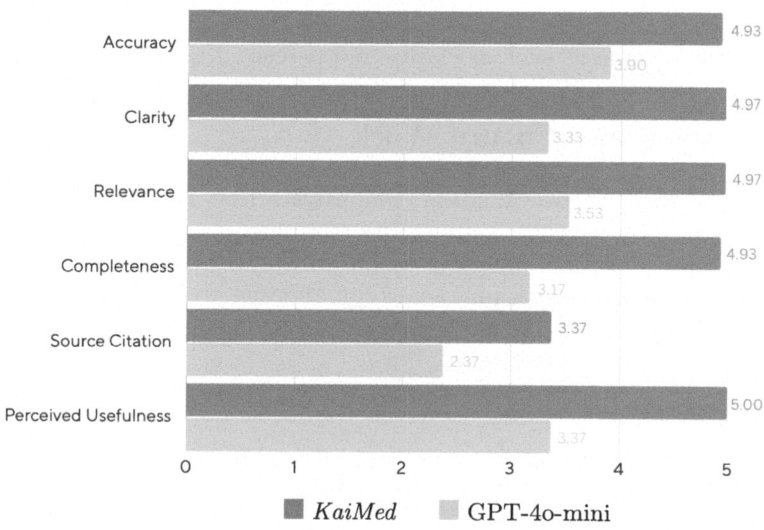

Fig. 2. Average QAMAI subscores (Accuracy, Clarity, Relevance, Completeness, Usefulness, Source Citation) across 30 IBD cases – *KaiMed* vs GPT-4o-mini baseline. ■ *KaiMed* ■ GPT-4o-mini.

As illustrated in Fig. 2, *KaiMed* consistently outperforms the GPT-4o-mini baseline across all QAMAI domains. These subscores represent the average results from a benchmark set of 30 clinically diverse IBD cases that were authored by domain experts based on published clinical trials and open-access datasets, covering a range of severity levels and therapeutic scenarios to ensure diversity and clinical realism.

6.4 Clinical Complexity and Agreement

In terms of clinical challenge (ACCS), both systems operate at the same high level of complexity. However, KaiMed exhibits lower disagreement scores (TDS), indicating more stable and grounded diagnostic outputs. This suggests that modular workflows and role-specific reasoning contribute to safer, more consistent decision-making.

6.5 Summary Insights

KaiMed delivers high-quality, **clinically relevant** outputs in complex IBD cases. The agent-based architecture enhances interpretability, consistency, and diagnostic precision compared to direct LLM prompting. While evaluation highlights strong performance in **clarity, relevance and usefulness** source citation mechanisms remain a target for improvement to ensure full traceability.

In conclusion, the *KaiMed* framework offers a robust and explainable clinical reasoning pipeline, validated through structured evaluation. It matches or exceeds baseline model performance across most metrics, particularly in usability-critical domains such as clarity and perceived usefulness.

7 Discussion and Future Work

The results of this initial evaluation demonstrate that **KaiMed** is capable of supporting clinically relevant, high-quality reasoning in complex IBD scenarios. Each agent contributes an explicit reasoning trace, including data sources and intermediate decisions, which physicians found easier to interpret compared to monolithic LLM outputs.

7.1 Key Strengths

- **Explainable reasoning**: Each decision path is traceable to a specific agent and evidence source allowing for transparent auditability.
- **Specialized task decomposition**: The use of role-specific agents ensures clinical logic is segmented and contextual, reflecting real-world care pathways.
- **Knowledge-aware orchestration**: Access to both structured (Neo4j) and unstructured (Qdrant) knowledge allows for robust, context-sensitive outputs.
- **Strong usability indicators**: High QAMAI scores across clarity, relevance, and usefulness suggest that the system is well-positioned to assist in clinical environments.

7.2 Current Scope and Limitations

While **KaiMed** has demonstrated strong performance in early clinical scenarios, the platform is still undergoing progressive validation and regulatory alignment:

- Although the system is currently validated on **Inflammatory Bowel Disease (IBD)**, expansion to other specialties is underway, and multi-domain validation is ongoing with clinicians in urology, chronic rhinosinusitis, and rare pediatric diseases.

- **Real-time integration with EMR/EHR systems** is not yet implemented, though the architecture supports it via modular API connectors.
- As with any system powered by large language models, **KaiMed** may be subject to occasional model variability or linguistic ambiguity, especially in edge cases.
- The platform is **not yet formally certified for clinical use under MDR or other regulatory frameworks**, though activities to address compliance and documentation are in progress.

These are not limitations in capability, but ongoing milestones on the path to robust, deployable clinical AI. Importantly, KaiMed has been developed under ethical guidelines, handling only anonymized or non-identifiable patient data. Any future integration with EHR systems will strictly comply with GDPR/HIPAA requirements, ensuring privacy and auditability.

7.3 Active Development Areas

Several extensions are already underway:

- **Cross-domain expansion**: New specialties—including urology, CRS (chronic rhinosinusitis), and rare pediatric conditions—are being actively modeled and tested using the same KG-driven, multi-agent architecture. This multi-specialty foundation enables not only broader clinical utility but also the emergence of cross-domain insights—such as shared therapies, overlapping symptoms, and underrecognized pharmacological interactions.
- **Clinical validation**: Collaborations with hospital partners are enabling iterative feedback and real-case testing to ensure relevance, safety, and adoption feasibility.
- **Citation & traceability improvements**: Agents are being upgraded to embed structured references, metadata, and publication links directly into their outputs—enhancing auditability and trust.
- **Benchmark alignment**: The evaluation strategy is evolving to align with reference frameworks such as *MultiMedQA* and *HealthBench*, enabling standardized comparison with other medical AI models.
- **Interface refinement**: Improvements to natural language interaction, agent explainability, and structured output formatting are focused on making the platform more usable in day-to-day clinical practice.

The system is currently accessible in a limited sandbox environment for selected institutional partners, supporting early experimentation and feedback collection.

KaiMed is not a prototype—it is an **operational architecture** built for real-world reasoning under uncertainty. Its goal is not to replace clinical expertise, but to *amplify it*—by making fragmented knowledge navigable, distributed evidence actionable, and complex decisions more transparent.

8 Conclusion

KaiMed introduces a hybrid AI framework designed to support clinical reasoning by combining symbolic knowledge graphs, semantic retrieval, and modular multi-agent coordination. It offers a transparent and adaptable approach to decision support, bridging structured knowledge with evolving scientific evidence.

Through its application to complex diagnostic tasks, **KaiMed** has demonstrated that structured, **explainable AI** can generate outputs that are not only accurate and clinically relevant but also aligned with real-world medical workflows. Its strength lies in its architecture: the ability to orchestrate specialized agents, blend heterogeneous data sources, and maintain full traceability sets it apart from traditional LLM-based systems.

More than a static decision tool, **KaiMed** is an **inference engine for discovery**—capable of connecting isolated clinical domains and surfacing **hidden relationships across specialties**, thereby supporting not just better decisions, but new insights.

While challenges such as citation formatting and broader validation remain, early results validate **KaiMed as a scalable, safe, and domain-extensible platform** for modern clinical AI. Ongoing development continues toward integration into hospital settings, expansion to new specialties, and alignment with open evaluation benchmarks.

KaiMed is not a final product—it is a **growing capability for the frontline of healthcare reasoning and scientific exploration**.

References

1. Graber, M.L.: The incidence of diagnostic error in medicine. BMJ Qual. Saf. **22**(Suppl. 2), ii21–ii27 (2013)
2. Lewis, P., et al.: Retrieval-augmented generation for knowledge-intensive NLP tasks. arXiv preprint arXiv:2005.11401 (2020)
3. Rotmensch, M., Halpern, Y., Tlimat, A., Horng, S., Sontag, D.: Learning a health knowledge graph from electronic medical records. Sci. Rep. **7**, 5994 (2017)
4. Singh, H., Meyer, A.N., Thomas, E.J.: The frequency of diagnostic errors in outpatient care. BMJ Qual. Saf. **23**(9), 727–731 (2014)
5. Sutton, R.T., Pincock, D., Baumgart, D.C., Sadowski, D.C., Fedorak, R.N., Kroeker, K.I.: An overview of clinical decision support systems: benefits, risks, and strategies for success. npj Digit. Med. **3**(1), 1–10 (2020)
6. Tang, H., Liu, J., Zhao, F., Wang, S., Zhang, Y.: MEDAGENT: a multi-agent collaboration framework for solving real-world medical problems. arXiv preprint arXiv:2410.04585 (2024)
7. Wang, Y., Kung, L., Byrd, T.A.: Big data analytics: understanding its capabilities and potential benefits for healthcare organizations. Technol. Forecast. Soc. Chang. **126**, 3–13 (2018)

8. Wang, Y., Zhang, J., Lin, X., Zhao, H., Chen, M.: Medkg-llm: enhancing medical reasoning of LLMs via medical knowledge graphs. arXiv preprint arXiv:2410.04660 (2024)
9. Zhu, Y., Zhang, Z., Wang, Q., Huang, X., Zhou, Y.: MultiMedQA: benchmarking medical reasoning capabilities of LLMs across tasks and specialties. arXiv preprint arXiv:2409.05556 (2024)

Comparing Different Positional Encodings for the Interpretation of Medical Images

Andrea Santomauro[1,2], Giorgio Leonardi[1], and Luigi Portinale[1(✉)]

[1] Computer Science Institute, DiSIT, University of Piemonte Orientale, Alessandria, Italy
{andrea.santomauro,giorgio.leonardi,luigi.portinale}@uniupo.it
[2] Lab of AI and Medical Informatics, DAIRI, AOUAL, Alessandria, Italy

Abstract. Traditional positional encoding (PE) methods in Vision Transformers (ViT) focus primarily on spatial information, but they may not adequately capture the complex geometric patterns intrinsic to medical images. To address this limitation, we have previously proposed a similarity-based positional encoding combining convolution operations and standard cosine similarity between image patches. In the present work we compare similarity-based PE with two traditional alternatives in ViT such as standard learned PE and rotatory PE. The goal is to show that, in addition to provide better classification accuracy of 2D images in different medical domains, the attention maps generated by similarity-based PE appears to be more meaningful than those generated by alternative encodings, focusing on the medical relevant part of the images. Finally, we also show the benefits of the proposed approach in dealing with 3D medical images, again in terms of classification performance. We validate our method on a set of six medical imaging datasets from MedMNIST which are benchmark datasets of medical images of various kinds, such as X-rays, histological samples, dermoscopic, ultrasounds and microscope images.

Keywords: Medical Image Classification · Positional Encoding · Vision Transformers

1 Introduction

In the present paper, we propose a novel perspective on learned positional encoding (PE) in Vision Transformers (ViT) with attention to medical images. We argue that these encodings may not merely learn "positions" in the traditional sense, but rather they are capturing high-level relationships and patterns within the visual data. This insight challenges the conventional understanding of positional encodings and opens up new avenues for improving ViT architectures.

In particular, by considering complex medical images such as X-rays, histological or dermoscopic ones, we can notice that particular diseases or findings are usually visible in form of geometric patterns, which can be properly

P. Bruno et al. (Eds.): HC_AIxIA_HYDRA 2025, CCIS 2830, pp. 78–89, 2026.
https://doi.org/10.1007/978-3-032-16708-8_6

extracted using convolutions. Building on these observations, we have previously proposed a new encoding method based on the computation of similarity measures between image patches, after applying convolution operations [1]. We show that this similarity-based encoding leads to improved performance and generalization across various computer vision tasks in medicine. In particular: we show the effectiveness of our approach through extensive experiments on medical benchmark datasets, showing improved performance compared to traditional positional encoding; we show that attention maps seem to focus on more informative region of the images, enhancing the model's explainability; finally, we show how the approach allows a seamless generalization to 3D-images (such as MRI scans) without the need of a specific pre-training phase on them.

The rest of the paper is organized as follows: in Sect. 2 we discuss related works on positional encoding; in Sect. 3 we provide the details of the proposed similarity-based positional encoding; in Sect. 4 we discuss the experimental setup and the obtained results. Finally, Sect. 5 is devoted to conclusion and future works.

2 Positional Encoding: Related Works

Positional Encoding (PE) is a key component of a Transfomer model, and has been introduced in [2] with the purpose of capturing ordering information in a model which is inherently permutation-invariant. In ViT, PE allows the model to take into consideration the position of the image patches. When the encoding is a learned representation of positional information then we talk about positional embedding[1]. We focus here on the most used task-independent approaches in the context of ViT: *standard learned positional encoding (SLPE)*, a widely used absolute encoding where a random matrix is combined with the patches and optimized during training [3]; *Rotatory Position Embedding (RoPE)*, addressing the limitations of fixed positional encoding by incorporating relative position information directly into the attention mechanism through rotational transformations in the embedding space [4]. Specifically, RoPE applies a position-dependent rotation to the query and key vectors, before computing attention scores; this has demonstrated a good performance in medical applications [5]. The main drawback of RoPE is that it must be applied directly to the query and key vectors before each attention layer, rather than being added once to the input embeddings. This requires an architectural change of the ViT model for the correct integration of the positional information, potentially complicating model implementation and making fine-tuning from a general Transformer architecture not suitable.

In the following, we will focus on the introduction, in a standard ViT architecture with a classification header, of an alternative PE mechanisms called *similarity-based PE (SimPE)*.

[1] In this paper we will focus only on learned positional information, thus we will use the terms enconding and embedding interchangeably.

3 Similarity Based Positional Encoding

As discussed in Sect. 2, most of the PE methods adopted in the context of ViT use a learned PE approach. Learned PE allows the model to implicitly capture the relationships between patches in a flexible way, by adapting the encoding to the task at hand and discovering representations that go beyond explicit spatial coordinates, such as semantic relationships and interactions that are spatially informed.

In medical image analysis, however, geometrical patterns (such as shapes, boundaries, and specific anatomical structures), often play a more crucial role than the general patch-to-patch correlation captured by learned PE, which is often unable to manage and to model these geometrical patterns. Based on this observation, we have previously proposed a new method for PE called similarity-based PE (SimPE), based on convolutional operations and cosine similarity between extracted features [1]. This approach guarantees that the overall ViT architecture has no need to be modified, and one can exploit pre-trained models for specific tasks, while fine-tuning just the PE blocks.

Figure 1 shows a graphical representation of the computation process of SimPE (see [1] for the details).

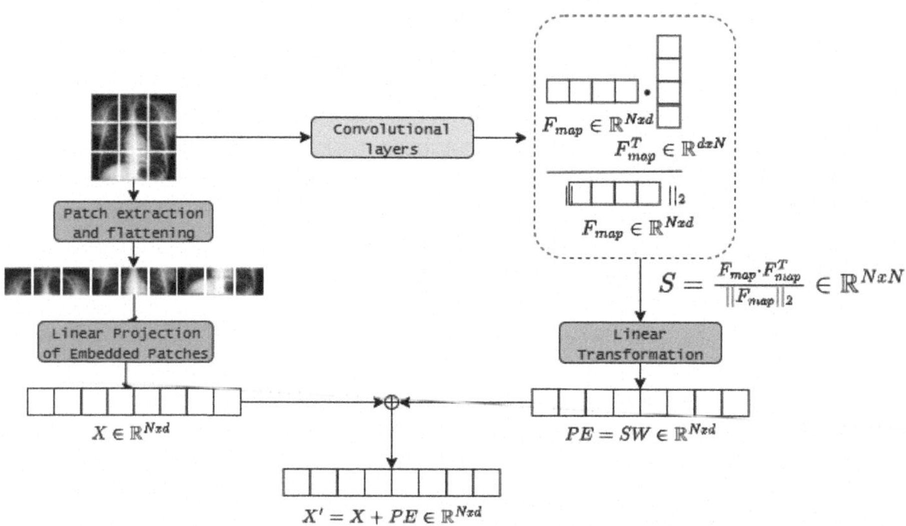

Fig. 1. Visual representation of SimPE; X' is the final embedding of the input image provided as input to the ViT architecture.

The learned convolutional filters extract geometrical information from the input images, which are essentials to medical image analysis. Through the usage of these geometrical features as encoding, we help the ViT architecture to learn patterns which can be useful for the specific task of medical image classification.

In the next section, we report the results we have obtained on a set of benchmark datasets by applying SimPE, and we compare them to the ones obtained with both SLPE and RoPE.

4 Experiments and Results

In order to compare SLPE and RoPE with the SimPE, we have defined a ViT architecture with fixed hyper-parameters and we have trained the network on specific medical datasets using the three encoding techniques, by comparing the results. As we report in the following, we tested two different ViT architectures, one without pre-training and another one pre-trained on ImageNet [6]. In particular, the architecture without pre-training has a number of transformer layers set to 4, the number of attention heads set to 4 as well, an embedding size set to 768 and an input size to the classification layer (MLP dimension) set to 256. The pre-trained architecture differs from the previous one in the number of layers and of attention heads (both set to 12) and in the MLP dimension set to 3072. For the fine-tuned model, we used the Adam optimizer with a learning rate of 1×10^{-3}, a CosineAnnealingLR scheduler, batch size of 512, input image size of 224×224, and gradient clipping at 1.0. Input images were normalized using mean [0.485, 0.456, 0.406] and standard deviation [0.229, 0.224, 0.225]. For the model trained from scratch, we used the same optimizer and normalization parameters, but we set the learning rate to 1×10^{-4} and the batch size to 256, keeping all other hyperparameters identical. We employed early stopping technique on validation accuracy in order to prevent overfitting, reduce computational cost and avoid manual epoch tuning.

We resort to 6 different datasets which are part of MedMNIST [7,8], representing different image classification tasks in different medical domains, and in particular: **PneumoniaMNIST**, a dataset of chest X-ray images, specifically designed to detect and classify pneumonia; **PathMNIST**, a dataset of pathology images of breast cancer tissue slides for the classification of different subtypes of breast cancer from microscope images; **DermaMNIST**, consisting of dermatological images (taken with a dermatoscope) aimed at classifying different types of skin lesions; **BreastMNIST**, a dataset derived from ultrasound images for the classification of breast cancer; **TissueMNIST**, a dataset that focuses on histological images from human tissue samples, containing tissue images from various organs, and to be classified into different cell types; **BloodMNIST**, a dataset of blood smear images for the classification of blood cells.

Some of the datasets are designed for binary classification and some of them for multi-class classification. An excerpt of images from some of such datasets is shown in Fig. 2.

4.1 Classification Results

In this section, we present a comparative analysis of the results obtained using SLPE, RoPE and SimPE. The performance of the model has been evaluated across the datasets previously described, under two training paradigms: training from scratch and fine-tuning with a model pre-trained on ImageNet. Table 1 summarizes the accuracy achieved on the benchmark splits provided by the MedMNIST dataset (see [7,8] for the details).

Table 1. Results in terms of accuracy and 95% confidence intervals on the MedMNIST benchmark split. Bold values show best results.

Training	Dataset	SLPE	RoPE	SimPE
Fine-tuning	BloodMNIST	87.16% ± 1.14	96.46% ± 0.97	**97.22% ± 0.35**
	BreastMNIST	73.07% ± 4.98	**85.89% ± 3.23**	83.13% ± 2.82
	DermaMNIST	67.83% ± 1.64	78.20% ± 1.64	**80.30% ± 1.22**
	PathMNIST	90.44% ± 1.79	90.14% ± 0.92	**98.14% ± 0.34**
	PneumoniaMNIST	85.96% ± 2.57	88.14% ± 1.52	**95.89% ± 0.76**
	TissueMNIST	55.61% ± 0.83	**65.62% ± 0.64**	60.01% ± 0.41
Training from scratch	BloodMNIST	83.95% ± 2.78	78.95% ± 2.66	**94.18% ± 2.76**
	BreastMNIST	73.01% ± 3.90	73.07% ± 3.81	**76.97% ± 3.44**
	DermaMNIST	70.97% ± 2.02	67.23% ± 1.47	**73.61% ± 0.98**
	PathMNIST	83.14% ± 1.97	63.87% ± 1.88	**88.53% ± 1.68**
	PneumoniaMNIST	85.89% ± 2.89	82.69% ± 2.04	**91.18% ± 0.71**
	TissueMNIST	50.87% ± 1.43	42.84% ± 0.78	**54.81% ± 0.49**

The results show that the proposed similarity-based PE consistently achieves higher accuracy across all benchmark datasets, regardless of the training paradigm employed (i.e. training from scratch or fine-tuning). For BloodMNIST, PneumoniaMNIST and PathMNIST the accuracy gap between SimPE and SLPE is larger with respect to the other datasets. This may be explained by the fact that these datasets contain more geometrical structure than the others, and since SimPE is explicitly designed to let the model recognize geometric shapes, this behavior is consistent. To show an example, Fig. 2 reports samples of images from BloodMNIST (2a), PneumoniaMNIST (2b) and PathMNIST (2c); among the tested datasets, they are those showing important geometric patterns useful to classify the image. In contrast, in other datasets such as DermaMNIST, where geometrical features are less present, the resulting performance is only slightly increased but overall comparable.

RoPE achieves slightly better performance on BreastMNIST and TissueMNIST while using fine-tuning, while the performance are worse than SimPE in all the other datasets. Moreover, in the model trained from scratch it is possible to notice that RoPE is consistently the worst model in terms of accuracy.

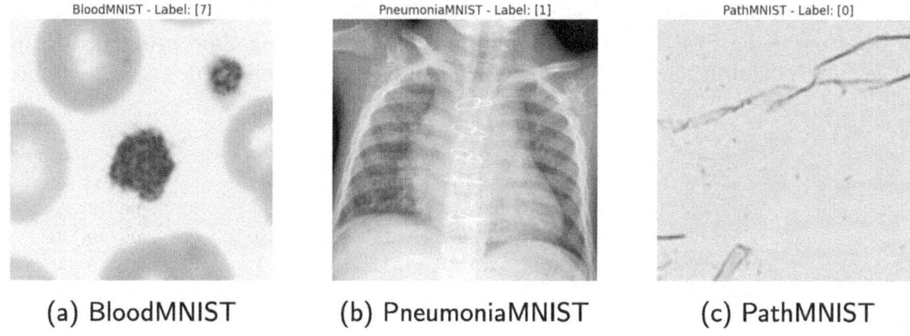

Fig. 2. Sample images from BloodMNIST, PneumoniaMNIST, and PathMNIST datasets.

In conclusion, fine-tuning enhances the generalization capability of all three encoding strategies, with important improvements for SimPE and RoPE. This suggests that the proposed encoding approach, coupled with pre-training, provides a robust feature representation, even if pre-training is very general (e.g., the ImageNet dataset) and not task-specific.

4.2 Training Time

In order to assess computational costs of traning, we have also measured the training time of the model under the different tested PE strategies. Table 2 presents the number of epochs required by the models (both fine-tuned and trained from scratch) to converge with different PE. Models using SimPE converges in general more quickly both in terms of number of epochs and of overall training time. RoPE shows the worst performance in terms of training efficiency, as it usually requirtes more time per epoch on average, and a larger number of epochs to trigger early-stopping. Exceptions are datasets PathMNIST in fine-tuning and BreastMNIST in training from scratch, where the overall training time is the shortest; however, the obtained final accuracy on the test set is better for SimPE with comparable training time (see Table 1). We can conclude that, SimPE can be considered a promising candidate for large-scale training on modern hardware[2].

4.3 Attention Maps Analysis

To better understand the impact of SimPE we have also analyzed the attention maps produced by the ViT architecture across various layers and heads. This qualitative evaluation aims to highlight how our method enhances the model's ability to capture and preserve meaningful geometric patterns in the

[2] All experiments have been performed on a single NVIDIA $A100$ GPU to ensure consistent hardware conditions.

Table 2. Total number of epochs before early stopping. The fourth column refers to training time using SLPE, the sixth column refers to training time using RoPE and the the eighth column refers to training time using SimPE. Bold values represents best results.

Training	Dataset	SLPE	Time(hh:mm:ss)	RoPE	Time(hh:mm:ss)	SimPE	Time(hh:mm:ss)
Fine-tuning	BloodMNIST	15	00 : 13 : 00	15	00 : 20 : 45	13	**00 : 11 : 55**
	BreastMNIST	18	00 : 00 : 54	35	00 : 01 : 10	10	**00 : 00 : 30**
	DermaMNIST	19	00 : 11 : 05	13	00 : 14 : 31	14	**00 : 08 : 10**
	PathMNIST	21	02 : 24 : 12	5	**00 : 37 : 10**	15	01 : 45 : 30
	PneumoniaMNIST	16	00 : 05 : 36	10	00 : 09 : 10	12	**00 : 04 : 24**
	TissueMNIST	21	04 : 30 : 57	48	08 : 28 : 48	15	**03 : 30 : 00**
Training from scratch	BloodMNIST	27	00 : 46 : 21	49	03 : 07 : 01	20	**00 : 35 : 20**
	BreastMNIST	25	00 : 13 : 45	40	**00 : 08 : 40**	22	00 : 12 : 28
	DermaMNIST	19	00 : 22 : 48	27	00 : 59 : 24	17	**00 : 21 : 15**
	PathMNIST	24	04 : 24 : 48	11	05 : 16 : 26	16	**03 : 22 : 16**
	PneumoniaMNIST	28	00 : 26 : 36	13	00 : 26 : 39	24	**00 : 24 : 48**
	TissueMNIST	24	09 : 52 : 24	52	45 : 19 : 36	22	**09 : 43 : 22**

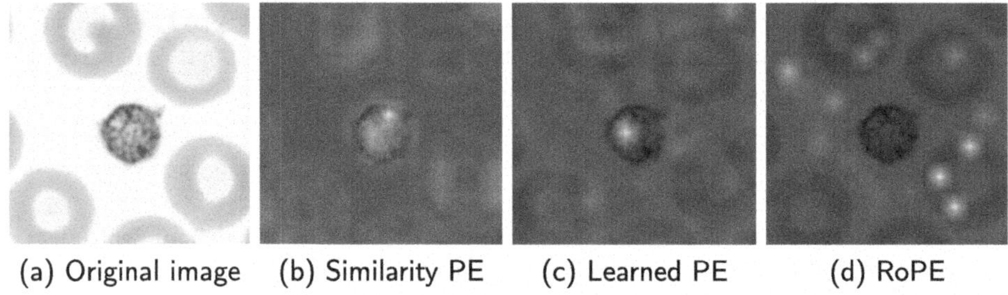

Fig. 3. BloodMNIST: Original image and attention maps using different positional encodings.

input images. Figures from 3 to 8 are examples showing that SimPE can capture geometric patterns more effectively and leads to attention distributions that are more spatially coherent and better aligned with the underlying anatomical or structural regions in the image. In the figures, the lighter the color, the higher the attention.

Figure 3a shows a platelet; it is evident that the activation pattern is much more coherent when using the SimPE. In contrast, SLPE produces a more diffuse attention across the entire image, while RoPE completely ignores the platelet (the circular, purplish region at the center).

Figure 4a depicts a malignant breast tumor; in this case, all three attention maps can be considered inadequate, as they focus on the surrounding tissue rather than the tumor region. Only RoPE shows a small area of activation over the tumor, but this result is not satisfactory in terms of clinical relevance.

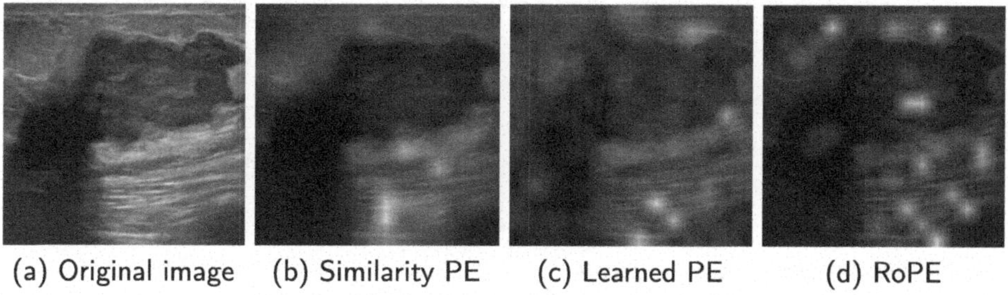

Fig. 4. BreastMNIST: Original image and attention maps using different positional encodings.

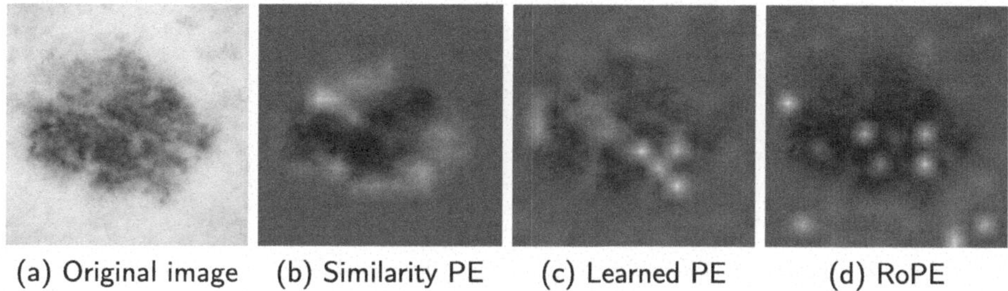

Fig. 5. DermaMNIST: Original image and attention maps using different positional encodings.

Figure 5a shows a melanoma; the attention map produced by RoPE focuses on regions that do not even contain the nevus and therefore lacks interpretability with respect to the outcome (melanoma). The attention map obtained using SLPE performs slightly better, as it correctly focuses on the nevus. However, the most accurate and clinically relevant result is achieved with SimPE, which precisely attends to the irregular borders of the melanoma—the very feature that clinicians rely on for diagnosis.

Figure 6a shows the epithelium of colorectal adenocarcinoma; the heatmap generated by SimPE highlights epithelial regions with high-grade dysplasia in a spatially coherent and anatomically plausible manner. Although features indicative of submucosal invasion are not present in this limited field of view, the model correctly classifies the sample as colorectal adenocarcinoma epithelium. All three attention maps highlight epithelial regions consistent with the label "colorectal adenocarcinoma epithelium". SimPE map shows a broad and anatomically plausible focus on dysplastic tissue, with homogeneous attention across the neoplastic epithelium. SLPE map presents a more fragmented attention pattern, with multiple sharp focal points but limited contextual integration. RoPE map displays sparse and highly localized activations, with reduced sensitivity to the overall epithelial structure.

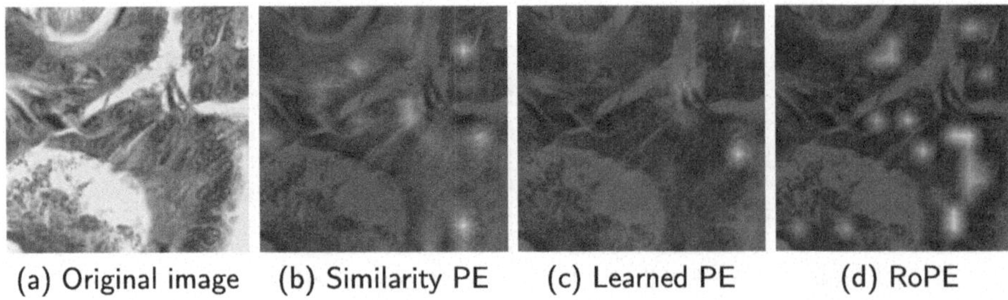

Fig. 6. PathMNIST: Original image and attention maps using different positional encodings.

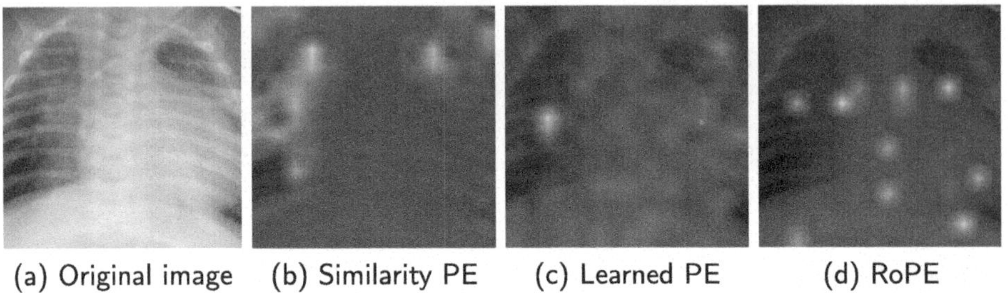

Fig. 7. PneumoniaMNIST: Original image and attention maps using different positional encodings.

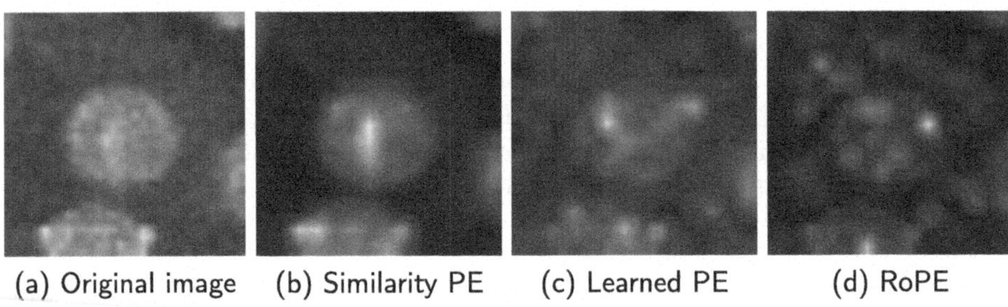

Fig. 8. TissueMNIST: Original image and attention maps using different positional encodings.

Figure 7a shows a patient with pneumonia; SimPE clearly focuses on the lung regions (both right and left), with some minor activations outside the lung area, yet the attention remains consistent with the classification. In contrast, the other two positional encodings produce highly diffuse attention maps, with no strongly activated regions in the heatmaps.

Lastly, Fig. 8a shows segments of the proximal tubule; the attention map generated by the SimPE precisely captures the geometric region of interest, whereas SLPE and RoPE encodings result in a highly diffuse attention and an almost entirely absent one respectively.

Table 3. Results on NoduleMNIST3D benchmark split using a pre-trained ViT on ImageNet

Encoding Type	Accuracy$\pm CI(95\%)$	Precision $\pm CI(95\%)$	Recall $\pm CI(95\%)$	F1$\pm CI(95\%)$
Learned PE	$79.35\% \pm 0.0$	1.0 ± 0.00	0.0 ± 0.0	0.0 ± 0.0
Similarity PE	$88.10\% \pm 0.01$	0.73 ± 0.021	0.69 ± 0.017	0.66 ± 0.019

4.4 Extension to 3D Medical Images

While ViTs have been extensively employed for 2D medical image analysis, their application to 3D medical imaging (e.g., MRI or PET scans) remains limited. Currently proposed methodologies usually adopt two main approaches for 3D medical image classification using ViTs:

- CNN Preprocessing: a CNN architecture is used to pre-process input images, before the ViT model. The resulting image embeddings are then projected into the ViT input dimensions to ensure computational compatibility.
- Multi-Slice Aggregation: multiple image slices are treated as individual images, extracting patches across all slices and passing them to the ViT model.

Both categories of approaches demonstrate to be effective across various tasks, including classification and segmentation. However, they suffer from significant computational limitations. The first approach needs the adoption of a complete CNN, substantially increasing the total parameter count. The second approach introduces a large number of patches, resulting in attention matrices that grow quadratically with respect to the input size, consequently escalating the memory consumption.

On the contrary, SimPE can be easily adapted to the case of 3D images by just substituting the convolutional layers of Fig. 1 into 3D convolutions. We have tested this idea on a 3D imaging dataset (again from MedMNIST) called NoduleMNIST3D [9], focusing on pulmonary nodule diagnosis in 3D computed tomography (CT) scans for potential lung cancer detection (binary classification). The dataset comprises 1,465 samples with a notable class imbalance: the training set contains 295 malignant nodules and 863 benign nodules, resulting in a malignant nodule ratio of 0.25 (a similar ratio is present in the test set).Each 3D sample has a standardized resolution of $28 \times 28 \times 28$ pixels; patch extraction employed a 3D convolutional layer with a kernel size and stride of 5, generating a total of 125 patches. We adapted the SimPE approach using 3D convolutions: a shallow CNN (with 3 layers) performs the feature extraction F_{map} from the original 3D input image (see Fig. 1), then we compute the cosine similarity matrix, project the result to the model's dimension, and finally use it as PE. We have performed experiments on the benchmark split provided by MedMNIST, comparing classification performance using both SLPE and SimPE, by leveraging a ViT pre-trained on ImageNet.

Table 3 shows the results where the positive class is the one representing malignant nodules. SLPE shows significant limitations, with a null recall, indicating a complete failure to correctly identify true positives (malignant nodules)[3]. Indeed, the model using SLPE actually classifies any nodule as a benign, resulting in an accuracy score equivalent to the benign nodule ratio present in the test set. In contrast, the use of similarity-based PE is able to suitably deal with the class imbalance problem, by avoiding the classification of every sample as negative. The reported high accuracy level, paired with consistent results in terms of precision and recall, shows a significant improvement of the classification results obtained using this approach.

5 Conclusion and Future Works

In this work we have experimentally analyzed similarity-based positional encoding in medical image analysis. The method shows superior performance in terms of classification accuracy when compared to standard learned PE and RoPE, particularly where images are characterized by distinct geometric structures and patterns, showing also a better efficiency in terms of training time. Moreover, a preliminary analysis of the attention maps generated with this enconding shows that regions related to the final classification/diagnosis are better recognized with respect to alternative techniques. Finally, extension to 3D images is straightforward, providing also in this case improved accuracy in classification results.

As future works, we plan to focus on comparing similarity-based PE also with task-specific positional encoding methods, such as those presented in [10], focusing on enhancing segmentation through long-range contextual learning for CT and MRI scans, or in [11] where a hierarchical PE adapted for volumetric medical images (PET, CT and MRI scans) is proposed.

Acknowledgment. Andrea Santomauro's PhD research is co-financed by ARLANIS REPLY.We also acknowledge the use of the Chameleon Cloud testbed [12] that has allowed us to perform all the experiments described in the present work. Source code used for the experimentation described in the paper can be found at https://github.com/andreascnz/similarity-pe

References

1. Leonardi, G., Portinale, L., Santomauro, A.:"Similarity-based positional encoding for enhanced classification in medical images. In: CEUR Proceedings 3880, 3rd AIxIA Workshop on Artificial Intelligence For Healthcare, 2024, pp. 182–188 (2024). https://ceur-ws.org/Vol-3880/paper16.pdf
2. Vaswani, A., et al.: Attention is all you need. In: 31st Conference on Neural Information Processing Systems (NIPS), Long Beach, CA, (2017). https://tinyurl.com/5463rwkz

[3] In this case, the value of precision is actually undefined and we can set it to 1 as usual, to indicate no "spurious" results for the positive class.

3. Dosovitskiy, A., et al.: An image is worth 16x16 words: Transformers for image recognition at scale. (2021). https://arxiv.org/abs/2010.11929
4. Su, J., Ahmed, M., Lu, Y., Pan, S., Bo, W., Liu, Y.: RoFormer: Enhanced transformer with rotary position embedding (2023). [Online]. Available: https://arxiv.org/abs/2104.09864
5. Li, Y., et al.: RoMedFormer: a rotary-embedding transformer foundation model for 3D genito-pelvic structure segmentation in MRI and CT (2025). https://arxiv.org/abs/2503.14304
6. Russakovsky, O., et al.: Imagenet large scale visual recognition challenge (2015). https://arxiv.org/abs/1409.0575
7. Yang, J., Shi, R., Ni, B.: MedMNIST classification decathlon: a lightweight automl benchmark for medical image analysis. In: IEEE 18th International Symposium on Biomedical Imaging (ISBI), pp. 191–195 (2021)
8. Yang, Z., et al.: MedMNIST v2-a large-scale lightweight benchmark for 2d and 3d biomedical image classification. Sci. Data **10**(1), 41 (2023)
9. Armato, S.G., McLennan, G., et al.: The lung image database consortium (LIDC) and image database resource initiative (IDRI): a completed reference databaseof lung nodules on CT scans. Med. Phys. **38**(2), 915–931 (2011)
10. Wang, L., et al.: UNetFormer: a UNet-like transformer for efficient semantic segmentation of remote sensing urban scene imagery. ISPRS J. Photogramm. Remote Sens. **190**, 196–214 (2022). https://www.sciencedirect.com/science/article/pii/S0924271622001654
11. Tang, Y., et al.: Self-supervised pre-training of swin transformers for 3D medical image analysis. In: 2022 IEEE/CVF Conference on Computer Vision and Pattern Recognition (CVPR), 2022, pp. 20 698–20 708 (2022)
12. Keahey, K., et al.: Lessons learned from the chameleon testbed. In: Proceedings of the 2020 USENIX Annual Technical Conference (USENIX ATC '20). USENIX Association, July 2020. [Online]. Available: https://chameleoncloud.org/

Short Communications

Designing a Multimodal Dataset for AI-Based Prognosis in STEMI

Simone Bartucci[2,3,4](✉), Edoardo De Rose[2], Alessandro Quarta[2,4], Rossella Quarta[1,5], Alessia Donata Camarda[2], Alberto Polimeni[5,6], and Francesco Calimeri[2,4]

[1] Division of Cardiology, Annunziata Hospital, Cosenza, Italy
[2] Department of Mathematics and Computer Science, University of Calabria, Arcavacata, Italy
[3] Department of Computer, Control and Management Engineering "Antonio Ruberti", Sapienza University of Rome, Rome, Italy
[4] DLVSystem Srl, Rende, Italy
simone.bartucci@uniroma1.it
[5] Department of Pharmacy, Health and Nutritional Sciences, University of Calabria, Arcavacata, Italy
[6] Division of Interventional Cardiology, Annunziata Hospital, Cosenza, Italy

Abstract. Despite advances in reperfusion therapy, ST-segment elevation myocardial infarction remains a leading cause of mortality in the general population. In this work, we present a multicenter multimodal dataset designed for AI-based 12-month prognostic stratification after STEMI. The cohort includes 822 patients with predischarge post-PCI (Percutaneous Coronary Intervention) 12-lead ECGs and comprehensive clinical, laboratory, echocardiographic, angiographic and pharmacological data, along with standardized acquisition and 12-month follow-up for major adverse cardiovascular events (MACE). Data were anonymized and harmonized, and a computer-vision pipeline has been designed to detect lead regions and extract analyzable signals.

To our knowledge, unlike other existing public datasets, this is the first multicenter dataset coupling predischarge ECGs with rich multimodal context and longitudinal outcomes in STEMI, enabling robust AI models for personalized risk prediction. This approach helps to bridge the gap between acute diagnosis and long-term risk stratification, with significant potential to improve clinical decision-making and patient outcomes.

Keywords: STEMI · ECG · Multimodal dataset

1 Introduction

Acute coronary syndromes (ACS) encompass a spectrum of conditions caused by acute myocardial ischemia, including unstable angina, nonâĂŞST-segment elevation myocardial infarction (NSTEMI), and ST-segment elevation myocardial

P. Bruno et al. (Eds.): HC_AIxIA_HYDRA 2025, CCIS 2830, pp. 93–98, 2026.
https://doi.org/10.1007/978-3-032-16708-8_7

infarction (STEMI), with the latter representing the most time-critical presentation and carrying the highest mortality risk [3]. Despite significant advances in reperfusion and secondary prevention, STEMI remains a major cause of morbidity, mortality, and healthcare resource utilization [1]. Careful post-discharge risk stratification and a person-centred approach are therefore essential to improve prognosis and quality of life in this population [13]. The resting 12-lead electrocardiogram (ECG) is the cornerstone for STEMI diagnosis and immediate reperfusion decision-making. Recently, it has been recognized that the ECG also carries prognostic information, reflecting myocardial injury and revascularization quality. In recent years, ECG has gained a new role beyond acute diagnosis: it may also contain prognostic information, reflecting the extent of myocardial injury and the quality of revascularization. In this context, Artificial Intelligence (AI), particularly Deep Learning (DL), has become a powerful tool for automated biomedical signal analysis. AI models can uncover subtle ECG patterns imperceptible to clinicians, improving diagnostic and prognostic accuracy in cardiovascular medicine. Ribeiro et al. [9] trained a deep network on over two million ECGs, outperforming cardiology residents in detecting abnormalities. More recently, Foundation Models (FMs) such as *ECG-FM* [6], a transformer pretrained on 1.5 million ECGs, have achieved strong performance in tasks like ejection fraction prediction and ECG interpretation, even with limited data. However, even FMs require a relevant reference dataset to address the inherent challenges of out-of-distribution (OOD) generalization, ensuring that their performance is reliable and clinically valid. This power is further amplified by integrating multimodal data, combining ECG signals with structured clinical information to improve diagnostic sensitivity and provide a more contextualized patient assessment. Despite these methodological advances, the development of clinically reliable DL models is critically hindered by the lack of large, representative, and rigorously annotated datasets. Publicly available ECG databases, often suffer from heterogeneous diagnostic labels, low STEMI prevalence leading to class imbalance, and variable signal quality. Furthermore, they frequently lack the complementary clinical data essential for robust multimodal modeling and often have limited demographic diversity, which compromises the generalizability of any resulting models. To address these limitations, we conducted a multi-centric observational study to develop a comprehensive, multi-parametric dataset; in this paper, we describe its design and features in detail. By ensuring standardized acquisition and complete clinical information, the dataset is intended not merely as a basis for classification experiments, but as a catalyst for the scientific community to develop AI tools genuinely applicable to the clinical context of ECG interpretation, particularly in STEMI. Furthermore, the primary motivation behind this work is to establish a solid groundwork for the development and validation of an AI-based risk score. The score would use predischarge post-PCI ECGs combined with extensive demographic, clinical, laboratory, echocardiographic, angiographic, and pharmacological data to predict 12-month Major Adverse Cardiovascular Events (MACE), defined as cardiovascular death, non-fatal myocardial infarction, non-fatal stroke, urgent coronary

Table 1. Summary of the main ECG datasets used in related works

INCART [5]	74 recordings, 12 leads. Holter-based recordings with limited annotations; primarily for arrhythmia research.
European ST-T [11]	90 recordings (79 patients), 2 leads. Suitable for ST-segment analysis; lacks full 12-lead coverage.
PTB-XL [12]	21,799 12-lead ECGs. Large-scale and balanced; lacks STEMI-specific labels and longitudinal data.
Chapman-Shaoxing [14]	45,152 10-second ECGs. Extensive dataset; low prevalence of acute events and no follow-up information.
CODE-15% [8]	345,779 ECGs (233,770 patients), 12 leads. Very large dataset; lacks STEMI-specific labels and detailed clinical outcomes.
ECG-Image-Kit [10]	21,801 synthetic ECG images. Fully synthetic; no additional clinical information available.
PMcardio [4]	6,000 images derived from PTB-XL. Image-based representation; lacks multimodal clinical data.

revascularization, and hospitalization for heart failure. By enabling more precise risk stratification, it is possible to guide personalized follow-up strategies, and ultimately reduce the incidence of MACE during the critical first year after a STEMI.

2 Related Works

Research on automatic ECG analysis has primarily relied on publicly available databases, many of which have been collected and distributed through PhysioNet [2], which for over two decades has served as the main open-access repository of physiological signals for the scientific community.

To improve clarity, we summarize the main ECG datasets used in prior work in Table 1. Historical datasets remain valuable but are limited by their small size, heterogeneous structure, and lack of comprehensive annotations. Modern large-scale databases offer a substantial number of ECGs with broader demographic coverage, but they often lack STEMI-specific labels, provide limited clinical annotations, and are devoid of longitudinal follow-up. More recently, ECG image-based resources have been introduced, though these are typically generated from pre-existing signal data and do not enrich the clinical spectrum.

Overall, while these resources significantly contributed to the advancements in automated ECG interpretation, they result inadequate for the targeted STEMI investigation. Current open-access repositories do not provide a multimodal foundation combining ECG with laboratory data, imaging, and long-term follow-ups, which is crucial for developing clinically relevant AI-driven prognostic tools.

3 Dataset Description

The dataset currently consists of a total of **822** (422+400) **electrocardiograms (ECGs)** collected from two high-volume Italian clinical centers, both serving as primary referral facilities within their regional STEMI network. A detailed description is reported in Table 2. All patients were admitted with a confirmed diagnosis of STEMI, and only those with a 12-lead ECG recorded at admission were considered, while we excluded poor-quality or incomplete ECG traces preventing reliable interpretation, missing essential clinical data or follow-up information. All files were standardized via preprocessing and converted into uniform formats for subsequent computational use.

Table 2. Summary of dataset features

Dataset size	822 patients from 2 different Hospitals
ECG acquisition	Standard 12-lead recordings (I, II, III, aVR, aVL, aVF, V1–V6), sampling frequency: 500 Hz, duration: 20 s
Center-specific differences	First Hospital: scanned millimeter-paper traces (grayscale or color), lower fidelity/resolution. Second Hospital: raw digital signals, consistently in color, higher fidelity/resolution.
Demographic & anthropometric data	Age, sex, weight, height, BMI
Clinical course	Date of coronary revascularization after STEMI diagnosis, total length of hospital stay
Clinical history (binary)	Family history of cardiovascular disease, smoking, arterial hypertension, diabetes mellitus, obesity, dyslipidemia, transient ischemic attack, stroke, previous acute coronary syndrome, chronic coronary syndrome, chronic kidney disease, peripheral artery disease, chronic obstructive pulmonary disease
Laboratory data (numeric)	Hemoglobin, glycated hemoglobin, creatinine (with eGFR), total cholesterol, HDL, LDL, triglycerides, C-reactive protein (CRP), peak troponin, peak BNP
Clinical & instrumental parameters	Systolic/diastolic blood pressure, heart rate, ejection fraction, number of diseased coronary vessels, number of implanted stents, location of culprit/other lesions (Syntax score). Presence of atrial fibrillation, bundle branch block, severe valvulopathy (binary). Coronary dominance (right/left/balanced).
Discharge therapy	List of prescribed drugs (up to 20 agents)
Follow-up data	Follow-up date, occurrence of major adverse cardiovascular events (death, hospitalization for heart failure, re-infarction, stroke, urgent coronary revascularization), and date of occurrence

4 Data Processing and ECG Signal Extraction

The ECG is the cornerstone for STEMI diagnosis and immediate reperfusion decisions, making its inclusion in our dataset of critical importance. Given the diverse cohorts from which we collected ECGs, a major challenge has been creating a unified dataset from the raw files, which vary widely in format and quality. Our collection includes both structured raw digital data and digitized images of varying resolutions and formats, which are unusable for computational analysis as they are. To address this, we are developing a robust pipeline to automate the extraction of analyzable time-series signals from these diverse sources. The core of this process leverages computer vision and object detection techniques.

Specifically, our pipeline is designed to address two main issues: (*i*) identifying the coordinates of the 12-lead regions within the image to create a precise bounding box, and (*ii*) removing artifacts and other sensitive information that could compromise patient anonymity. To achieve this, the data is first subjected to a preprocessing stage. This stage includes Optical Character Recognition (OCR) to identify and remove any text, followed by image normalization. These initial steps help standardize the dataset, preparing it for subsequent analysis. We then leverage the potential of a novel framework for generating synthetic ECGs [7]. This framework provides a robust method for obtaining the coordinates of the lead regions and their corresponding names. By fine-tuning the model, our goal is to accurately identify the regions of interest in the ECG and discard any artifacts, thus ensuring a clean and consistent dataset of standardized digital ECG images for AI-based analysis.

5 Ethics and Data Availability

The study protocol was approved by the local ethics committees of both hospitals, and informed consent was obtained in accordance with national and international regulations. This manuscript reports preliminary results from ongoing work, and the dataset used in this study is currently being compiled. Once completed, it will be made available upon reasonable request to the corresponding author and shared under a Data Use Agreement with the participating hospitals. In the meantime, the dataset can already be accessed on request for academic purposes.

6 Conclusions

We have introduced a multicenter and multimodal dataset dedicated to STEMI patients, which integrates predischarge post-PCI ECGs with comprehensive clinical, laboratory, echocardiographic, angiographic, and pharmacological information, along with 12-month follow-up for major adverse cardiovascular events (MACE). Unlike existing public resources, this dataset provides standardized and richly annotated data, establishing a robust foundation for the development of clinically reliable AI models. By enabling the combination of ECG-derived features with multimodal patient information, this resource offers a unique opportunity to bridge the gap between acute diagnosis and long-term prognostic assessment. Such integration has the potential to support personalized risk stratification, guide follow-up strategies, and ultimately improve patient outcomes in the critical first year after STEMI. As already stated, this is a report of an ongoing work; besides full release, we aim to expand the dataset with additional centers and broader demographic diversity, further enhancing its representativeness and applicability to real-world clinical settings.

Acknowledgements. This work has been carried out while Simone Bartucci was enrolled in the Italian National Doctorate on Artificial Intelligence run by Sapienza University of Rome in collaboration with Università della Calabria.

References

1. Akbar, U.A., et al.: Young adults undergoing percutaneous coronary intervention for myocardial infarction in the united states, 2011-2023. Am. J. Cardiol. (2025)
2. Alday, E.A.P., et al.: Classification of 12-lead ecgs: the physionet/computing in cardiology challenge 2020. Physiol. Meas. **41**(12), 124003 (2020)
3. Byrne, R.A., et al.: 2023 esc guidelines for the management of acute coronary syndromes: developed by the task force on the management of acute coronary syndromes of the european society of cardiology (esc). Eur. Heart J. Acute Cardiovasc. Care **13**(1), 55–161 (2024)
4. Iring, A., Krešnáková, V., Hojcka, M., Boza, V., Rafajdus, A., Vavrik, B.: A diverse ecg database for evaluating digitization solutions, Pmcardio ecg image database (pm-ecg-id) (2024)
5. Llamedo, M., Martínez, J.P.: Heartbeat classification using feature selection driven by database generalization criteria. IEEE Trans. Biomed. Eng. **58**(3), 616–625 (2010)
6. McKeen, K., Masood, S., Toma, A., Rubin, B., Wang, B.: Ecg-fm: An open electrocardiogram foundation model. arXiv preprint arXiv:2408.05178 (2024)
7. Rahimi, M., Karbasi, R., Vahabie, A.-H.: An open-source python framework and synthetic ECG image datasets for digitization, lead and lead name detection, and overlapping signal segmentation. CoRR, abs/ arXiv: 2506.06315 (2025)
8. Ribeiro, A.H., et al.: Code-15%: A large scale annotated dataset of 12-lead ecgs. Zenodo, Jun **9**, 10–5281 (2021)
9. Ribeiro, A.H., et al.: Automatic diagnosis of the 12-lead ecg using a deep neural network. Nat. Commun. **11**(1), 1760 (2020)
10. Shivashankara, K.K., Shervedani, A.M., Clifford, G.D., Reyna, M.A., Sameni, R., et al.: Ecg-image-kit: a synthetic image generation toolbox to facilitate deep learning-based electrocardiogram digitization. Physiol. Meas. **45**(5), 055019 (2024)
11. Taddei, A.: The european st-t database: standard for evaluating systems for the analysis of st-t changes in ambulatory electrocardiography. Eur. Heart J. **13**(9), 1164–1172 (1992)
12. Wagner, P., et al.: Ptb-xl, a large publicly available electrocardiography dataset. Sci. Data **7**(1), 1–15 (2020)
13. Wang, C., et al.: The effect of follow-up reexamination on the long-term prognosis of patients with acute coronary syndrome undergoing coronary angiography. BMC Med. **23**(1), 1–13 (2025)
14. Zheng, J., Zhang, J., Danioko, S., Yao, H., Guo, H., Rakovski, C.: A 12-lead electrocardiogram database for arrhythmia research covering more than 10,000 patients. Sci. Data **7**(1), 48 (2020)

Automatic Explainable Progress Prediction of Wet Age-Related Macular Degeneration

Riccardo Fidanza[1], Daniele Meli[1](✉), and Emilia Maggio[2]

[1] Department of Computer Science, University of Verona, Verona, Italy
daniele.meli@univr.it

[2] Ophthalmology Unit, IRCCS Sacro Cuore Don Calabria Hospital Verona, Verona, Italy

Abstract. Wet age-related macular degeneration (wAMD) is an aggressive pathology representing a leading cause of central vision loss in the elderly population. Currently, diagnosis and treatment evaluation rely on clinical experts visually interpreting tomography scans to identify pathological features for decision-making, a process that is time-consuming and subject to inter-observer variability.

Stemming from the success of artificial intelligence (AI) in medicine, this paper proposes two main contributions. First, we address the **novel task of automatic diagnosis and monitoring of the treatment outcome for wAMD**. We adopt a **unique and novel dataset** containing recordings from 275 patients over different years of treatment. We show that different **AI models significantly outperform the recall (measuring misclassified wAMD worsening) of human evaluation (+20% at least)**. As a second contribution, we perform an **explainability study** on the trained AI models, evidencing that the **relevant features guiding the predictions are indeed a smaller subset and clinically relevant**. Our results pave the way towards **trustable automatic diagnosis and treatment evaluation for wAMD and related pathologies**, reducing significantly the effort required from clinicians.

Keywords: Explainable AI · Ophthalmology · Computer-assisted medicine

1 Introduction

Age-related macular degeneration (AMD), and especially its wet version (wAMD), is one of the leading causes of irreversible central vision loss in older adults, especially in developed countries [3]. Despite advances in treatments (notably anti-VEGF drug injections that can slow disease progression), wAMD remains a major cause of severe vision impairment. Clinicians typically analyze optical coherence tomography (OCT) scans of the eyes of the patients, in order

P. Bruno et al. (Eds.): HC_AIxIA_HYDRA 2025, CCIS 2830, pp. 99–104, 2026.
https://doi.org/10.1007/978-3-032-16708-8_8

to identify relevant features which can support the diagnosis and the evaluation of treatment response [2]. However, this process is time-consuming, error-prone, and requires a significant effort [5]. Artificial intelligence (AI) has shown promising results in the detection of different types of wAMD [6]. However, one fundamental unanswered question is whether AI can also support the evaluation of treatment outcome, reducing the burden for the clinician.

This paper provides two contributions. First, we consider the **novel task of automatic prediction of wAMD progression after treatment**. To this aim, we use a **unique and novel dataset** collected at IRCCS Sacro Cuore Don Calabria Hospital in Verona (Italy), consisting of the historical treatment data of 235 patients across multiple years of monitoring, annotated with 90 standard clinical features. We then compare different AI models at predicting the status of wAMD, also in view of the standard performance by clinicians in literature. Secondly, we employ *explainable AI (XAI)* techniques to highlight relevant features for the trained models, and **analyze both the clinical importance and the contribution of these features to the classification performance**.

2 Novel wAMD Dataset

Our novel dataset[1] consists of 325 observations, each representing a single eye affected by AMD. These observations were collected from 275 patients under treatment for wAMD monitored at IRCCS Sacro Cuore Don Calabria Hospital in Verona (Italy), with some patients contributing data from both eyes. Each sample is described by 90 features annotated by clinicians, providing a comprehensive and heterogeneous profile of both the eye and the patientâĂŹs overall medical context. Among the 90 available numerical features, notable ones include the duration of the follow-up period (FU); the best corrected visual acuity (BCVA), measured at various time points during treatment; the ellipsoid zone (EZ), external limiting membrane (ELM) and thickness (CT) of the retina in the macular area, the intraretinal (IRF) and subretinal fluids (SRF); the neovascular lesion area (NLA).

3 Methodology

In this section, we present the main methods for explainable wAMD progress classification.

3.1 Data Preprocessing

To ensure data quality and usability, the dataset underwent a thorough cleaning process. First, the presence of missing values (NaNs) was carefully examined across all features. Features with a high percentage of missing data (greater than 10%) were removed entirely to avoid introducing bias or noise, reducing the total

[1] **The dataset was collected with patients' consent and anonymized.**

number of features from 90 to 63. For features with a low percentage of missing values, imputation was performed using the mode (i.e., the most frequent value) of each respective feature, given the mostly categorical/discrete nature of most features. Finally, categorical variables were encoded into numerical representations to enable the application of machine learning classification algorithms.

3.2 AI Models

Different AI models were selected to leverage different strengths in handling the dataset's characteristics, such as feature heterogeneity, nonlinearity and interpretability. Hyperparameter tuning was performed via grid search and cross validation based on the accuracy metric.

We selected the following AI models as the most popular in the body of literature in other ophthalmologic classification tasks [1,6]: **decision tree (DT)** and **Random Forest (RF)**, tree-based models chosen for their interpretability and ability to handle nonlinear relationships, categorical data and numerical data without normalization; **linear and nonlinear support vector classifier (SVC)**, selected for their efficiency and performance at class separation; **logistic regression (LR)** for interpretability as a baseline model; an **artificial neural network (ANN)** consisting of 2 fully connected layers with ReLU activations to capture complex inter-feature dependencies, and a dropout rate of 0.5 to mitigate overfitting.

3.3 Explainability Analysis

To identify the most informative features and reduce dimensionality, recursive feature elimination with cross-validation (RFECV) was employed. This method recursively removes the least important features based on feature importance scores provided by an estimator and evaluates model performance at each step using cross-validation. In this case, a Random Forest classifier was used as the underlying estimator due to its ability to provide reliable and interpretable feature importance rankings. RFECV automatically selects the optimal number of features by maximizing the cross-validated accuracy score. This process not only enhances the generalization of the model, but also offers valuable insights into which features contribute the most to the classification task.

4 Classification Results

We trained the classification models with 5-fold cross-validation, and evaluated them according to precision, recall, F1-score and accuracy. Since the dataset is slightly imbalanced, with approximately 64.3% negative (i.e., worsened wAMD) points vs. 35.7% positive entries (i.e., improved wAMD), we report median and IQR, and also evaluate ROC curves.

Table 1 and Fig. 1a show the results obtained using the full dataset of 63 features (after data cleaning).

Table 1. Classification performance with the full 63 features (Table 2 left).

Model	Accuracy		Precision		Recall		F1 Score	
	Median	IQR	Median	IQR	Median	IQR	Median	IQR
Decision Tree	0.9231	0.0154	0.9242	0.0050	0.9231	0.0154	0.9234	0.0168
Random Forest	**0.9692**	**0.0154**	**0.9692**	**0.0159**	**0.9692**	**0.0154**	**0.9689**	**0.0152**
Nonlinear SVM	0.8923	0.0154	0.8979	0.0141	0.8923	0.0154	0.8927	0.0159
Logistic Regression	0.9231	0.0308	0.9290	0.0315	0.9231	0.0308	0.9240	0.0311
ANN	0.9385	0.0615	0.9286	0.0581	0.9512	0.0584	0.9359	0.0602

All models demonstrate good performance in the classification task, with comparable metrics and especially **very high recall with respect to known clinical performance** [4] ($> 89\%$ vs. 62%). **The recall identifies the number of misclassified wAMD worsening instances**. In particular, the RF classifier demonstrates a clear distinction by attaining the highest median accuracy and the lowest variability across metrics, thereby evidencing its superior robustness and reliability.

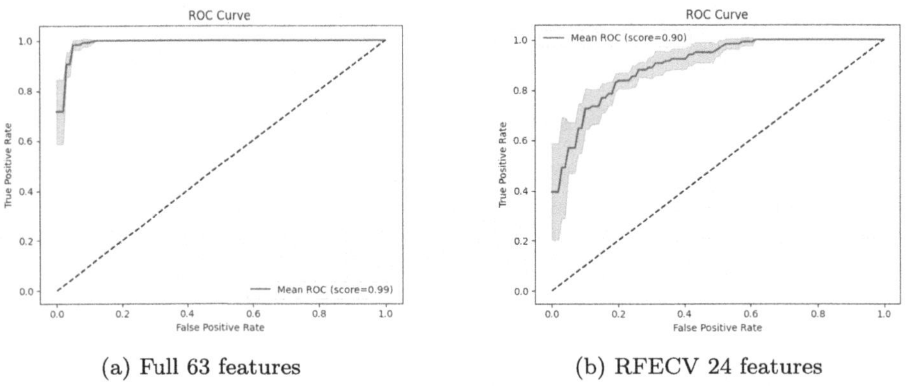

(a) Full 63 features (b) RFECV 24 features

Fig. 1. ROC curves.

5 Explainability Results

We apply RFECV to the best-performing RF classifier, in order to highlight the relevant features behind its high scores and gain interesting clinical outcomes.

Table 2 (**left**) shows the top-5% important features. **Two clinical experts agree on the well-known relevance of these features in the ophthalmologic literature, evidencing the trustworthy and reliable decision-making process behind the AI model.**

Table 2. Selected features from the full dataset with their importances.

Feature	Importance
EZ last visit	0.2456
BCVA 8 years	0.2378
BCVA 7 years	0.1935
ELM last visit	0.1379
BCVA 6 years	0.0724
FU (years)	0.0596
BCVA 5 years	0.0533

Feature	Importance
BCVA 4 years	0.1978
NLA	0.1361
BCVA 3 years	0.1297
BCVA 6 years	0.0905
BCVA 2 years	0.0755
Final CT	0.0616
BCVA 1 years	0.0609
Predom Persistent IRF	0.0587

In order to gain deeper clinical insights, Table 2 (**right**) reports the results of RFECV (top-5%) when applied to the RF classifier, but *excluding the well-known relevant features reported on the left of Table* 2. **The clinicians also acknowledge the relevance of these features (24 total), though usually not considered in the available medical literature, hence representing an advancement in clinical knowledge.**

Table 3. Classification performance with 24 RFECV features (Table 2. right).

Model	Accuracy		Precision		Recall		F1 Score	
	Median	IQR	Median	IQR	Median	IQR	Median	IQR
Decision Tree	0.7692	0.0462	0.7870	0.0249	0.7692	0.0462	0.7703	0.0373
Random Forest	**0.8462**	**0.0308**	**0.8445**	**0.0352**	**0.8462**	**0.0308**	**0.8404**	**0.0368**
Nonlinear SVM	0.8154	0.0308	0.8251	0.0211	0.8154	0.0308	0.8051	0.0275
Logistic Regression	0.8154	0.0154	0.8271	0.0056	0.8154	0.0154	0.8182	0.0134
ANN	0.7077	0.0923	0.7833	0.1340	0.6005	0.1160	0.6038	0.1958

In order to further validate this finding, in Table 3 and Fig. 1b we report the performance of the AI classifiers *considering only the newly discovered relevant features of Table* 2 (right). Compared to the results obtained in Table 1, the performance decreases by approximately 10% over all metrics, remaining well above the state-of-the-art human capabilities (**RF achieves 85% vs. 62% recall** [4]). Moreover, the ANN results much more sensitive to the changes in the feature set, showing its lower robustness and interpretability.

Overall, our findings indicate that the **AI models rely on clinically-relevant features** (Table 2), and that **a limited set of features (24/63) usually not reported in established ophthalmologic literature have an important impact on classification accuracy** (Table 3), still consistently outperforming humans.

6 Conclusion

This paper addresses the **novel and crucial problem of automatic wAMD treatment outcome evaluation with AI**. The results on **our unique dataset containing records of 235 patients** evidence that **AI models (especially Random Forests) significantly outperform human capacities (96% vs. 62% recall** [4]). Moreover, our XAI study shows that the **AI model relies its predictions on clinically-relevant features**. More specifically, some of these features are well-known to the ophthalmologic community, evidencing the trustability of AI for this application. On the other hand, **a subset of other automatically extracted 24/63 features is recognized by the clinicians to advance the current medical knowledge**, while yielding slightly worse classification performance (**still well above the human performance, 85% vs. 62% recall**). **This potentially significantly shrinks the range of features to be annotated from OCT scans, relaxing the effort from the clinicians.**

This paper represents a preliminary, yet fundamental step towards the adoption of trustworthy AI for the diagnosis and monitoring of wAMD and related pathologies. In the future we plan to address several limitations of this work. First, we will enrich our unique dataset to solve some imbalance problem, and make it available to the research community. Moreover, we will investigate the problem of predicting the wAMD evolution after treatment starting directly from OCT scans, thus not requiring any dataset annotation.

References

1. Desai, R.J., Wang, S.V., Vaduganathan, M., Evers, T., Schneeweiss, S.: Comparison of machine learning methods with traditional models for use of administrative claims with electronic medical records to predict heart failure outcomes. JAMA Netw. Open **3**(1), e1918962–e1918962 (2020)
2. Hu, Y., et al.: Amd-sd: an optical coherence tomography image dataset for wet amd lesions segmentation. Sci. Data **11**(1), 1014 (2024)
3. Kansagara, D., Gleitsmann, K., Gillingham, M., O'Neil, M., Saha, S.: Nutritional supplements for age-related macular degeneration: A systematic review. Tech. rep., Department of Veterans Affairs (US), Washington (DC) (Jan 2012), https://www.ncbi.nlm.nih.gov/books/NBK84266/, vA Evidence-based Synthesis Program Reports
4. Liefers, B., et al.: Quantification of key retinal features in early and late age-related macular degeneration using deep learning. Am. J. Ophthalmol. **226**, 1–12 (2021)
5. Mete, M., Iacovello, D., Maggio, E.: Novel diagnosis and therapeutics approaches in retina diseases (2024)
6. Wang, Z., Keane, P.A., Chiang, M., Cheung, C.Y., Wong, T.Y., Ting, D.S.W.: Artificial intelligence and deep learning in ophthalmology. Artifi. Intell. Med. 1519–1552 (2022)

Explaining Medical Time Series Classification Through Boundary-Aware Feature Analysis

Christel Sirocchi[1](✉) and Damiano Verda[2]

[1] Department Artificial Intelligence in Biomedical Engineering, Friedrich-Alexander Universität Erlangen-Nürnberg, Erlangen, Germany
christel.sirocchi@fau.de

[2] Rulex Innovation Labs, Genova, Italy
damiano.verda@rulex.ai

Abstract. Borderline clinical cases, characterised by highly similar patient profiles but divergent outcomes, pose a persistent challenge in medical decision-making. Laboratory data from electronic health records can help trace temporal trajectories of disease progression and uncover subtle differences between such cases. However, their sparse, irregular, and asynchronous nature complicates analysis and calls for tailored methods. Recent efforts in modelling such data have primarily relied on deep learning architectures, which typically prioritise overall performance and often lack interpretability, particularly in difficult boundary cases. This study introduces a methodology to identify features and criteria associated with divergent outcomes in borderline cases. Medical time series are summarised into interpretable statistics and pairwise distances are computed to identify similar admissions with either the same or different outcomes. Feature-wise differences within these pairs are then used to train monotonic gradient boosting models that highlight key discriminative factors. Applied to hospital mortality prediction in two ICU cohorts, the approach shows that features relevant in borderline cases differ from those emphasised by models trained on all admissions. Rule extraction from shallow monotonic trees yields interpretable patterns associated with outcome divergence. These findings suggest that the proposed framework can contribute to the refinement of clinical guidelines and strengthen decision support in uncertain scenarios. The method implementation is openly available at: https://github.com/ChristelSirocchi/TS-XAI.

Keywords: Laboratory data · Time series · Feature importance · Rule extraction · Tree ensemble

1 Introduction

Longitudinal laboratory data in electronic health records provide a continuous readout of a patient's pathophysiological state, offering insights into disease pro-

P. Bruno et al. (Eds.): HC_AIxIA_HYDRA 2025, CCIS 2830, pp. 105–119, 2026.
https://doi.org/10.1007/978-3-032-16708-8_9

gression and recovery. Their sparse, irregular, and asynchronous nature, however, poses significant challenges that require tailored analytical approaches [12]. Recent advances in deep learning, particularly transformer- and autoencoder-based architectures, have shown promise in learning effective representations of laboratory time series and predicting clinical outcomes [17]. Despite these successes, such models often require large, high-quality datasets and struggle with sparse, noisy, or imbalanced data, while their complex architecture limits interpretability and reduces trust among end users [10]. In contrast, traditional tree ensemble methods such as random forests and gradient boosting often outperform deep learning on real-world datasets and provide readily available feature importance scores, making them particularly attractive in clinical contexts [6].

A further limitation of current medical machine learning frameworks is that standard performance metrics typically treat all samples equally, even though some cases are inherently more difficult to predict. Clinical guidelines acknowledge this uncertainty, as they do not always provide definitive recommendations but are intended to support clinician expertise. Some patients, therefore, fall within the so-called clinical *grey zone*, where the optimal course of action is uncertain and left to clinician discretion [15]. Straightforward cases are generally well managed by existing medical protocols and decision support systems, so machine learning efforts should prioritise understanding and improving outcomes for patients in this *grey zone* [13]. In this context, beyond building accurate predictive models for borderline cases, analysing the criteria that drive these outcomes is even more valuable. Such analysis can deepen understanding of underlying mechanisms, potentially guiding updates to clinical protocols [9]. Explainable artificial intelligence has made significant contributions toward model interpretability, offering global explanations through rule extraction to summarise model behaviour, or local explanations through counterfactuals to explore decision boundaries [3,14]. Although these methods have recently been adapted for time series models, a focus on borderline medical cases is lacking.

In this study, we focus on boundary cases characterised by highly similar temporal trajectories but divergent clinical outcomes. Medical time series are summarised into intuitive statistics, and pairwise distances are computed to identify similar admissions with either matching or differing outcomes. Feature-wise differences within these pairs are then used to train monotonic gradient boosting models that identify key discriminative features in these challenging cases. This approach provides interpretable insights that may support medical decision-making and guideline refinement. The full method implementation, including code to reproduce all analyses, is publicly available at https://github.com/ChristelSirocchi/TS-XAI.

2 Methodology Overview

The proposed methodology aims to uncover the features and criteria that can discriminate ICU admissions with similar temporal progression but different clinical outcomes. An overview of the steps is presented in Fig. 1 and explained below, while the implementation and design choices are detailed in Sect. 3. The input of the method consists of medical time series, typically multivariate, sparse, and irregularly sampled, along with the corresponding clinical target.

Time series featurisation. Laboratory time series are summarised using descriptive statistics across multiple temporal segments, prioritising metrics that are both informative and interpretable for clinicians (e.g., range rather than coefficient of variation).

Distance computation. Time series are discretised, standardised, imputed, and concatenated across features to provide admission-level vector representations. Pairwise distances between admissions are computed to quantify similarity in temporal patterns.

Pair selection. Admission pairs with distances below a specified quantile are identified as having highly similar trajectories. From this subset, two groups are formed: pairs with shared outcomes and pairs with differing outcomes.

Paired dataset construction. For each selected pair, absolute differences between their time series summary statistics are computed, and a binary target is assigned to indicate whether their outcomes match or diverge.

Constrained tree ensemble learning. A supervised tree-based classifier is trained on the paired dataset to distinguish, among admissions with similar temporal trajectories, those with the same versus different outcomes. Monotonicity constraints are enforced on all features to align with the intuition that greater differences between time series features should not imply an increased probability of the same outcome.

Feature importance analysis. Feature importance scores are extracted to identify key features associated with diverging outcomes. For comparison, a classifier with the same architecture is trained on the original summary features without monotonic constraints, and the importances from both models are contrasted to highlight features most relevant to borderline cases.

Rule extraction. Rules are extracted from a single tree trained with monotonic constraints to identify thresholds that may influence outcomes in boundary cases. These rules provide criteria for detecting changes in patient profiles that could signal or precede condition deterioration.

3 Experimental Setup

Datasets. The proposed approach is evaluated on medical time series derived from two real-world EHR datasets, the PhysioNet Challenge [5] and MIMIC-III [8], following the setup in [16]. In both datasets, the target task is in-hospital mortality prediction based on the first 48 h of ICU stay.

The **PhysioNet Challenge** dataset comprises 34 clinical laboratory variables across 11988 ICU stays of adult patients, of which 1707 resulted in in-hospital death. **MIMIC-III** is a publicly available database containing 58976 ICU admissions from the Beth Israel Deaconess Medical Center, classified as *elective*, *emergency*, *newborn*, or *urgent*. Due to differing mortality rates (10%

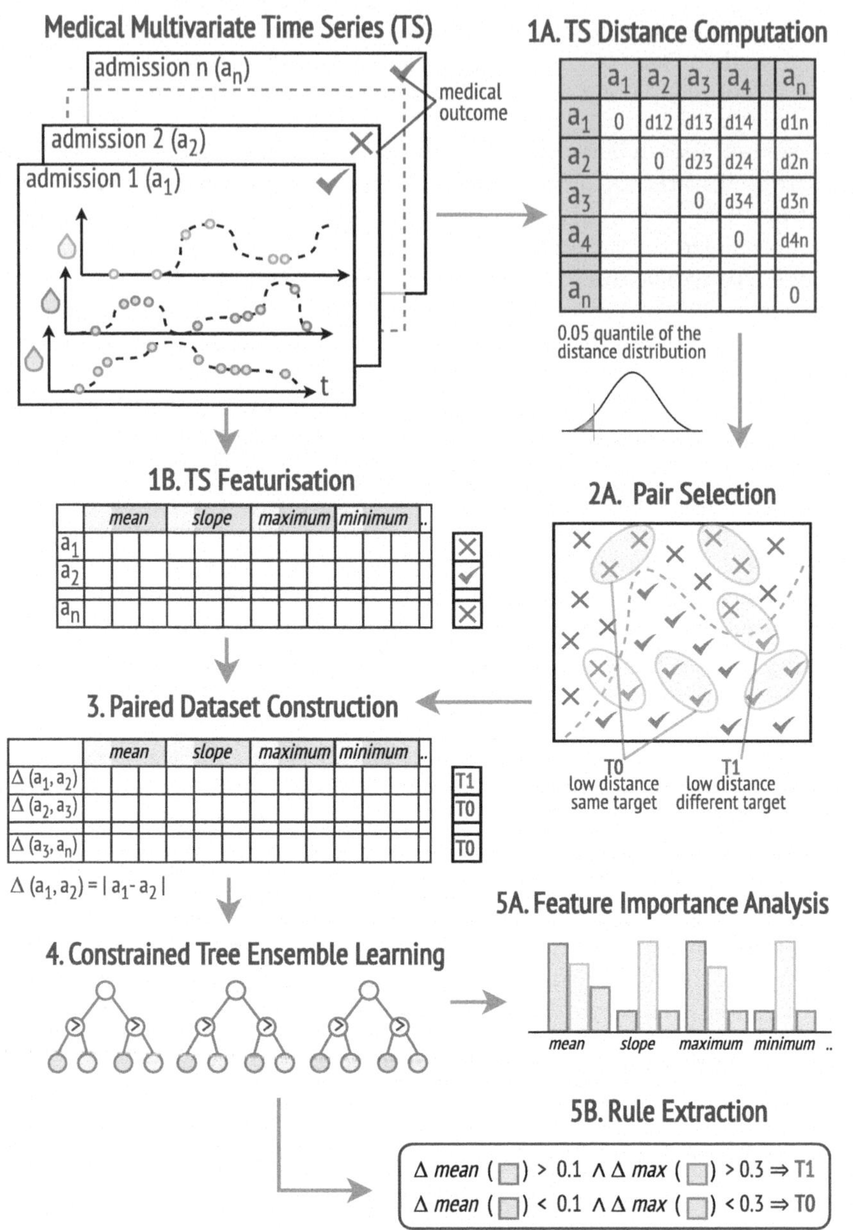

Fig. 1. Overview of the proposed methodology.

in *emergency* and *urgent* vs 2% and 0.3% in *elective* and *newborn*), we focus on *emergency* admissions, comprising 37813 stays. Retaining only the last admission per patient yields 25064 stays. Following preprocessing steps in [11], 12 physiological variables are extracted (feature lists are provided in Appendix A).

Only laboratory measurements are used in both datasets, while demographic and anthropometric data (e.g., age, gender, height, weight) are excluded. Urine output is represented as a cumulative sum, as recommended in [7]. Outliers are removed by excluding values with a *z-score* greater than 5. To eliminate extremely sparse records, admissions reporting fewer than half of the variables are discarded, resulting in 11587 stays for PhysioNet (1675 positive, 9912 negative) and 24720 for MIMIC-III (3072 positive, 21648 negative), with positive cases accounting for 14.4% and 12.4% of admissions, respectively.

Time Series Featurisation. For each admission and laboratory test, summary statistics are computed over three temporal segments: the full 48-h window (*all*), the first 24 h, and the last 24 h. Within each segment, count, mean, standard deviation, minimum, maximum, and the slope of a fitted linear regression are derived. If measurements are available in both 24-h segments, the difference between the second and the first segment (*diff*) is also included. First and last observed values are also recorded for each series.

Distance Computation. For each admission, laboratory measurements are discretised into hourly intervals over the first 48 h of the ICU stay, with values averaged within each 1-hour window. Discretised values are standardised by subtracting the mean and dividing by the standard deviation of the respective feature. Missing hourly values are imputed through linear interpolation along the time axis, followed by forward- and backward-filling at the boundaries. For time series with no observed values, remaining missing values are imputed using k-nearest neighbour imputation ($k = 5$). Preprocessed time series of all features within an admission are concatenated into a single vector representation, from which pairwise distances between admissions are computed. The distance metrics considered include Euclidean, Chebyshev, cityblock, cosine, correlation, and Canberra (computed using `scipy`[1]), as well as Dynamic Time Warping (DTW), computed with the fast C-based implementation in `dtaidistance`[2].

Pair Selection. Pair selection is guided by the computed pairwise distances between admissions. Only pairs with distances below a specified percentile threshold (set to 5%) are retained. From this subset, two categories are defined: *different-target pairs*, consisting of admissions with low distance but differing clinical outcomes (target label 1), and *same-target pairs*, comprising admissions with low distance and identical outcomes (target label 0). To prevent any single admission from being overrepresented and disproportionately influencing downstream analyses, a greedy selection algorithm is applied to both groups. This procedure restricts each admission to at most N selected pairs (here $N = 3$) by iterating through pairs in ascending order of distance and selecting only those for which neither admission has reached the limit. Further details on the pairs selected at each step are provided in Table 3 (Appendix B).

[1] https://scipy.org/.

[2] https://dtaidistance.readthedocs.io/.

Paired Dataset Construction. The paired feature dataset is derived from the selected admission pairs and the precomputed time series summary statistics by taking, for each pair, the absolute difference between the corresponding feature vectors. The binary target, defined as above, indicates whether the pair shares the same outcome (0) or differs in outcome (1). This pairwise feature representation is subsequently used for model training.

Constrained Tree Ensemble Learning. The constructed pairwise feature dataset is used to train a binary classifier that distinguishes between same-outcome and different-outcome pairs. An XGBoost classifier is trained using 5-fold stratified cross-validation, where stratification is performed across three groups: pairs with differing outcomes, pairs where both admissions result in survival, and pairs where both admissions result in death (to account for the fact that the latter are typically underrepresented within the same-outcome group). To address class imbalance, the majority class is undersampled in the training set. Hyperparameters are optimised within each training fold via grid search, using the ROC AUC score as the objective metric. The final configuration used for evaluation is: `n_estimators` = 100, `max_depth` = 10, `learning_rate` = 0.01, `subsample` = 0.8, `colsample_bytree` = 0.8. Monotonicity constraints are enforced for each feature, ensuring that an increase in any feature difference cannot lead to a decreased probability of a different outcome (target label 1). Feature importances are extracted from the trained models for subsequent analysis.

For comparison, an XGBoost classifier is also trained on the original dataframe of time series features under the same training conditions but without monotonicity constraints. Feature importances from this model are extracted and compared to those obtained from the paired feature dataset.

For rule extraction, a single shallow decision tree is trained with monotonic constraints on all features, using maximum depths ranging from 3 to 6, on a single 80-20 split. The tree with the highest ROC AUC score is selected and rules are extracted from the tree with antecedents formed by the conjunction of conditions at nodes along the path from root to leaf, and the consequent corresponding to the outcome predicted at the leaf.

4 Results

4.1 Classification Performance

The monotonic XGBoost models trained on the paired dataset, constructed from admission pairs selected using each of the seven distance metrics, demonstrate overall satisfactory performance in the challenging task of predicting whether pairs with similar temporal trajectories have the same or different clinical outcomes. Performance is generally comparable across the various distances, with the highest AUC ROC scores reaching 0.721 for PhysioNet 2012 and 0.729 for MIMIC-III, as shown in Table 1.

Table 1. Performance metrics (averaged over 5 folds of cross-validation) for XGBoost classifiers trained with monotonic constraints on the paired dataset, using pairs selected based on various distance metrics.

	Physionet 2012			MIMIC-III		
	AUC ROC	AUC PR	Recall	AUC ROC	AUC PR	Recall
	Paired dataset					
Euclidean	**0.721**	0.345	0.685	**0.729**	0.404	0.614
Chebyshev	0.713	0.376	0.690	**0.729**	0.422	0.618
Cityblock	**0.721**	0.356	0.665	0.717	0.403	0.596
Correlation	0.711	0.387	0.717	0.711	0.397	0.601
Cosine	0.712	0.391	0.714	0.712	0.394	0.595
Canberra	0.715	0.390	0.690	0.705	0.388	0.568
DTW	0.717	0.342	0.685	0.680	0.321	0.611

Models trained on the Euclidean-based dataset achieve one of the top two AUC ROC scores in both datasets, making this distance the preferred choice for downstream analyses (although results in Sect. 4.2 indicate that analyses using other distances yield similar insights). Notably, DTW, a time-series-specific metric with high computational cost, does not provide a clear advantage over the more efficient and interpretable Euclidean distance. This is likely because preprocessing reduces the variability of the originally sparse and irregular time series, limiting the alignment flexibility that DTW is designed to exploit.

The same XGB model trained on the original dataset of time series features without constraints achieves higher predictive accuracy [PhysioNet: AUC ROC = 0.848, AUC PR = 0.480, Recall = 0.795; MIMIC-III: AUC ROC = 0.852, AUC PR = 0.534, Recall = 0.773]. This is expected, as the original model is trained on all admissions, many of which are easier to classify. By contrast, the paired dataset approach focuses on borderline cases that are inherently more difficult to distinguish, making the results of the two settings not comparable.

4.2 Feature Importance Analysis

XGBoost models trained on the original dataset and the constructed paired dataset display distinct patterns of feature importance. This indicates that while certain features are generally informative for predicting clinical outcomes, different sets of features become more predictive in borderline cases, where admissions with similar trajectories present divergent outcomes. Figure 2 compares feature importance scores between models trained on the original and paired datasets, averaged across all summary statistics for each laboratory test. In both datasets, the (Total) Glasgow Coma Score (GCS and TGCS) consistently emerges as a key discriminatory feature in borderline cases. Respiratory rate (RR), blood oxygenation measures (SaO2 in PhysioNet, SpO2 in MIMIC), and systolic blood pressure (NISysABP and SysABP in PhysioNet, SBP in MIMIC) also gain importance in predicting such cases. Glucose is more predictive across both datasets, while blood urea nitrogen (BUN) stands out in PhysioNet. In contrast, features such as heart rate (HR), pH, and urine output appear less informative in these threshold cases. Models trained on paired datasets constructed using different distance metrics yield similar feature importance profiles (Fig. 2). This suggests that the choice of a distance metric, while affecting pair selection, may not substantially alter the resulting clinical insights.

An in-depth analysis of feature importance for individual summary statistics, shown in Fig. 3 for the Euclidean paired dataset, reveals that each selected statistic (min, max, mean, standard deviation, range, slope) and each time window (first 24 h, last 24 h, difference between the two, entire series) is most relevant for at least some features. For example, blood oxygenation measures (SaO2 and SpO2) receive the highest importance scores for statistics that capture variability, particularly range and standard deviation, followed by min and max, while mean values have low importance. This can also be appreciated in the temporal progression of these features for borderline admissions (low-distance, different-outcome pairs) shown in Fig. 3, where patients who died in hospital do not exhibit markedly different average values but show greater fluctuation around the mean, especially in the PhysioNet dataset.

For the Glasgow Coma Score, the last recorded value and the maximum, either across the full series or within the last 24 h, are most predictive in both datasets. Feature trajectories in borderline cases show that patients with in-hospital mortality tend to have a consistently low score, whereas patients who survive either start with a higher score (as seen more clearly in MIMIC-III) or show improvement over time (as observed in PhysioNet). This highlights the importance of the maximum score reached, particularly in the final 24 h.

For respiratory rate, both the mean and range are highly predictive. In both datasets, patients who do not survive tend to have higher average respiratory rates and greater variability, further confirming that features capturing both level and fluctuation carry strong predictive value in borderline cases.

4.3 Rule Extraction

To better understand the criteria associated with diverging outcomes, rules were extracted from a shallow decision tree trained with monotonic constraints on the paired Euclidean dataset for PhysioNet (with 19.5% different-target pairs). The tree, limited to depth 5 for rule readability, achieved good predictive performance (AUC ROC of 0.685) and yielded 32 root-to-leaf rules, of which 10 predicted positive outcomes. Table 2 displays rules with coverage greater than 1%, with conditions ordered from left to right according to their position in the tree.

The maximum value of the Glasgow Coma Scale (GCS) in the last 24 h appears at the root node, confirming its status as the most predictive feature. The split threshold at zero suggests that even small differences in this feature are strongly associated with divergent outcomes, highlighting the clinical relevance of monitoring GCS closely during this period. In the left subtree, where the last 24-hour maximum GCS is equal across pairs, additional features influence

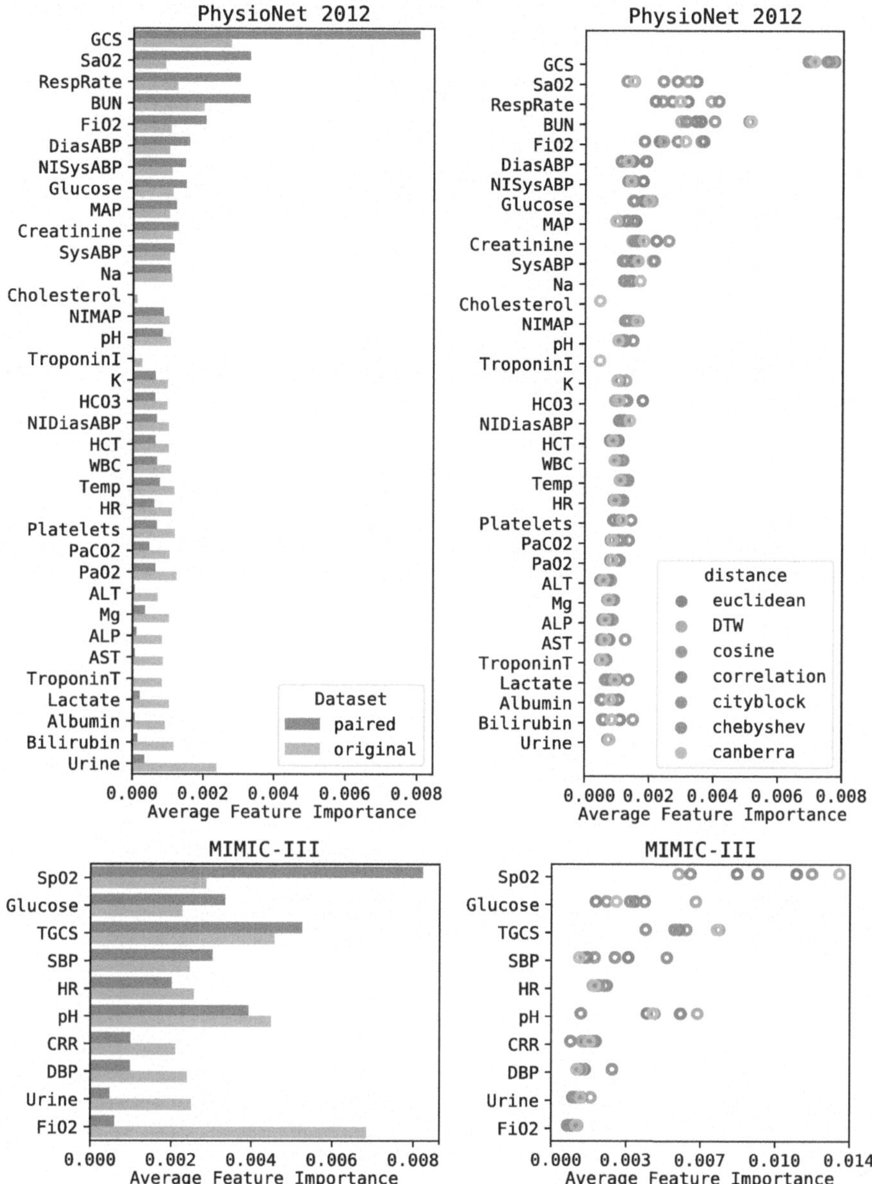

Fig. 2. *Left panel*: Feature importance for XGBoost trained on the original time series dataset and on the paired dataset constructed using Euclidean distance. Importance scores are averaged across all summary statistics for each laboratory test. *Right panel*: Feature importance for XGBoost trained on paired datasets constructed using each of the seven distance metrics, averaged over lab tests.

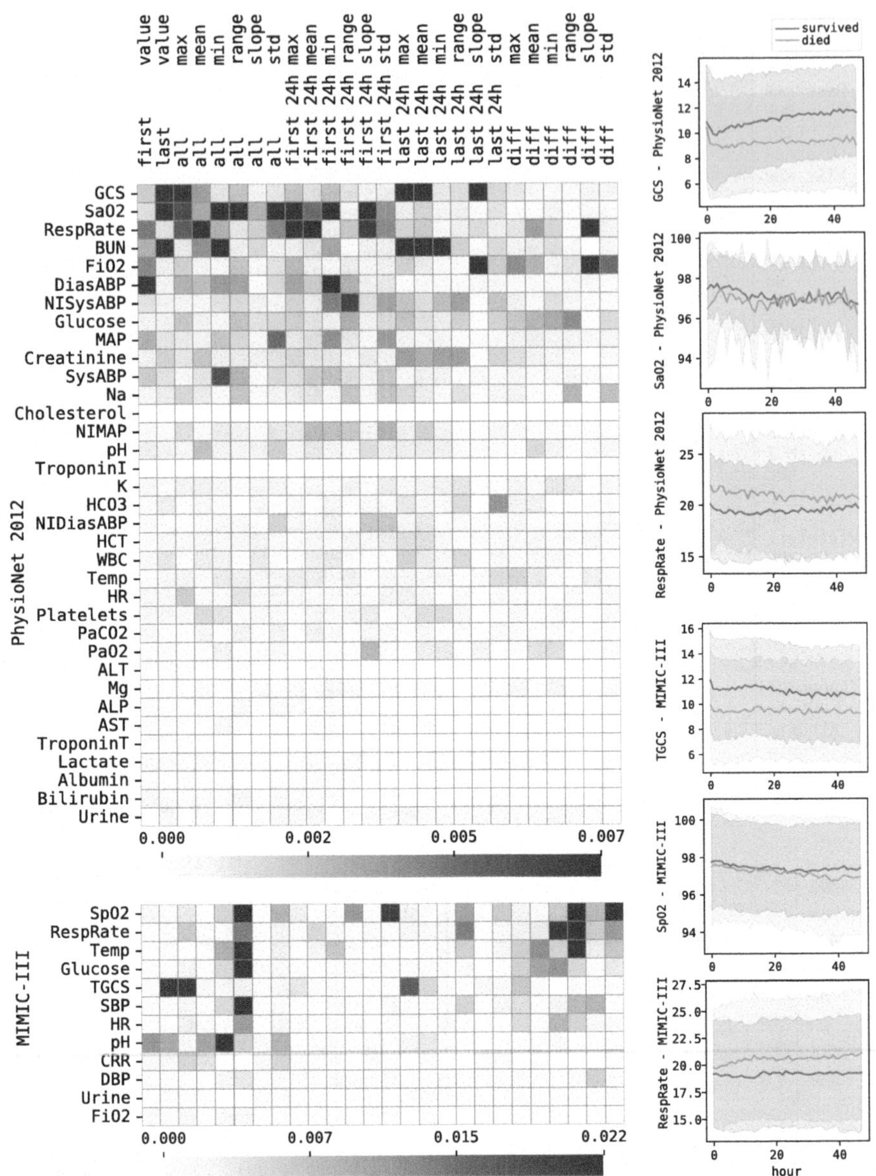

Fig. 3. *Left panel*: Feature importance scores from XGBoost models trained on the paired dataset constructed using Euclidean distance, shown for each summary statistic and laboratory test. *Right panel*: Temporal progression of top features for admissions in low-distance, different-outcome pairs, illustrating how surviving patients evolve differently from patients who died in hospital with respect to these relevant features.

Table 2. Conditions of rules predicting a positive target (similar admission pairs with differing outcomes), extracted from a decision tree trained with monotonicity constraints on the paired Physionet dataset, along with the rule accuracy.

Condition 1	Condition 2	Condition 3	Condition 4	Condition 5	accuracy
Δ last24h max GCS > 0	Δ last24h max BUN > 9	Δ first24h mean GCS > 4.3	Δ last24h max pH > 0.1	Δ max HCT > 0.2	0.64
Δ last24h max GCS ≤ 0	Δ last value BUN > 18	Δ first24h min GCS > 0	Δ last24h max HR > 31	Δ all slope Creat. > 0.002	0.67
Δ last24h max GCS ≤ 0	Δ last value BUN > 18	Δ first24h min GCS > 0	Δ last24h max HR ≤ 31	Δ all max GCS > 0	0.76
Δ last24h max GCS ≤ 0	Δ last value BUN > 18	Δ first24h min GCS ≤ 0	Δ last value BUN > 24	Δ max HR > 29	0.59
Δ last24h max GCS ≤ 0	Δ last value BUN ≤ 18	Δ first24h mean SysABP ≤ 26.8	Δ all max GCS > 0	Δ range pH > 0.1	0.41

outcomes, including other statistics of GCS (e.g., first 24-hour minimum, overall maximum), as well as indicators of kidney function (e.g., BUN, Creatinine) and circulatory stability (e.g., heart rate, systolic arterial blood pressure).

For BUN, identified as important in the previous analysis, relevant thresholds include a difference of 18 mg/dL in the last recorded value and a difference of 9 mg/dL in the last 24-hour maximum value. While heart rate did not stand out in feature analysis, large differences, such as a difference exceeding 30 bpm in the last 24-hour maximum value, still influenced outcomes within specific rule paths. This suggests that while features like GCS and BUN contribute broadly to outcome divergence, with low-threshold splits at higher tree levels, others, such as heart rate, may only be relevant in more specific contexts, reflected by deeper nodes and higher thresholds. Overall, rule-based analysis can clarify not only which features are critical but also the specific value ranges within which these variables should be monitored to mitigate the risk of adverse outcomes.

5 Limitations and Future Work

The proposed framework was designed with simplicity, interpretability, and data efficiency in mind. Methods requiring large datasets or extensive pretraining were deliberately avoided to ensure applicability in challenging data settings. Nevertheless, several limitations remain and suggest directions for future work.

In the pipeline, time series distances were computed on discretised and imputed vectors, prioritising efficiency over expressiveness. Recent transformer- and autoencoder-based approaches have shown promise in deriving compact embeddings directly from raw time series [4], which could serve as an alternative basis for similarity computation. Additionally, distance metrics tailored to time series, such as those based on wavelets or local pattern matching, may provide complementary perspectives and could be seamlessly integrated into the pipeline [1]. Notably, although distances were computed across all features and time points, not all are equally informative. Focusing on predictive subsets of features or temporal segments could produce more meaningful distances that better capture clinically relevant intra-individual temporal variation.

Time series featurisation relied on a small set of intuitive, clinically relevant statistics. Although this supports interpretability, it limits the model's ability to capture complex temporal patterns. Future work will incorporate a broader set of descriptive features, including autocorrelation-based and spectral measures [2].

Demonstrated on a binary in-hospital mortality prediction task, the approach extends to a wider range of outcomes, including multi-class and continuous targets such as length of stay or treatment response. Integration of additional modalities, including demographics and prior diagnoses, represents another straightforward extension. Admissions with insufficient laboratory measurements were excluded, and only the last ICU stay for emergency admissions in MIMIC-III was analysed to avoid bias from multiple same-patient stays. Extending the analysis to include repeated stays and other admission types, such as elective and neonatal cases, would increase generalisability.

The pipeline employs minimal manual tuning by setting robust defaults, such as selecting the lowest 5% of pairwise distances and capping the number of admission occurrences in selected pairs to 3. Preliminary experiments with alternative values (e.g., 1%, 2%, or 10% distance thresholds, and 3, 5, or 10 allowed occurrences) yielded comparable results. Nevertheless, a systematic assessment of parameter sensitivity and optimisation remains to be conducted.

Finally, although the feature importance and rule extraction analyses were consistent with medical knowledge, they have not been validated by clinicians, which will be addressed in future work. Expert feedback could also be incorporated within a human-in-the-loop framework, allowing clinicians to evaluate the extracted insights in terms of novelty, utility, and adherence to clinical protocols.

6 Conclusions

This study presents a methodology designed to identify features and criteria that differentiate clinically similar ICU admissions with distinct outcomes, focusing on borderline cases that pose significant challenges in clinical decision making. By summarising time series laboratory data into interpretable statistics, computing similarity-based admission pairs, and applying constrained tree ensemble learning to feature differences between paired admissions, the approach highlights factors associated with outcome divergence. The method was applied to hospital mortality prediction in two cohorts, revealing that features most predictive overall often differ from those relevant at the boundary, while also identifying common discriminative patterns across cohorts. These findings offer novel insights into patient trajectories and have the potential to inform and support healthcare professionals in complex decision scenarios. Future work will extend this framework to other medical outcomes and explore integration with advanced time series representations to enhance robustness and applicability.

Acknowledgements. This work was supported by the Emerging Talents Initiative (FAUeti) of Friedrich-Alexander-Universität Erlangen-Nürnberg.

Appendix A: EHR Datasets Features

(See Table 3).

PhysioNet Challenge 2012	MIMIC-III
34 available variables	12 variables extracted as in [11]
Albumin (Albumin)	Arterial pH (pH)
Alkaline phosphatase (ALP)	Capillary refill rate (CRR)
Alanine transaminase (ALT)	Diastolic blood pressure (DBP)
Aspartate transaminase (AST)	Fraction of inspired O_2 (FiO2)
Bilirubin (Bilirubin)	Serum glucose (Glucose)
Blood urea nitrogen (BUN)	Heart rate (HR)
Cholesterol	Oxygen saturation (SpO2)
Serum creatinine (Creatinine)	Respiratory rate (RespRate)
Invasive diastolic arterial blood pressure (DiasABP)	Systolic blood pressure (SBP)
Fractional inspired O_2 (FiO2)	Temperature (Temp)
Glasgow Coma Score (GCS)	Total Glasgow Coma Score (TGCS)
Serum glucose (Glucose)	Urine output (Urine)
Serum bicarbonate (HCO3)	
Hematocrit (HCT)	
Heart rate (HR)	
Serum potassium (K)	
Lactate (Lactate)	
Serum magnesium (Mg)	
Invasive mean arterial blood pressure (MAP)	
Mechanical ventilation respiration (MechVent)	
Serum sodium (Na)	
Non-invasive diastolic arterial blood pressure (NIDiasABP)	
Non-invasive mean arterial blood pressure (NIMAP)	
Non-invasive systolic arterial blood pressure (NISysABP)	
Partial pressure of arterial CO_2 ($PaCO_2$)	
Partial pressure of arterial O_2 (PaO2)	
Arterial pH (pH)	
Platelets	
Respiratory rate (RespRate)	
O_2 saturation in haemoglobin (SaO2)	
Invasive systolic arterial blood pressure (SysABP)	
Temperature (Temp)	
Troponin-I (TropI)	
Troponin-T (TropT)	
Urine output (Urine)	
White blood cell count (WBC)	

Appendix B: Paired Dataset Construction

Table 3. Pair counts at successive filtering steps for MIMIC-III and PhysioNet datasets across distance metrics. Columns report total number of pairs, same-outcome pairs, and different-outcome pairs.

	1. all admission pairs			2. after quantile filtering			3. after greedy filtering		
distance	all pairs	same-outcome	different-outcome	all pairs	same-outcome	different-outcome	all pairs	same-outcome	different-outcome
MIMIC-III									
canberra	305,526,840	66,502,656	239,024,184	15,276,331	2,141,738	13,134,593	43,665	8,878	34,787
chebyshev	305,526,840	66,502,656	239,024,184	15,238,536	1,716,038	13,522,498	34,043	6,501	27,542
cityblock	305,526,840	66,502,656	239,024,184	15,276,339	1,521,468	13,754,871	40,015	7,724	32,291
correlation	305,526,840	66,502,656	239,024,184	15,276,339	1,945,850	13,330,489	43,018	8,844	34,174
cosine	305,526,840	66,502,656	239,024,184	15,276,339	1,931,354	13,344,985	43,225	8,852	34,373
dtw	305,526,840	66,502,656	239,024,184	15,276,335	1,844,074	13,432,261	41,477	7,820	33,657
euclidean	305,526,840	66,502,656	239,024,184	15,276,329	1,501,738	13,774,591	37,821	7,153	30,668
PhysioNet									
canberra	67,123,491	16,602,600	50,520,891	3,356,172	437,085	2,919,087	20,127	4,631	15,496
chebyshev	67,123,491	16,602,600	50,520,891	2,822,247	408,505	2,413,742	15,727	3,395	12,332
cityblock	67,123,491	16,602,600	50,520,891	3,356,172	258,944	3,097,228	15,587	3,066	12,521
correlation	67,123,491	16,602,600	50,520,891	3,356,174	499,736	2,856,438	21,929	5,016	16,913
cosine	67,123,491	16,602,600	50,520,891	3,356,172	497,227	2,858,945	21,977	5,018	16,959
dtw	67,123,491	16,602,600	50,520,891	3,356,173	267,969	3,088,204	15,776	3,081	12,695
euclidean	67,123,491	16,602,600	50,520,891	3,356,173	265,452	3,090,721	15,062	2,934	12,128

References

1. Abanda, A., Mori, U., Lozano, J.A.: A review on distance based time series classification. Data Min. Knowl. Disc. **33**(2), 378–412 (2019)
2. Baydogan, M.G., Runger, G.: Time series representation and similarity based on local autopatterns. Data Min. Knowl. Disc. **30**, 476–509 (2016)
3. Ciatto, G., Sabbatini, F., Agiollo, A., Magnini, M., Omicini, A.: Symbolic knowledge extraction and injection with sub-symbolic predictors: a systematic literature review. ACM Comput. Surv. **56**(6), 1–35 (2024)
4. Ghahremani, Y., Metsis, V.: Time series embedding methods for classification tasks: a review. arXiv preprint arXiv:2501.13392 (2025)
5. Goldberger, A.L., et al.: Physiobank, physiotoolkit, and physionet: components of a new research resource for complex physiologic signals. Circulation **101**(23), e215–e220 (2000)
6. Grinsztajn, L., Oyallon, E., Varoquaux, G.: Why do tree-based models still outperform deep learning on typical tabular data? In: Koyejo, S., Mohamed, S., Agarwal, A., Belgrave, D., Cho, K., Oh, A. (eds.) Advances in Neural Information Processing Systems. vol. 35, pp. 507–520. Curran Associates, Inc. (2022)

7. Johnson, A.E., Kramer, A.A., Clifford, G.D.: Data preprocessing and mortality prediction: the physionet/cinc 2012 challenge revisited. In: Computing in Cardiology 2014. pp. 157–160. IEEE (2014)
8. Johnson, A.E., et al.: Mimic-iii, a freely accessible critical care database. Sci. Data **3**(1), 1–9 (2016)
9. Leiser, F., Rank, S., Schmidt-Kraepelin, M., Thiebes, S., Sunyaev, A.: Medical informed machine learning: a scoping review and future research directions. Artif. Intell. Med. **145**, 102676 (2023)
10. Piccialli, F., Di Somma, V., Giampaolo, F., Cuomo, S., Fortino, G.: A survey on deep learning in medicine: why, how and when? Information Fusion **66**, 111–137 (2021)
11. Shukla, S.N., Marlin, B.: Interpolation-prediction networks for irregularly sampled time series. In: International Conference on Learning Representations (2019)
12. Shukla, S.N., Marlin, B.: Multi-time attention networks for irregularly sampled time series. In: International Conference on Learning Representations (2021)
13. Sirocchi, C., Bogliolo, A., Montagna, S.: Medical-informed machine learning: integrating prior knowledge into medical decision systems. BMC Med. Inform. Decis. Mak. **24**(Suppl 4), 186 (2024)
14. Spinnato, F., Guidotti, R., Monreale, A., Nanni, M., Pedreschi, D., Giannotti, F.: Understanding any time series classifier with a subsequence-based explainer. ACM Trans. Knowl. Discov. Data **18**(2), 1–34 (2023)
15. Sutton, R.T., Pincock, D., Baumgart, D.C., Sadowski, D.C., Fedorak, R.N., Kroeker, K.I.: An overview of clinical decision support systems: benefits, risks, and strategies for success. NPJ Digital Med. **3**(1), 17 (2020)
16. Tipirneni, S., Reddy, C.K.: Self-supervised transformer for sparse and irregularly sampled multivariate clinical time-series. ACM Trans. Knowl. Discov. Data (TKDD) **16**(6), 1–17 (2022)
17. Zhou, H.Y., et al.: A transformer-based representation-learning model with unified processing of multimodal input for clinical diagnostics. Nat. Biomed. Eng. **7**(6), 743–755 (2023)

A Logic-Based Framework for Inferring Medical Events (Extended Abstract)

Yvon K. Awuklu[1,2,3(✉)], Meghyn Bienvenu[1], Katsumi Inoue[4], Vianney Jouhet[2,3], and Fleur Mougin[3]

[1] Univ. Bordeaux, CNRS, Bordeaux INP, LaBRI, Talence UMR 5800, 33400, France
{kokou-yvon.awuklu,meghyn.bienvenu}@u-bordeaux.fr

[2] CHU de Bordeaux, Service d'Information Médicale, Bordeaux 33000, France
vianney.jouhet@chu-bordeaux.fr

[3] Univ. Bordeaux, INSERM, BPH, U1219, Bordeaux 33000, France
fleur.mougin@u-bordeaux.fr

[4] National Institute of Informatics, Tokyo, Japan
inoue@nii.ac.jp

Abstract. We give a brief overview of our recent work on developing a novel logic-based framework for inferring high-level temporally extended events from timestamped clinical data and background knowledge. The framework specifies existence and termination conditions for simple events and derives meta-events by combining them. To address data imperfections, we introduce confidence annotations, consistency constraints, and a repair mechanism that selects preferred consistent event sets. While reasoning in the general setting is intractable, we identify useful fragments with polynomial-time data complexity. A prototype system, CASPER, implements the approach using answer set programming. Applied to two healthcare use cases, CASPER achieved feasible runtimes and produced clinically plausible inferences, demonstrating both computational feasibility and medical relevance. Although developed for healthcare applications, the framework is generic and can be reused in other domains.

Keywords: Medical informatics · Temporal event detection · Temporal reasoning · Answer set programming

1 Introduction

The adoption of electronic health records (EHRs) has significantly improved access to vast amounts of clinical data, but this data is inherently complex, imperfect, and strongly temporal [4,17]. In practice, EHRs record sequences of time-stamped observations–such as test results, diagnoses, or treatments–that implicitly refer to underlying clinical events (e.g., a disease episode or a therapeutic intervention) [11], yet these events are not explicitly documented and are usually inferred by physicians. Uncovering such latent events is crucial to obtain

P. Bruno et al. (Eds.): HC_AIxIA_HYDRA 2025, CCIS 2830, pp. 120–125, 2026.
https://doi.org/10.1007/978-3-032-16708-8_10

explicit, interpretable, and clinically useful representations. On the other hand, given the overwhelming volume of raw observations, it is essential to shift from low-level data toward higher-level, event-based representations that align with clinical reasoning and enable transparency by tracing inferred events back to the original observations. A wide range of approaches have been proposed for temporal reasoning [1,5,15], including automata-based systems [9,12], machine learning methods [14,16], and logic-based formalisms [3,13,18]. Logic-based methods are particularly suitable for clinical domains, as they provide formal semantics, enable modular integration of knowledge, and support explainable reasoning. However, to the best of our knowledge, no existing framework mirrors clinical reasoning while explicitly accounting for imperfect data.

In this paper, we provide an overview of our recent proposal of a new logic-based framework that address this gap by inferring high-level temporally extended events, incorporating confidence levels and a repair mechanism to handle data imperfections. Though designed with clinical applications in mind, the framework is sufficiently generic to apply in other domains.

2 A Logic-Based Framework for Event Detection

The aim of our framework is to infer high-level temporally extended events such as $\mathsf{AntibioTherapy}(p, d, [t_1, t_2])$ stating that patient p receives antibiotic d during the time period $[t_1, t_2]$, from temporal observations and expert knowledge. The key challenge is not recognizing that an observation indicates an event, but rather determining its interval boundaries. To this end, users specify: (i) *existence conditions*, which indicate that an event is ongoing at timepoint t (e.g. the observation $\mathsf{DrugAdmin}(p, d, t)$ implies therapy with d at t), and (ii) optional *termination conditions*, indicating when an event ends (e.g. $\mathsf{DrugStopNotification}(p, d, t)$).

2.1 Simple Events

We use the term *simple event* to refer to events for which we can define existence conditions (and optionally termination conditions) in terms of data predicates, without reference to other events. Two types are distinguished: persistent and non-persistent simple events.

Persistent Simple Events. Once initiated, persistent events continue until a termination condition is met (similar to the principle of inertia in reasoning about actions).

Example 1. Tyrosine kinase inhibitor (TKI) therapy is used in specific cases of lung cancer, which is intended to be taken for life unless it leads to toxicity or proves ineffective, in which case a patient is switched to another TKI drug. We thus model TKI therapy (TKITh) as a persistent simple event as follows:

$$\mathsf{exists}(\mathsf{TKITh}(p, d), t) \leftarrow \mathsf{Adm}(p, d, t) \wedge \mathrm{TKI}(d)$$
$$\mathsf{ends}(\mathsf{TKITh}(p, d), t) \leftarrow \mathsf{Adm}(p, d', t) \wedge \mathrm{TKI}(d') \wedge \mathrm{TKI}(d) \wedge d' \neq d$$

Non-persistent Simple Events. This kind of simple event requires repeated evidence to continue. The time intervals associated with the event are built by grouping together timepoints satisfying existence conditions, if they are sufficiently close (with 'closeness' being determined by a provided *time window*), ending an event when a termination condition is reached, or when there are no further timepoints in the vicinity that satisfy existence conditions.

Example 2. For the simple event AntibioTherapy (shortened to ABTh), we could use the following rules:

$$\mathsf{exists}(\mathsf{ABTh}(p,d),t) \leftarrow \mathsf{Adm}(p,d,t) \wedge \mathsf{AB}(d)$$
$$\mathsf{ends}(\mathsf{ABTh}(p,d),t) \leftarrow \mathsf{Stop}(p,d,t) \wedge \mathsf{AB}(d)$$
$$\mathsf{window}(\mathsf{ABTh}(p,d),48) \leftarrow \mathsf{P}(p) \wedge \mathsf{AB}(d)$$

The existence condition looks for administrations (Adm) of an antibiotic (AB) drug. The termination rule applies when there is a drug stop notification (Stop). A fixed window of 48 h is defined, but one could use multiple rules with different windows to e.g. differentiate by the class of antibiotics.

2.2 Meta-Events

Our framework also supports *meta-events*, defined using rules that may refer to simple events and possibly other meta-events. Such higher-level events allow one e.g. to group disease episodes or identify concurrent conditions or treatments. They also make it possible to present events at different levels of abstraction (e.g. DrugTherapy generalizes AntibioTherapy).

2.3 Confidence Levels and Repairs

Because existence and termination rules are rarely both complete and fully accurate, event facts are annotated with *confidence levels* reflecting rule reliability (e.g. specific diagnostic codes outrank generic ones). To ensure consistency despite imperfect data, we apply two kinds of constraints: *temporal constraints* (prohibiting overlapping intervals of the same event) and *domain-specific constraints.* A repair mechanism is then applied to select consistent sets of events. Our first notion of repair considers the inclusion-maximal consistent sets of facts, in line with the subset repairs previously investigated for databases and knowledge bases [6,7]. In addition, we introduce preferred repairs, which give priority to retaining facts with higher confidence levels, following the spirit of the $\subseteq_P$-repairs proposed in [8].

2.4 Complexity Considerations

From a computational perspective, the inference of simple and meta-events can be computed in PTIME in data complexity. However, when domain constraints and confidence-based repairs are taken into account, reasoning may become intractable in the general case. However, we can identify practically relevant tractable fragments, such as when only temporal constraints are considered and termination rules share a single confidence level.

3 CASPER System

We have implemented core components of our framework using Answer Set Programming (ASP), chosen for its declarative style and expressive power. The prototype system CASPER for Clinical ASP-based Event Recognition (see Fig. 1), currently implements the tractable fragment of our framework, which proves sufficient for the use cases addressed in this work.

CASPER takes as input: (i) event rules, expressed in ASP-Core-2 with head predicates `exists`, `exists_pers` (existence conditions for persistent events), `terminates`, `pt_window` (provided time window), and `m_event`; (ii) atemporal facts (e.g. `tki(ceritinib)`); and (iii) observation facts encoded using the `obs` predicates, e.g. `obs(has_adm, p, d, t)` (note the reified predicate name).

CASPER is composed of five interacting ASP modules. The *expansion module* computes non-persistent simple events facts from the input facts, `exists` and `terminates` rules, by expanding intervals iteratively and pruning non-maximal intervals. The *linear module* computes persistent simple events facts from the input facts and `exists_pers` and `terminates` rules. The *temporal predicate module* defines standard temporal relations between intervals, such as Allen interval relations [2], interval manipulation predicates (e.g. to compute the intersect function), and further helper predicates that simplify rule writing, such as `start` and `end` which identify the earliest/latest timepoints of a given event. These defined predicates can be used in the bodies of meta-event rules, while additional helper predicates, internal to CASPER, are provided by the *auxiliary module*. Finally, the *temporal repair module* computes the set of repairs or the preferred repair.

Depending on user options, CASPER passes the required ASP programs and facts to the Clingo[1] ASP system [10], which produces *stable model(s)*.

Evaluation. We evaluated our approach on two real-world use cases using data from the Bordeaux University Hospital Clinical Data Warehouse: (i) a lung cancer use case, targeting six clinical events of interest, and (ii) an infection use case, focused on antibiotic therapy in pulmonary and urinary infections, targeting five events. In both cases, rules were developed in close collaboration with physicians. Confidence levels were manually assigned according to rule reliability, with 1 denoting maximal confidence. These levels were carefully determined based on semantics, the granularity of the clinical observations (e.g., prescription data are less reliable than administration data when reconstructing a therapy), and physician expertise. For the lung cancer use case, evaluation consisted of four physicians annotating 30 randomly selected patient records to identify the same clinical events that CASPER had to infer. For the infection use case, evaluation was performed by a single domain expert who assessed the quality of CASPER's

[1] https://potassco.org/clingo/.

inferences. CASPER processed 322 lung cancer patients individually, using as input 16 event rules, 497 atemporal facts, and between 3 and 815 observation facts per patient. For the infection use case, 443 patients were processed individually, with 14 event rules, 587 atemporal facts, and between 9 and 4,015 observation facts per patient. Despite the heterogeneity of patient records, runtimes remained practical: from 0.11 to 123.97 s, with an average of 1.36 s for the lung cancer use case and 1.32 s for the infection use case. Domain experts judged the inferred events clinically plausible. These preliminary results underline the practical relevance of the approach.

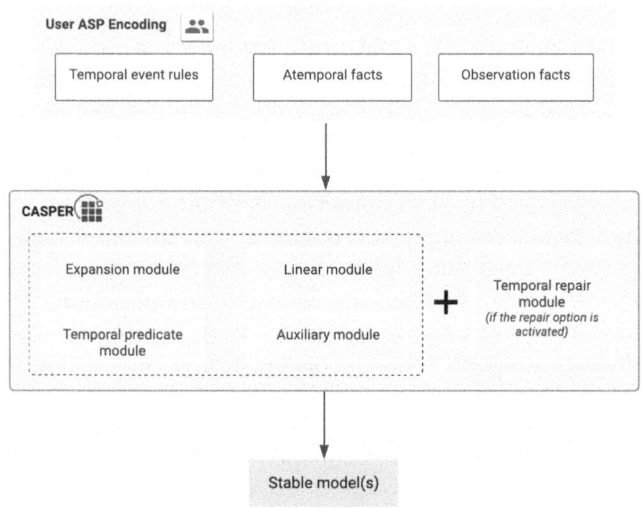

Fig. 1. Overview of the CASPER system architecture.

4 Conclusion and Future Work

We introduced an expressive logical framework for inferring temporally extended events, based on the specification of simple events through existence and termination conditions combined with temporal windows. The framework further incorporates confidence levels, constraints, and a repair mechanism to address uncertainty in event detection. While reasoning in the full framework is intractable, we identified restricted fragments with more favorable complexity. Future work will refine these fragments, extend the complexity analysis to additional reasoning tasks such as temporal query answering, and improve usability by developing a domain-specific language with templates for common medical events. We also plan to explore how medical ontologies can support the (semi-)automatic generation of domain constraints and facts and event rule conditions.

Acknowledgments. This work was partially supported by the ANR AI Chair INTENDED (ANR-19-CHIA-0014) and JST CREST Grant Number JPMJCR22D3.

References

1. Alevizos, E., Skarlatidis, A., Artikis, A., Paliouras, G.: Complex event recognition under uncertainty: a short survey. Proc. of EDBT/ICDT **1330**, 7 (2015)
2. Allen, J.F.: Maintaining knowledge about temporal intervals **26**(11) (1983)
3. Artikis, A., Sergot, M., Paliouras, G.: An event calculus for event recognition. IEEE Trans. Knowl. Data Eng. **27**(4), 895–908 (2015)
4. Awuklu, Y.K., Mougin, F., Griffier, R., Bienvenu, M., Jouhet, V.: Ontology-driven identification of inconsistencies in clinical data: a case study in lung cancer phenotyping. J. Biomed. Inform. **165**, 104808 (2025)
5. Batsakis, S., Petrakis, E.G.M., Tachmazidis, I., Antoniou, G.: Temporal Representation and Reasoning in OWL 2. Semantic Web **8**(6), 981–1000 (2017)
6. Bertossi, L.E.: Database Repairing and Consistent Query Answering. Synthesis Lectures on Data Management, Morgan & Claypool Publishers (2011)
7. Bienvenu, M., Bourgaux, C.: Inconsistency-tolerant querying of description logic knowledge bases. In: Pan, J.Z., et al. (eds.) Reasoning Web 2016. LNCS, vol. 9885, pp. 156–202. Springer, Cham (2017). https://doi.org/10.1007/978-3-319-49493-7_5
8. Bienvenu, M., Bourgaux, C., Goasdoué, F.: Querying inconsistent description logic knowledge bases under preferred repair semantics. In: Proceedings of AAAI (2014)
9. Bucchi, M., Grez, A., Quintana, A., Riveros, C., Vansummeren, S.: CORE: a complex event recognition engine. Proc. VLDB Endow. **15**(9), 1951–1964 (2022)
10. Gebser, M., Kaminski, R., Kaufmann, B., Schaub, T.: Multi-shot ASP solving with clingo. Theory Pract. Log. Program. **19**(1), 27–82 (2019)
11. Hripcsak, G., Albers, D.J.: Next-generation phenotyping of electronic health records. J. Am. Med. Inform. Assoc. **20**(1), 117–121 (2013)
12. Katzouris, N., Paliouras, G.: Answer set automata: a learnable pattern specification framework for complex event recognition. In: ECAI 2023, pp. 1223–1230. IOS Press (2023)
13. Mantenoglou, P., Artikis, A., Paliouras, G.: Online probabilistic interval-based event calculus. In: ECAI 2020, pp. 2624–2631. IOS Press (2020)
14. Michelioudakis, E., Artikis, A., Paliouras, G.: Semi-supervised online structure learning for composite event recognition. Mach. Learn. **108**(7), 1085–1110 (2019)
15. Morveli-Espinoza, M., Nieves, J.C., Tacla, C.A.: Handling temporality in human activity reasoning. J. Intell. Fuzzy Syst. **42**(5), 4387–4398 (2022)
16. Ntoulias, E., Alevizos, E., Artikis, A., Akasiadis, C., Koumparos, A.: Online fleet monitoring with scalable event recognition and forecasting. GeoInformatica **26**(4), 613–644 (2022)
17. Tsai, C.H., Eghdam, A., Davoody, N., Wright, G., Flowerday, S., Koch, S.: Effects of electronic health record implementation and barriers to adoption and use: a scoping review and qualitative analysis of the content. Life (Basel) **10**(12), 327 (2020)
18. Tsilionis, E., Artikis, A., Paliouras, G.: A tensor-based formalization of the event calculus. In: Proceedings of the Thirty-Third International Joint Conference on Artificial Intelligence. pp. 3584–3592. International Joint Conferences on Artificial Intelligence Organization, Jeju, South Korea (Aug 2024)

When ‘Scarce’ Becomes ‘*Too* Scarce’: The Rare Diseases Drama

Alice Bernasconi[1(✉)], Federico Pirola[2], Alessio Zanga[1,2], and Antonio Balordi[3]

[1] Evaluative Epidemiology Unit, Department of Epidemiology and Data Science, Fondazione IRCCS Istituto Nazionale dei Tumori, Milan, Italy
alice.bernasconi@istitutotumori.mi.it

[2] Models and Algorithms for Data and Text Mining Laboratory (MADLab), Department of Informatics, Systems and Communication (DISCo), University of Milano-Bicocca, Milan, Italy

[3] CASD - Italian Defense University, Rome, Italy

Abstract. Rare diseases pose unique methodological challenges for causal questions, where data scarcity is not incidental but inherent. We present a case study on the external validation of a causal Bayesian network (BN) developed to investigate cardiovascular diseases (CVDs) in adolescent and young adult female breast cancer survivors. Despite strong internal performance, external validation across multiple Italian regions revealed scenarios where the model's predictions collapsed into complete uncertainty. These included: (i) circumstances in which shifts in missingness and selection mechanisms made the original model parameters inappropriate (ii) unobserved infrequent treatments in training data; and (iii) novel treatment combinations emerging from evolving clinical protocols. We discuss the implications of these findings, emphasizing the need for including informative priors, making timely model updates, and explicit uncertainty quantification. Our experience underscores that in rare disease research, robust causal modeling demands critical scrutiny, adaptive learning, and the indispensable role of human revision. These lessons could be broadly applicable to other domains where data are scarce, emphasizing that methodological rigor and adaptability are as crucial as the models themselves.

Keywords: Rare diseases · Data scarcity · Causal models · Uncertainty

1 Introduction

When dealing with *rare diseases*, *scarcity* is not just a background condition: it is the main character. Samples are small, events are few, and the gaps in knowledge are wide. Causal questions in medicine are often tackled with whatever data are at hand. As Hernán reminds us: *“If a causal question is important, analyze your*

P. Bruno et al. (Eds.): HC_AIxIA_HYDRA 2025, CCIS 2830, pp. 126–131, 2026.
https://doi.org/10.1007/978-3-032-16708-8_11

data, publish your estimates, encourage others to do the same, and then meta-analyze. The alternative is an unanswered question" [1]. Yet here lies the drama: in rare diseases, even pooling every dataset in sight may leave us facing large and stubborn uncertainty. Data scarcity may arise when the dataset is (too) small, unbalanced, or incomplete to sustain reliable causal estimation. It is not just inconvenient: it can be an insurmountable barrier.

Artificial intelligence (AI) offers some promising tools to navigate this terrain, like Bayesian networks (BNs). These AI tools are able to break complex systems into conditional dependencies, making causal relationships explicit [2,3]. They can also integrate prior expert knowledge (a valuable asset when data are scarce) and update as new evidence arrives. But when prior knowledge is itself incomplete or uncertain, these tools may produce weak or misleading causal graphs. External validation through new cohorts can help, but it is often expensive, slow, and, in some cases, insufficient to meaningfully reduce uncertainty [4,5].

In this discussion paper, we critically examine some possible limitations and pitfalls of building causal BNs in the rare disease context, where both data and prior knowledge may be too scarce. We will do that through a real-world application: the external validation of a causal BN to study rare diseases, i.e. cardiovascular diseases (CVDs) in adolescent and young adult (AYA, 15–39 years old) female breast cancer (BC) survivors [6].

2 Background

The causal BN model was developed using data from two distinct real-world observational cohorts of AYA BC survivors living in the Lombardy region in Italy: a population-based cohort (PBC) and a clinic-based cohort (CBC). The PBC was identified through Italian population-based cancer registries (CRs), which were asked to select AYA cases (i.e. patients aged 15 to 39 at BC diagnosis) and link them to multiple administrative datasets (hospital discharge records, outpatient visits, and drug prescription flows) to enable long-term CVD identification. This cohort included 1,037 BC patients diagnosed between 2009 and 2014. Information on treatments, CVD diagnoses, and major cardiovascular risk factors was extracted from these administrative sources. The PBC provided substantial advantages, including a large sample size and the ability to track patients for long-term outcomes. However, it lacked detailed cancer-related variables and treatment information that are potentially crucial for understanding CVD development and are essential for causal inference. To address this gap, we collected an additional retrospective single-institution CBC comprising 339 AYA BC patients diagnosed between 2011 and 2019. Patients in the CBC were identified through a clinical BC registry, and detailed information on BC treatments and prognostic factors was obtained from clinical charts.

The use of these two heterogeneous datasets introduced two major methodological challenges: *i) Selection bias*, due to differences in patient distributions between the PBC and CBC and *ii) Missing not at random* data, which can bias causal estimates if not explicitly modeled. To overcome these issues, we designed the structure of a causal BN that integrates selection diagrams, missingness graphs, and expert prior knowledge. The modeling process began with an expert-informed causal graph, which was then refined through a Structural Expectation-Maximization algorithm to jointly update the graph structure and parameter estimates. This approach allowed the final model to balance expert insights with empirical evidence [7]. For training and internal validation, the combined dataset (PBC + CBC) was split as follows: training set âĂŞ all 339 CBC patients plus 623 PBC patients (approximately 70% of the total sample); validation set – the remaining 413 PBC patients (approximately 30%). The CBC was excluded from the validation phase due to the absence of the main outcome of interest for that cohort. In the end, according to our experimental results, the model showed very good predictive performances, in the internal validation setting, in predicting the target variable (i.e. CVD within 5 years after BC diagnosis) with AUC around 88% [8]. However, it is also important to mention that, due to the rarity of the outcome in this population (<5% of AYA with BC developed a CVD within 5-years) the model suffered from strong class imbalance, resulting in a true positive rate around 70%.

To make our results transportable from a one-region-only sample to the entire italian population of AYA with BC, we started a new population-based data collection in 4 additional CRs located in different italian regions: Veneto (N = 952), Apulia (N = 554), Tuscany (N = 335) and Friuli Venezia Giulia (N = 105). These PBCs meet the same selection criteria as the original PBC. The marginal distribution of all the variables in all five PBCs, including missing values, is shown in Supplementary Material Table @reftab:supspstable. Despite the good predictive performance of the model (AUC > 70%) observed in the validation cohorts - with the exception of the Apulian cohort, where some variable coding issues were detected - we identified several instances in which the model exhibited complete uncertainty in its predictions. For this reason, in Sect. 3, we highlighted the main limitations and potential pitfalls of the current model, illustrating them through three examples drawn from the external validation results.

3 The Uncertainty Behind the Model

To facilitate the reader's understanding of the narrative across the three proposed scenarios, we included Fig. 1, which highlights the nodes and their relationships within the original graph.

1. **Dealing with shifts in selection and missingness mechanisms**
   As described in Sect. 2, the conditional probability tables (CPTs) of the Bayesian network were learned from the data of the two study cohorts (PBC+CBC). However, each of these cohorts suffered from missing-not-at-random patterns due to a selection mechanism. In the CBC, cardiovascular events (i.e., the outcome of major interest) were systematically missing, whereas in the population-based cohort, many cancer prognostic factors (i.e., the ones in yellow in Fig. 1) were not available. Learning from these data therefore yielded CPTs for the PBC that were essentially random with respect to

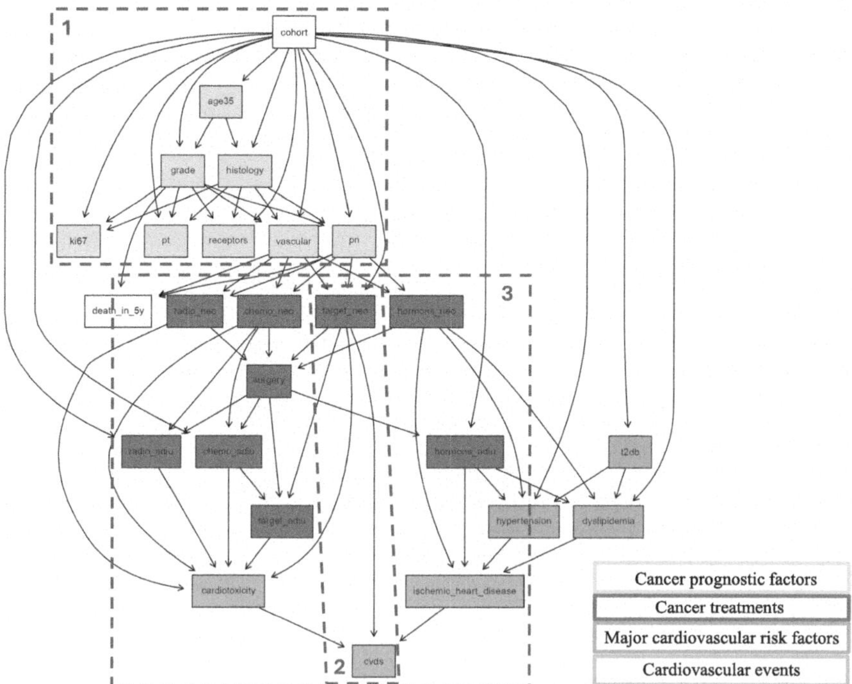

Fig. 1. Graphical illustration of the proposed scenarios according to the BN structure.

these factors, owing to the absence of information on which to base the estimation. In the new validation cohorts, which are also population-based, some of these prognostic variables are collected, albeit with a high proportion of missing values (see Supplementary Material Table @reftab:supspstable). The use of the original model's CPTs for these validation cohorts is thus inappropriate, since the selection mechanism governing the original data is different from that of the validation sets.
How can this issue be addressed? One potential approach could be to reconstruct the CPTs of the PBC - currently random - by simulating a distribution shift from the clinical cohort, using the partially observed distributions in the new validation cohorts as guidance [9].

2. **Unobserved rare treatments** In the training cohorts, we observed that neo-adjuvant targeted therapy (i.e., administered prior to surgery) was an extremely infrequent treatment option. Specifically, it was recorded for only a few patients in the CBC and for none in the patients in the PBC. Consequently, the outcome of interest (whether it occurred or not) was never observed among patients receiving this treatment in the training data due to the systematic missingness in both training cohorts. As a result, the model remains entirely agnostic to the risk associated with these patients and can only produce random guesses when such cases appear in the vali-

dation cohorts. In this context, introducing an informative prior distribution derived from the scientific literature (when available) becomes essential to complete the missing portion of the corresponding CPT [10]. This is particularly relevant when the available data concern a small, under-represented patient subgroup (as in our use-case) where direct evidence is scarce but prior knowledge can help produce more reliable estimates.
3. **Unexpected combination of treatments**
   In the external validation cohorts, we identified treatment combinations that had not been previously observed in the training cohorts, because they were not included with the treatment guidelines. Such occurrences are not uncommon in the medical domain, where therapeutic protocols may change over time, introducing novel treatment patterns. While it is possible to address these shifts by simulating plausible scenarios, these simulations may not always be realistic or materialize in the specific use case. In this context, it becomes essential not only to acquire new data but also to update the model by retraining it on the combined data, thereby ensuring that its predictions remain valid under evolving clinical practices [11].

4 Conclusions

In conclusion, with this work we wish to send a message to (young) researchers venturing into the demanding task of answering causal questions in the realm of rare diseases: your work is as complex as it is valuable, and the evidence you will produce will be essential in narrowing, even slightly, the gap between 'Scarce' and 'too *Scarce*'. So, please, *be brave!*
In addition to Hernán's recommendations, and drawing from the experience done in this work, we would like to offer a few simple yet crucial tips:

1. *be relentlessly critical* - scrutinize your data, your models (don't just train it - question it); sometimes the most treacherous pitfalls are hidden behind the façade of outstanding performance;
2. *embrace uncertainty* - it is not necessarily an enemy, and when acknowledged and quantified, it becomes a powerful ally in interpreting results and better guiding future decisions;
3. never forget to *put the human in the loop* - artificial intelligence achieves its full potential only when guided by human judgment, especially when data alone cannot tell the whole story.

Acknowledgments. This work was possible thanks to the data collected in the *ROSANNA validation working group*: *Friuli-Venezia-Giulia CR* (Ettore Bidoli, Luigino Dal Maso, Federica Toffolutti, Fabiola Giudici), *Apulia CR* (Danila Bruno, Rossella Bruni, Cinzia Tanzarella, Francesco Cuccaro, Vanna Burgio), *Trapani-Agrigento CR* (Tiziana Scuderi, Giovanna Fantaci), *Tuscany CR* (Giulia Bertini, Adele Caldarella, Gianfranco Manneschi, Federico Pirona), *Palermo CR* (Walter Mazzucco, Rosalba Amodio, Maurizio Zarcone), *Veneto CR* (Alessandra Andreotti, Stefano Guzzinati, Manuel Zorzi).

This work is part of an *AIRC* 2020 project, grant number 24864, titled *"pRedicting cardiOvascular diSeAses iN adolescent and young breast caNcer pAtients (ROSANNA)"*.

The work of Federico Pirola was funded by the National Plan for NRRP Complementary Investments - project n. PNC0000003 - AdvaNced Technologies for Human-centrEd Medicine (ANTHEM).

The work of Alessio Zanga was partially supported by the MUR under the grant "Dipartimenti di Eccellenza 2023-2027" of the Department of Informatics, Systems and Communication (DISCo), University of Milano-Bicocca, Milan, Italy.

References

1. Hernán, M.A.: Causal analyses of existing databases: no power calculations required. J. Clin. Epidemiol. **144**, 203–205 (2022)
2. Pearl, J.: Causality, 2nd edn. Cambridge University Press, Cambridge (2009)
3. Koller, D., Friedman, N.: Probabilistic graphical models: principles and techniques. MIT Press, Cambridge (2009)
4. Bareinboim, E., Pearl, J.: Causal inference and the data-fusion problem. Proc. Natl. Acad. Sci. **113**(27), 7345–7352 (2016)
5. Riley, R.D., Ensor, J., Snell, K.I.E., et al.: External validation of clinical prediction models using big datasets from e-health records or ipd meta-analysis: opportunities and challenges. BMJ **353**, i3140 (2016)
6. Bernasconi, A., Zanga, A., Lucas, P.J.F., Scutari, M., Stella, F.: Towards a transportable causal network model based on observational healthcare data. In: Calimeri, F., Dragoni, M., Stella, F. (eds.) Proceedings of the 2nd AIxIA Workshop on Artificial Intelligence for Healthcare (HC@AIxIA 2023), co-located with the 22nd International Conference of the Italian Association for Artificial Intelligence (AIxIA 2023). CEUR Workshop Proceedings, vol. 3578. CEUR-WS.org (2023). https://ceur-ws.org/Vol-3578/paper7.pdf
7. Bernasconi, A., Zanga, A., Lucas, P.J.F., Scutari, M., Trama, A., Stella, F.: A causal network model to estimate the cardiotoxic effect of oncological treatments in young breast cancer survivors. Progress Artif. Intell. (2024)
8. Bernasconi, A., et al.: The ada working group: from real-world data to causally interpretable models: a bayesian network to predict cardiovascular diseases in adolescents and young adults with breast cancer. Cancers **16**(21), 3643 (2024)
9. Pearl, J., Bareinboim, E.: External validity: from do-calculus to transportability across populations. Stat. Sci. **29**(4), 579–595 (2014)
10. Constantinou, A.C., Fenton, N., Neil, M.: Integrating expert knowledge with data in bayesian networks: Preserving data-driven expectations when the expert variables remain unobserved. Expert Syst. Appl. **56**, 197–208 (2016)
11. Friedman, N., Goldszmidt, M.: Sequential update of Bayesian network structure (2013)

Application of Nonlinear Autoregressive Neural Network for Prediction of HIV Infections in Poland

Marek Landowski[1(✉)] and Anna Landowska[2]

[1] Faculty of Computer Science and Telecommunications, Maritime University of Szczecin, Waly Chrobrego 1-2, 70-500 Szczecin, Poland
m.landowski@pm.szczecin.pl

[2] Institute of Spatial Management and Socio-Economic Geography, University of Szczecin, Mickiewicza 64, 71-101 Szczecin, Poland
anna.landowska@usz.edu.pl

Abstract. The article presents the application of a nonlinear autoregressive neural network to predict the HIV infection rate in Poland. The prediction was made using neural network models with three training functions: Levenberg-Marquardt, Bayesian Regularization, and BFGS Quasi-Newton. Real data was used to predict the HIV infection rate. Due to lower testability during the COVID-19 pandemic, these data indicated a lower infection rate during this period. This fact did not significantly affect the prediction using the NAR neural network. The prediction results obtained using the NAR neural network, linear regression and exponential smoothing methods were compared. The presented research is important due to the increasing number of HIV infections worldwide. The use of artificial neural networks to predict the infection rate can help locate places that require intensified preventive measures.

Keywords: Nonlinear Autoregressive Neural Network · HIV Infection Rate · Data Mining · Artificial Intelligence

1 Introduction

Artificial neural networks are a type of information processing systems that partially reproduce the biological operation of the real nervous system. The schemes of artificial neurons and mathematical models are based on the biological dependencies of human neurons. Artificial neural networks are widely used to solve many problems, e.g. clustering, data fitting, pattern recognition, time series prediction and many others.

Time series prediction is an important task that is still relevant and analyzed in the scientific literature. For example, in [9], the authors use dendritic neuron model to detect transmission trends of the COVID-19 pandemic. In [10], the authors propose to use grey-informed neural network (GINN) for time series forecasting. They show in the article that the model generates reliable forecasts

P. Bruno et al. (Eds.): HC_AIxIA_HYDRA 2025, CCIS 2830, pp. 132–137, 2026.
https://doi.org/10.1007/978-3-032-16708-8_12

and predicts patterns occurring in the real world. The authors of [3] propose a model called Hypergraph Recurrent Neural Networks for time series forecasting. This model exploits the connections not only between pairs of time series but also beyond them. In the work [2] the authors use NAR neural network to predict financial time series and additionally apply Kalman filter to improve the model accuracy. In [8] the application of NAR neural network to assess groundwater destruction caused by unconventional gas leakage from abandoned wells in the ground is described. Neural networks are also used to study the effects of antiretroviral therapy in HIV-infected patients [4,7].

In this article, a nonlinear autoregressive (NAR) neural network was used to forecast time series of HIV infections among Poles. The authors' motivation to undertake this type of research is the fact that the HIV infection rate values are disturbed in the analyzed period by the approximately two-year period of the COVID-19 pandemic. During this period, people were isolated and not as many tests were performed as in other years. For this reason, the prediction of time series values may be burdened with error. The authors showed that NAR neural networks are able to make predictions also in the case when part of the analyzed period has declining values.

The use of the NAR neural network to predict the HIV infection rate can help identify places where there is a high increase in infections. By locating areas at risk of a large increase in HIV infections, it is possible to intensify information activities or other preventive steps.

The aim of the work is to demonstrate that it is possible to forecast the HIV infection rate using the NAR neural network.

The rest of the paper is organized as follows. Section 2 presents the methods used in the study. Section 3 describes the analyzed data. Section 4 gives the prediction result obtained by the applied NAR neural network training method and their comparison with the prediction using linear regression and exponential smoothing methods. The last Sect. 5 contains the final conclusions.

2 Method

A nonlinear autoregressive neural network (NAR) was used to predict the HIV infection rate in Poland. The NAR neural network can train itself to be able to predict time series values based on previous observations. In this work, tests were carried out on three training functions: Levenberg-Marquardt, Bayesian Regularization and BFGS Quasi-Newton to train the NAR neural network.

The accuracy of the model, i.e. the difference between the output values and the network response, was checked using statistics: the mean squared error $MSE = \frac{1}{n}\sum_{i=1}^{n}(y_i - \hat{y}_i)^2$, the correlation coefficient $r = \frac{1}{n-1}\sum_{i=1}^{n}\left(\frac{y_i-\bar{y}}{\sigma_y}\right)\left(\frac{\hat{y}_i-\bar{\hat{y}}}{\sigma_{\hat{y}}}\right)$, and the coefficient of determination $R^2 = 1 - \sum_{i=1}^{n}(y_i - \hat{y}_i)^2 / \sum_{i=1}^{n}(y_i - \bar{y}_i)^2$, where y_i is a target value, $\hat{y}_i$ is output value ($i = 1, \ldots, n$), $\bar{y}$ and $\bar{\hat{y}}$ are means of y_i and $\hat{y}_i$, σ_y and $\sigma_{\hat{y}}$ are standard deviations of y_i and $\hat{y}_i$, respectively, [5,6].

3 Data Description

The data used for the study were taken from the website of the National Institute of Public Health in Poland (https://wwwold.pzh.gov.pl/oldpage/epimeld/hiv_aids/index.htm). The data concern the number of HIV infections in Poland in the years 1996-2024 recorded by the Polish Institute of Hygiene. Before using them for prediction with a neural network, they were normalized to the interval $[0,1]$ using the min-max norm $y* = \frac{y-\min(y)}{\max(y)-\min(y)}$, where y is the value of the time series under consideration and $y*$ is the normalized value, [1].

4 Application of NAR Neural Network to Prediction

This section presents the results of HIV infection value prediction using NAR neural network. Three training functions Levenberg-Marquardt, Bayesian Regularization and BFGS Quasi-Newton were used to train the neural network.

For the model with the Levenberg-Marquardt training function, the best results were obtained with 7 neurons in the hidden layer and feedback delays of 4 periods. For the model with Bayesian regularization, 10 neurons in the hidden layer were used, and feedback delays of 4 periods were also assumed. For the third model with the BFGS Quasi-Newton training function, the best results were obtained for 13 neurons in the hidden layer and feedback delays of 3 periods.

The results presented in Table 1 indicate that the best fit is the neural network model with the Levenberg-Marquardt training function. In this case, the MSE error values are the lowest, for the training and testing samples, respectively, are 1.5563e-3 and 2.1631e-3. The correlation coefficient is also high for the training and testing samples, respectively, are 0.9816 and 0.9689.

Analyzing the results between the NAR prediction of the neural network using Bayesian Regularization or BFGS Quasi-Newton training functions, the MSE error values is lower for the Bayesian Regularization training function. In this case, the MSE error for the training samples is 6.9533e-3 and 1.0847e-2, respectively. While the prediction results MSE error using the Bayesian Regularization training function for the test samples is higher than for BFGS Quasi-Newton training function, they are 7.8814e-2 and 3.3316e-2, respectively.

Let us consider the correlation coefficient value for the prediction results of the neural network using the Bayesian Regularization or BFGS Quasi-Newton training function. For the training sample, a higher r value was obtained using the Bayesian Regularization function, which is $r = 0.9385$, in this case for the BFGS Quasi-Newton training function $r= 0.9150$. However, for the test sample, the situation is similar. A higher value of the correlation coefficient was obtained for the prediction using the Bayesian Regularization learning function, it is $r = 0.9530$, than for the prediction using the BFGS Quasi-Newton learning function ($r = 0.9256$).

Analyzing the value of the coefficient of determination R^2, we clearly conclude that the appropriate prediction model is the one obtained using the NAR neural network with the Levenberg-Marquardt training function. In this case, for the training sample $R^2 = 0.9621$, while for the testing sample $R^2 = 0.7222$. The obtained R^2 values indicate a high level of correlation between the empirical values and the theoretical values obtained from the model. For the remaining models, the coefficient of determination is lower.

Table 1. Comparison of results by training function

Training function	Data	MSE	r	R^2
Levenberg-Marquardt	Training	1.5563e-3	0.9816	0.9621
	Test	2.1631e-3	0.9689	0.7222
Bayesian Regularization	Training	6.9533e-3	0.9385	0.8803
	Test	7.8814e-2	0.9530	0.0145
BFGS Quasi-Newton	Training	1.0847e-2	0.9150	0.8363
	Test	3.3316e-2	0.9256	0.4361

Figure 1 shows graph containing marked neural network response, target values and error between target and output. The COVID-19 pandemic period covering the years 2020-2021 is visible, where due to the lockdown significantly fewer tests were performed than in other years. The results in individual graphs depend on the training function used.

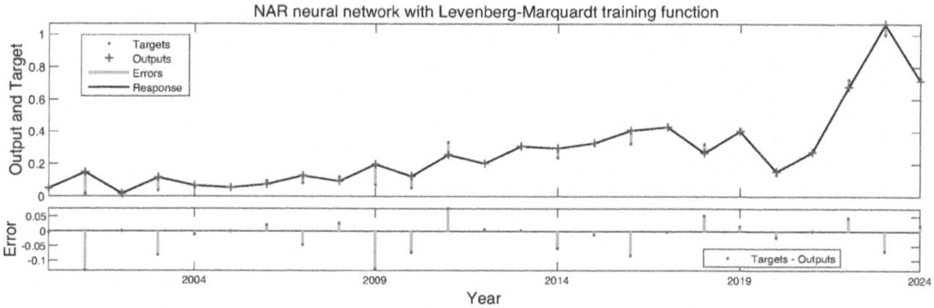

Fig. 1. Results generated by NAR neural network with Levenberg-Marquardt training function for HIV infection prediction.

To compare the results, also predictions were performed using linear regression and exponential smoothing without a seasonal component, taking into account the linear, exponential and decay trend. The MSE error values are higher than for prediction using the NAR neural network model with the Levenberg-Marquardt learning function. The obtained correlation coefficient r also indicates that prediction using the neural network gives more accurate results.

The coefficient of determination R^2 indicate a lower fit of the prediction values obtained using linear regression and exponential smoothing to the empirical data than in the case of the model obtained using the NAR neural network with the Levenberg-Marquardt training function.

The MSE error, correlation coefficient r and coefficient of determination R^2 of predictions are presented in Table 2.

Table 2. Results of prediction by linear regression and exponential smoothing without a seasonal component

Method	MSE	r	R^2
Linear regression	2.0707e-2	0.8082	0.6533
Exponential smoothing, linear trend	2.8428e-2	0.8355	0.5199
Exponential smoothing, exponential trend	2.0893e-2	0.8548	0.6471
Exponential smoothing, decaying trend	4.7937e-2	0.8491	0.1904

Figure 2 presents graphs of real and predictions data on HIV infections from 1996 to 2024 and 5 years predictions (2025-2029) using the NAR neural network with the Levenberg-Marquardt learning function, linear regression and exponential smoothing without a seasonal component, taking into account the linear, exponential and decaying trend. The predicted normalized HIV infection rates for 2025-2029 generated by the NAR neural network are 1.0190, 1.1930, 1.4096, 1.4732, and 1.5451, respectively.

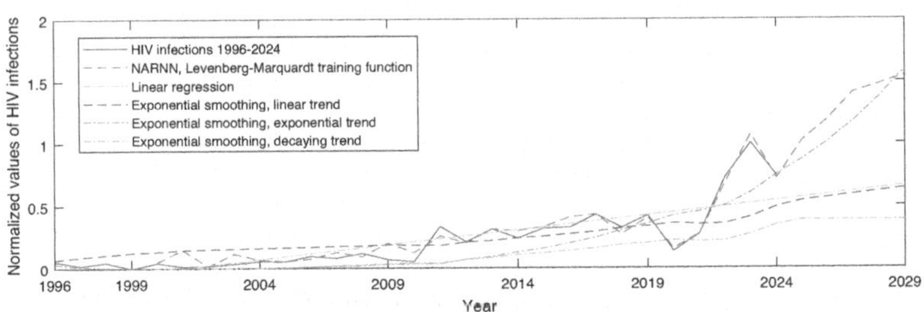

Fig. 2. HIV infections in Poland (1996-2024) and predictions (1996-2029) using the NAR neural network with the Levenberg-Marquardt learning function, linear regression, exponential smoothing without a seasonal component, taking into account the linear, exponential and decaying trend.

The exponential smoothing prediction with an exponential trend shows a strong increase starting in 2028. This indicates that the prediction beyond 5 years in this situation may be inaccurate. The model obtained using an artificial neural network not only has parameters (MSE, r, R^2) that indicate a better fit of the empirical data to the obtained prediction, but also does not show a strong increase after 2028.

5 Conclusions

The article presents the application of nonlinear autoregressive (NAR) neural network to predict the HIV infection rate in Poland. The obtained results indicate the possibility of predicting the HIV infection rate. Tests were conducted using three training functions: Levenberg-Marquardt, Bayesian Regularization and BFGS Quasi-Newton. The best prediction results were obtained for the neural network model with the Levenberg-Marquard training function. The obtained prediction results were compared with the linear regression and the exponential smoothing method without a seasonal component, with three development trends. The MSE error, correlation coefficient r and coefficient of determination R^2 showed that the prediction model obtained using the NAR neural network with the Levenberg-Marquardt learning function best describes the analyzed empirical data. It was shown that the use of NAR neural network allows for the prediction of the infection rate, and therefore also the location of places most at risk of an increase in HIV infection. Such information can help in the rapid implementation of preventive measures. Further research will focus on comparing other types of neural networks for the prediction of HIV infections.

References

1. Benhar, H., Idri, A., Fernandez-Aleman, J.L.: Data preprocessing for heart disease classification: a systematic literature review. Comput. Methods Programs Biomed. **197**, 105635 (2020)
2. Benrhmach, G., Namir, K., Namir, A., Bouyaghroumni, J.: Nonlinear autoregressive neural network and extended kalman filters for prediction of financial time series. J. Appl. Math. **2020**(5057801), 1–6 (2020)
3. Chen, H., Rossi, R.A., Mahadik, K., Kim, S., Eldardiry, H.: Hypergraph neural networks for time-series forecasting. In: 2023 IEEE International Conference on Big Data (BigData), pp. 1076–1080. IEEE, Sorrento, Italy (2023)
4. Das, B., Kutsal, M., Das, R.: Effective prediction of drug - target interaction on hiv using deep graph neural networks. Chemom. Intell. Lab. Syst. **230**, 104676 (2022)
5. Fisher, R.A.: Statistical Methods for Research Workers, 13th edn. Hafner, New York (1958)
6. Kendall, M.G.: The Advanced Theory of Statistics, 4th edn. Macmillan, New York (1979)
7. Lew, C.: Neural network modeling of hiv acute and chronic phases with and without antiretroviral intervention. In: 2022 Fourth International Conference on Transdisciplinary AI (TransAI), pp. 47–54. IEEE, Laguna Hills, CA, USA (2022)
8. Taherdangkoo, R., Tatomir, A., Taherdangkoo, M., Qiu, P., Sauter, M.: Nonlinear autoregressive neural networks to predict hydraulic fracturing fluid leakage into shallow groundwater. Water **12**(841), 1–14 (2020)
9. Tang, C., Todo, Y., Kodera, S., Sun, R., Shimada, A., Hirata, A.: A novel multivariate time series forecasting dendritic neuron model for covid-19 pandemic transmission tendency. Neural Netw. **179**, 106527 (2024)
10. Xie, W., Zhao, R., Xu, Z., Liang, T.: Grey-informed neural network for time-series forecasting., pp. 1–18. arXiv:2403.15027 (2024)

SEDformer: Path Signatures and Transformers to Predict Newborns Movement Symmetry

Philippe Rambaud[1,2](✉), Arpad Rimmel[2], Imen Trabelsi[3], Justine Zini[4,5], Alexandra Wodecki[6,7], Emmanuelle Motte Signoret[5,6,7], François Jouen[3], Joanna Tomasik[2], and Jean Bergounioux[4,6]

[1] SogetiLabs, Capgemini, Paris, France
philippe.rambaud.perso@gmail.com
[2] CNRS, Laboratoire interdisciplinaire des sciences du numérique, Université Paris-Saclay, 91405 Orsay, France
[3] CHArt, EPHE, Université PSL, Paris 8, UPEC, CY, 75014 Paris, France
[4] Université Paris-Saclay, UVSQ, 2IC UMR 1173, AP-HP, CHU Raymond Poincaré, 92380 Garches, France
[5] Neonatal Intensive Care Unit, CHI Poissy St Germain, 78300 Poissy, France
[6] Université Paris-Saclay, UVSQ, UFR Simone Veil Santé, 78180 Montigny le Bretonneux, France
[7] Université Paris-Saclay, UVSQ, INRAE, BREED, 78350 Jouy-en-Josas, France

Abstract. In pediatric healthcare, the accurate prediction of movement symmetry in newborns is crucial as a foundational component for future automated screening systems. The long-term goal is to develop anomaly detection tools that can identify deviations from normal movement patterns by comparing observed data with model predictions. However, achieving this objective first requires robust forecasting models capable of accurately capturing the complex dynamics of typical infant movement. Traditional time series forecasting methods often struggle to capture the complex, non-linear dependencies present in real-world temporal data, particularly in the context of infantile movement patterns. To address these challenges, we introduce the *Signature Enhanced Decomposition Transformer* (SEDformer), which integrates path signatures from rough path theory into the FEDformer architecture by replacing Fourier transforms with signature-based operations. Our experiments demonstrate that SEDformer achieves superior forecasting performance compared to FEDformer on a specialized dataset of infantile movement patterns. While the current study focuses on prediction accuracy evaluation against this baseline model, these results establish the foundation for future anomaly detection applications in early screening of motor development issues.

Keywords: Time series forecasting · Path signatures · Transformers · Infant movement analysis · Healthcare applications

P. Bruno et al. (Eds.): HC_AIxIA_HYDRA 2025, CCIS 2830, pp. 138–151, 2026.
https://doi.org/10.1007/978-3-032-16708-8_13

1 Introduction

1.1 Infant Motricity Symmetry

Monitoring the symmetry of movement in newborns is crucial for early detection of neurodevelopmental disorders. Asymmetries in spontaneous movements can serve as early indicators of conditions such as cerebral palsy (CP) and autism spectrum disorders (ASD) [12].

Traditional approaches rely on expert assessment of movement patterns, which is time-intensive and subject to inter-observer variability. An alternative approach is to develop computational models that learn the characteristics of typical movement patterns from healthy populations, and subsequently detect anomalies by measuring deviations from predicted normal behavior. This anomaly detection paradigm enables automated screening tools that can flag cases requiring professional examination, rather than attempting direct pathological classification.

Early identification of such asymmetries allows for timely interventions, which are essential for improving long-term developmental outcomes. Tools like the General Movement Assessment (GMA) have been validated for predicting early infantile CP, highlighting the importance of assessing movement patterns in high-risk infants [1].

1.2 Challenges in Time Series Forecasting

Time series forecasting is a critical area of research with widespread applications in healthcare, particularly in the context of monitoring infant movement symmetry. Accurate forecasting models enable better decision making, resource allocation, and strategic planning in pediatric healthcare. Traditional methods for time series forecasting, such as AutoRegressive Integrated Moving Average (ARIMA) and exponential smoothing, have been extensively used but often struggle to capture the complex, nonlinear temporal dependencies and long-range correlations present in real-world data [24].

Real-world time-series data on infant movement often exhibit intricate patterns due to factors such as developmental milestones, growth spurts, and individual variability. Capturing these patterns requires models that can handle nonlinearity and long-term dependencies. Traditional statistical models are limited in this regard, and while they perform well on linear and stationary data, their effectiveness diminishes with increasing data complexity and forecasting horizon.

Recent advances in deep learning have introduced Transformer-based architectures, which have shown significant promise in addressing the limitations of traditional models. Transformers, originally developed for natural language processing tasks, utilize self-attention mechanisms to capture long-range dependencies in sequential data. Models like the Informer [25] and the Fourier Enhanced Decomposition Transformer (FEDformer) [27] have adapted Transformers for time-series forecasting. FEDformer, in particular, leverages Fourier transforms to decompose time series data into frequency components, enhancing the model's ability to capture periodic patterns. However, the reliance on Fourier-based techniques may limit the model's capacity to capture nonlinear temporal dependencies and higher-order dynamics, especially in long-term forecasting scenarios.

In the context of infant movement symmetry, these advanced models could provide valuable insights into developmental trajectories, enabling early detection of neurodevelopmental disorders and timely interventions.

1.3 Introduction of Path Signatures

To address the challenges of capturing nonlinear temporal dependencies and higher-order dynamics in infant movement data, we introduce the concept of path signatures from rough path theory [10] into the Transformer architecture. Path signatures provide a powerful mathematical framework for encoding complex, high-dimensional temporal data by capturing the effects of a path up to a certain order. By incorporating path signatures, we aim to model subtle, nonlinear interactions within time series data that are not adequately addressed by traditional Fourier-based methods. This integration allows the model to capture higher-order temporal dynamics, enhancing its ability to understand intricate patterns over extended periods, which is crucial for accurate forecasting and early detection of neurodevelopmental disorders in infants.

1.4 Our Contributions

We introduce SEDformer, an adaptation of FEDformer designed to improve time series forecasting through path signature integration. Our main contributions are:

- SEDformer architecture: integration of path signatures into the FEDformer decomposition framework to capture nonlinear temporal dependencies in infant movement patterns.
- Comparative evaluation against FEDformer on benchmark datasets, demonstrating that SEDformer maintains competitive performance while introducing enhanced mathematical foundations.
- Performance validation on our specialized infant movement dataset, where SEDformer significantly outperforms FEDformer, establishing improved forecasting accuracy as a foundation for future anomaly detection applications.

1.5 Overview

Section 2 describes the datasets used in this study, which include videos of spontaneous motricity in newborns, and the preprocessing steps. Next, we present the SEDformer model in detail, including its theoretical foundations and implementation. Section 4 outlines the evaluation methodology, the experimental setup, and the results obtained. In Sect. 5, we discuss the implications of our findings, the limitations of the study, and potential directions for future research. Finally, we draw conclusions by summarizing the main contributions and emphasizing the significance of SEDformer in advancing time series forecasting.

2 Related Works

2.1 Transformers for Time Series Forecasting

Transformers, initially introduced for natural language processing tasks [21], have been adapted for time series forecasting due to their ability to capture long-range dependencies through self-attention mechanisms. Several Transformer-based models have been developed specifically for time series forecasting, each enhancing different aspects of the original architecture.

Informer [25] introduces a ProbSparse self-attention mechanism to handle long sequences efficiently, making it suitable for long-term forecasting tasks. The Autoformer [22] incorporates a decomposition architecture with auto-correlation mechanisms to better capture periodic patterns and long-term dependencies. The Temporal Fusion Transformer (TFT) [9] enhances interpretability and accuracy in multi-horizon forecasting by integrating gating mechanisms and variable selection networks to handle both static and time-varying covariates. The FEDformer [27] leverages frequency enhanced decomposition techniques, using Fourier and wavelet transforms to capture both global and local temporal patterns.

2.2 Path Signatures in Machine Learning

Path signatures, originating from rough path theory [11], provide a mathematical framework for encoding complex, high-dimensional temporal data through iterated integrals. They offer a unique representation of the evolution of data over time, capturing essential information about the path without redundancy.

Computational tools like the `iisignature` library [15] and `Signatory` [6] have facilitated the integration of path signatures into machine learning pipelines. Applications of path signatures include online character recognition [4], where modeling pen trajectories achieved state-of-the-art results, and physiological signal analysis [23], improving the prediction of patient outcomes.

Integrating path signatures with deep learning models has shown potential in enhancing feature extraction from sequential data. Kidger and Lyons [5] demonstrated that deep signature transforms could capture hierarchical features in time series, improving performance on classification and regression tasks. Perez Arribas and Roberts [13] combined signature kernels with Gaussian processes to scale sparse models on sequential data, achieving improved predictive performance.

Recent work has begun exploring the integration of path signatures with Transformer architectures. SigFormer [19] demonstrates the potential of signature-enhanced Transformers for financial applications, particularly in deep hedging strategies. Similarly, Li et al. [8] employed path signature features within Transformer modules for gesture recognition, showing promising results in sequential pattern recognition tasks. These specialized architectures highlight the potential for signature-Transformer integration, though systematic evaluation across diverse time series forecasting tasks remains limited.

Given this emerging landscape, our approach focuses on adapting the well-established FEDformer architecture [27] to incorporate path signatures. This provides a solid baseline for evaluating signature-enhanced forecasting before systematic comparison with these specialized architectures, which represents an important direction for future comprehensive benchmarking studies.

3 SEDformer

This section will cover the motivation for using FEDformer as the baseline model, the rationale for incorporating path signatures, and how the Frequency Enhanced Block (FEB) and Frequency Enhanced Attention (FEA) blocks have been adapted to leverage these signatures. A complete illustration of SEDformer is depicted in Fig. 1. For more detailed information concerning global architecture or Mixture-of-Experts Decomposition blocks, refer to the original FEDformer article [26].

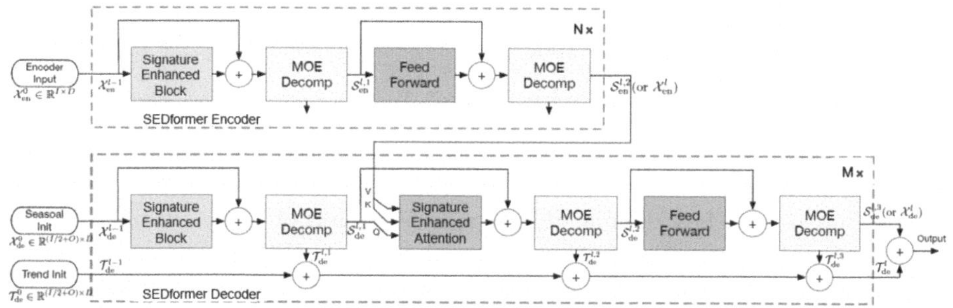

Fig. 1. SEDformer Structure. The SEDformer (a variation of FEDformer) consists of N encoders and M decoders. The Signature Enhanced Block (SEB, green blocks) and Signature Enhanced Attention (SEA, red blocks) are used to perform representation learning in the signature domain. The Mixture Of Experts Decomposition Blocks (MOEDecomp, yellow blocks) are used to extract seasonal-trend patterns from the input data. (Color figure online)

3.1 Motivation for Using FEDformer as Baseline

FEDformer is a state-of-the-art model for time series forecasting, incorporating Transformer architecture with Fourier decomposition techniques. By decomposing time series data into trend and seasonal components, FEDformer can capture long-term dependencies and recurring patterns, making it highly suitable for applications where periodic variations are essential for analysis. However, while the Fourier transform captures frequency-based patterns effectively, it has limitations when applied to complex, non-linear signals [16].

3.2 Limitations of Fourier Transforms and Motivation for Path Signatures

To overcome the limitations of Fourier-based frequency analysis, we incorporate path signatures—a mathematical tool from rough path theory—into the model. Path signatures provide a rich, non-linear description of sequential data by encoding higher-order interactions and capturing the geometric properties of a path. For a path $\gamma : [0, T] \to \mathbb{R}^d$, the path signature of order n is given by:

$$S^n(\gamma) = \int_{0 \leq t_1 \leq \cdots \leq t_n \leq T} d\gamma(t_1) \otimes \cdots \otimes d\gamma(t_n),$$

where this iterated integral encodes the interactions up to the n-th order. In practice, the signature is often truncated at order N, producing the truncated signature series:

$$S(\gamma) = \left(1, S^1(\gamma), S^2(\gamma), \ldots, S^N(\gamma)\right).$$

This representation captures the temporal ordering and higher-order dependencies, providing a richer feature set for complex signals, where both frequency and structural order are essential.

3.3 Signature Enhanced Block (SEB)

The Signature Enhanced Block (SEB) is a key component of SEDformer (green blocks in Fig. 1), designed to replace the Fast Fourier Transform (FFT) blocks used in FEDformer. The SEB transforms the input data using path signatures to capture non-linear temporal dependencies and complex patterns within the data. The steps of the SEB are:

1. **Linear Projection**: The input time series data $\mathbf{x} \in \mathbb{R}^{N \times D}$ is first linearly projected using a weight matrix $\mathbf{w} \in \mathbb{R}^{D \times D}$, resulting in $\mathbf{q} = \mathbf{x} \cdot \mathbf{w}$.
2. **Signature Transform**: The projected data $\mathbf{q}$ is transformed using path signatures computed via the Signatory library [6]. Each sequence in $\mathbf{q}$ is treated as a discrete path, and the signature transform captures its higher-order geometric features, resulting in $\mathbf{S} \in \mathbb{R}^{N \times M}$ where M represents the signature dimension determined by the truncation depth.
3. **Weight Matrix Application**: The signature matrix $\mathbf{S}$ is processed using a parameterized weight matrix $\mathbf{R} \in \mathbb{R}^{M \times M}$. The production operator $\odot$ is defined as:

$$\mathbf{Y}_{m,d_o} = \sum_{d_i=0}^{M} \mathbf{S}_{m,d_i} \cdot \mathbf{R}_{d_i,d_o}.$$

   where d_i and d_o are the input and output dimensions, respectively.
4. **Inverse Signature Transform**: The result $\mathbf{Y}$ is transformed back using the inverse signature transform, which reconstructs a path from its signature representation. We employ the insertion method [3] originally introduced by

Chang and Lyons [2], which solves a linear optimization problem to approximate the path derivatives. This method reconstructs a piecewise linear path with depth + 1 points that approximates the original sequence the signature was computed from.

3.4 Signature Enhanced Attention (SEA)

The Signature Enhanced Attention (SEA) mechanism is an extension of the attention mechanism used in FEDformer (red blocks in Fig. 1). In SEA, the input data is first transformed using path signatures before applying the attention mechanism. This transformation allows SEA to capture richer and more complex interactions between different parts of the time series data.

The process involves the following steps:

1. **Queries, Keys, and Values**: The input queries $\mathbf{q}$, keys $\mathbf{k}$, and values $\mathbf{v}$ are obtained from the decoder and encoder, respectively. These are defined as:

$$\mathbf{q} = \mathbf{x}_{en} \cdot \mathbf{w}_q, \quad \mathbf{k} = \mathbf{x}_{de} \cdot \mathbf{w}_k, \quad \mathbf{v} = \mathbf{x}_{de} \cdot \mathbf{w}_v,$$

   where $\mathbf{w}_q, \mathbf{w}_k, \mathbf{w}_v \in \mathbb{R}^{D \times D}$.
2. **Signature Transform**: The queries, keys, and values are transformed using path signatures as described above, resulting in signature representations $\tilde{\mathbf{Q}}, \tilde{\mathbf{K}}, \tilde{\mathbf{V}} \in \mathbb{R}^{L \times M}$ that encode higher-order interactions within each sequence.
3. **Attention Mechanism**: The signature-enhanced attention mechanism is then applied as:

$$\text{SEA}(\mathbf{q}, \mathbf{k}, \mathbf{v}) = \text{InverseSignature}(\sigma(\tilde{\mathbf{Q}} \cdot \tilde{\mathbf{K}}^\top) \cdot \tilde{\mathbf{V}}),$$

   where σ is the activation function, which can be either softmax or tanh.
4. **Inverse Signature Transform**: The attention result is transformed back using the inverse signature transform via the insertion method [3], reconstructing the attended sequence from its signature representation.

4 Material and Method

4.1 AiMotherNeo Dataset

To present the clinical application of our model, we introduce the AiMotherNeo dataset. Designed to address a specific clinical need, this dataset consists of videos capturing the spontaneous motor activity of newborns and infants. Although distinct from the BabyGarches dataset mentioned in previous work [14], AiMotherNeo shares similar characteristics, such as the use of video recordings and a focus on spontaneous motricity. Importantly, AiMotherNeo comprises entirely new video data, specifically tailored to evaluate and demonstrate the capabilities of our model in a clinical context.

The dataset includes 91 videos with an average duration of 1 min and 54 s, capturing the spontaneous motor activity of newborns in their first days of life. The data were collected between September and December 2024, with videos recorded at a frame rate of 15 frames per second. Pose estimation is performed using a dedicated method based on AlphaPose [18] to obtain the coordinates of 12 body joints. These values are normalized between -1 and 1, with the center of the body serving as the origin. Figure 2 illustrates an example of pose estimation applied to a newborn.

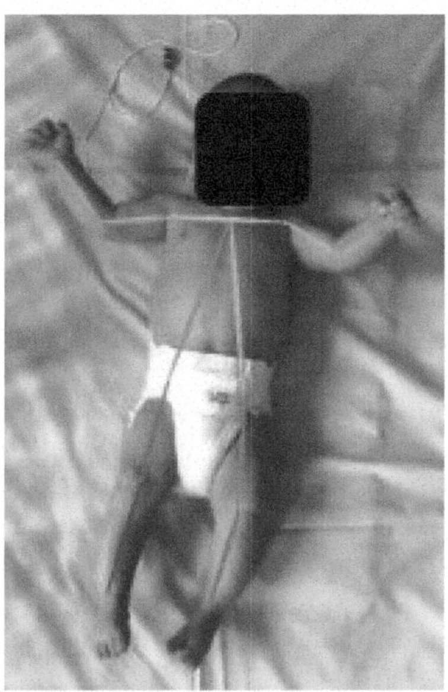

Fig. 2. Example output from the infant-adapted pose estimation model. The detected joints are displayed as a skeleton overlaid on the input image.

We then measure the quantity of displacement for each joint from one frame to the next to assess upper/lower and left/right symmetry. For each frame, we derive 26 values: 12 joints with x and y coordinates, and the corresponding symmetry values for upper/lower and left/right symmetry. This dataset provides a rich source of information for evaluating the performance of our SEDformer model in predicting movement symmetry in infants, highlighting its potential for early detection of motor development issues.

4.2 Evaluation Process

Firstly, we evaluated SEDformer against FEDformer on our specialized clinical dataset, AiMotherNeo. We performed 10 runs with 5-fold cross-validation stratified by patients to ensure robustness and prevent temporal data leakage.

This stratification ensures that each fold contains videos from different patients, preventing the model from learning patient-specific patterns that could lead to overly optimistic performance estimates. For this evaluation, we used an input length of 60 time steps (equivalent to 4 s) and a prediction horizon of 15 time steps (equivalent to 1 s). Given the limited size of our clinical dataset, we opted for robust cross-validation rather than maintaining a separate test set. This approach maximizes the available training data while providing reliable performance estimates through multiple validation folds. The prediction horizon of 1 s was chosen as technically sufficient for capturing movement deviations rather than being driven by specific clinical requirements. Hyperparameter tuning was conducted to select the optimal parameters for each model. Additionally, early stopping was implemented to halt training once the model's performance on the validation set ceased to improve, ensuring efficient training and preventing overfitting. The performance was quantified using MSE.

Secondly, to assess the generalizability of the proposed SEDformer model beyond its specialized clinical application, we conducted a comprehensive comparison against the FEDformer model. This evaluation aimed to determine whether SEDformer, while optimized for a specific clinical use case, maintains robust performance across a broader range of scenarios. We used the same datasets and experimental protocols as in the original FEDformer study, including six publicly available multivariate time series datasets—ETTm2 [25], Exchange [7], Traffic [17], Electricity [20], Weather[1], and ILI[2]—to ensure a consistent benchmarking scenario. By replicating the original benchmark settings of FEDformer, we compared SEDformer's accuracy at the established prediction horizons. Standard evaluation metrics such as Mean Squared Error (MSE) and Mean Absolute Error (MAE) were used to quantify the performance gains of SEDformer over FEDformer, demonstrating its versatility and effectiveness in diverse contexts.

4.3 Computational Resources and Training Setup

The training of the SEDformer model was conducted on a cluster of 4 GPUs (NVIDIA Tesla V100 with 32 GiB of RAM). The implementation was based on the original FEDformer code, written in PyTorch. Additionally, we used the Signatory library to compute the path signatures and make them exploitable on the GPU. This setup ensured efficient and scalable computation of path signatures, crucial for capturing non-linear interactions within the time series data.

5 Results

In Fig. 3, the validation linear and logarithmic loss curves for SEDformer, FEDformer-f, and FEDformer-w over 40 epochs are presented on AiMother-Neo dataset. The final mean validation loss values are: SEDformer achieved a

[1] https://www.bgc-jena.mpg.de/wetter/.

[2] https://gis.cdc.gov/grasp/fluview/fluportaldashboard.html.

mean validation loss of 0.148 ± 0.21, FEDformer-f achieved 0.297 ± 0.34, and FEDformer-w achieved 0.288 ± 0.33. The shaded areas in the figures represent the 95% confidence interval across multiple runs and cross-validation folds.

SEDformer consistently demonstrated superior performance compared to both FEDformer-f and FEDformer-w, as evidenced by the lower validation loss values. This indicates that the integration of path signatures into the FEDformer architecture enhances the model's ability to capture complex temporal dependencies and non-linear dynamics in the clinical dataset. The results highlight the potential of SEDformer for accurate and reliable movement symmetry prediction in pediatric healthcare applications.

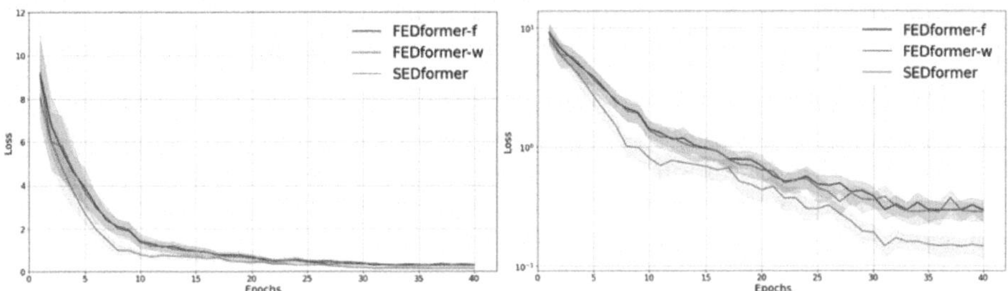

Fig. 3. Validation loss curves for SEDformer (green), FEDformer-f (blue), and FEDformer-w (orange) over 40 epochs on the AiMotherNeo dataset. The curves are presented on both a linear and a logarithmic scale. The final mean validation loss values are: SEDformer (0.148 ± 0.21), FEDformer-f (0.297 ± 0.34), and FEDformer-w (0.288 ± 0.33). The shaded areas represent the 95% confidence interval across 10 runs and 5 cross-validation folds. (Color figure online)

In Table 1, we replicate the benchmark setting used by FEDformer to evaluate the general performance of SEDformer across various datasets and prediction horizons. This evaluation aims to demonstrate that, while SEDformer is designed for a specific clinical application, it maintains competitive accuracy in broader contexts, considering the same input lengths and prediction horizons as in the original FEDformer paper. In the original benchmark setting (Table 1), SEDformer performs on par with both FEDformer-f and FEDformer-w. This similarity across multiple datasets and prediction lengths demonstrates that incorporating path signatures does not compromise accuracy. For example, on the Exchange dataset at a prediction length of 96, SEDformer achieves an MSE of 0.147, closely aligning with FEDformer-f (0.148) and FEDformer-w (0.139). Similar trends are observed for intermediate horizons on Traffic, Electricity, and Weather, reinforcing that SEDformer remains comparable to the state-of-the-art FEDformer variants under standard benchmark conditions.

In conclusion, SEDformer demonstrates strong performance in our specialized clinical application for predicting movement symmetry, significantly outperforming FEDformer. This highlights its enhanced capability to handle complex,

Table 1. Multivariate long-term series forecasting results on six datasets with input length $I = 96$ and prediction length $O \in \{96, 192, 336, 720\}$. For the ILI dataset, we use input length $I = 36$ and prediction length $O \in \{24, 36, 48, 60\}$. For the sake of clarity, we do not report standard deviations (no significant differences were observed). A lower MSE indicates better performance, and the best results are highlighted in bold.

Methods	Metric	ETTm2				Exchange				Traffic				Electricity				Weather				ILI			
		96	192	336	720	96	192	336	720	96	192	336	720	96	192	336	720	96	192	336	720	24	36	48	60
FEDformer-f	MSE	**0.203**	**0.269**	**0.325**	**0.421**	0.148	0.271	0.460	1.195	0.587	0.604	0.621	0.626	0.193	0.201	0.214	0.246	**0.217**	**0.276**	**0.339**	**0.403**	3.228	2.679	2.622	2.857
	MAE	**0.287**	**0.328**	**0.366**	**0.415**	0.278	0.380	0.500	0.841	0.366	0.373	0.383	0.382	0.308	0.315	0.329	0.355	0.396	0.336	**0.380**	**0.428**	1.260	1.080	1.078	1.157
FEDformer-w	MSE	0.204	0.316	0.359	0.433	**0.139**	**0.256**	**0.426**	1.090	**0.562**	**0.562**	**0.570**	**0.596**	**0.183**	**0.195**	**0.212**	**0.231**	0.227	0.295	0.381	0.424	**2.203**	**2.272**	**2.209**	2.545
	MAE	0.288	0.363	0.387	0.423	0.276	**0.369**	**0.464**	0.800	**0.349**	**0.346**	**0.323**	**0.368**	**0.297**	**0.308**	0.313	0.343	**0.304**	0.363	0.416	0.434	**0.963**	**0.976**	**0.981**	**1.061**
SEDformer (**our**)	MSE	0.243	0.331	0.368	0.436	0.147	0.268	0.453	**1.188**	0.591	0.603	0.624	0.631	0.187	0.196	0.214	0.237	0.231	0.284	0.353	0.409	2.455	2.476	2.471	**2.521**
	MAE	0.301	0.377	0.394	0.425	**0.272**	0.371	0.483	**0.789**	0.371	0.381	0.384	0.383	0.299	0.311	**0.312**	**0.339**	0.309	**0.334**	0.3391	0.443	1.117	1.132	1.140	1.139

non-stationary data, making it particularly well-suited for improving predictive accuracy in clinical settings. Furthermore, SEDformer maintains robust performance on the original benchmark datasets, matching the accuracy of FEDformer. This indicates that the integration of path signatures does not compromise its effectiveness in broader applications, ensuring reliability across diverse scenarios. Thus, SEDformer paves the way for more effective and personalized healthcare interventions while remaining a versatile tool for general time series forecasting.

6 Conclusion

We introduced SEDformer, a Transformer-based model integrating path signatures to enhance time series forecasting capabilities for clinical applications. By leveraging the mathematical framework of path signatures alongside the frequency decomposition strengths of FEDformer, SEDformer demonstrated superior ability to capture complex temporal dependencies in infant movement data. Our experiments showed that SEDformer maintains comparable performance to FEDformer on standard benchmark datasets while slightly outperforming it on our specialized clinical dataset of infant movement patterns.

The enhanced forecasting accuracy achieved by SEDformer on infant movement data establishes a crucial foundation for future anomaly detection applications in pediatric healthcare. By accurately modeling normal movement patterns, the improved predictions enable more sensitive detection of deviations that may indicate motor development issues. This represents a critical step toward automated screening tools that can flag cases requiring professional examination, potentially enabling earlier interventions in neurodevelopmental disorders.

The successful integration of path signatures into the FEDformer architecture demonstrates the potential of advanced mathematical frameworks to enhance deep learning models for healthcare applications. While this study focused on forecasting evaluation, the superior performance on clinical data validates the approach as a stepping stone toward comprehensive anomaly detection systems for pediatric motor assessment.

7 Future Works

While SEDformer shows promising results in modeling complex temporal dependencies, several future research directions remain. The primary next step involves developing the complete anomaly detection pipeline that leverages SEDformer's enhanced forecasting capabilities, including threshold mechanisms for identifying deviations from predicted normal behavior and establishing clinical workflows for professional review of flagged cases.

A critical technical direction is comprehensive comparison with the broader state-of-the-art in time series forecasting, particularly other approaches that integrate path signatures within Transformer architectures. While our current evaluation against FEDformer provides a solid baseline, systematic benchmarking against specialized signature-based neural networks and alternative signature-enhanced Transformer variants will better position our contribution within the evolving landscape of signature-based deep learning.

One avenue is to optimize the use of path signatures, such as employing adaptive signature truncation methods to enhance computational efficiency and model interpretability. Additionally, extending the application of SEDformer to other clinical datasets, different types of movement data, and broader motor indicators such as movement variability and temporal coordination patterns could provide comprehensive motor development screening capabilities.

Future clinical validation across multiple sites and diverse populations will be essential for translating these forecasting improvements into clinically validated tools for early detection and intervention in infant motor development disorders.

Acknowledgments. The authors would like to thank the team from the maternity ward of CHI Poissy-St-Germain-en-Laye (France) for the dedication to collect the data: L. Bertheleu, A. Carpentier, M. Duval, K. Guerbert, M. Guerin, K. Lafferrere, N. Liege, C. Mateu, M. Renoncourt. Also, this research was supported by Axa Mécénat Insurance Mutuals.

Disclosure of Interests. The authors have no competing interests to declare that are relevant to the content of this article.

References

1. Battisti, O., et al.: Interests of observing archaic reflexes and general movements in newborns and infants. Case Rep. **7**(4), 1–8 (2014)
2. Chang, J., Lyons, T.: Insertion algorithm for inverting the signature of a path. arXiv preprint arXiv:1907.08423 (2019)
3. Fermanian, A., Chang, J., Lyons, T., Biau, G.: The insertion method to invert the signature of a path. arXiv preprint arXiv:2304.01862 (2023)
4. Graham, B.: Sparse arrays of signatures for online character recognition. arXiv preprint arXiv:1308.0371 (2013)
5. Kidger, P., Lyons, T.: Deep signatures. In: Advances in Neural Information Processing Systems, vol. 33, pp. 3099–3110 (2020)

6. Kidger, P., Lyons, T.: Signatory: Differentiable computations of the signature and logsignature transforms. arXiv preprint arXiv:2001.00706 (2020)
7. Lai, G., Chang, W.C., Yang, Y., Liu, H.: Modeling long-and short-term temporal patterns with deep neural networks. In: The 41st international ACM SIGIR conference on research and development in information retrieval, pp. 95–104 (2018)
8. Li, C., Zhang, X., Liao, L., Jin, L., Yang, W.: Skeleton-based gesture recognition using several fully connected layers with path signature features and temporal transformer module. In: Proceedings of the AAAI conference on artificial intelligence, vol. 33, pp. 8585–8592 (2019)
9. Lim, B., Murena, P.A., Salimbeni, H.: Temporal fusion transformers for interpretable multi-horizon time series forecasting. Int. J. Forecasting (2021). https://www.sciencedirect.com/science/article/pii/S0169207021000762
10. Lyons, T.: Rough paths, signatures and the modeling of functions on streams. In: Proceedings of the International Congress of Mathematicians (ICM), vol. 1, pp. 163–184. Korean Mathematical Society (2014). https://arxiv.org/abs/1405.4537
11. Lyons, T.: Rough paths, signatures and the modeling of functions on streams. In: Proceedings of the International Congress of Mathematicians, vol. 1, pp. 163–184 (2014)
12. Menier, I., Soulier: Warning signs and identification of motor abnormalities in infants in early life. Kinésithérapie, la Revue 558, 13–20 (2014). https://michele-forestier.fr/wp-content/uploads/2022/04/Anomalies-motrices-du-nouveau-ne
13. Arribas, P.I., Roberts, S.: SigGPDE: Scaling sparse gaussian processes on sequential data. arXiv preprint arXiv:2006.07238 (2020)
14. Rambaud, P., et al.: Binary classification vs. anomaly detection on imbalanced tabular medical datasets. In: 2023 Congress in Computer Science, Computer Engineering and Applied Computing (CSCE), pp. 01–05. IEEE (2023)
15. Reizenstein, J., Graham, B.: The `iisignature` library: Efficient calculation of iterated-integral signatures and log signatures. arXiv preprint arXiv:1802.08252 (2018)
16. Sifuzzaman, M., Islam, M.R., Ali, M.Z.: Application of wavelet transform and its advantages compared to fourier transform (2009)
17. Song, C., Lin, Y., Guo, S., Wan, H.: Spatial-temporal synchronous graph convolutional networks: a new framework for spatial-temporal network data forecasting. In: Proceedings of the AAAI conference on artificial intelligence, vol. 34, pp. 914–921 (2020)
18. Taleb, A., et al.: Improve pose estimation model performance with unlabeled data. In: 2023 Congress in Computer Science, Computer Engineering and Applied Computing (CSCE), pp. 1316–1321. IEEE (2023)
19. Tong, A., Cuchiero, C., Lee, J., Salvi, C., Teichmann, J.: Sigformer: Signature transformers for deep hedging. In: Proceedings of the Fourth ACM International Conference on AI in Finance, pp. 462–470 (2023)
20. Trindade, A.: Electricityloaddiagrams20112014, UCI machine learning repository (2015). https://doi.org/10.24432/C58C86
21. Vaswani, A., et al.: Attention is all you need. In: Advances in Neural Information Processing Systems, vol. 30, pp. 5998–6008 (2017)
22. Wu, N., Zhou, H., Zhang, S., Bao, J.: Autoformer: Decomposition transformers with auto-correlation for long-term series forecasting. arXiv preprint arXiv:2106.13008 (2021). https://arxiv.org/abs/2106.13008
23. Yang, W., Lyons, T., Ni, H.: Leveraging the path signature framework in healthcare analytics. In: Proceedings of the Machine Learning for Healthcare Conference, pp. 143–156 (2017)

24. Zhang, G.P.: Time series forecasting using a hybrid arima and neural network model. Neurocomputing **50**, 159–175 (2003)
25. Zhou, H., et al.: Informer: Beyond efficient transformer for long sequence time-series forecasting. AAAI (2021). https://arxiv.org/abs/2012.07436
26. Zhou, T., et al.: FEDformer: Frequency enhanced decomposed transformer for long-term series forecasting. In: Proceedings of the 39th International Conference on Machine Learning, pp. 27268–27286. PMLR (2022). https://arxiv.org/abs/2201.12740
27. Zhou, T., et al.: FEDformer: Frequency enhanced decomposed transformer for long-term series forecasting. In: Proceedings of the 39th International Conference on Machine Learning, pp. 27268–27286 (2022)

LLM-Assisted Conformance Checking for Medical Processes

Giorgio Leonardi, Stefania Montani(✉), and Manuel Striani

Computer Science Institute, DISIT, University of Piemonte Orientale, Alessandria, Italy
{giorgio.leonardi,stefania.montani,manuel.striani}@uniupo.it

Abstract. Clinical guidelines serve as normative process models for healthcare organizations but are often presented in unstructured, textual formats. This lack of formalization hinders the use of traditional conformance checking algorithms, which require structured, machine-readable process descriptions. In this study, we address this challenge by: (i) employing a Large Language Model (LLM) to extract normative rules from textual guidelines; (ii) assessing and quantifying the conformance of patient event logs to these rules; and (iii) using this framework to evaluate the quality of process models generated by various process discovery algorithms, based on their conformance to the extracted rules. In the paper, we present the approach, which represents the first step of a larger and more ambitious project, and its first results in the domain of stroke care.

Keywords: Process Mining · Large Language Models · Conformance checking · Medical Applications

1 Introduction

Conformance checking is a core task in Process Mining [3], aimed at verifying whether an organization's actual behavior aligns with its normative processes. The actual behavior is recorded in the event log, a set of process traces [26] capturing the activities performed during daily operations, each with a time stamp. In healthcare, a trace corresponds to the ordered sequence of activities executed for a patient during hospital stay. In the medical context, normative behavior is typically specified by a clinical guideline.

Conformance checking algorithms require both an event log and a formal, machine-interpretable representation of the normative process—often a graphical control-flow model in a dedicated modeling language, convertible into a Petri Net [12]. However, such formalizations are seldom available in healthcare, where clinical guidelines are expressed as lengthy, complex natural-language documents. While approaches exist for creating Computer Interpretable Guidelines (CIGs) [11], they demand substantial knowledge acquisition effort.

P. Bruno et al. (Eds.): HC_AIxIA_HYDRA 2025, CCIS 2830, pp. 152–163, 2026.
https://doi.org/10.1007/978-3-032-16708-8_14

In this work, we propose a Large Language Model (LLM)-assisted approach for supporting medical conformance checking by verifying patient traces without requiring a CIG.

Specifically, our contributions are:

1. Using an LLM to extract normative behaviors from a textual guideline, and formalize them into executable rules;
2. Assessing patient trace conformance to these rules by computing the *Trace Conformance Indicator* ($\mathcal{TCI}$), a measure[1] which quantifies the percentage of log traces satisfying the rules;
3. Leveraging the approach to evaluate process discovery algorithms [3], first by mining a process model from the event log through the algorithm under evaluation, and then by assessing its compliance by introducing the *Path Conformance Indicator* ($\mathcal{PCI}$), a measure which quantifies the percentage of model paths satisfying the rules.

$\mathcal{TCI}$ allows physicians and administrators to quickly identify compliance issues or bottlenecks in a real world event log. $\mathcal{PCI}$ offers a new criterion for comparing process discovery algorithms, complementing existing measures [10]: according to this dimension, the best-performing miner is the one whose $\mathcal{PCI}$ is closest to the $\mathcal{TCI}$ for the same log, indicating alignment between the model and the underlying log data with respect to normative rules.

We show some first results of our approach in the stroke care domain, verifying hospital compliance to the normative indications, and assessing different process mining algorithms.

It is worth mentioning that this work is just a first step towards the realization of a larger and more ambitious project, as discussed in more detail the concluding section.

2 Related Works

In process mining literature (see, e.g., [14]), conformance checking methods fall into three main categories: *log replay algorithms*, *trace alignment algorithms*, and *constraint-based conformance checking*. *Log replay algorithms* re-execute each event log trace on the given normative model. If the model is a Petri Net, a token-based technique [29] is applied, where extra tokens are generated to bypass dead ends and complete the replay; conformance is then evaluated based on the number of superfluous tokens. More generally, when the model is not a Petri Net, the fitness [23] (i.e., the ratio of replayable traces to the total number of traces) provides a conformance measure. *Trace alignment algorithms* detect deviations at the activity level, identifying asynchronous moves where the trace and model cannot proceed in sync. Each such move is assigned a cost, and an optimal alignment minimizing this cost is computed [5]. This method offers higher precision than log replay but is more computationally intensive, as the

[1] similar to what is called "support" in pattern mining.

number of possible alignments grows quickly with large logs. *Constraint-based conformance checking* (e.g., [9]) expresses process logic as rules and verifies trace compliance with them. Our approach belongs to this family, with the notable distinction that, to our knowledge, no prior work in this area uses an LLM to extract rules from a free-text normative model.

Large Language Models (LLMs) such as BERT [13] and OpenAI GPT-5 *Thinking* [24] have greatly advanced NLP capabilities [20], enabling new applications in process mining. The survey in [6] summarizes recent uses of LLMs in this field. LLMs have been employed to generate natural language descriptions from event logs or process models [7,21], and even from visual representations like dotted charts [25]. Techniques such as abstraction [7] and advanced prompt engineering [21] have been adopted to help users better understand processes. They have also been used to answer natural language queries for process analysis, such as identifying performance bottlenecks or fairness issues [25]. Another application is process model extraction from textual documents, enhanced with prompt engineering, error handling, and code generation [22]. In [17], LLMs are applied to mine imperative or declarative process models from text and to assess process suitability for robotic automation—surpassing earlier NLP methods limited to specific tasks. Interactive refinement of generated models is also supported in [22]. LLMs have additionally been used for SQL query generation to filter or analyze event logs stored in databases [19]. Note that, with respect to declarative process mining, our goal is more specific and narrower: we do not aim at mining an entire process model in the declarative form, and also the knowledge acquisition effort is smaller. Moreover, only the paper in [7] has addressed conformance checking, but results for medical data were unsatisfactory, and no method for extracting rules from domain knowledge was provided.

3 LLM-Assisted Conformance Checking

The system, implemented in Python v3.12.3 leveraging the PM4Py library [8], and integrating OpenAI's GPT-5 *Thinking* API[2] [24] along with the Anthropic's Claude AI Opus 4.1 for coding[3], works as illustrated in Fig. 1:

1. *Rule Detection*: The clinical guideline, provided as natural language text, is processed by a Python module that sends an HTTP-REST request to the GPT-5 *Thinking* API. The LLM extracts candidate rules in natural language.
2. *Rule Checking*: A domain expert reviews the extracted rules, validating them against medical knowledge.
3. *Rule Formalization*: The validated rules, together with an example trace from the event log, are passed to the Anthropic's Claude Opus 4.1 model (optimized for code generation), which converts them into executable Python scripts.
4. *Trace Conformance Checking*: The event log is evaluated against the formalized rules, computing the $\mathcal{TCI}$ (percentage of compliant traces for each rule).

[2] https://platform.openai.com/docs/api-reference/introduction.

[3] https://www.anthropic.com/solutions/coding.

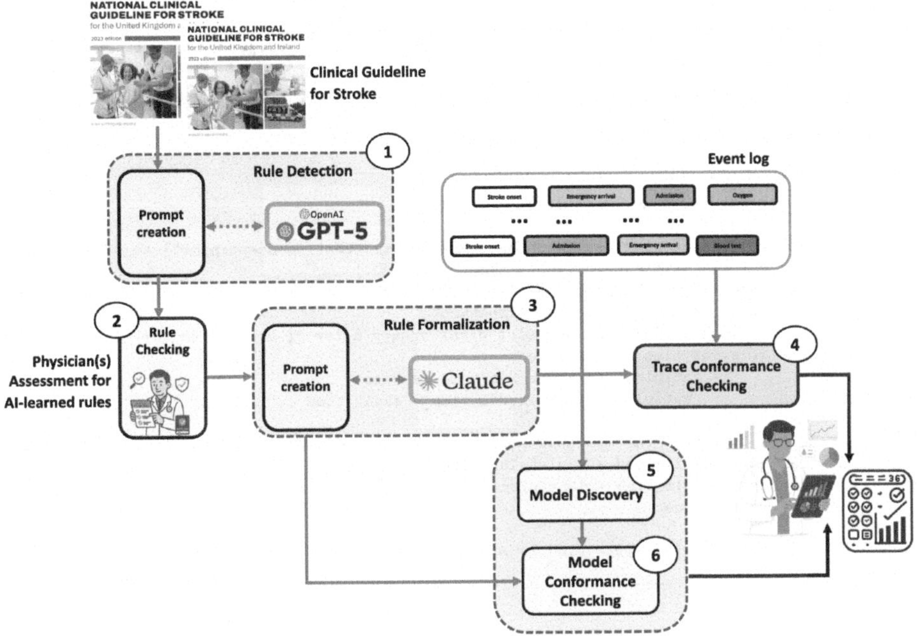

Fig. 1. Tool architecture (circled numbers indicate workflow steps).

5. *Model Discovery*: Various process discovery algorithms (e.g., Heuristic Miner [30]) are applied to the event log, producing Petri Net models.
6. *Model Conformance Checking*: Each discovered model is checked against the rules to compute the $\mathcal{PCI}$ (percentage of compliant paths). The model whose $\mathcal{PCI}$ is closest to the $\mathcal{TCI}$ from step 4 is considered the most aligned with the normative behavior.

In Trace Conformance Checking (step 4), we begin by identifying an *anchor activity* (typically, the diagnostic or therapeutic procedure at hand) explicitly mentioned in the rule. For example, consider **Rule 1** (see Sect. 4 for more details), which states that patients treated with thrombolysis should undergo antiplatelet therapy after 24 h. Here, the anchor activity is thrombolysis, a key, life-saving treatment procedure. Rules may include additional activities and temporal constraints (as in this example), but the anchor activity determines the relevant scope: in this example, only traces containing thrombolysis are evaluated, while all others are excluded. After identifying all traces containing the anchor activity at hand, these traces are collected into a set, and the $\mathcal{TCI}$ is calculated as the percentage of traces in this set that fulfill the given rule. Figure 2 shows the Python implementation, automatically generated by the Anthropic's Claude Opus 4.1 model (step 3), for checking **Rule 1**.

In the Model Conformance Checking step (step 6), the models under analysis are represented as Petri Nets, a well-established and extensively studied process

```
1  import pm4py
2  from datetime import datetime, timedelta
3  from pm4py.objects.log.importer.xes import importer as xes_importer
4
5  # Rule: IF thrombolysis before (Antiplatelet after 24 hours) THEN compliance
6  def rule_1_compliance(trace):
7      thrombolysis_time = None
8      antiplatelet_after_24h_time = None
9
10     # find thrombolysis and antiplatelet events
11     for event in trace:
12         if event["concept:name"] == "thrombolysis" or event["concept:name"] == "TPA":
13             thrombolysis_time = event["time:timestamp"]
14         elif event["concept:name"] == "antiplatelet":
15             event_time = event["time:timestamp"]
16             # Check if this antiplatelet event occurs after 24 hours from thrombolysis
17             if event_time is not None:
18                 if antiplatelet_after_24h_time is None:
19                     antiplatelet_after_24h_time = event_time
20
21     # Check compliance: thrombolysis must occur before antiplatelet (that occurs after 24h)
22     if thrombolysis_time and antiplatelet_after_24h_time:
23         if thrombolysis_time < (antiplatelet_after_24h_time + (timedelta(hours=24))):
24             return True
25
26     # If no antiplatelet after 24h, or no thrombolysis, rule doesn't apply
27     return False
```

Fig. 2. Python code generated with Anthropic's Claude Opus 4.1 for **Rule 1**.

modeling language capable of representing concurrency. Petri Nets combine an intuitive graphical notation with formal execution semantics, enabling the application of numerous analysis techniques [4,18,27]. As in the previous case, the first move is to locate all paths in the process model that include the anchor activity specified in the rule, which determines the scope of the check. To identify these paths while respecting Petri Net semantics, we perform an unfolding step to generate an occurrence net—a structure without cycles, self-conflicts, or backward conflicts. Following [15], we construct a finite prefix of the unfolding that fully captures all reachable states. We then traverse this occurrence net to collect the set of paths to be considered. The $\mathcal{PCI}$, which represents the percentage of paths within the set that comply with a given rule, is then calculated. To carry out this computation, we utilize a method[4] provided by the open-source Python library PM4Py [8], which enriches the process model with temporal performance data. This data, aggregated as an average, is derived through trace replay. Consequently, the enhanced model indicates the mean traversal times along each path segment, which is essential for checking whether rules with temporal constraints are fulfilled by the path under analysis. It is important to highlight that during the model conformance checking phase, the exploration of the process model may reveal paths that do not appear in any of the actual recorded traces. This outcome is anticipated and, to some extent, beneficial. In fact, real-world processes rarely have event logs that capture every possible execution scenario,

[4] https://pm4py-source.readthedocs.io/en/latest/pm4py.objects.petri.html.

making it necessary for the process model to generalize beyond the observed behavior. This generalization allows the model to represent more behaviors than those explicitly documented in the event log. Nevertheless, the extent of this generalization depends solely on the process mining algorithm used [2], and is independent of our conformance checking method.

4 Experiments

We performed our experiments within the domain of stroke management, as a first step of a larger applicative project. Stroke is a critical medical condition characterized by insufficient blood flow to the brain, which can result in cell death. This may occur due to ischemia—caused by thrombosis or embolism leading to a lack of glucose and oxygen—or due to hemorrhage. Consequently, the patient's life is endangered during the acute phase, and stroke survivors often face serious complications that can cause permanent disability. Stroke is the leading cause of adult disability in both the United States and Europe, and ranks as the second leading cause of death globally.

In line with step 1 of our architecture, in this first experiment we queried OpenAI's GPT-5 *Thinking* using the natural language prompt: "Extract and formalize rules from $< text >$ by using if-then semantics", where $< text >$ corresponds to the emergency phase management section of a recently published stroke clinical guideline [1]. This aligns with the "direct provision of insights" paradigm described in [6]. The emergency phase section of the guideline contains 109,905 characters including spaces. OpenAI's GPT-5 *Thinking* produced a set of rules, dealing with initial assessment/diagnostics, or with immediate interventions. All rules are expressed as simple IF-THEN statements, and were easy and fast to check by the human expert. In the following, we will focus on two rules (one referring to immediate interventions, and one referring to initial diagnostics).

Rule 1 is a specific rule referring to thrombolysis, a life-saving procedure and the primary intervention for preserving physical and cognitive functions after stroke. This critical procedure must be administered under specific conditions and must be followed by proper therapies within precise time frames. In particular, **Rule 1** dictates that all patients who underwent thrombolysis must receive antiplatelets after 24 h. The rule thus involves a temporal constraint, and does not refer to all patients, but only to those who were eligible for this treatment; it is also worth noting that not all the hospitals are equipped for thrombolysis.

Rule 2, on the other hand, is very general. It states that all patients affected by stroke should be investigated by means of a CT scan within 3 h from stroke onset: this time, the rule, which involves a temporal constraint as well, applies to all patients, and must be respect at every healthcare center.

In step 2 of our approach (see Fig. 1), our medical collaborator reviewed these rules. The rules were deemed both semantically accurate—faithfully reflecting the medical knowledge in the guideline—and clinically relevant, as their application is necessary for delivering correct and timely patient care. According to the expert, the extracted rules were free from hallucinations or inaccuracies. During the rule formalization phase (step 3 in our architecture), the rules were translated into a computer-interpretable format. Figure 2 shows the Python code for **Rule 1**.

We then analyzed an event log collected from nine different hospitals located in Northern Italy, totaling 313 traces (the relatively small number is justified by the fact that thrombolysis is applied to a minority of patients)[5].

On average, the traces contain 17 activities each (further statistics are reported in Table 1).

Following step 4 of the architecture depicted in Fig. 1, we computed the Trace Conformance Indicator ($\mathcal{TCI}$). Table 2 presents in the first row the average results obtained for **Rule 1** and **Rule 2**, introduced earlier, on the nine hospitals.

Table 1. Statistics on numbers of trace activities

Traces length statistics	
Mean	17
Standard Deviation	3
Minimum	12
Maximum	22

Table 3, on the other hand, shows the $\mathcal{TCI}$ values in two specific hospitals, that we wish to analyse in further detail: as it can be observed, both hospitals operate well on thrombolysis patients, administering antiplatelets on time. Hospital H2, however, experiences significant problems in guaranteeing TC scan within 3 h: this issue may be due to a limited availability of imaging equipment, a fact that often poses an organizational bottleneck. The $\mathcal{TCI}$ value may serve as an actionable insight for hospital administrators, pointing to the need to increase the availability of imaging devices and/or reconsider patient scheduling priorities.

Table 2. Average $\mathcal{TCI}$ and $\mathcal{PCI}$ values on **Rule 1** and **Rule 2** for a set of Italian hospitals. Row 2 shows the $\mathcal{PCI}$ values obtained by Heuristic Miner, while row 3 refers to Inductive Miner

Average values	Rule 1	Rule 2
$\mathcal{TCI}$	95%	95%
$\mathcal{PCI}$ HM	99%	100%
$\mathcal{PCI}$ IM	78%	100%

[5] All data originate from a research project conducted with a group of hospitals in Northern Italy, approved by ethical committees. Data processing ensured the use of a common vocabulary, and of a common structure in event logs. However, due to privacy constraints, patient data cannot be publicly shared.

Table 3. Trace conformance indicator ($\mathcal{TCI}$) on **Rule 1** and **Rule 2** for two different hospitals

Hospital	$\mathcal{TCI}$ **Rule 1**	$\mathcal{TCI}$ **Rule 2**
H1	98%	96%
H2	100%	60%

Subsequent steps of the architecture (Fig. 1) involve generating process models through various discovery algorithms (step 5) and calculating the Path Conformance Indicator ($\mathcal{PCI}$) for each (step 6).

We propose to adopt $\mathcal{PCI}$ as a novel metric (to complement existing measures such as Fitness, Precision, Generalization, and Simplicity [10]) that aids in comparing mining algorithm performance. A $\mathcal{PCI}$ value close to the $\mathcal{TCI}$ measured on the same event log would indicate that the miner preserved much of the event log's ability in respecting the normative behavior.

The following tables present $\mathcal{PCI}$ values for the two rules above, computed on two distinct model sets: the first set (Table 4) contains the models mined using the Heuristic Miner algorithm [30] for the two hospitals we are examining in detail; the second set (Table 5) derives from the Inductive Miner algorithm [16]. The two algorithms were chosen as they are very well known and largely exploited in practice [3]; both were run using default parameters. For ease of comparison, $\mathcal{TCI}$ values are also shown in brackets. The best outcomes - where $\mathcal{PCI}$ closely matches $\mathcal{TCI}$ and outperforms/equals the other miner - are highlighted in bold.

Table 4. Path conformance indicator ($\mathcal{PCI}$) on **Rule 1** and **Rule 2** for two different hospitals models, mined by the Heuristic Miner algorithm.

Hospital	$\mathcal{PCI}$ **vs. (**$\mathcal{TCI}$**) Rule 1**	$\mathcal{PCI}$ **vs. (**$\mathcal{TCI}$**) Rule 2**
H1	**99%** vs. (98%)	**100%** vs. (96%)
H2	**100%** vs. (100%)	**79%** vs. (60%)

Table 5. Path conformance indicator ($\mathcal{PCI}$) on **Rule 1** and **Rule 2** for two different hospitals models, mined by the Inductive Miner algorithm

Hospital	$\mathcal{PCI}$ **vs. (**$\mathcal{TCI}$**) Rule 1**	$\mathcal{PCI}$ **vs. (**$\mathcal{TCI}$**) Rule 2**
H1	95% vs. (98%)	**100%** vs. (96%)
H2	**100%** vs. (100%)	100% vs. (60%)

Based on the $\mathcal{PCI}$ values and their proximity to the $\mathcal{TCI}$, the study on these two hospitals shows that Heuristic Miner is more accurate than Inductive Miner. The same conclusion can be drawn by observing the average results on all the Italian hospitals, shown in Table 2.

Interestingly, Heuristic Miner is recognized for its suitability to handle noisy logs - such as those in medical contexts - and has been already effectively applied in medical process mining [28]. The findings reported in the tables above thus reinforce previous results and offer a positive validation for our study. Of course, a more complete comparison can be conducted considering the other existing evaluation measures, such as, e.g., Fitness [10]. Additional experiments involving such measures, more patient logs and more miners will further evaluate the usefulness of our approach. Looking ahead, in fact, we intend to expand the current tests by considering a larger set of rules and a broader range of mining algorithms. Moreover, we plan to apply this approach across different application domains.

5 Conclusion

In this paper, we have proposed an LLM-assisted method to aid conformance checking in medical process mining. Our contribution is innovative along several dimensions: (i) it employs an LLM to extract normative behaviors from textual clinical guidelines and formalize them into computer-interpretable rules; although this task is relatively straightforward and potentially applicable to other domains, to the best of our knowledge, this is the first approach of its kind in medicine; (ii) it assesses the conformance of patient traces against the extracted rules, quantifying it through the $\mathcal{TCI}$. The $\mathcal{TCI}$ enables evaluation of how closely a hospital's actual behavior aligns with the guideline, offering a quality assessment perspective without requiring a time-consuming formalization of the guideline itself; (iii) it measures the conformance of process models to these rules, providing a new dimension to compare different discovered process models (and thus different mining algorithms) based on their adherence to prescribed normative behavior.

Our experiments within the stroke management domain have shed light on the quality of processes implemented by a set of hospitals in Northern Italy, suggesting that some healthcare centers may face bottlenecks in accessing imaging equipment, which is time critical. Furthermore, our results confirm the strong performance of Heuristic Miner as a process discovery algorithm in this medical context, reinforcing findings previously reported [28].

It is worth mentioning that this work is just a first step towards the realization of a larger project, which will imply a continuous collaboration with medical experts. In particular, we plan to:

- adopt an LLM-assisted approach also to extract patient traces from free text discharge letters, thus significantly enlarging the available event logs;
- extend the rule conformance experiments to the new event logs, and to other sections of the guideline; if these sections produce more complex rules, possibly harder to verify by domain experts, we will consider finer prompting strategies;
- develop an education facility, testing the capability of non-expert physicians in learning the guideline and identifying non-conformant traces with respect

to it, and supporting them through the LLM-assisted approach in case of need.

Last but not least, we plan to explore rule extraction using other LLMs, especially those trained specifically on healthcare data, such as Google's Med-Gemini[6] [31]. We aim to evaluate whether Med-Gemini can extract a greater number of rules, able to better cover guideline indications, to be tested on the extended event logs that will be available in the future.

References

1. National clinical guideline for stroke for the UK and Ireland. London: Intercollegiate stroke working party. https://www.strokeguideline.org, Accessed 08 Apr 2025
2. van der Aalst, W.M.P., et al.: Process mining: a two-step approach to balance between underfitting and overfitting. Softw. Syst. Model. **9**(1), 87–111 (2010)
3. van der Aalst, W.M.P.: Process Mining - Data Science in Action. 2nd edn. Springer (2016). https://doi.org/10.1007/978-3-662-49851-4
4. van der Aalst, W.M.P., Stahl, C.: Modeling Business Processes - A Petri Net-Oriented Approach. Cooperative Information Systems series, MIT Press (2011). http://mitpress.mit.edu/books/modeling-business-processes
5. Adriansyah, A., et al.: Alignment based precision checking. In: Rosa, M.L., Soffer, P. (eds.) Business Process Management Workshops - BPM 2012 International Workshops, Tallinn, Estonia, September 3, 2012. Revised Papers. Lecture Notes in Business Information Processing, vol. 132, pp. 137–149. Springer (2012). https://doi.org/10.1007/978-3-642-36285-9_15
6. Berti, A., Kourani, H., Hafke, H., Li, C.Y., Schuster, D.: Evaluating large language models in process mining: capabilities, benchmarks, and evaluation strategies (2024)
7. Berti, A., Schuster, D., van der Aalst, W.M.P.: Abstractions, scenarios, and prompt definitions for process mining with LLMs: a case study. In: Weerdt, J.D., Pufahl, L. (eds.) Business Process Management Workshops - BPM 2023 International Workshops, Utrecht, The Netherlands, September 11–15, 2023, Revised Selected Papers. Lecture Notes in Business Information Processing, vol. 492, pp. 427–439. Springer (2023). https://doi.org/10.1007/978-3-031-50974-2_32
8. Berti, A., van Zelst, S., Schuster, D.: Pm4py: A process mining library for python. Software Impacts **17**, 100556 (2023). https://doi.org/10.1016/j.simpa.2023.100556, https://www.sciencedirect.com/science/article/pii/S2665963823000933
9. Borrego, D., Barba, I.: Conformance checking and diagnosis for declarative business process models in data-aware scenarios. Expert Syst. Appl. **41**(11), 5340–5352 (2014). https://doi.org/10.1016/J.ESWA.2014.03.010
10. Buijs, J.C.A.M., van Dongen, B.F., van der Aalst, W.M.P.: On the role of fitness, precision, generalization and simplicity in process discovery. In: Meersman, R., et al. (eds.) On the Move to Meaningful Internet Systems: OTM 2012, Confederated International Conferences: CoopIS, DOA-SVI, and ODBASE 2012, Rome, Italy, September 10–14, 2012. Proceedings, Part I, Lecture Notes in Computer Science, vol. 7565, pp. 305–322. Springer (2012). https://doi.org/10.1007/978-3-642-33606-5_19

[6] https://research.google/blog/advancing-medical-ai-with-med-gemini/.

11. de Clercq, P.A., Kaiser, K., Hasman, A.: Computer-interpretable guideline formalisms. In: ten Teije, A., Miksch, S., Lucas, P.J.F. (eds.) Computer-based Medical Guidelines and Protocols: A Primer and Current Trends, Studies in Health Technology and Informatics, vol. 139, pp. 22–43. IOS Press (2008). https://doi.org/10.3233/978-1-58603-873-1-22
12. Desel, J., Reisig, W., Rozenberg, G. (eds.): Lectures on Concurrency and Petri Nets, Advances in Petri Nets [This tutorial volume originates from the 4th Advanced Course on Petri Nets, ACPN 2003, held in Eichstätt, Germany in September 2003. In addition to lectures given at ACPN 2003, additional chapters have been commissioned], Lecture Notes in Computer Science, vol. 3098. Springer (2004). https://doi.org/10.1007/B98282
13. Devlin, J., Chang, M.W., Lee, K., Toutanova, K.: BERT: Pre-training of deep bidirectional transformers for language understanding. In: Burstein, J., Doran, C., Solorio, T. (eds.) Proceedings of the 2019 Conference of the North American Chapter of the Association for Computational Linguistics: Human Language Technologies, Volume 1 (Long and Short Papers), pp. 4171–4186. Association for Computational Linguistics, Minneapolis, Minnesota (2019). https://doi.org/10.18653/v1/N19-1423, https://aclanthology.org/N19-1423
14. Dunzer, S., Stierle, M., Matzner, M., Baier, S.: Conformance checking: a state-of-the-art literature review. In: Betz, S. (ed.) Proceedings of the 11th International Conference on Subject-Oriented Business Process Management, S-BPM ONE 2019, Seville, Spain, June 26–28, 2019, pp. 4:1–4:10. ACM (2019). https://doi.org/10.1145/3329007.3329014
15. Esparza, J., Römer, S., Vogler, W.: An improvement of McMillan's unfolding algorithm. Formal Methods Syst. Des. **20**(3), 285–310 (2002). https://doi.org/10.1023/A:1014746130920
16. Ghawi, R.: Process discovery using inductive miner and decomposition. CoRR abs/1610.07989 (2016). http://arxiv.org/abs/1610.07989
17. Grohs, M., Abb, L., Elsayed, N., Rehse, J.R.: Large language models can accomplish business process management tasks (2023)
18. Jensen, K., Kristensen, L.M.: Coloured Petri Nets - Modelling and Validation of Concurrent Systems. Springer (2009). https://doi.org/10.1007/B95112
19. Jessen, U., Sroka, M., Fahland, D.: Chit-chat or deep talk: Prompt engineering for process mining (2023)
20. Khurana, D., Koli, A., Khatter, K., Singh, S.: Natural language processing: state of the art, current trends and challenges. Multim. Tools Appl. **82**(3), 3713–3744 (2023). https://doi.org/10.1007/S11042-022-13428-4
21. Kourani, H., et al.: Leveraging large language models for enhanced process model comprehension (2024), https://arxiv.org/abs/2408.08892
22. Kourani, H., Berti, A., Schuster, D., van der Aalst, W.M.: PromoAI: Process modeling with generative AI. In: Proceedings of the Thirty-Third International Joint Conference on Artificial Intelligence. International Joint Conferences on Artificial Intelligence Organization (2024)
23. Leemans, S.J.J., Fahland, D., van der Aalst, W.M.P.: Scalable process discovery and conformance checking. **17**, 599–631 (2018). https://doi.org/10.1007/S10270-016-0545-X
24. OpenAI: Introducing GPT-5 (2025). https://openai.com/index/introducing-gpt-5/, Accessed 18 Aug 2025
25. Qafari, M.S., van der Aalst, W.: Fairness-aware process mining. In: Panetto, H., Debruyne, C., Hepp, M., Lewis, D., Ardagna, C.A., Meersman, R. (eds.) On

the Move to Meaningful Internet Systems: OTM 2019 Conferences, pp. 182–192. Springer International Publishing, Cham (2019)
26. Reichert, M., Weber, B.: Enabling Flexibility in Process-Aware Information Systems - Challenges, Methods, Technologies. Springer (2012). https://doi.org/10.1007/978-3-642-30409-5
27. Reisig, W., Rozenberg, G. (eds.): Lectures on Petri Nets I: Basic Models, Advances in Petri Nets, the volumes are based on the Advanced Course on Petri Nets, held in Dagstuhl, September 1996, Lecture Notes in Computer Science, vol. 1491. Springer (1998). https://doi.org/10.1007/3-540-65306-6
28. Rojas, E., Munoz-Gama, J., Sepúlveda, M., Capurro, D.: Process mining in healthcare: a literature review. J. Biomed. Inform. **61**, 224–236 (2016). https://doi.org/10.1016/j.jbi.2016.04.007, https://www.sciencedirect.com/science/article/pii/S1532046416300296
29. Rozinat, A., van der Aalst, W.M.P.: Conformance checking of processes based on monitoring real behavior. Inf. Syst. **33**(1), 64–95 (2008). https://doi.org/10.1016/J.IS.2007.07.001
30. Weijters, A.J., van Der Aalst, W.M., De Medeiros, A.A.: Process mining with the HeuristicsMiner algorithm. Technische Universiteit Eindhoven (2006)
31. Yang, L., et al.: Advancing multimodal medical capabilities of Gemini (2024). https://arxiv.org/abs/2405.03162

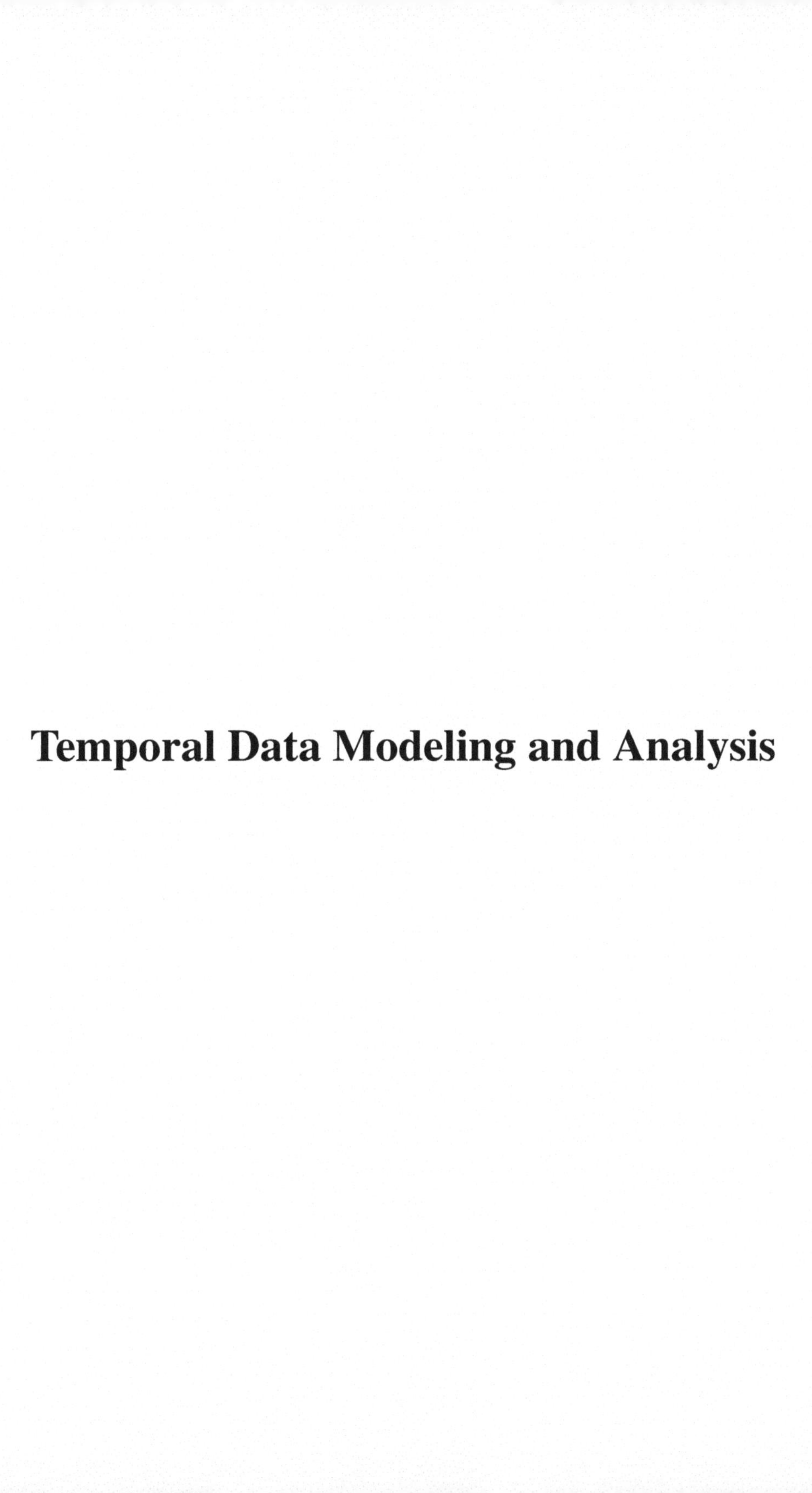

Temporal Data Modeling and Analysis

LUME-DBN: Full Bayesian Learning of DBNs from Incomplete Data in Intensive Care

Federico Pirola[1(✉)], Fabio Stella[1,3,4], and Marco Grzegorczyk[2]

[1] Department of Informatics, Systems and Communication, University of Milano-Bicocca, Milano, Italy
f.pirola17@campus.unimib.it

[2] Department of Science and Engineering, University of Groningen, Groningen, Netherlands

[3] BReCHS – Bicocca Research Centre in Health Services, Milano, Italy

[4] Bicocca Bioinformatics Biostatistics and Bioimaging Centre - B4, Vedano al Lambro, MB, Italy

Abstract. Dynamic Bayesian networks (DBNs) are increasingly used in healthcare due to their ability to model complex temporal relationships in patient data while maintaining interpretability, an essential feature for clinical decision-making. However, existing approaches to handling missing data in longitudinal clinical datasets are largely derived from static Bayesian networks literature, failing to properly account for the temporal nature of the data. This gap limits the ability to quantify uncertainty over time, which is particularly critical in settings such as intensive care, where understanding the temporal dynamics is fundamental for model trustworthiness and applicability across diverse patient groups. Despite the potential of DBNs, a full Bayesian framework that integrates missing data handling remains underdeveloped. In this work, we propose a novel Gibbs sampling-based method for learning DBNs from incomplete data. Our method treats each missing value as an unknown parameter following a Gaussian distribution. At each iteration, the unobserved values are sampled from their full conditional distributions, allowing for principled imputation and uncertainty estimation. We evaluate our method on both simulated datasets and real-world intensive care data from critically ill patients. Compared to standard model-agnostic techniques such as MICE, our Bayesian approach demonstrates superior reconstruction accuracy and convergence properties. These results highlight the clinical relevance of incorporating full Bayesian inference in temporal models, providing more reliable imputations and offering deeper insight into model behavior. Our approach supports safer and more informed clinical decision-making, particularly in settings where missing data are frequent and potentially impactful.

Keywords: Dynamic Bayesian Networks · Missing Data · Bayesian methods · Intensive Care

P. Bruno et al. (Eds.): HC_AIxIA_HYDRA 2025, CCIS 2830, pp. 167–181, 2026.
https://doi.org/10.1007/978-3-032-16708-8_15

1 Introduction

In intensive care units (ICUs), timely and accurate assessment of a patient's evolving condition is critical for guiding interventions. Bayesian networks (BNs) provide a principled way to represent complex dependencies among physiological variables under uncertainty, and dynamic Bayesian networks (DBNs) extend this capability to temporal domains by explicitly modeling multivariate interactions over time. DBNs have been applied to predict organ failure trajectories [1], forecast physiological changes and mortality risk [2], demonstrating their value in integrating heterogeneous ICU time-series data and delivering interpretable decision support in the setting of severe patients care.

However, ICU data are often plagued by missing values, irregular sampling, and measurement biases, which can significantly impair predictive performance and the reliability of the inferred temporal relationships. Traditional imputation or frequentist approaches may fail to fully account for the uncertainty introduced by missingness, potentially leading to biased parameter estimates or convergence to suboptimal solutions. A fully Bayesian approach to missing data imputation in DBNs addresses these challenges by explicitly modeling uncertainty in network structures, parameters and missing values. In this work we propose a Markov Chain Monte Carlo (MCMC) based missing values sampling strategy which naturally accommodates suboptimal local solutions during training, mitigating the risk of convergence to local minima, and efficiently working in case of extensive missingness.

The rest of the manuscript is organized as follows. In Sect. 2, we review the literature on both static and dynamic Bayesian networks learning from incomplete data. Section 3 introduces a Bayesian formulation of DBNs and the implementation of our method. Section 4 evaluates convergence and network reconstruction effectiveness in simulated scenarios characterized by different sample sizes and missingness rates. Section 5 introduces the ICU data employed, describes the preprocessing pipeline adopted to avoid potential systematic missingness and reports the reconstructed networks obtained through our approach. Section 6 concludes by wrapping up the results obtained in both simulated and real-world settings and illustrates the future directions of research.

2 Related Works

The presence of missing values represents a central issue in Artificial Intelligence, significantly influencing model effectiveness and generalizability. Several methods have been developed to handle missing data when learning static BNs from incomplete datasets. A widely used approach is the structural expectation-maximization (SEM) algorithm [3]. In its Hard EM variant, the most practical version, an expectation (E) step imputes missing values using the current model, followed by a maximization (M) step that updates parameters and a structural move (S), iterating until convergence. Despite their effectiveness to work in the context of limited data, such methods always follow the current best local moves and impute missing values based on the best model at each step, which can underestimate uncertainty and lead to convergence to local optima.

Bayesian approaches have recently emerged to overcome these limitations. Recently, [4] proposed a sampling-based MCMC method that jointly infers structure, parameters, and missing values. Unlike classical score-based or constraint-based structure learning methods, which greedily optimize toward local improvements, these techniques can escape local minima and yield more accurate network reconstructions [4].

Despite these progresses, missing data in DBNs is often still handled using model-agnostic methods such as Multiple Imputation by Chained Equations (MICE) or mean imputation, or temporal adaptations of frequentist approaches as SEM [1,2].

Since sampling-based MCMC methods have proven effective in static settings, we aim to extend them to DBNs by designing a Gibbs sampling step for recursive missing data imputation. A key insight is that the full conditional distribution (FCD) of missing values in this setting remains tractable, enabling efficient MCMC-based inference, a point we develop further in the methodological section.

3 Methods

3.1 DBNs and Bayesian Linear Regressions

DBNs present a popular and valid approach to model the temporal evolution of multivariate continuous time series.[1] They factorize the joint distribution of all variables across time into a product of conditional distributions for each node given its parents in the previous time slice [5]. Assuming no instantaneous effects, i.e., variables at time t do not influence other variables at the same time point, there is no need to impose an acyclicity constraint as in static BNs. Under these assumptions, a DBN could be framed as k independent Bayesian linear regression (BLRs) models [6]. A DBN is characterized by its structure, consisting of k nodes (variables) $\{X_1, \ldots, X_k\}$ connected through edges, and its parameters, which specify the BLRs. An edge $X_i \rightarrow X_j$ indicates a temporal dependency, namely, variable X_i at time $t-1$ directly influences variable X_j at time t.[2] The parameters, instead, are given in the form of BLRs as in Eq. 1.

$$x_i^t = \beta_0^{(i)} + \sum_{j:(X_j^{t-1} \in \pi_{(i)})} \beta_j^{(i)} x_j^{t-1} + \epsilon_i^t \quad (t = 1, \ldots, T) \tag{1}$$

x_i^t is the realization of variable X_i at time t, $\beta_0^{(i)}$ is the intercept of the linear regression model and the vector $\beta^{(i)} = [\beta_1^{(i)}, \ldots, \beta_{|\pi_{(i)}|}^{(i)}]$ represents the

[1] For simplicity, throughout the paper we refer to Gaussian DBNs simply as DBNs, although discrete or mixed variants also exist.

[2] For a given edge $X_i \rightarrow X_j$, we define X_i as the parent of X_j and X_j as the child of X_i. The set of the incoming edges for a node X_i define its parent set $\pi_{(i)}$..

ordered linear coefficients associated with the parents of X_i^t in $\pi_{(i)}$. Finally, ϵ_i^t is a Gaussian-distributed error term with mean 0.

3.2 Conditional Likelihoods and Prior Distributions

To learn a DBN from data, we consider a group of N samples $\{s_1, \ldots, s_N\}$ observed at $T+1$ equally spaced time points $\{0, 1, \ldots, T\}$, where each sample is described by a set of k variables $\mathcal{X} = \{X_1, \ldots, X_k\}$. This results in a dataset $\mathcal{D}$ of dimensions $(N, k, T+1)$, representing realizations of $\mathcal{X}$ across both the sample and the time domain. Since in DBN we assume the first Markov order, namely $\mathcal{X}^{t+1} \perp\!\!\!\perp \mathcal{X}^{t-1} \mid \mathcal{X}^t$, we could then rewrite $\mathcal{D}$ in its lagged form $\mathcal{D}_{\mathcal{L}}$ to easily learn the actual model from data. $\mathcal{D}_{\mathcal{L}}$ would then be of dimensions $(N \cdot T, 2k)$ [5]. In Eq. 2 we define the conditional Gaussian likelihood for a variable X_i^t.

$$X_i^t \mid (\mathcal{X}^{t-1}, \beta^{(i)}, \sigma^{2(i)}, \pi_{(i)}) \sim \mathcal{N}\Big(\mathcal{X}_{[\pi_{(i)}]}^{t-1} \beta^{(i)}, \sigma^{2(i)} I\Big). \tag{2}$$

The regression coefficients $\beta^{(i)}$ quantify the linear effect of parent variables $\mathcal{X}_{[\pi_{(i)}]}$ at time $t-1$ on X_i^t, while $\pi_{(i)}$ defines the current parent set for variable X_i at time t, and the noise parameter $\sigma^{2^{(i)}}$ capture unexplained variability.

Since we are working in a full Bayesian framework, all the parameters have their own prior distribution and we impose conjugate priors. The regression coefficients follow a Gaussian prior $\beta^{(i)} \sim N(\mu_{(i)}, \sigma^{2^{(i)}} \delta^{2^{(i)}} I)$, where $\delta^{2^{(i)}}$ express uncertainty over the parameters $\beta^{(i)}$. The noise and uncertainty terms are assumed to follow Inverse-Gamma distributions, $\sigma^{2^{(i)}} \sim \text{Inv-Gamma}(a, b)$ and $\delta^{2^{(i)}} \sim \text{Inv-Gamma}(\alpha_\delta, \beta_\delta)$ respectively. Finally, a Poisson prior $|\pi_{(i)}| \sim \text{Poisson}(\lambda)$ over the parent set size is set, encouraging simpler network structures with fewer parents, controlling model complexity. Depending on the application a fan-in restriction could be imposed too, limiting the maximum number of parents per variable. The detailed derivations of the closed-form solutions for the parameters FCDs and the marginal likelihoods can be found in [6].

3.3 A Gibbs Step for Missing Data Imputation

We design a unified imputation step that updates missing values jointly across all regression models in which they appear. We adopt a Gibbs move, sampling from the full conditional distributions (FCDs) of the missing values. Here for a matter of simplicity we assume uniform priors over the missing values domain, though Gaussian priors would also be possible. Then, a missing value for a variable X_i at time t contributes to:

- Its own conditional likelihood: $P(X_i^t \mid \pi_{(i)})$
- The conditional likelihoods of all its children (X_j^{t+1}): $P(X_j^{t+1} \mid \pi_{(j)})$

For the local Markov property of a DBN, all nodes are conditionally independent to their non-descendants given their parents [5]. Indeed, for the property of conditional Gaussian distribution, the product of independent conditional Gaussians is also a Gaussian [7]. It follows that the FCD of each missing value is a univariate Gaussian distribution, thus we can efficiently sample the missing values, enabling a robust Gibbs sampling procedure.

In Supplementary Material A we show the derivation of the missing values' FCDs in an incremental way. We start out by computing the FCD of single missing values in three simple cases and then we illustrate how the derivation of the missing's FCD extends to the general case with more complex Markov blankets.[3]

In Eq. 3 we report the FCD for a general missing value $x^t_{i[MIS]}$ over a random variable X_i at a certain time $t > 0$. The FCD is a univariate Gaussian distribution with a closed form whose structure remains unchanged regardless the size of its Markov blanket. The noise term σ^{2^*} is a weighted combination of the precisions $(1/\sigma^2)$ from the conditional likelihood of X^t_i and from the likelihoods of the children X^{t+1}_j. The mean term μ^* is determined by the conditional mean μ^t_i, the isolated contribution $\beta^{(j)}_i$ of X^t_i adjusted by the other parents contributions $\mu^{(j)}_{\{-i\}}{}^{(t+1)}$, and the observed values of the children x^{t+1}_j.

$$P(x^t_{i[MIS]} \mid \cdot) = \mathcal{N}(\mu^*, \sigma^{2^*}) \tag{3}$$

$$\text{where:} \quad \sigma^{2^*} = \left(\frac{1}{\sigma^{2(i)}} + \sum_{j:\,(X^t_i \in \pi_{(j)})} \frac{(\beta^{(j)}_i)^2}{\sigma^{2(j)}} \right)^{-1},$$

$$\mu^* = \sigma^{2^*} \cdot \left(\frac{\mu^t_i}{\sigma^{2(i)}} + \sum_{j:\,(X^t_i \in \pi_{(j)})} \beta^{(j)}_i \frac{\left(x^{t+1}_j - \mu^{(j)}_{\{-i\}}{}^{(t+1)}\right)}{\sigma^{2(j)}} \right),$$

$$\mu^{(j)}_{\{-i\}}{}^{(t+1)} = \sum_{m \neq i:(X^t_m \in \pi_{(j)})} x^t_m \beta^{(j)}_m.$$

3.4 Learning DBNs from Incomplete Data

When data contain missing values, DBN learning procedure can no longer be framed as k independent BLRs, unless the data are first imputed to obtain a complete dataset, which seems suboptimal. Since any variable may serve as both a response and a covariate, independent imputations per regression would assign inconsistent values to the same missing value and violate the DBN factorization.

Therefore, we combine the Gibbs sampling step for missing data imputation from Sect. 3.3 with the MCMC sampling scheme designed for learning DBNs in case of complete data from [6]. We refer to the resulting MCMC scheme for learning DBNs from incomplete data as Latent Uncertainty Modeling via

[3] The *Markov blanket* of a variable X_i is the set of its parents, its children, and variables sharing children with it. Conditioned on its Markov blanket, X_i is independent from all other variables in the network.

MCMC Estimation in DBNs (LUME-DBN). LUME-DBN is characterized by an iterative procedure sampling the DBN structure, its parameters and the missing values in consecutive steps.

For the parameter and structural moves, we refer to [6], which illustrates the DBN learning procedure in case of fully observed data. In Supplementary Material B, we provide the detailed Gibbs sampling step for parameter updates sampling from the FCDs and the Metropolis-Hasting step for updating parent sets in each BLR built on marginal likelihoods.

Missing values are, instead, updated jointly across the network once every E_M epochs, where E_M is chosen based on application-dependent factors such as missingness rate and convergence time. Conditional on the current structure and parameters, each missing entry is independent across samples, but strictly dependent on the observed trajectory of the corresponding sample. As detailed in Eq. 3, the FCDs are shown to be time-invariant with respect to the DBN's parameters, allowing us to derive efficient index sets and making the imputation step computationally feasible even under high missingness. Supplementary Material B shows also the entire implementation of LUME-DBN, deriving posterior samples for the structure, the parameters and the missing values.

3.5 Convergence Diagnostics and DBN Reconstruction Evaluation

After running independent simulations, we obtain a set of posterior samples for the parent sets (binary arc indicators) and the missing values. Since our method focuses on network reconstruction in the context of incomplete data, we want to ensure that both the parent sets, thus the DBN structure, and the missing values converge to the right solutions.

To assess convergence we employ the potential scale reduction factor (PSRF) [8] at each epoch separately for both arc indicators and missing values. A detailed description of PSRF for DBNs arcs is reported in [6]. Let Φ_e denote, for epoch e, the proportion of posterior samples with PSRF < 1.1. Convergence is declared when Φ_e consistently reaches 1 over successive epochs.

To evaluate the proposed Gibbs imputation procedure, we compare it in terms of network reconstruction accuracy with two baselines model-agnostic methods for handling missing values in DBN learning. MICE [1] is applied to the original dataset before temporal lagging, regressing each incomplete variable on all the others iteratively using linear models until convergence. Because of the time-lag of all interactions, the original MICE algorithm could result suboptimal in our setting, thus, we implemented *Temporal MICE*, a new variant that uses lagged predictors to predict the missing values.

We discard the first S samples prior to convergence (burn-in) and then thin the chain by retaining only every 5th sample to reduce autocorrelation. Then, we compute the averaged inclusion probabilities, namely the average probabilities of each potential parent in each linear regression model, obtained by averaging the posterior arc indicators across epochs and replicates. The result is a matrix where each row is associated with the probability of the parents for a given outcome variable at time t. This matrix is then compared with the original adjacency matrix of the data-generating DBN for each competing method. Model performances are quantified using the area under the precision–recall curve (AUC–PR), where the precision–recall curve plots the trade-off between the proportion of predicted arcs that are correct (precision) and the proportion of true arcs that are recovered (recall) [9]. Higher values of AUC–PR indicate better reconstruction accuracy.

4 Synthetic Data Generation and Performance Evaluation

To assess the performance of LUME-DBN, we generate synthetic temporal data from given DBNs. A total of ten independent DBN structures with 10 nodes each are randomly sampled, with each structure constrained to have a maximum of five parents per node. To ensure acyclicity and maintain the faithfulness condition—that is, the compatibility between the model parameters and the underlying graph structure—a random topological ordering of the nodes is imposed during the structure generation process.

Conditional dependencies are modeled using linear Gaussian relationships. For each node, regression coefficients corresponding to its parents are independently drawn from a Uniform distribution over the interval $[0.2, 0.8]$, and the noise variance is fixed at $\sigma^2 = 1$. Together, the structure, coefficients, and variance parameters fully specify each DBN.

For each of the ten DBNs, multiple time series are simulated with three different lengths $T = \{50, 100, 200\}$, to evaluate the impact of the number of time frames on structural reconstruction accuracy.[4] To evaluate the robustness of the method to missing data, missing values are introduced randomly at four levels of missingness: $\{10\%, 20\%, 30\%, 40\%\}$. The incomplete datasets at each missingness level are generated by randomly removing data entries according to a Bernoulli distribution with success probability equal to the specified missingness rate.

We assess convergence of both DBN structure and imputed missing values, averaged over 10 simulated DBNs with time series length $T = 100$. At each epoch e, for each missingness level, the convergence diagnostic Φ_e described in Sect. 3.5, is tracked. In Supplementary Material C we show that structure convergence occurs within 1.5k epochs for all missingness rates, whereas missing values require up to 5k epochs at 40% missingness. Convergence time increases with missingness, with 10% missingness resembling the fully observed case and 30–40% missingness producing more unstable structure learning. Still, in all settings convergence is ultimately achieved within $S = 5k$ epochs, thus we discard the first S posterior samples to ensure the stationarity of the distribution.

[4] We also conducted ablation experiments varying sample sizes, maximum number of parents and linear coefficients ranges; the experimental setting reported was chosen to avoid trivially easy or infeasible cases while still covering a broad spectrum of different settings.

We then run five independent simulations of 20k epochs for each experimental condition. Missing values are imputed every $E_M = 10$ iterations, with initial imputation given by the mean at time t. This value of E_M guarantees faster converge time compared to an update of the missing values at every single epoch. A fan-in restriction is imposed by randomly initializing the covariate sets with at most five parents. Noise ${\sigma^2}^{(i)}$ and uncertainty ${\delta^2}^{(i)}$ parameters are initialized to 1, linear coefficients $\beta^{(i)}$ to 0, and the Poisson prior parameter is set to $\lambda = 1$. All experiments were implemented in R, and the full code of LUME-DBN algorithm is publicly available at https://doi.org/10.5281/zenodo.17544061.

In Fig. 1 the results are shown aggregated for sample sizes and missingness rates. Confidence bars show the variability across different DBN models, whereas p-values of the paired t-test show the significance of the differences between each DBN's AUC-PR for LUME-DBN and for the baseline methods.

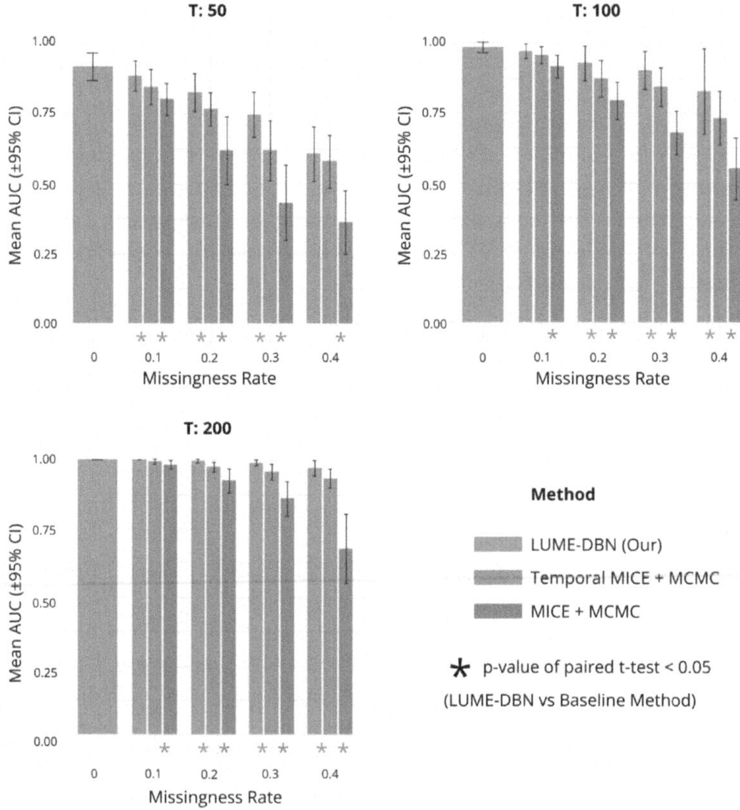

Fig. 1. Area Under the Precision-Recall Curve for different experimental settings (sample sizes, missingness rates and imputation methods). The p-values of the paired t-test LUME-DBN AUC vs Baseline Method AUC are computed for each experimental condition, highlighting p-values < 0.05 with colored '$\star$' based on the baseline method. Confidence bars represent the 95% confidence intervals for each experimental setting.

The average AUC-PR on the complete data is reported to evaluate the impact of missingness in all the settings.

Across all settings, MICE consistently shows the worst performance, completely losing effectiveness once missingness exceeds 20% reflecting its inefficiency when applied in the context of temporal data. Temporal MICE performs better, but remains significantly inferior to LUME-DBN across all sample sizes and missingness rates over 10%, as it is applied before the actual learning phase. In contrast, LUME-DBN proves more effective, particularly at high missingness levels, highlighting its superior ability to handle missing data, while not losing much compared to the fully observed case, especially for larger sample sizes.

5 A Case Study in Intensive Care

5.1 PhysioNet Data Description and Preprocessing

To validate our approach in the context of real-world intensive care data, we employ the PhysioNet 2012 Challenge dataset [10], a large-scale database comprising records from over 20,000 adult patients admitted to intensive care units (ICUs) across multiple hospitals. The dataset includes rich temporal and static information routinely collected in the ICU. All patients included in the dataset were hospitalized for at least 48 h, and data collection covers the first 48 h of ICU stay, with variables recorded at varying sampling frequencies.

Since our approach is designed to manage only random missing values, knowing the systematic missingness due to patients' conditions we apply two consecutive preprocessing steps. First, we restrict our analysis on patients with severe clinical conditions, identified by a Sequential Organ Failure Assessment (SOFA) score greater than 12, consistent with thresholds used in clinical literature to define critical illness [11]. Secondly, we stratify patients into four subgroups according to the ICU admission due to the diverse missingness rate per class, as described in Table 1. In such a way, assuming unconfoundness due to external reasons, we could consider missingness distribution as random conditional to the current model [12].

To handle the heterogeneity in measurement frequencies, we discretize the temporal data into 6-hour intervals, balancing high- and low-frequency signals following previous works on ICU monitoring and ensuring the tractability of missing value imputation based on the previous simulation results [13]. Following this, we apply a feature selection step based on missingness rates: variables with more than 40% missing values in any ICU subgroup are excluded. This results in a final set of 11 clinical variables retained for analysis. The final set is comprised of vital signs, blood measurements, physiological features and a brain damage indicator, each described by temporal observations at $T = 9$ time points.

Since variables differed in scale and variance, we standardized them using observed values before learning. Experiments are first runned with local standardization (per ICU group), then repeated with global standardization (entire dataset) to appreciate the impact of standardization on the entire learning procedure. In Supplementary Material D we report the descriptive statistics of the included variables and the missingness rates by group.

Table 1. Descriptions of ICU subgroups included in the study along with the number of patients per group.

Group	Description	# Patients
MICU	Medical ICU: Patients having medical conditions requiring intensive monitoring and treatment (i.e. Sepsis, Pneumonia, ...).	34
SICU	Surgical ICU: Post-operative patients recovering from non-cardiac surgeries (abdominal, vascular, orthopedic, or general surgeries). Monitored to avoid bleeding, infection, or organ dysfunction post-surgery.	104
CCU	Coronary Care Unit: Patients in intensive care for acute cardiac events and conditions like Myocardial infarction, Arrhythmias or Acute heart failure, which do not need surgeries.	114
CSRU	Cardiac Surgery Recovery Unit: Patients recovering from cardiac surgeries (i.e., Coronary artery bypass grafting, valve replacements, aortic repairs). Under observation to ensure hemodynamic stability and recovery after major heart operations.	62

5.2 Convergence Diagnostics and Reconstructed DBNs

Having demonstrated the superior reconstruction accuracy of LUME-DBN, we apply it to the ICU data. Supplementary Material C reports the convergence of missing values and DBN structures, which is consistently reached within 5k epochs across all ICU groups. We then proceed under the same experimental conditions used in the simulations (missing values and parameter initialization, prior distributions, and burn-in restriction) for each ICU group, limiting the maximum number of parents to 5. Since no reference network is available for the real data, the validation of the method focuses on differences between the networks learned across groups and under different standardization strategies.

In Fig. 2 we report the reconstructed network structures obtained by applying a threshold of 0.8 to the inclusion probabilities averaged over the posterior samples to compare the reconstructed networks for the different groups. Supported by multiple surveys of critical care from the clinical literature [14,15], we highlight the following commonalities and differences between different ICU groups in terms of temporal dynamics:

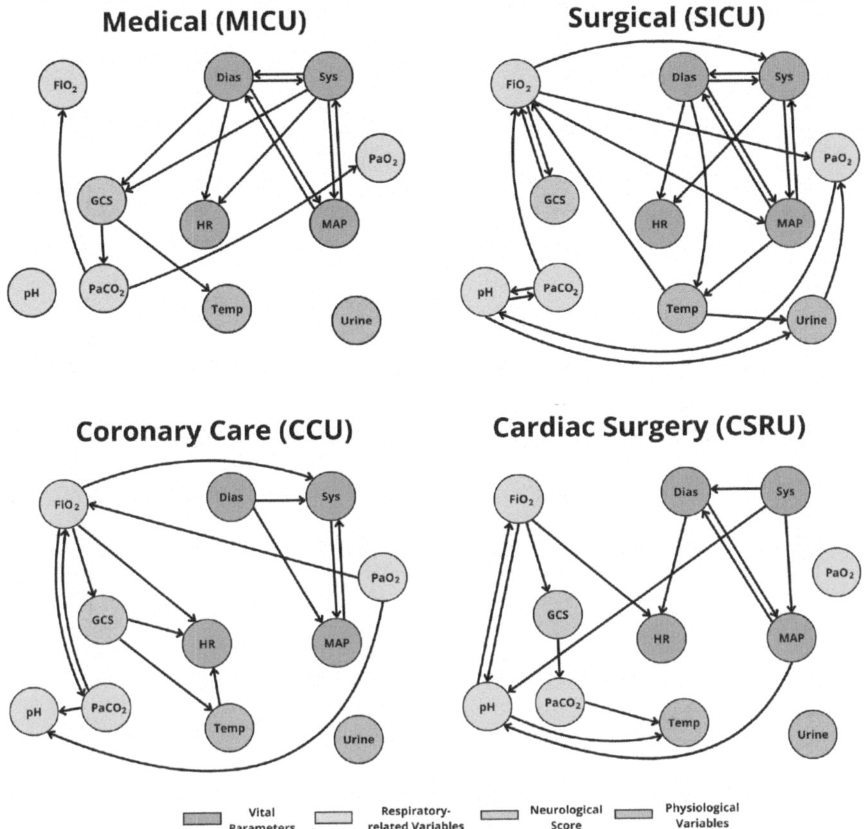

Fig. 2. Reconstructed DBNs for each ICU type, averaged over five independent simulations after local data standardization. A threshold of 0.8 is applied to the averaged inclusion probabilities. Arcs are meant to represent temporal relationships with a single temporal lag, namely between nodes at time $t-1$ and nodes at time t.

- **Self-regulatory loops:** Pressure parameters (MAP, Sys, Dias) were closely interrelated, reflecting the coordinated regulation of arterial blood pressure. Similarly, respiratory-related variables (FiO_2, $PaCO_2$, PaO_2, pH) were strongly connected, highlighting the integrated control of oxygenation, ventilation, and acid–base balance in all kind of ICUs.
- **Neurological interactions:** Reduced consciousness increased heart rate in coronary care patients ($GCS \rightarrow HR$) and was linked to higher oxygen requirements in non-medical patients ($GCS \leftrightarrow FiO_2$), reflecting autonomic and respiratory coupling.
- **Hemodynamic effects:** Blood pressure strongly influenced consciousness ($Dias, MAP \rightarrow GCS$) in medical patients, underlining the importance of maintaining cerebral perfusion during shocks.

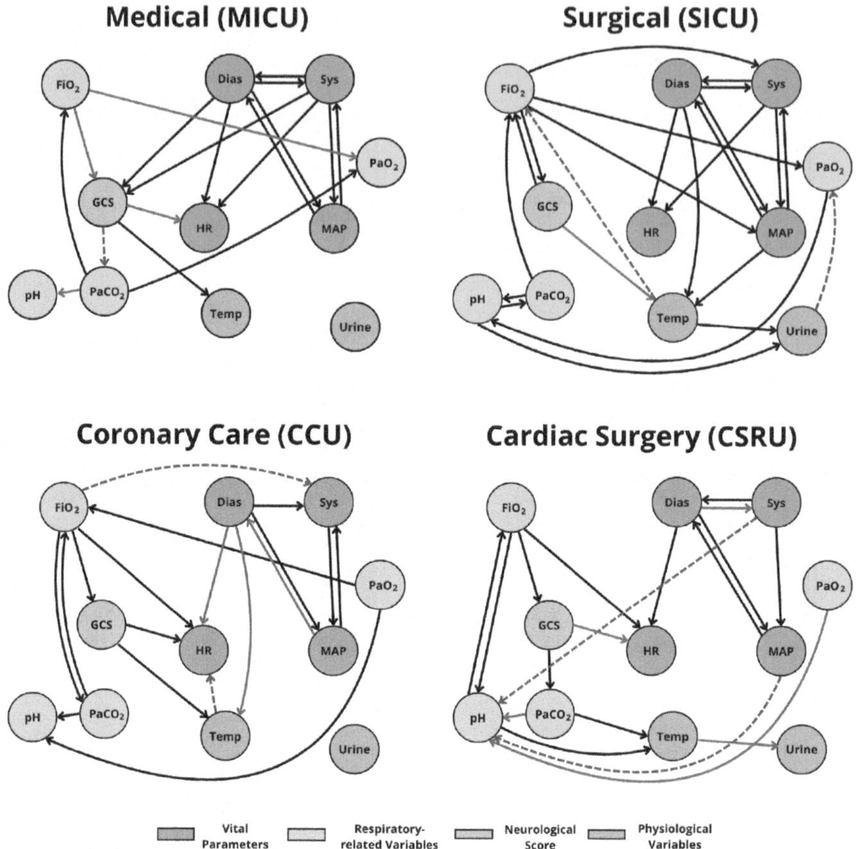

Fig. 3. Reconstructed DBNs for each ICU type (MICU, SICU, CCU, CSRU), averaged over five independent simulations for two different data standardization techniques. A threshold of 0.8 is applied to generate the network structures. Arcs are meant to represent temporal relationship with a single temporal lag, namely between nodes at time $t-1$ and nodes at time t. Green arcs are present just in the context of global standardization, red dotted arcs are present in local standardization per ICU group only and black arcs are common to the two settings. (Color figure online)

- **Thermoregulatory dynamics:** In surgical recovery, body temperature changes affected urine output ($Temp \rightarrow Urine$) and were also shaped by pressure and metabolic disturbances ($pH, PaCO_2 \rightarrow Temp$) after bypass. This highlights the sensitivity of thermoregulation to hemodynamic and metabolic conditions during post-operative care.
- **Cardiorespiratory feedbacks:** In coronary care and post-surgical patients, low oxygen levels triggered compensatory increases in heart rate ($FiO_2 \rightarrow HR$), consistent with hypoxia-driven cardiac responses.

Figure 3 also reports a comparison between the two standardization techniques (local and global). With a global standardization, the networks exhibit more commonalities, likely reflecting the uncertainty associated with small sample sizes and the interpretation of relationships as deviations from group-specific means. Certain temporal relationships appeared highly dependent on local standardization and are not well supported by clinical evidence, such as the influence of pressure parameters (Sys, MAP) on pH in CSRU patients or the effect of body temperature on FiO_2 levels in SICU patients. These findings highlight the need to incorporate prior clinical knowledge to guide and validate model inference.

6 Conclusions and Research Directions

In this work we have proposed LUME-DBN, a novel method to learn DBNs from incomplete data positioned in a full Bayesian framework. We have derived the FCDs for missing values and showed they are tractable. Indeed we have employed them in the sampling-based imputation step to recover DBNs' structures. Our work highlights:

- The convergence behaviour and effectiveness of LUME-DBN in learning DBN structures from both simulated and real-world ICU data, demonstrating superior reconstruction accuracy compared to model-agnostic methods.
- Significant improvements in terms of model interpretability due to its capacity of explicitly encoding uncertainty over the models, parameters and missing values' spaces.
- The potential for future extensions due to the Bayesian nature of the model, opening the possibility of incorporating prior clinical knowledge towards an expert-informed learning and improving the clinical relevance of the findings.

We also plan to compare our approach against classical frequentist approaches, but since DBN libraries do not yet support structure learning from incomplete data, dedicated development building on static BN libraries such as *bnlearn* [16] will be required. An evaluation of the overall computation time required by the single steps of LUME-DBN will also be carried out, assessing how much time could be spared by parallelizing part of each module.

Another extension we have in mind is the integration of methods to manage Missing Not At Random (MNAR) patterns, which are frequent in clinical data due to unmodeled external factors. While methods combining BNs with missingness graphs have shown effectiveness in capturing MNAR mechanisms [17], their applicability in temporal settings remain unexplored. Morover, extending these methods to continuous domains poses an additional challenge, as it requires dealing with mixed variable types. To address these complexities, we plan to investigate approaches based on logistic distributions, drawing inspiration from the global-optimization strategy of LiM [18].

We also aim to generalize our approach to non-homogeneous DBNs (NH-DBNs) to capture non-stationary relationships across time and patient groups.

Specifically we plan to extend the method to globally coupled NH-DBNs, characterized by a shared structure among time and/or groups of patients, with deviations only in parameter distributions [19,20]. Such modeling is key to representing evolving treatment effects in intensive care.

Supplementary Material

Supplementary material, including demonstrations, pseudocodes, and additional figures, is available at https://doi.org/10.5281/zenodo.17543666.

Acknowledgments. This work is funded by the National National Plan for NRRP Complementary Investments (Project n. PNC0000003 - AdvaNced Technologies for Human-centrEd Medicine (ANTHEM)), and by the MUR under the grant "Dipartimenti di Eccellenza 2023–2027" of the Department of Informatics, Systems and Communication (DISCo), University of Milano-Bicocca, Milan, Italy.

References

1. Sandri, M., Berchialla, P., Baldi, I., Gregori, D., De Blasi, R.A.: Dynamic Bayesian networks to predict sequences of organ failures in patients admitted to ICU. J. Biomed. Inform. **48**, 106–113 (2014)
2. Chen, Q., et al.: Dynamic Bayesian network for predicting physiological changes, organ dysfunctions and mortality risk in critical trauma patients. BMC Med. Inform. Decis. Mak. **22**(1), 119 (2022)
3. Ruggieri, A., Stranieri, F., Stella, F., Scutari, M.: Hard and soft EM in Bayesian network learning from incomplete data. Algorithms **13**(12), 329 (2020)
4. Grzegorczyk, M.: Being Bayesian about learning gaussian Bayesian networks from incomplete data. Int. J. Approximate Reasoning **147**, 1–22 (2023)
5. Ghahramani, Z.: Learning dynamic Bayesian networks. Lect. Notes Comput. Sci. **1387**, 168–197 (1998)
6. Grzegorczyk, M., Husmeier, D.: Modelling non-homogeneous dynamic Bayesian networks with piecewise linear regression models. In: Balding, D.J., Moltke, I., Marioni, J., (eds.) Handbook of Statistical Genomics, vol. 2, pp. 899–931. John Wiley and Sons (2019)
7. Bishop, C.M.: Pattern Recognition and Machine Learning. Springer (2006)
8. Gelman, A., Rubin, D.B.: Inference from iterative simulation using multiple sequences. Stat. Sci. **7**(4), 457–472 (1992)
9. Saito, T., Rehmsmeier, M.: The precision–recall plot is more informative than the roc plot when evaluating binary classifiers on imbalanced datasets. PLoS ONE **10**(3), e0118432 (2015)
10. Goldberger, A.L., et al.: PhysioNet 2012 challenge dataset (2012)
11. Jean-Louis, V., et al.: The sofa (sepsis-related organ failure assessment) score to describe organ dysfunction/failure. Intensive Care Med. **22**(7), 707–710 (1996)
12. Rubin, D.B.: Inference and missing data. Biometrika **63**(3), 581–592 (1976)
13. Zhao, Y., Zhang, Y., Zhang, Y., Zhang, Y., Zhang, Y.: Temporal clustering of critical illness events on medical wards. JAMA Intern. Med. **179**(9), 1237–1244 (2019)
14. Pinsky, M.R., et al.: Effective hemodynamic monitoring. Critical Care **26** (2022)

15. Kreit, J.: Respiratory–cardiovascular interactions during mechanical ventilation: physiology and clinical implications. Compr. Physiol. **12**(3), 3425–3448 (2022)
16. Scutari, M.: Learning Bayesian networks with the bnlearn R package. Stat. Softw. **35**, 10 (2010)
17. Liu, Y., Constantinou, A.C.: Greedy structure learning from data that contain systematic missing values. Mach. Learn. **111**(10), 3867–3896 (2022)
18. Zeng, Y., Shimizu, S., Matsui, H., Sun, F.: Causal discovery for linear mixed data. In: Proceedings of the First Conference on Causal Learning and Reasoning (CLeaR 2022), vol. 77 of Proceedings of Machine Learning Research, pp. 994–1009 (2022)
19. Shafiee, K., Heberle, A.M., Thedieck, K., Grzegorczyk, M.: Partially non-homogeneous dynamic Bayesian networks based on Bayesian regression models with partitioned design matrices. Bioinformatics **35**(12), 2108–2117 (2019)
20. Zhang, J., Hu, C., Zhang, Q.: Constructing a gene regulatory network based on a nonhomogeneous dynamic Bayesian network. Electronics **11**(18), 2936 (2022)

Using Temporal Features to Improve Accuracy in Multivariate Pattern Analysis (MVPA) of M/EEG Data

Fateheh Barazesh Morgani(✉), Erin Goddard, and Gustavo Batista

University of New South Wales (UNSW), Sydney, Australia
{f.barazesh_morgani,erin.goddard,g.batista}@unsw.edu.au

Abstract. Multivariate Pattern Analysis (MVPA), or 'brain decoding' methods, have become a popular approach for analyzing time series brain recordings such as magnetoencephalography (MEG) and electroencephalography (EEG) to address experimental questions in cognitive neuroscience. Currently, the most common approach is to epoch data relative to an event of interest (e.g., stimulus onset) and apply the classification analyses to relative time points individually. This approach reveals how neural information unfolds over time but neglects any information that may be present in the temporal dynamics of brain activity. In this work, we employ several time series methods (classifiers that incorporate temporal information) with varying time window durations to analyze MEG and EEG data and compare their utility for revealing the temporal dynamics of neural information. As the window duration increases, classifier accuracy improves, but the results become less precise regarding the timing of neural information. We found that a window of ~20 ms resulted in accurate classifiers while maintaining the temporal precision of the results. We also tested time series classifiers based on convolutional kernels, which often outperform simpler methods in benchmark datasets. However, these did not yield better performance in our datasets. Our results suggest that using a brief window, rather than a single time point, could lead to improved sensitivity for MVPA methods to detect neural representations from MEG and/or EEG data.

Keywords: Multivariate Pattern Analysis · Time series Classification · Magnetoencephalography · Electroencephalography

1 Introduction

Multivariate pattern analysis (MVPA) has become a standard approach in cognitive neuroscience to extract information from high-dimensional neuroimaging signals. Applied to time series modalities like MEG and EEG, it enables tracking representational dynamics on millisecond timescales. MVPA [1] encompasses a range of methods for analyzing neuroimaging data. In MVPA, machine learning classifiers are used to identify brain activity patterns associated with participants' experiences (e.g., stimulus) or their internal state (e.g., decision or task)

P. Bruno et al. (Eds.): HC_AIxIA_HYDRA 2025, CCIS 2830, pp. 182–195, 2026.
https://doi.org/10.1007/978-3-032-16708-8_16

(Fig. 1-A). Brain responses are recorded using M/EEG, and activation levels across experimental conditions are represented as patterns in a high-dimensional space. A classifier is trained on a subset of data to associate these patterns with specific conditions, then tested on unseen data. Successful generalization to new data indicates that brain responses contain condition-specific information (Fig. 1-B). Training and testing classifiers at each time point independently reveals when information about a stimulus or task becomes detectable, enabling the temporal mapping of sensory and cognitive processes [1]. However, most studies have relied on conventional classifiers that ignore temporal structure, despite M/EEG being inherently a multidimensional time series.

In this paper, we extend MVPA with time series classifiers to improve decoding accuracy, i.e., predicting experimental conditions from neural data. Unlike conventional methods that treat each time point in isolation, time series classifiers leverage the temporal context provided by neural activations that occur before and after a given moment. We systematically evaluate three approaches for time series classification and benchmark their performance on three M/EEG datasets, collected by our research group and external collaborators.

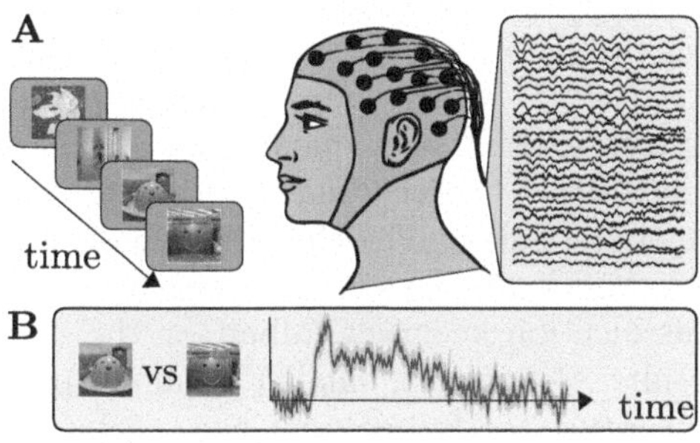

Fig. 1. MVPA in cognitive neuroscience.

Previous attempts to incorporate temporal information into MVPA have primarily relied on averaging strategies to improve the signal-to-noise ratio (e.g., [2,3]. However, they found that performance gains were marginal, with slight variations across window sizes. These findings demonstrate that temporal smoothing can offer incremental benefits, but may not fully utilize the temporal structure inherent in M/EEG signals. Our experiments demonstrate that incorporating time series classifiers into MVPA improves its sensitivity compared to traditional methods.

This paper is organized as follows. Section 1 introduces the background and related work. Section 2 describes the datasets and preprocessing. Section 3 details the methodology. Section 4 presents and discusses results, and Sect. 5 concludes and provides directions for future work.

1.1 Background and Problem Formulation

We begin with a formal notation for time series. A time series $T = (t_1, t_2, \ldots, t_m)$ is an ordered sequence of m data points. If each point $t_i \in \mathbb{R}$, the series is called *univariate*, whereas if $t_i \in \mathbb{R}^d$ is a d-dimensional vector capturing multiple variables at each time step, it is termed *multivariate*. In this work, we focus on multivariate time series.

To capture local temporal patterns, a sliding window extracts subsequences of length l from a time series T of length m:

$$S_{i,l} = (t_i, t_{i+1}, \ldots, t_{i+l-1}), \quad 1 \leq i \leq m - l + 1. \tag{1}$$

A time series classifier can be formally defined as a function $f : \mathcal{T} \rightarrow \mathcal{Y}$ that maps an entire time series to a class label from a set of classes $\mathcal{Y} = \{1, \ldots, c\}$. While this formulation is standard in time series classification, it is not directly applicable to MVPA, where the objective is to track how discriminative information unfolds over time. In this context, classification is not performed on whole sequences but on temporally localized portions of the data (Fig. 1). To address this, we define *time series MVPA* as the application of a subsequence classifier $g : \mathcal{S} \rightarrow \mathcal{Y}$, which maps a subsequence to a class label. A sliding window is used to extract subsequences across the signal, each of which is classified independently. The decoding accuracy of these subsequences is then evaluated as a function of time. The choice of window length l plays a crucial role in this analysis: larger windows capture richer contextual information and tend to improve classification accuracy, albeit at the expense of the temporal precision of the results. Conversely, smaller windows preserve temporal resolution but may fail to capture the full context necessary for robust decoding [3]. Thus, the window length introduces a trade-off between sensitivity and temporal specificity that must be carefully balanced in practice.

This work focuses on M/EEG data, typically organized into *channels*, *trials*, and *time points*. Each channel corresponds to a sensor or electrode (typically ~64–128 electrodes for EEG, ~150–300 sensors for MEG). Trials capture repetitions of experimental conditions (e.g., viewing a stimulus or making a decision), often several hundred per condition across sessions. Within each trial, signals are sampled at high temporal resolution (e.g., 1000 Hz), yielding hundreds to thousands of time points defined relative to task events, such as stimulus onset or a participant's behavioral response (e.g., decision time).

1.2 Related Work

This section reviews the time series classification approaches considered in this work. Middlehurst et al. [4] extended the taxonomy of Bagnall et al. [5], originally based on the type of discriminatory features exploited, to incorporate recent developments, refining the categories into distance–, feature–, interval–, shapelet–, dictionary–, convolution–, deep learning–based, and hybrid approaches.

In this paper, we focus on distance-based, feature-based, and convolution-based methods, which demonstrated the strongest performance in preliminary experiments with M/EEG data. While recent advances in multivariate time series classification have centered on deep learning models, particularly those leveraging attention mechanisms, we found that such models did not yield competitive accuracy in our setting. We attribute this to the limited size of M/EEG datasets, which are inherently constrained by the practical challenges of collecting human data over long experimental sessions. These limitations underscore the need for approaches that strike a balance between expressive power and data efficiency, motivating our focus on classical yet robust methods in this study.

Distance-Based. These methods utilize a distance function to calculate the similarity between time series. This work employs a different approach, using distance to compute a feature vector representation. This approach begins by computing a distance matrix that contains pairwise distances between all time series training samples, as illustrated in Equation (2). Each row of this matrix then serves as a feature vector representing a time series, which is subsequently used as input to a standard classifier [6].

$$\begin{bmatrix} D(TS_1, TS_1) & D(TS_1, TS_2) & \cdots & D(TS_1, TS_n) \\ \vdots & \vdots & \ddots & \vdots \\ D(TS_n, TS_1) & D(TS_n, TS_2) & \cdots & D(TS_n, TS_n) \end{bmatrix} = \begin{bmatrix} C_1 \\ \vdots \\ C_n \end{bmatrix} \tag{2}$$

Paparrizos et al. [7] present a taxonomy of time series distance measures across seven categories. Lock-step measures compare the i-th points of two series and, with $O(m)$ complexity (m is the series length), are widely applied. In this work, we use Euclidean distance, the most common lock-step measure, to transform time series into feature vectors.

Distance measures for multivariate time series extend those for univariate data to quantify dissimilarity between two sequences [7]. For example, the Euclidean distance, shown in Equation (3), is computed by summing the squared differences across all time points and dimensions and then taking the square root.

$$d(X, Y) = \sqrt{\sum_{j=1}^{d} \sum_{i=1}^{n} (x_{i,j} - y_{i,j})^2} \tag{3}$$

Distance-based time series classification represents each series as a feature vector of its distances from other series, allowing standard classifiers to be applied. The k-Nearest Neighbor method leverages these distances, with 1-NN being popular for its simplicity and strong performance [8].

Gudmundsson et al. [9] first explored integrating time series distance measures with classifiers beyond k-NN, combining Support Vector Machines (SVMs) with Dynamic Time Warping. Building on this, Kate [10] studied extensively using various distance measures as SVM input features for time series classification.

Feature-Based. These techniques extract summary statistical features from time series, converting each series into a single vector to enable standard classifiers to handle temporal data [4]. The Highly Comparative Time Series Analysis (HCTSA) toolbox [11] generates over 7,700 time series features. Lubba et al. [12]

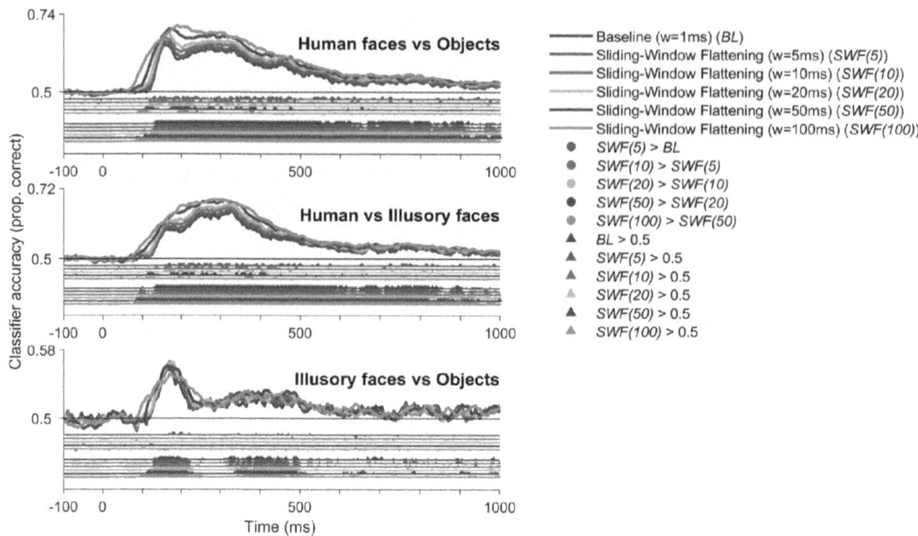

Fig. 2. Classification accuracy and temporal precision for Sliding-window flattening across three category pairs of the Pareidolia-MEG dataset. Dots below the x-axis show Bayes Factor results: colored dots mark above-chance or above-baseline performance (small dots: moderate evidence, $BF > 3$; large dots: strong evidence, $BF > 10$); Small gray dots mark moderate evidence for chance or no baseline difference ($BF < 0.3$). (Color figure online)

selected the 22 most discriminative features, called canonical time series characteristics (Catch22)[1], representing a compact and informative subset. Here, we use Catch22 as our feature-based approach for time series classification.

Convolution-Based. This approach applies convolutions between time series and specialized kernels, short subseries patterns that capture discriminative features. Each kernel produces an activation map via a sliding dot product. These maps are then summarized into feature vectors for classification [4].

Convolution (cross-correlation) applies a kernel ω of length l to a time series T via a sliding dot product, producing an activation map M, where the value at the i-th position is:

$$M_i = (T_{i,l} * \omega) = \sum_{j=0}^{l-1} T_{i+j} \cdot \omega_j \tag{4}$$

The Random Convolutional Kernel Transform (ROCKET) was proposed by Dempster et al. [13]. It generates thousands of randomly parameterized convolutional kernels. Each kernel applies two pooling operations—maximum value and proportion of positive values—and the resulting features are concatenated to form a $2k$-dimensional feature vector for k kernels.

[1] https://github.com/DynamicsAndNeuralSystems/catch22.

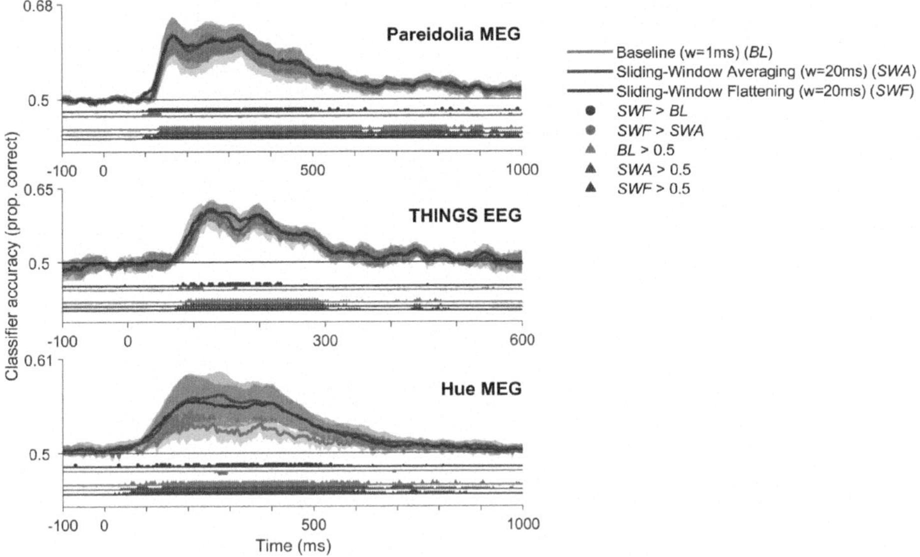

Fig. 3. Comparison of classifier performance for baseline methods across datasets (conventions as in Fig. 2). Sliding-window flattening outperforms Baseline 1 ms throughout post-stimulus. On Pareidolia-MEG and THINGS-EEG, it also exceeds Sliding-window averaging early on, while on Hue-MEG, averaging briefly outperforms flattening.

MiniROCKET[2] [14] is a faster variant of ROCKET, improving speed by over an order of magnitude while maintaining accuracy. It simplifies the method by using mostly fixed kernels and only the proportion of positive values for pooling, discarding maximum value extraction. Using 10,000 kernels, MiniROCKET efficiently generates 10,000 features.

2 Datasets

We evaluate various time series classification methods on three M/EEG datasets: *Pareidolia-MEG*, *THINGS-EEG*, and *Hue-MEG*. In each case, we performed pairwise classification of stimulus categories, since this matches the approaches used in the original works, where the patterns of relative classifier accuracy across different pairs are used to infer the brain's representation of the stimuli.

2.1 Pareidolia MEG

The first dataset contains MEG recordings (from a 160 sensor system) of brain responses to illusory faces, from [15]. Humans possess remarkable face detection and recognition abilities, supported by specialized cortical regions. This sensitive system can produce false positives, triggering the perception of faces in inanimate objects, such as trees or fruit—a phenomenon known as face pareidolia.

[2] https://github.com/angus924/minirocket.

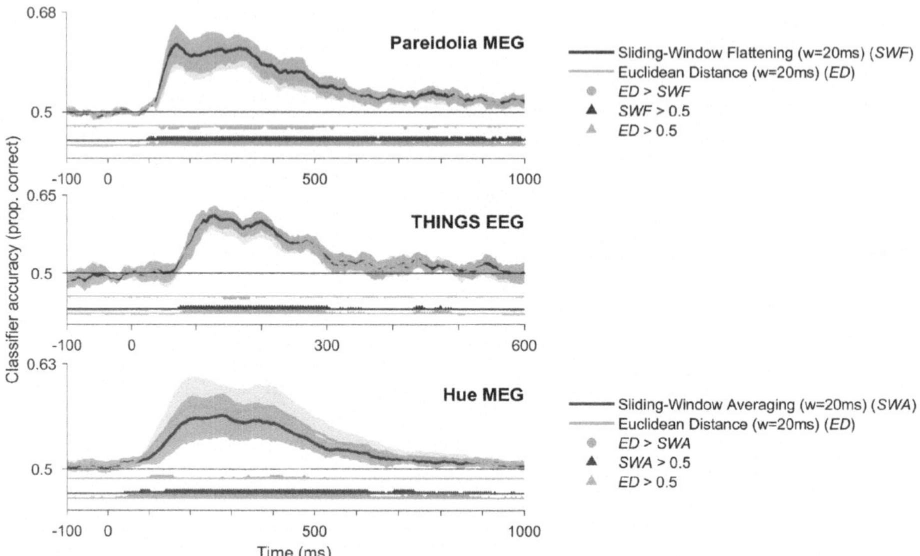

Fig. 4. Comparison of classifier performance for Euclidean Distance across datasets (conventions as in Fig. 2). On Pareidolia-MEG, Sliding-window flattening outperforms Euclidean Distance throughout post-stimulus, whereas on THINGS-EEG this advantage is brief. On Hue-MEG, Euclidean Distance outperforms Sliding-window averaging.

21 participants viewed 96 visual stimuli divided into three categories: 32 illusory faces, 32 matched non-face objects, and 32 human faces. Stimuli were presented in random order across six runs per participant, each containing four repetitions of all 96 stimuli, yielding a total of 2,304 trials (24 repetitions per stimulus).

The original study implemented cross-decoding using leave-one-exemplar-out cross-validation, where a linear discriminant analysis classifier was trained to distinguish between two categories (e.g., human faces vs. objects) using all exemplars except one from each category, then tested on the held-out exemplars. For our analysis, we used MEG recordings from the 9 participants for which head shape information was available. We calculated pairwise classification performance across the three stimulus categories using the same cross-validation scheme, meaning that all trials corresponding to the held-out stimulus exemplar were excluded from training and used for testing, but employed a ridge regression classifier instead.

2.2 THINGS EEG

The second dataset contains EEG recordings (from a 64-channel system) of brain responses to a systematic collection of objects and concepts designed to understand how the human brain categorizes and represents objects, from [16]. The full dataset comprises EEG recordings from 50 participants who viewed 22,248 images depicting 1,854 object concepts, each presented twice. In separate validation data, a further 200 images were repeated 12 times across 12 sequences. The original study employs a leave-one-sequence-out cross-validation procedure and trains a regularized linear discriminant classifier to discriminate between images.

We used the validation data with 12 repeats per image, as it is most similar to a traditional M/EEG design. To improve computational efficiency, we reduced the dataset by selecting EEG recordings from 10 participants for 20 object concepts, using 200 validation images (10 per concept), making it comparable in size to the other datasets. Pairwise classification performance was then computed using a ridge regression classifier with the same cross-validation scheme, ensuring that all trials from the held-out sequence were excluded to prevent image overlap between training and testing.

2.3 Hue MEG

The third dataset contains MEG responses (275-sensor system) to 14 different hues from 8 participants [17], designed to investigate how neural responses to color evolve over time. Stimuli were large circular blobs presented 84 times in counterbalanced order across two tasks: color categorization and color discriminability. Linear SVM classifiers were trained to discriminate stimulus hue within each task using leave-one-trial-out cross-validation.

In our study, we used MEG responses from 8 participants to 14 hues and computed pairwise classification, combining data from both tasks. We used the same cross-validation to split training and test data and a ridge regression classifier to compute accuracy.

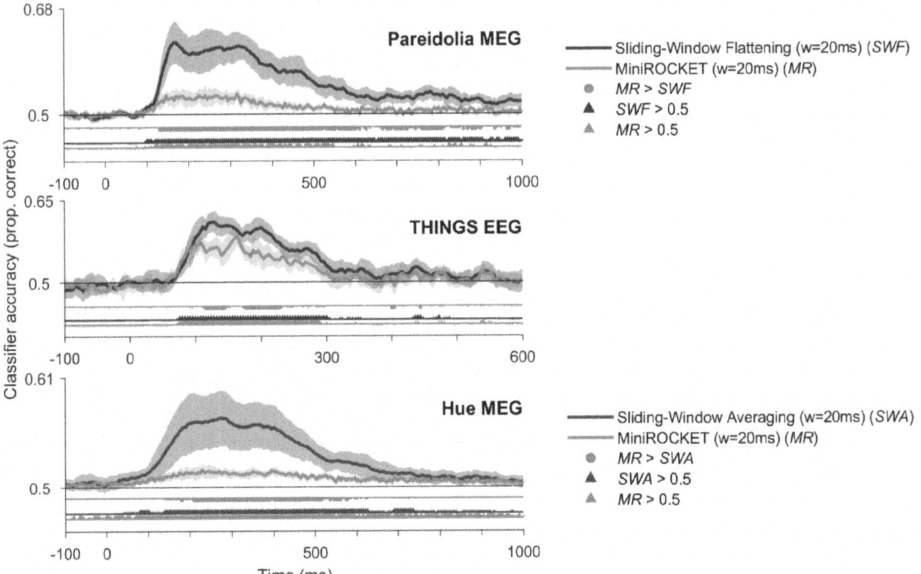

Fig. 5. Comparison of classifier performance for MiniROCKET across datasets (conventions as in Fig. 2). Sliding-window methods consistently outperform MiniROCKET.

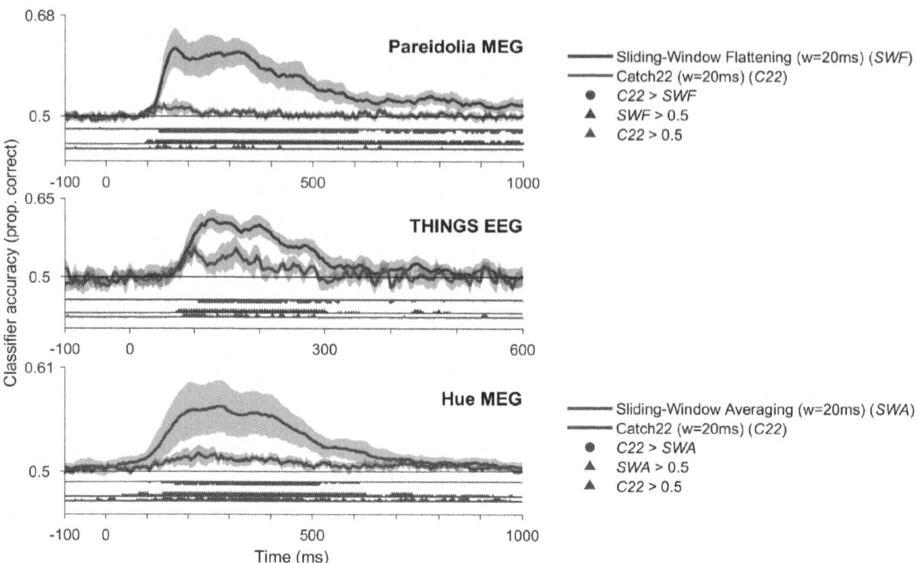

Fig. 6. Comparison of classifier performance for Catch22 across datasets (conventions as in Fig. 2). Sliding-window methods consistently outperform Catch22.

2.4 Data Preprocessing

Preprocessing of M/EEG data was performed using Brainstorm ([18], http://neuroimage.usc.edu/brainstorm), as described previously for the Hue-MEG data [17]. All M/EEG functional data were notch filtered to remove line frequency interference (50, 100, 150, and 200 Hz for THINGS and Pareidolia data, acquired in Australia, and 60, 120 and 180 Hz for Hue data, acquired in Canada), then bandpass filtered (0.2–200 Hz, using an even-order linear phase FIR filter). For MEG data (Pareidolia and Hue), cardiac and eye blink artifacts were removed using signal space projection (SSP) [19]. For THINGS-EEG data, eye blink artifacts were removed using independent component analysis (ICA) [20]. In each case, 1000 Hz functional data were extracted for each trial: from -100 to 1000 ms (MEG) or 600 ms (EEG) relative to stimulus onset. After epoching, whole-head EEG data were used in subsequent analyses.

For MEG data, we applied a further step, using minimum norm source reconstruction of the trial data to correct for participant movement between recordings during the same session. This is described elsewhere for the Hue-MEG dataset [17]. For the Pareidolia-MEG dataset, we employed a similar procedure, but since anatomical MRI images were unavailable, we created individual head models from head shape data, as in [21]. In source reconstruction, the recordings of 160 or 275 sensors are used to estimate responses from 15,000 cortical sources. To reduce this redundancy, we transformed the source-reconstructed data using principal component analysis (PCA), retaining data from the first n components that accounted for 99.99% of the variance across sources.

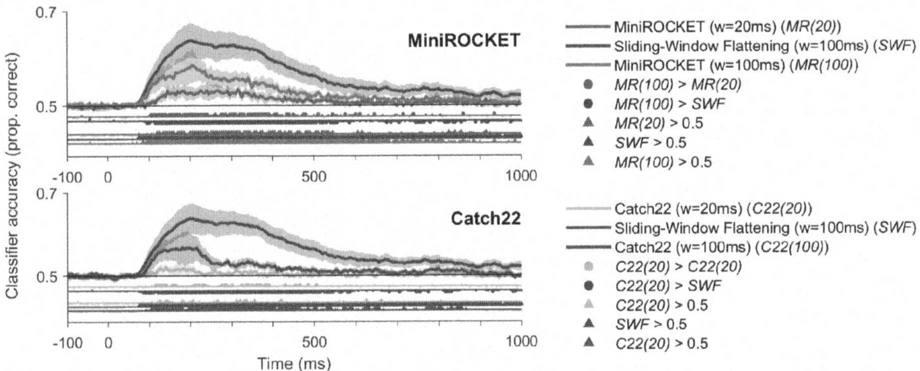

Fig. 7. Classifier performance of MiniROCKET and Catch22 on Pareidolia-MEG with longer time windows (conventions as in Fig. 2). Both methods perform better at 100 ms compared to 20 ms, but Sliding-window flattening (100 ms) still outperforms them.

3 Methodology

We evaluate six decoding approaches: three baselines that do not explicitly model temporal dependencies, and three time series classifiers that capture sequential structure. All methods operate on M/EEG trials that are aligned to stimulus onset and are evaluated using sliding windows of varying durations.

Baseline 1 ms. The standard MVPA approach applies classification independently at each time point, ignoring temporal context.

Sliding-window averaging. Averages samples within a brief temporal segment to compute summary features (here, the mean). This preserves dimensionality but collapses temporal dynamics into static values [5,22].

Sliding-window flattening. Concatenates all samples within a window into the classifier input (e.g., a 20 ms window with 150 channels yields 150×20 features). This increases dimensionality and allows richer local dynamics to be captured, though without encoding temporal order [1].

These baselines illustrate complementary trade-offs: pointwise decoding neglects temporal information, averaging incorporates context but discards dynamics, and flattening captures more temporal features without sequential order.

To overcome these limitations, we additionally assess three established families of time series classifiers, distance-based, feature-based, and convolution-based, which have been shown to perform strongly in prior benchmarks [4]. These methods explicitly model the order and dependencies among time points, designed to capture discriminative temporal patterns in MEG/EEG signals.

For all approaches, we employ `RidgeClassifierCV`, a linear classifier with L_2 regularization, from `sklearn.linear_model`. Regularization strength is selected automatically via cross-validation across a logarithmic grid of parameters ($\alpha \in$

$(-3, 3, 10)$). This yields a favorable bias–variance trade-off, typically outperforming 1-NN while training more efficiently than SVMs in our setting.

4 Experiments and Results

To support reproducible research, we created a public repository[3]. Our classifiers were trained to separate pairwise categories of images in the Pareidolia-MEG and THINGS-EEG datasets, as well as hue pairs in the Hue-MEG dataset. We assess three baseline methods and three time series classification methods—Euclidean Distance, MiniROCKET, and Catch22—with different window lengths.

We treated the time window length as a hyperparameter. We evaluated the classification accuracy and temporal precision across different time window sizes ($t = 5, 10, 20, 50, 100$ ms) for Sliding-window flattening on three category pairs of the Pareidolia-MEG dataset (Human faces vs. Objects, Human faces vs. Illusory faces, and Illusory faces vs. Objects). Figure 2 shows that classification accuracy increases with larger windows for Human faces vs. Objects and Human faces vs. Illusory faces. For Illusory faces vs. Objects, accuracy rises for windows of 5, 10, and 20 ms, but decreases for 50 and 100 ms. Additionally, as the window of time increases, there is a decrease in temporal precision with which the results can be used to draw inferences regarding the underlying neural processes. This is seen in Fig. 2 where the different dynamics or shapes of decoding accuracy curves across classifications become less distinct for the longest windows. Overall, a window of approximately 20 ms provides an effective balance between maximizing accuracy and preserving temporal precision.

Here, we used a Bayes Factor [23], which quantifies how much more likely the data are under one hypothesis (e.g., H_1) than another (e.g., H_0). It provides a continuous measure of evidence, unlike the traditional frequentist approach.

Next, we compare the average pairwise classification accuracy of the three baseline methods using a 20 ms sliding window across all datasets. As shown in Fig. 3, Sliding-window flattening achieves the highest accuracy for the Pareidolia-MEG and THINGS-EEG datasets, while Sliding-window averaging performs best for the Hue-MEG dataset. These baselines are therefore selected for subsequent comparisons with time series classification methods.

We then evaluate three time series methods—Euclidean Distance (Fig. 4), MiniROCKET (Fig. 5), and Catch22 (Fig. 6)—with a 20 ms sliding window, and compare them against their best baselines. Based on Fig. 4, Sliding-window flattening outperforms Euclidean Distance on the Pareidolia-MEG and THINGS-EEG datasets, whereas Euclidean Distance surpasses Sliding-window averaging on the Hue-MEG dataset. Furthermore, as shown in Figs. 5 and 6, baseline methods significantly outperform MiniROCKET and Catch22, suggesting that these time series approaches may require longer time windows to be more effective.

To test whether the MiniROCKET and Catch22 approaches can outperform the baseline methods at longer time windows, we compared classifier accuracy using 20-ms and 100-ms windows for both methods on the Pareidolia-MEG

[3] https://github.com/F-Barazesh-Morgani/MVPA_TemporalFeatures.

dataset. As shown in Fig. 7, although MiniROCKET and Catch22 with 100 ms windows outperform their 20 ms counterparts, Sliding-window flattening with a 100 ms window still outperforms both, even at 100 ms.

5 Conclusion and Future Work

The results of computing the average pairwise classification accuracy across stimuli in the Pareidolia-MEG, THINGS-EEG, and Hue-MEG datasets demonstrate that using a brief time window—as in Sliding-window flattening, which incorporates multiple adjacent time points as input features—enables the classifier to capture richer temporal dynamics compared to traditional single-time-point approaches (Baseline 1 ms). This strategy enhances the sensitivity of MVPA methods for detecting neural representations in both MEG and EEG data across all three datasets. However, Sliding-window flattening does not account for the temporal order of observations within each window.

To address this limitation and model the sequential structure of the data, we employed three time series classification methods—representing distance-based, feature-based, and convolution-based approaches—that explicitly capture dependencies among time points in dynamic brain signals.

Among these, we found that applying Euclidean distance with a 20 ms window to transform the time series into feature vectors improved the sensitivity of MVPA compared to traditional methods (Baseline 1 ms), which compute classifier accuracy at individual time points. This improvement was observed across all three datasets, and in the Hue-MEG dataset, the Euclidean distance method even outperformed Sliding-window flattening and averaging.

While methods like MiniROCKET and Catch22 often outperform simpler approaches in other domains (e.g., gesture recognition), they did not yield better performance in our analysis when using a 20 ms window. These methods typically benefit from longer time windows, but extending the window length would compromise temporal precision, which is critical for our research goals.

As future work, we will explore deep learning methods such as LSTMs, RNNs, TCNs, and Transformers, combined with data augmentation, to better capture temporal dependencies and dynamic patterns in M/EEG data.

Disclosure of Interests. The authors have no competing interests to declare that are relevant to the content of this article.

References

1. Grootswagers, T., Wardle, S.G., Carlson, T.A.: Decoding dynamic brain patterns from evoked responses: a tutorial on multivariate pattern analysis applied to time series neuroimaging data. J. Cogn. Neurosci. **29**(4), 677–697 (2017)
2. Ashton, K., et al.: Time-resolved multivariate pattern analysis of infant EEG data: a practical tutorial. Dev. Cogn. Neurosci. **52**, 101044 (2022)

3. Wu, H., et al.: Decoding n400m evoked component: a tutorial on multivariate pattern analysis for op-meg data. Brain Sci. **12**(5), 1–19 (2022)
4. Middlehurst, M., Schäfer, P., Bagnall, A.: Bake off redux: a review and experimental evaluation of recent time series classification algorithms. Data Min. Knowl. Discov. (2023)
5. Bagnall, A., Lines, J., Bostrom, A., Large, J., Keogh, E.: The great time series classification bake off: a review and experimental evaluation of recent algorithmic advances. Data Min. Knowl. Discov. **31**(3), 606–660 (2017)
6. Abanda, A., Mori, U., Lozano, J.A.: A review on distance based time series classification. Data Min. Knowl. Discov. **33**(2), 378–412 (2019)
7. Paparrizos, J., et al.: A survey on time series distance measures. ACM Comput. Surv. **55**(4) 2023
8. Ding, H., Trajcevski, G., Scheuermann, P., Wang, X., Keogh, E.: Querying and mining of time series data: experimental comparison of representations and distance measures. Proc. VLDB Endow. **1**(2), 1542–1552 (2008)
9. Gudmundsson, S., Runarsson, T.P., Sigurdsson, S.: Support vector machines and dynamic time warping for time series. In: Proceedings of the Joint Conference Neural Networks (IEEE World Congress on Computational Intellignce), pp. 2772–2776. IEEE (2008)
10. Kate, R.J.: Using dynamic time warping distances as features for improved time series classification. Data Min. Knowl. Discov. **30**(2), 283–312 (2016)
11. Fulcher, B.D., Jones, N.S.: hctsa: a computational framework for automated time series phenotyping using massive feature extraction. Cell Syst. **5**(5), 527-531.e3 (2017)
12. Lubba, C.H., et al.: catch22: canonical time series characteristics selected through highly comparative time series analysis. Data Min. Knowl. Discov. **33**(6), 1821–1852 (2019)
13. Dempster, A., Petitjean, F., Webb, G.: Rocket: exceptionally fast and accurate time series classification using random convolutional kernels. Data Min. Knowl. Discov. **34**, 1454–1495 (2020)
14. Dempster, A., Schmidt, D.F., Webb, G.I.: Minirocket: a very fast (almost) deterministic transform for time series classification. In: Proceedings of the ACM SIGKDD International Conference on Knowledge Discovery and Data Mining, pp. 248–257. ACM (2021)
15. Wardle, S.G., Taubert, J., Teichmann, L., Baker, C.I.: Rapid and dynamic processing of face pareidolia in the human brain. Nat. Commun. **11**, 4518 (2020)
16. Grootswagers, T., Zhou, I., Robinson, A.K., Hebart, M.N., Carlson, T.A.: Human EEG recordings for 1,854 concepts presented in rapid serial visual presentation streams. Sci. Data **9**(1), 3 (2022)
17. Goddard, E., Mullen, K.T.: Temporal evolution of color representations measured with magnetoencephalography reveals a "coarse to fine" dynamic. J. Cogn. Neurosci. 1–25 (2025)
18. Tadel, F., Baillet, S., Mosher, J.C., Pantazis, D., Leahy, R.M.: Brainstorm: a user-friendly application for MEG/EEG analysis. Comput. Intell. Neurosci. **2011**, 879716 (2011)
19. Uusitalo, M.A., Ilmoniemi, R.J.: Signal-space projection method for separating MEG or EEG into components. Med. Biol. Eng. Comput. **35**(2), 135–140 (1997)
20. Ablin, P., Cardoso, J., Gramfort, A.: Faster independent component analysis by preconditioning with Hessian approximations. IEEE Trans. Sign. Process. **66**(15), 4040–4049 (2018)

21. Goddard, E., Carlson, T.A., Woolgar, A.: Spatial and feature-selective attention have distinct, interacting, effects on population-level tuning. **34**(2), 290–312
22. Fulcher, B.D., Jones, N.S.: Highly comparative feature-based time series classification. IEEE Trans. Knowl. Data Eng. **26**(12), 3026–3037 (2014)
23. Kass, R.E., Raftery, A.E.: Bayes factors. J. Am. Stat. Assoc. **90**(430), 773–795 (1995)

Relevance-Aware Thresholding in Online Conformal Prediction for Time Series

Théo Dupuy[1(✉)], Binbin Xu[1], Stéphane Perrey[2], Jacky Montmain[1], and Abdelhak Imoussaten[1]

[1] EuroMov Digital Health in Motion, Univ Montpellier, IMT Mines Ales, Ales, France
theo.dupuy@mines-ales.fr
[2] EuroMov Digital Health in Motion, Univ Montpellier, IMT Mines Ales, Montpellier, France

Abstract. Uncertainty quantification has received considerable interest in recent works in Machine Learning. In particular, Conformal Prediction (CP) gains ground in this field. For the case of time series, Online Conformal Prediction (OCP) becomes an option to address the problem of data distribution shift over time. Indeed, the idea of OCP is to update a threshold of some quantity (whether the miscoverage level or the quantile) based on the distribution observation. To evaluate the performance of OCP methods, two key aspects are typically considered: the coverage validity and the prediction interval width minimization. Recently, new OCP methods have emerged, offering long-run coverage guarantees and producing more informative intervals. However, during the threshold update step, most of these methods focus solely on the validity of the prediction intervals – that is, whether the ground truth falls inside or outside the interval – without accounting for their relevance. In this paper, we aim to leverage this overlooked aspect. Specifically, we propose enhancing the threshold update step by replacing the binary evaluation (inside/outside) with a broader class of functions that quantify the relevance of the prediction interval using the ground truth. This approach helps prevent abrupt threshold changes, potentially resulting in narrower prediction intervals. Indeed, experimental results on real-world datasets suggest that these functions can produce tighter intervals compared to existing OCP methods while maintaining coverage validity.

1 Introduction

Machine learning algorithms are increasingly applied in sensitive fields such as health, sport, finance, education, etc. Consequently, significant effort is being devoted to trustworthy AI, and more specifically to explainable and robust AI. Among the available approaches, uncertainty quantification is an effective way to develop more robust models. Indeed, cautious prediction methods have the advantage of providing information about the uncertainty related to an output. They also allow the Decision Makers (DMs) to incorporate their preferences in

P. Bruno et al. (Eds.): HC_AIxIA_HYDRA 2025, CCIS 2830, pp. 196–217, 2026.
https://doi.org/10.1007/978-3-032-16708-8_17

order to minimize risk [11]. Various methods have been introduced to address this global need of uncertainty quantification. One method that stands out from the rest is *Conformal Prediction* (CP) [9]. Indeed, Conformal Prediction (CP) offers the key advantage of ensuring the targeted coverage regardless of the predictor's quality.

This paper focuses on time series data, which are commonly found in sensitive applications. In such contexts, forecasts should incorporate uncertainty quantification to better support DMs. Classical methods such as *AutoRegressive*, *Moving Average*, and *ARIMA* (AutoRegressive Integrated Moving Average) models [7] are commonly used to forecast time series. However, these methods do not include an uncertainty quantification component. CP could have been a suitable candidate for incorporating uncertainty quantification into time series forecasting. Nevertheless, the theoretical coverage guarantee of CP, which relies on the assumption of data exchangeability [9,16], does not hold in the context of time series. Moreover, classical CP has limitations in the presence of data distribution shifts, which are common in time series. In order to overcome the shortcomings of classical CP, methods such as weighted CP [6,14,15] or *Adaptive Conformal Inference* (ACI) [10,20] were introduced. In this paper, we build on the ACI approach, where prediction intervals are adjusted based on coverage errors, without relying on specific assumptions about the time series. Specifically, in the ACI framework, online prediction is performed: at each time step, a prediction interval is produced, then the ground truth is revealed. Based on the observed prediction error, the confidence level (or miscoverage rate α) is updated and used to compute the interval for the next time step. The main drawback of this method is that it often produces uninformative intervals. New approaches [1,2,18,19] have emerged that consider updating the quantile threshold q, which regulates the size of the prediction interval, rather than changing the confidence placed on it. These approaches have demonstrated significant results both theoretically, by maintaining the targeted coverage, and empirically, by providing reasonably tight prediction subsets. Note that these two criteria are essential to evaluate these methods. Throughout this paper, we will refer to all these online methods as *Online Conformal Prediction* (OCP).

However, when updating the threshold q_t, most of these OCP methods consider only a binary notion of error: whether the ground truth lies within the prediction subset or not. Our approach seeks to address this limitation by fully leveraging the revealed ground truth. Specifically, to evaluate a prediction subset with respect to the ground truth, we favour the notion of relevance over the traditional concept of error. This newly introduced relevance feedback relies on the distance between the ground truth and the bounds of the prediction interval. We argue that this approach leads to improved performance of several OCP methods concerning the size of the prediction subsets. Based on this proposition, our contributions are the following:

- We propose a family of customizable functions, each with specific characteristics, to incorporate the concept of relevance during threshold update in OCP methods.

- We enhance the state-of-the-art OCP methods by introducing the proposed functions and then analyze how this modification impacts the validity, i.e. the long-run coverage guarantees, and improves the efficiency, i.e. minimal width of the intervals, of the original OCP methods.
- We show, on real-world datasets, that the modified OCP methods achieve better or competitive validity and efficiency compared to the original ones.

Our code, including all experiments and methods used, is available on GitHub.

Notations. In the sequel, we use the following notations: $[\![a,b]\!] = \{a, a+1, \dots, b\}$; $\mathbb{1}$ denotes the indicator function; $\mathbb{R}_+^*$ denotes the set of strictly positive real numbers (excluding 0); ∇f denotes the gradient of the function f; $\lceil \cdot \rceil$ denotes the ceiling function; α refers to miscoverage level and $1-\alpha$ refers to nominal level or confidence level.

2 Background

In this section, we introduce all the problem setup and the OCP methods that we will use in Sect. 3.

Conformal Prediction (CP). There are a lot of techniques that use the general formalisation of CP, as described in [3]. We can, for example, mention *Split Conformal Prediction* (SCP) [13] or *jacknife+* [5]. We briefly explain SCP in the context of regression tasks. Let us consider n observations $(X_i, Y_i)_{i \in [\![1,n]\!]} \in \mathcal{X} \times \mathcal{Y}$ and a regressor ζ that maps $\mathcal{X}$ to $\mathcal{Y}$. For SCP method, this training set of size n is split into two subsets T and C_{al}: T is used for the proper training of the regressor ζ and C_{al} is used for the calibration (in this example, let m be the size of C_{al}). Then, this trained regressor ζ is used to predict the values $\widehat{Y}_{i \in [\![1,m]\!]}$ of the calibration subset C_{al}, i.e. $\widehat{Y}_i = \zeta(X_i)$. Thus, $\forall i \in [\![1,m]\!]$ the non-conformity scores $s(X_i, Y_i)$ can be computed. A classic choice for $s(X_i, Y_i)$ is $s(X_i, Y_i) = |Y_i - \widehat{Y}_i|$. We denote by q_α the $1-\alpha$ quantile of these non-conformity scores. Finally, for a test sample X_{test}, $\widehat{Y}_{test}$ is predicted with ζ and, using the scores $|Y_i - \widehat{Y}_i|$, the algorithm outputs the interval $\widehat{C}(X_{test}) = [\widehat{Y}_{test} \pm q_\alpha]$. The more general formalisation of the output of SCP is $\widehat{C}(X_{test}) = \{Y \in \mathcal{Y};\ s(X_{test}, Y) \leq q_\alpha\}$. Note that, if the test point and the calibration set are exchangeable, $1-\alpha \leq \mathbb{P}(Y_{test} \in \widehat{C}(X_{test})) \leq 1-\alpha+\frac{1}{m+1}$ holds [9,16] where Y_{test} is the ground truth associated to X_{test}.

Online Conformal Prediction (OCP). OCP is a special setting for CP when exchangeability doesn't hold. It allows to tackle the case of predicting values online. The idea is to predict the next value based on the ground truths of the previous time step (which have been revealed). Thus, $(X_t, Y_t)_{t \geq 1}$ are collected online. At time t we want to output a prediction subset $\widehat{C}_t$ for the unknown ground truth Y_t based on $(X_{t'}, Y_{t'})_{t'<t} \in \mathcal{X} \times \mathcal{Y}$.

Usually, in the context of OCP, the subset $\widehat{C}_t$ is expressed as follows:

$$\widehat{C}_t(X_t) = \{Y \in \mathcal{Y};\ s(X_t, Y) \leq q_t\}. \tag{1}$$

In the OCP setting, authors typically update either the miscoverage level α_t or the threshold q_t, as they are dependent on each other. In the following, let $s_t = s(X_t, Y_t)$. As an example, we present the two methods used in the following sections:

- In PID [1], the update is the following:

$$\begin{aligned} q_{t+1} = \hat{s}_t + \eta \cdot (\mathbb{1}\{Y_t \notin \widehat{C}_t\} - \alpha) \\ + r_t \left(\sum_{i=1}^{t} (\mathbb{1}\{Y_i \notin \widehat{C}_i\} - \alpha) \right). \end{aligned} \tag{2}$$

  with $\hat{s}_t$ being a scorecaster and r_t a saturation function. Thus, r_t respects the following property:

$$\begin{aligned} x \geq c \cdot h(t) \implies r_t(x) \geq b, \\ x \leq -c \cdot h(t) \implies r_t(x) \leq -b. \end{aligned} \tag{3}$$

  for constants $b, c > 0$, and a sub-linear, non-negative, non-decreasing function h. Furthers details on this method are provided in Appendix B.1.
- In ECI [18], the authors propose the following update depending on a smoothing function g:

$$q_{t+1} = q_t + \eta[\mathbb{1}\{Y_t \notin \widehat{C}_t\} - \alpha + (s_t - q_t)\nabla g(s_t - q_t)]. \tag{4}$$

This idea of smoothing is closely related to our work, and we analyze how it differs in Appendix B.2. Several other update strategies have been proposed, and some of them are presented in Appendix B.3.

To assess the performance of OCP methods, two criteria are considered: validity, defined as the long-run coverage property:

$$\lim_{T \to +\infty} \frac{1}{T} \sum_{t=1}^{T} \mathbb{1}\{Y_t \notin \widehat{C}_t\} = \alpha, \tag{5}$$

and efficiency, which aims at minimizing the size of the prediction subsets.

3 Methodology

The core idea of this paper is to estimate the relevance of the prediction subset $\widehat{C}_t$ using the distance between the ground truth Y_t and the bounds of $\widehat{C}_t$, in order to reduce the prediction interval size while maintaining the validity. To approximate this distance, we use the quantity $s_t - q_t$ (see Appendix C.1 for details). Then, we use this relevance estimation for the prediction of $\widehat{C}_{t+1}$ through the value q_{t+1} which has been updated. In the state of the art of OCP methods, only the quantity $\mathbb{1}\{Y_t \notin \widehat{C}_t\}$ is used to evaluate the prediction subset. This leads to a substantial loss of information. To illustrate, consider two prediction subsets,

$\widehat{C}^1 = [0, 6]$ and $\widehat{C}^2 = [0, 2]$, with a ground truth of 6.1. Using the indicator function, both intervals are treated as equally erroneous, although this is not the case. In this paper, we introduce a family of functions to quantify relevance and address this limitation.

The introduced family of functions are used within two OCP methods. The choice of these OCP methods is arbitrary but the idea of relevance-awareness remains general for all OCP methods. In the following, we introduce and refer to the sigmoid function as: $\sigma(x) = \frac{1}{1+\exp(-x)}$.

Presentation of the Proposed Functions. To meet the relevance and error tracking requirements, the new functions should satisfy the following constraints:

1. **Indicator function behaviour:** We want the functions to have a range in $[0, 1]$. It allows a behaviour close with that of the indicator function.
2. **Scale independence:** Moreover, we want to avoid a scale dependency.
3. **Static state:** We also want to have $f(0) = \alpha$ in order to allow the OCP methods to leave the threshold unchanged when the correct choice has already been made.

We set $\Omega = \{\omega \in (\mathbb{R}_+^*)^l;\ \sum_{i=1}^{l} \omega_i = 1\}$. Based on the constraints 1, 2 and 3, we propose the following family of functions: $\forall(\omega, v) \in \Omega \times (\mathbb{R}_+^*)^l$,

$$f_{\omega,v,\mu_t}(s_t - q_t) = \sum_{i=1}^{l} \omega_i.\sigma\left(\frac{v_i}{\mu_t}.(s_t - q_t) - \ln\left(\frac{1-\alpha}{\alpha}\right)\right). \tag{6}$$

with $l \geq 1$, $\mu_t = \frac{1}{T_w}|\sum_{i=\max(t-T_w,1)}^{t-1}(s_i - q_i)|$ and T_w being the window size.

Further details regarding the construction of these functions are provided in Appendix C.2.

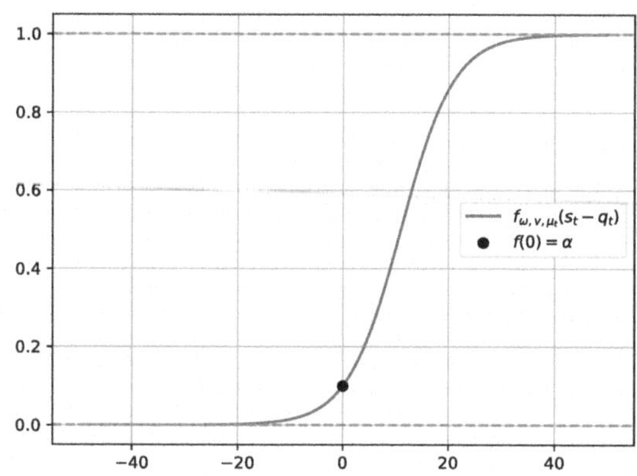

Fig. 1. f_{ω,v,μ_t} with $\alpha = 0.1, \omega = 1, v = 4$ $(l = 1)$ and $\mu_t = 20$.

Note that the summation is introduced to enable the DMs to precisely parametrize the functions according to their respective domains.

As explained earlier, these functions are used at time t to quantify the relevance of the prediction interval $\widehat{C}_t$. Then, the quantity $f_{\omega,v,\mu_t} - \alpha$ is incorporated into the computation of q_{t+1} which determines the size of the next prediction interval $\widehat{C}_{t+1}$. Thus, as one can see in Fig. 1, for $s_t - q_t > 0$ (i.e. the ground truth is outside the interval), the quantity f_{ω,v,μ_t} will increase until 1 when $s_t - q_t$ grows. This means that the more the ground truth is far from the interval, the more we will increase q_{t+1} and the larger the next interval will be. On the other side (i.e. $s_t - q_t < 0$ and the ground truth is inside the interval), the more the ground truth is far from the bounds the more we will decrease q_{t+1} and the tighter the next interval will be.

Moreover, given that f_{ω,v,μ_t} depends on μ_t, it allows the function to adapt its behaviour dynamically based on the previous errors. Indeed, intuitively, if μ_t (i.e., the mean of the distances over the last steps) is large, we should avoid penalizing too heavily when the current error $s_t - q_t$ is smaller. This behaviour can be adapted through the parameters ω and v.

Parametrization of the Proposed Functions. As shown in Eq. (6), the functions are customizable, enabling their behaviour to be tailored according to the DMs' preferences and field experience. Thus, in this part, we will analyse this behaviour with respect to the values of the vectors v and ω.

Firstly, we analyse the impact of the parameter v. Intuitively, this parameter guides how quickly the function approaches its horizontal asymptotes. Indeed, if $v \to 0$, $f_{\omega,v,\mu_t} \to \alpha$ and if $v \to \infty$ the function will behave as the indicator function. Figure 2 shows the curve of f for different values of v.

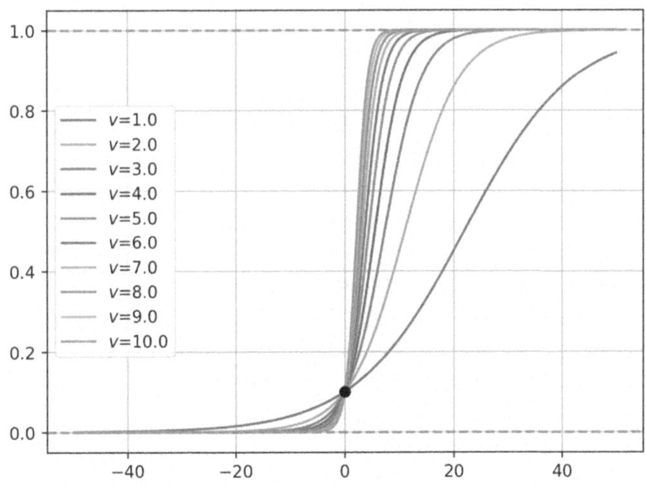

Fig. 2. Plots of f_{ω,v,μ_t} with $\alpha = 0.1, \omega = 1$ ($l = 1$) and $\mu_t = 10$.

This could help the DMs decide how they want to penalize the errors of the OCP methods. Hence, the DMs can choose the value of v based on their decision preferences and expertise.

Secondly, we note that, the parameter ω has an impact if and only if $l > 1$ and $\exists(i,j) \in [\![1,l]\!]^2;\ v_i \neq v_j$. Otherwise, the sum could be gathered as a single sigmoid function. Thus, in this part, we will respect these conditions to show the impact of ω.

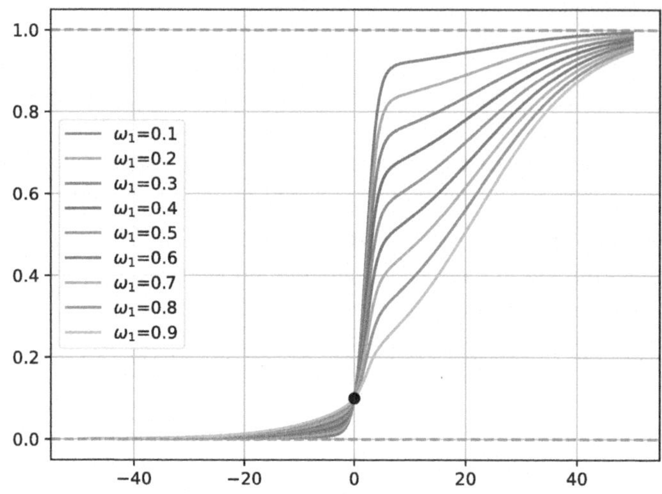

Fig. 3. Plots of f_{ω,v,μ_t} with $\alpha = 0.1, v_1 = 1, v_2 = 10$ and $\mu_t = 10$.

In Fig. 3, we show an example with $l = 2$ and with parameters v_i enough different to observe the behaviour due to ω. Indeed, choosing very distinct v_i allows to avoid a behaviour close to what we could expect with $l = 1$. Thus, the parameter ω, combined with the parameter v, is designed to offer an additional way to create the most suitable function shape for the specific case the DMs face. Indeed, with this parameter, you can add a plateau to the function. This can help the DMs if, for example, for their application, they know that the errors between 10 and 20 have almost the same impact but beyond they want to penalize more. Note that, the parameters ω and v could depend on time. Hence, the DMs can change the desire behaviour dynamically. A few reflections on the selection process are presented in Appendix C.3.

In the following, we introduce the modified OCP methods that we tested in Sect. 4:

Modifications of PID Update Rule. In this part, we consider the modification of the PID (Equation (2)) with the proposed functions. We also consider the impact that it will have on the long-run coverage (Equation (5)). We introduce the following updates:

- In the first update (Equation (7)), we replace all the occurrences of the quantity $\mathbb{1}\{Y_t \notin \widehat{C}_t\}$ by the proposed function:

$$q_{t+1} = \hat{s}_t + \eta \cdot (f_{\omega,v,\mu_t}(s_t - q_t) - \alpha) + r_t\left(\sum_{i=1}^{t}(f_{\omega,v,\mu_i}(s_i - q_i) - \alpha)\right). \tag{7}$$

- In the second one (Equation (8)), we just replace the occurrence in the saturation function:

$$q_{t+1} = \hat{s}_t + \eta \cdot (\mathbb{1}\{Y_t \notin \widehat{C}_t\} - \alpha) + r_t\left(\sum_{i=1}^{t}(f_{\omega,v,\mu_i}(s_i - q_i) - \alpha)\right). \tag{8}$$

- In the last update rule (Equation (9)), we just replace the occurrence outside the saturation function:

$$q_{t+1} = \hat{s}_t + \eta \cdot (f_{\omega,v,\mu_t}(s_t - q_t) - \alpha) + r_t\left(\sum_{i=1}^{t}(\mathbb{1}\{Y_i \notin \widehat{C}_i\} - \alpha)\right). \tag{9}$$

The following theorems state the long-run coverage of the three modified PID updates. The proofs are given in Appendix A.

Theorem 1. *Let $(s_i)_{i\in\mathbb{N}^*}$ be any sequence of numbers in $[-\frac{b}{2}, \frac{b}{2}]$, where $b > 0$, and may be infinite. Assume that r_t is a saturation function following the Eq.* (3).

Then, the update (9) *satisfies the long-run coverage given in Eq.* (5).

Theorem 2. *Let $(s_i)_{i\in\mathbb{N}^*}$ be any sequence of numbers in $[-\frac{b}{2}, \frac{b}{2}]$, where $b > 0$, and may be infinite. Assume that r_t is a saturation function following the Eq.* (3).

Then, if there exists $T' \in \mathbb{N}^*$ such that $\forall T \geq T'$, $|\sum_{i=1}^{T}(\mathbb{1}\{Y_i \notin \widehat{C}_i\} - \alpha)| \leq |\sum_{i=1}^{T}(f_{\omega,v,\mu_i}(s_i - q_i) - \alpha)|$, the updates (7) *and* (8) *satisfy the long-run coverage given in Eq.* (5)

We notice that the last assumption of Theorem 2 (about the existence of T') could be pretty strong. Indeed, given that the values taken by f_{ω,v,μ_t} are often around α, the sum $\sum_{i=1}^{T}(f_{\omega,v,\mu_i}(s_i - q_i) - \alpha)$ can be very small.

Modification of ECI Update Rule. Equation (10) modifies the update of Eq. (4):

$$q_{t+1} = q_t + \eta[\mathbb{1}\{Y_t \notin \widehat{C}_t\} - \alpha + (s_t - q_t)\nabla f_{\omega,v,\mu_t}(s_t - q_t)]. \tag{10}$$

For the following theorem, we notice that $|\nabla f_{\omega,v,\mu_t}|$ and $|x \cdot \nabla f_{\omega,v,\mu_t}(x)|$ are bounded, i.e. there exists $M, U > 0$ such as $\forall x \in \mathbb{R}, |\nabla f_{\omega,v,\mu_t}(x)| \leq M$ and $|x \cdot \nabla f_{\omega,v,\mu_t}(x)| \leq U$ [18].

Theorem 3. *Let $(s_i)_{i\in\mathbb{N}^*}$ be any sequence of numbers. We assume that $\forall i \in \mathbb{N}^*$ there exists B such that $s_i \in [0, B]$. We set $N = \lceil\frac{1}{\alpha}\rceil$. Assume that $\eta > N.B$, $M < \frac{\min(\eta, N^2)}{2N^2[B+\eta(1-\alpha+U)]}$.*

Then, the update (10) *satisfies the long-run coverage given in Eq.* (5).

4 Results

In this section, we compare the modified ECI and PID methods to their respective original versions to illustrate how the proposed functions can improve their results. Thus, the purpose is not to perform a comparison between the original OCP methods because it has already been done in the original papers. Once again, our approach to relevance-awareness is global, and the selection of the OCP methods we chose to modify and test remains subjective. As a justification, we selected PID and ECI because they represent the most recent state-of-the-art methods and because their use of three terms makes them more elaborate.

To compare the methods performance, we consider the following criteria: the global coverage, the average size and the median width of the prediction intervals. We report the last two criteria, acknowledging that evaluating interval width, even when an error occurs, can be debated; however, this choice enables a fair comparison with state-of-the-art OCP methods that use the same evaluation protocol.

Firstly, we present the experiment setup, including the datasets, regressors, and parameter configurations. Note that, most of these choices align with those in PID [1] and ECI [18] propositions to ensure meaningful and consistent comparisons.

Datasets and Regressors. We use the following datasets:

- The stock price of *Amazon*, *Google* and *Microsoft* [12].
- The temperature in Delhi [17].

As for the regressors, we use basic time series forecasters:

- The *AutoRegressive* (AR) model [7] with $p = 3$.
- The *Theta* model [4] with $\theta = 2$.

General Implementation. For all the experiments conducted, the regressors are trained using the most recent 365 data points, meaning the training dataset follows a sliding window as forecasting progresses. Furthermore, we use the score $s_t = |Y_t - \widehat{Y}_t|$ along with symmetric prediction intervals, resulting in $\widehat{C}_t = [\widehat{Y}_t \pm q_t]$.

General Parameters. We choose a confidence level $1 - \alpha = 90\%$ and $T_w = 100$ for the computation of μ_t. We use $\eta = 0.005$ for the learning rate and initialize $q_1 = 0$. We fixed these parameters to classical values in order to isolate and evaluate the impact of the proposed functions. Note that the parameters η and q_1 play a crucial role in convergence – particularly for ECI, for which we reserve the right to use a different learning rate. The complete set of parameters used in our experiments is available on the GitHub repository.

4.1 PID Vs Modified PID.

In this part, we take $\hat{s}_t = q_t$ to facilitate the computation. Note that in the PID paper, the authors show how a real scorecaster can impact the results. In this section, we specifically focus on the modified PID update rule presented in Eq. (9). In the following, we refer to this update as a modified PID. Additional results, including those based on Eqs. (7) and (8), are presented in Appendix D.1.

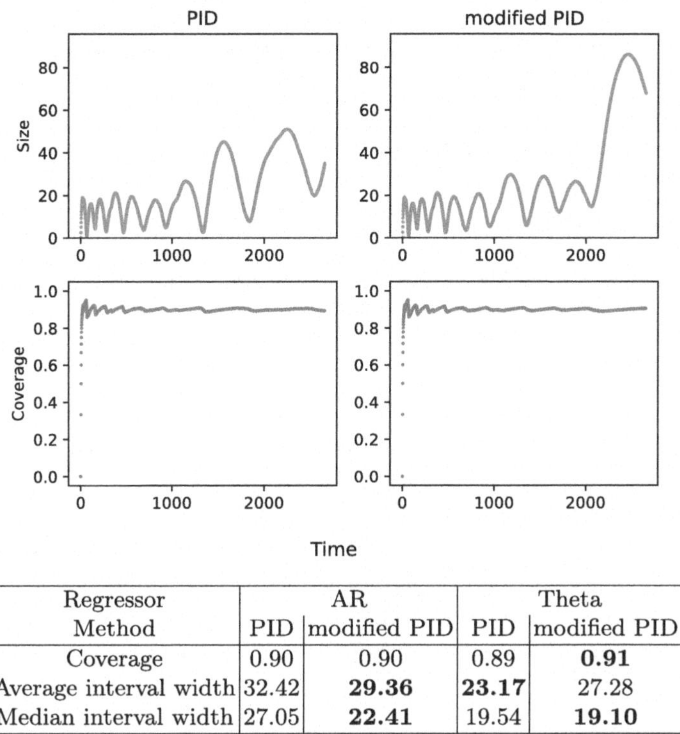

Regressor	AR		Theta	
Method	PID	modified PID	PID	modified PID
Coverage	0.90	0.90	0.89	**0.91**
Average interval width	32.42	**29.36**	**23.17**	27.28
Median interval width	27.05	**22.41**	19.54	**19.10**

Fig. 4. PID vs modified PID performances on the *Amazon* stock price dataset. The plots show *Theta* as the regressor.

In the table of Fig. 4, we observe that the modified PID update leads to a reduction in both the average interval width and the median interval width when using the AR regressor. However, for the *Theta* regressor, while the median interval width and coverage improve, the average interval width increases slightly. As shown in the graph of Fig. 4, this higher average size is primarily due to a sharp increase at the end of the series. This could be related to a distribution shift – visible in Fig. 6 of Appendix E – which may have caused a degradation in the regressor's performance.

Table 1. PID vs modified PID performances on the *Google* stock price dataset.

Regressor	AR		Theta	
Method	PID	modified PID	PID	modified PID
Coverage	**0.91**	0.90	0.91	0.91
Average interval width	43.75	**34.96**	38.61	**35.48**
Median interval width	39.44	**35.14**	31.97	**27.85**

In Table 1, we also observe improved performances, particularly in terms of interval width, while maintaining the targeted coverage. This improvement can be attributed to the enhanced stability provided by using the notion of relevance instead of the traditional concept of error.

4.2 ECI Vs Modified ECI

In this part, we compare the original ECI method (Equation (4) with the modified version introduced in Eq. (10). For the original ECI, we use the sigmoid function with $\lambda = 1$, as specified in the original paper [18]. Additional results are presented in Appendix D.2.

Table 2. ECI vs modified ECI performances on the *Microsoft* stock price dataset.

Regressor	AR		Theta	
Method	ECI	modified ECI	ECI	modified ECI
Coverage	0.83	**0.90**	0.82	**0.90**
Average interval width	**1.32**	1.72	**1.31**	1.70
Median interval width	**1.29**	1.58	**1.27**	1.62

Table 3. ECI vs modified ECI performances on the temperature dataset.

Regressor	AR		Theta	
Method	ECI	modified ECI	ECI	modified ECI
Coverage	0.78	**0.90**	0.78	**0.90**
Average interval width	**3.73**	5.32	**3.71**	5.41
Median interval width	**3.76**	5.38	**3.78**	5.49

First of all, as shown in Table 2 and Table 3, we observe that the original ECI update struggles to achieve the expected coverage. These results differ from those reported in [18], despite using the learning rate that yields the best coverage in our setting (this setting has been described in Sect. 4). To ensure a fair comparison, the results for the modified ECI and the original ECI updates are obtained using the same learning rate, while only adjusting the parameter v (with $\omega = 1$ at this stage) for the modified ECI update. We frequently observe this coverage issue with the original ECI update. A possible explanation is discussed in Appendix B.2.

Regarding the results, both methods demonstrate strong performances. In particular, the evolution of the prediction interval sizes is well controlled, with smooth adjustments rather than abrupt changes, as illustrated in Fig. 5. However, the favourable results in terms of interval size for the original ECI update should be interpreted with caution, as the targeted coverage level is not achieved.

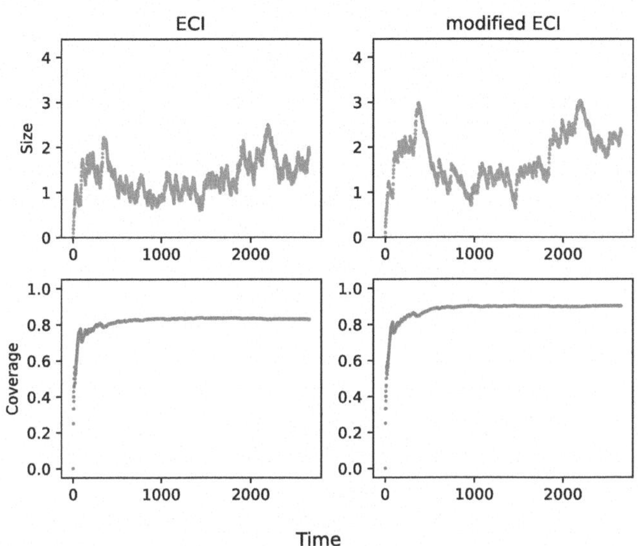

Fig. 5. ECI vs modified ECI on the Microsoft stock price dataset (AR regressor).

Finally, we report the results presented in [18], obtained using their standard ECI update and experimental setting (Table 4):

Table 4. Results of the original ECI method as reported in [18].

	AR			Theta		
Dataset	Coverage	Avg width	Med width	Coverage	Avg width	Med width
Amazon	0.895	17.12	12.73	0.897	17.46	12.49
Google	0.897	19.95	17.19	0.896	30.92	29.53
Temperature	0.901	6.39	6.10	0.90	6.41	6.27

The results for the *Microsoft* stock price dataset are not provided in their paper. Comparing with our results of the modified ECI method (Tables 3, 9, 10), we observe the following:

- ***Amazon***: The performance is comparable overall, with the original ECI showing a slight advantage in median interval width.
- ***Google***: Our modified ECI method performs significantly better with the *Theta* regressor, while the original ECI performs slightly better with the AR model.
- **Temperature**: Our method outperforms ECI across all metrics, demonstrating a clear improvement.

5 Conclusion

Our work introduces the idea of using the distance between the ground truth and the bounds of the prediction interval to quantify the relevance of this interval for the next prediction. This notion of relevance is then incorporated into state-of-the-art OCP updates, aiming to avoid overly abrupt threshold changes. This approach contributes to reducing the width of the prediction intervals. While maintaining long-run coverage remains a fundamental requirement, we emphasize the crucial role of interval width in decision-making processes.

This work contributes to the current effort to implement trustworthy AI systems with regard to the sensitive applications in which they will be used. This paper is all the more important given the problem of distribution shift of time series which is very common in these applications.

Many perspectives have to be considered for this work. First, one needs to study and optimize the hyper-parameters of the proposed function to reduce, even more, the prediction interval sizes. Moreover, it could be interesting to understand the links between the parametrization of our functions and DMs' expertise. Also, the choice of μ_t to fulfil the constraint about scale independence is not unique. Indeed, this is the choice that we did in this paper but future researches may be conducted about the impact that this parameter has on the algorithm outputs.

Acknowledgement. This work is supported by the European Union's HORIZON Research and Innovation Programme, grant agreement No 101120657, project ENFIELD (European Lighthouse to Manifest Trustworthy and Green AI).

A Proofs

In the theorem and the proofs, we use the same notations and the same structure as presented in the respective original papers to facilitate the understanding for the readers.

General information for proofs of theorems 1 and 2: For these proofs, two updates are introduced:

$$q_{t+1} = r_t \left(\sum_{i=1}^{t} (A_i - \alpha) \right) \tag{11}$$

$$q_{t+1} = \hat{q}_{t+1} + r_t \left(\sum_{i=1}^{t} (A_i - \alpha) \right) \tag{12}$$

with $\hat{q}_{t+1}$ being any function of the past: x_i, y_i, q_i for $i \leq t$. Moreover, $\forall i \leq t$, $A_i = \mathbb{1}\{Y_i \notin \widehat{C}_i\}$ for theorem 1 and $A_i = f_{\omega,v,\mu_i}(s_i - q_i)$ for theorem 2.

The structure of the proofs is the following:

1. we prove the long-run coverage for the update in Eq. (11) with $(s_i)_{i \in \mathbb{N}^*}$ being any sequence of numbers in $[-b, b]$.
2. we apply the point 1 on $q'_{t+1} = q_{t+1} - \hat{q}_{t+1}$ with $(s_i)_{i \in \mathbb{N}^*}$ being any sequence of numbers in $[-\frac{b}{2}, \frac{b}{2}]$ and $(\hat{q}_i)_{i \in \mathbb{N}^*}$ any sequence of numbers in $[-\frac{b}{2}, \frac{b}{2}]$. This leads to the fact that the update in Eq. (12) satisfies the long-run coverage.

Thus, proving the point 1 is enough to prove the results of theorems 1 and 2.

Theorem 1. Given that, in this update, we don't change anything on the saturation function part, this proof is the same as the one in the paper [1] and whose structure is presented above.

Theorem 2. We introduce the update:

$$q_{T+1} = r_T \left(\sum_{i=1}^{T} (f_{\omega,v,\mu_i}(s_i - q_i) - \alpha) \right). \tag{13}$$

We want to prove that, by using the update (13), we have:

$$\forall T \in \mathbb{N}^*, \left| \frac{1}{T} \sum_{i=1}^{T} (f_{\omega,v,\mu_i} - \alpha) \right| \leq \frac{c.h(T) + 1}{T}$$

We proceed by induction for both sides of the inequation. Let's show the idea with the upper bound:

For T=1, we have $f_{\omega,v,\mu_1}(s_1 - q_1) - \alpha \leq 1 - \alpha \leq c.h(1) + 1 - \alpha \leq c.h(1) + 1$ given that $c > 0$ and h is non-negative.

Let $T \in \mathbb{N}^*$. To facilitate the lecture, we set

$$E_T = \sum_{i=1}^{T} (f_{\omega,v,\mu_i}(s_i - q_i) - \alpha)$$

We assume that $E_T \leq c.h(T) + 1$. (induction hypothesis)

- If $E_T \leq c.h(T)$.
  We have,
$$\begin{aligned}E_{T+1} &= E_T + f_{\omega,v,\mu_{T+1}}(s_{T+1} - q_{T+1}) - \alpha \\ &\leq E_T + 1 - \alpha \leq c.h(T) + 1 - \alpha \\ &\leq c.h(T+1) + 1 - \alpha \text{ (h is non-decreasing)} \\ &\leq c.h(T+1) + 1\end{aligned}$$

- If $E_T > c.h(T)$.
  Using the properties of the saturation function r_T (Equation (3)), we have $r_T\,(E_T) \geq b$ then $q_{T+1} \geq b \geq s_{T+1}$. Thus $s_{T+1} - q_{T+1} \leq 0$ and we have $f_{\omega,v,T+1}(s_{T+1} - q_{T+1}) \leq \alpha$ by construction of f.
$$\begin{aligned}E_{T+1} &= E_T + f_{\omega,v,\mu_{T+1}}(s_{T+1} - q_{T+1}) - \alpha \\ &\leq E_T \leq c.h(T) + 1 \\ &\leq c.h(T+1) + 1 \text{ (h is non-decreasing)}\end{aligned}$$

Doing the same thing with the lower bound, we proved that

$$\forall T \in \mathbb{N}^*,\ |\frac{1}{T}\sum_{i=1}^{T}(f_{\omega,v,\mu_i}(s_i - q_i) - \alpha)| \leq \frac{c.h(T) + 1}{T}.$$

Thus, if there exists $T' \in \mathbb{N}^*$ such that $\forall T \geq T'$, $|\sum_{i=1}^{T}(\mathbb{1}\{Y_i \notin \widehat{C}_i\} - \alpha)| \leq |\sum_{i=1}^{T}(f_{\omega,v,\mu_i}(s_i - q_i) - \alpha)|$, we have the long-run coverage of the update of Eq. (13) because h is sub-linear. Using the same idea as presented in result 2, we obtain the desired result.

Theorem 3. Notice that for the Eq. (10), the proofs, from the original ECI paper hold. Indeed, the function f_{ω,v,μ_t} respects the condition of the paper (moreover, μ_t doesn't depend on q_t which doesn't change the original expression of ECI in Eq. (4)).

B Existing methods

B.1 Details on Conformal PID

In *Conformal PID* [1], the authors use ideas from control theory to propose their algorithm. Thus, they propose the following update:

$$\begin{aligned}q_{t+1} = \hat{s}_t &+ \eta \cdot (\mathbb{1}\{Y_t \notin \widehat{C}_t\} - \alpha) \\ &+ r_t\left(\sum_{i=1}^{t}(\mathbb{1}\{Y_i \notin \widehat{C}_i\} - \alpha)\right).\end{aligned} \tag{14}$$

with $\hat{s}_t$ being a scorecaster and r_t a saturation function as described in Eq. (3). The scorecaster is trained on previous non-conformity scores and outputs a prediction for the quantile of the next score. In fact, it's designed to capture the trend in the score distribution. A special case for the scorecaster is to take $\hat{s}_t = q_t$, the authors call this update *conformal PI control.* The authors propose to take the following saturation function r_t:

$$r_t(x) = \frac{K_I \cdot \tan(x \cdot \log(t))}{t \cdot C_{sat}}. \tag{15}$$

where it is set $\tan(x) = \text{sign}(x) \cdot \infty$ for $x \notin [-\pi/2, \pi/2]$, and where $C_{sat}, K_I > 0$ are constants.

B.2 Discussion on ECI

Comparison with ECI. In this paper we estimate the relevance of a prediction interval using the distance between the ground truth and the bounds of this interval. During our experimentations, an idea, comparable to ours, appeared in ECI [18] under the term of smoothing. Nevertheless, our work differs from ECI for, at least, three reasons:

1. First of all, we propose a general idea that could be generalized to all the OCP methods.
2. In ECI, the authors use the sigmoid function $\sigma(\lambda \cdot x)$. They set, in almost all the experiments, $\lambda = 1$. With this function they have $\sigma(0) = 0.5$ whereas, we propose a family of functions for which $f_{\omega,v,\mu_t}(0) = \alpha$. Indeed, when $s_t = q_t$ (i.e. the ground truth is equal to one of the interval bounds) the prediction subset is optimal. Thus, with $f_{\omega,v,\mu_t}(0) = \alpha$ we impose not to change anything based on the last prediction.
3. The functions f_{ω,v,μ_t} try to consider the scale of the dataset which is a crucial aspect. Indeed, let's take the two following cases:
   - First, we have a dataset where, usually, the targeted values range between 0 and 10. Let's say at time t, the algorithm outputs the interval $\widehat{C_t} = [5, 7]$ whereas the ground truth is 8.
   - Second, we have a dataset where, usually, the targeted values range between 0 and 1. Let's say at time t, the algorithm outputs the interval $\widehat{C}_t = [0.5, 0.7]$ whereas the ground truth is 0.8.

   We agree that we are doing the same error in both cases. Nevertheless, with the update chosen in ECI (without scale dependency), the first case will be more penalized (i.e., in this case, the value of $\sigma(s_t - q_t)$ is closer to 1). The functions f_{ω,v,μ_t} are designed to avoid this kind of behaviour including the value μ_t in their expressions.

Remark on ECI. As a remark, we note that the proof of the long-run coverage in ECI (and reused for Theorem 3) assumes $\eta > N.B$. This strong assumption, which implies high learning rates, likely contributes significantly to the long-run coverage result. Indeed, the proof relies on the fact that a mistake made at time t will be followed by, at least, $N - 1$ steps with no mistakes (i.e. $\forall i \in [\![1, N-1]\!], Y_{t+i} \in \hat{C}_{t+i}$). While this fact holds, in the OCP setting, making an error with a large learning rate considerably enlarge q_t, which in turn can artificially ensure these mistake-free steps. Hence, the significance of this result (under such an assumption) is debatable. This observation is further supported by experiments, which show that the long-run coverage is strongly dependent on the choice of the learning rate.

B.3 Other OCP Methods

In this section, we introduce a few OCP methods:

- In ACI [10], we still have a calibration subset to compute the $1-\alpha$ quantile q. Thus, at time t, $\widehat{C}_t(X_t)$ is computed with Eq. (1) then Y_t is revealed and used to update the miscoverage level α for the next prediction as follows:

$$\alpha_{t+1} = \alpha_t + \gamma\left(\alpha - \mathbb{1}\{Y_t \notin \widehat{C}_t(X_t)\}\right). \tag{16}$$

  ACI was the first OCP method introduced. This idea has since been reused and improved in various ways.
- To keep a constant miscoverage level, an idea is to update the threshold q_t used to compute the prediction interval (Equation (1)). A common way to proceed is to use, at time t the *Online sub-Gradient Descent* (OGD) on the quantile loss. This results in the update:

$$q_{t+1} = q_t + \eta(\mathbb{1}\{Y_t \notin \widehat{C}_t\} - \alpha). \tag{17}$$

  where $\eta > 0$ is a learning rate and could be constant or time-dependent. In [2], the authors use the learning rate $\eta_t = t^{-\frac{1}{2}-\epsilon}$ with $\epsilon = 0.1$.

C Details on the proposed functions

C.1 The distance $s_t - q_t$

From the outset, we refer to the distance between the ground truth and the bounds of the prediction interval as a means to estimate the relevance of a prediction interval. As shown in Eq. (6), we choose to use the quantity $s_t - q_t$ to estimate this distance. Indeed, using the non-conformity score $s_t = |\hat{Y}_t - Y_t|$ and symmetric prediction intervals, we have $\widehat{C}_t = [\hat{Y}_t \pm q_t]$, and thus the quantity $s_t - q_t$ is exactly the distance between the ground truth and the bounds of the interval. Indeed:

- if $\hat{Y}_t \geq Y_t$: $s_t - q_t = (\hat{Y}_t - q_t) - Y_t$
- if $Y_t \geq \hat{Y}_t$: $s_t - q_t = Y_t - (\hat{Y}_t + q_t)$

This is the case in our study setting. In all other cases, this quantity $s_t - q_t$ still serves as a useful indicator to capture the trend of this distance.

C.2 Construction of the proposed functions

To respect the constraint 1, our idea is to use the sigmoid function because it has, by definition, a range in [0, 1]. It avoids the use of min or max operators to constrain the proposed functions. Moreover, in order to satisfy the constraint 2, we consider a sigmoid function $\sigma(a.x + b)$ with a being inversely proportional to $\frac{1}{T_w}|\sum_{i=t-T_w}^{t}(s_i - q_i)|$ and with T_w being a window size. Indeed, it will produce a kind of rescaling of the input. In addition, the goal is to enable the function to recognize what occurred in the previous steps and adapt its behaviour accordingly. Furthermore, to satisfy the constraint 3, it is necessary to set a non-null value to b. Besides, to provide a precise customisation we will consider a sum of sigmoid functions. Indeed, this is possible according to the universal approximation theorem [8].

Thus, at time t, our family of functions takes the following form:

$$\forall(\omega, v) \in (\mathbb{R}_+^*)^l \times (\mathbb{R}_+^*)^l,\ g_{\omega,v,\mu_t}(x) = \sum_{i=1}^{l} \omega_i \cdot \sigma\left(\frac{v_i}{\mu_t} \cdot x + b_i\right). \tag{18}$$

with $l \geq 1$ and $\mu_t = \frac{1}{T_w}|\sum_{i=\max(t-T_w,1)}^{t-1}(s_i - q_i)|$.

Using this form, let us now examine the constraints in detail:

- First we set $\Omega = \{\omega \in (\mathbb{R}_+^*)^l; \sum_{i=1}^{l} \omega_i = 1\}$. To satisfy constraint 1, we impose $\omega \in \Omega$.
- From constraint 3, it follows that:

$$\sum_{i=1}^{l} \omega_i \cdot \sigma(b_i) = \alpha. \tag{19}$$

To reduce the expression, we set $b_1 = b_2 = ... = b_l$. Thus, with Eq. (19), we obtain:

$$\forall i \in [\![1, l]\!],\ b_i = -\ln\left(\frac{1-\alpha}{\alpha}\right). \tag{20}$$

Finally, using the Eqs. (18) and (20), we obtain the family of functions of Eq. (6).

C.3 Discussion on the parametrization

For now, the parameters are chosen empirically. The next step is to develop a method for translating the DMs' knowledge – regarding the context, dataset, chosen regressor, and selected OCP method – into appropriate values for the parameters ω and v. For example, if the DMs know that the chosen regressor performs poorly, they are aware that a trade-off must be made between coverage and interval size. If they prioritize coverage over interval tightness, they would prefer assigning a large value to v – and conversely, a smaller value if they favour narrower intervals over higher coverage. These different possibilities, stemming from the DMs' domain knowledge, merit further in-depth investigation.

D Additional results

D.1 PID results

In this section, we continue to use $1 - \alpha = 90\%$, $\eta = 0.005$, $q_1 = 0$ and $T_w = 100$ for the computation of μ_t.

Using update (9)**.** We present the remaining results from Sect. 4.1, namely the results for the *Microsoft* stock price dataset and the temperature dataset (Table 5).

Table 5. PID vs modified PID performances on the *Microsoft* stock price dataset.

Regressor	AR		Theta	
Method	PID	modified PID	PID	modified PID
Coverage	0.90	0.90	0.89	**0.90**
Average interval width	4.50	**3.70**	4.00	**3.91**
Median interval width	3.56	**2.91**	2.97	**2.81**

Table 6. PID vs modified PID performances on the temperature dataset.

Regressor	AR		Theta	
Method	PID	modified PID	PID	modified PID
Coverage	0.90	0.90	0.90	**0.91**
Average interval width	9.41	**9.04**	10.88	**7.38**
Median interval width	9.52	**8.83**	9.40	**7.30**

Using Updates (7) **and** (8)**.** We present the results for the *Amazon* stock price dataset and temperature dataset. In the following, half PID refers to the update of Eq. (8) and full PID refers to the update of Eq. (7) (Table 6).

Table 7. PID vs half PID vs full PID performances on the *Amazon* stock price dataset.

Regressor	AR			Theta		
Method	PID	half PID	full PID	PID	half PID	full PID
Coverage	**0.90**	0.89	0.89	0.89	0.89	0.89
Average interval width	32.42	25.21	**23.80**	**23.17**	31.96	29.60
Median interval width	27.05	**18.42**	18.69	**19.54**	**19.54**	22.45

Table 8. PID vs half PID vs full PID performances on the temperature dataset.

Regressor	AR			Theta		
Method	PID	half PID	full PID	PID	half PID	full PID
Coverage	**0.90**	**0.90**	0.89	0.90	0.90	0.90
Average interval width	9.41	**7.87**	8.06	10.88	**7.62**	9.70
Median interval width	9.52	7.67	**7.20**	9.40	**7.73**	8.22

As presented in Tables 7 and 8, both updates can perform well (especially half PID). Nevertheless, as discussed following Theorem 2, the coverage guarantee relies on an assumption that is highly dependent on the choice of parameters ω and v.

D.2 ECI results

In this section, we continue to use $1 - \alpha = 90\%$, $q_1 = 0$ and $T_w = 100$ for the computation of μ_t. However, as explained in Sect. 4.2, for the ECI update, we use the optimal learning rate selected from a predefined set of values.

Table 9. ECI vs modified ECI performances on the *Google* stock price dataset.

Regressor	AR		Theta	
Method	ECI	modified ECI	ECI	modified ECI
Coverage	0.84	**0.90**	0.84	**0.90**
Average interval width	**17.34**	20.10	**17.52**	20.05
Median interval width	**15.50**	18.49	**15.32**	18.22

Table 10. ECI vs modified ECI performances on the *Amazon* stock price dataset.

Regressor	AR		Theta	
Method	ECI	modified ECI	ECI	modified ECI
Coverage	0.83	**0.90**	0.82	**0.90**
Average interval width	**14.94**	17.67	**14.77**	17.50
Median interval width	**11.08**	14.32	**11.02**	14.28

E *Amazon* stock price dataset

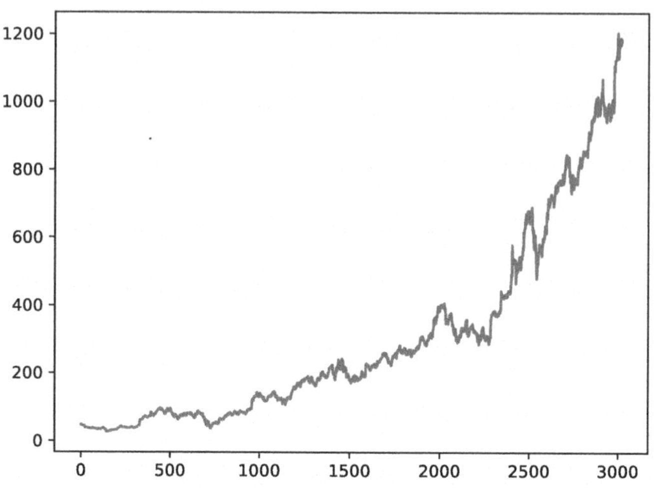

Fig. 6. Evolution of *Amazon* stock price over time

In Fig. 6, we observe a distribution shift around time step 2300. The increase in interval size appears around time step 2000 in Fig. 4. However, the change actually occurs around the same time in the original timeline because the first 365 points are not forecasted (as they are used to initialize the training).

References

1. Angelopoulos, A., Candes, E., Tibshirani, R.J.: Conformal PID Control for Time Series Prediction. In: Oh, A., Naumann, T., Globerson, A., Saenko, K., Hardt, M., Levine, S. (eds.) Advances in Neural Information Processing Systems. vol. 36, pp. 23047–23074. Curran Associates, Inc. (2023)
2. Angelopoulos, A.N., Barber, R., Bates, S.: Online conformal prediction with decaying step sizes. In: Salakhutdinov, R., et al. (eds.) Proceedings of the 41st International Conference on Machine Learning, PMLR, vol. 235, pp. 1616–1630 (2024). https://proceedings.mlr.press/v235/angelopoulos24a.html
3. Angelopoulos, A.N., Bates, S.: A Gentle Introduction to Conformal Prediction and Distribution-Free Uncertainty Quantification (Dec 2022). https://doi.org/10.48550/arXiv.2107.07511, arXiv:2107.07511
4. Assimakopoulos, V., Nikolopoulos, K.: The theta model: a decomposition approach to forecasting. Int. J. Forecast. **16**(4), 521–530 (2000)
5. Barber, R.F., Candes, E.J., Ramdas, A., Tibshirani, R.J.: Predictive inference with the jackknife+ (May 2020). https://doi.org/10.48550/arXiv.1905.02928
6. Barber, R.F., Candes, E.J., Ramdas, A., Tibshirani, R.J.: Conformal prediction beyond exchangeability (Mar 2023). https://doi.org/10.48550/arXiv.2202.13415, http://arxiv.org/abs/2202.13415, arXiv:2202.13415 [stat]

7. Box, G.E.P., Jenkins, G.M.: Time Series Analysis: Forecasting and Control, 1st edn. Holden-Day, San Francisco (1970)
8. Cybenko, G.: Approximation by superpositions of a sigmoidal function. Math. Contr., Signals Syst. **2**(4) (1989)
9. Gammerman, A., Vapnik, V., Vovk, V.: Learning by transduction. In: Proceedings of the Fourteenth Conference on Uncertainty in Artificial Intelligence. Morgan Kaufmann, San Francisco, CA (1998)
10. Gibbs, I., Candes, E.: Adaptive conformal inference under distribution shift. In: Advances in Neural Information Processing Systems, vol. 34, pp. 1660–1672. Curran Associates, Inc. (2021)
11. Jacquin, L., Imoussaten, A., Trousset, F., Didier, P., Montmain, J.: Control of waste fragment sorting process based on MIR imaging coupled with cautious classification. Resour., Conserv. Recycl. **168**, art. 105258 (May 2021). https://doi.org/10.1016/j.resconrec.2020.105258
12. Nguyen, C.: S&p 500 stock data. https://www.kaggle.com/datasets/camnugent/sandp500 (2018)
13. Papadopoulos, H., Proedrou, K., Vovk, V., Gammerman, A.: Inductive Confidence Machines for Regression. In: Elomaa, T., Mannila, H., Toivonen, H. (eds.) Machine Learning: ECML 2002, pp. 345–356. Springer, Berlin, Heidelberg (2002). https://doi.org/10.1007/3-540-36755-1_29
14. Prinster, D., Stanton, S.D., Liu, A., Saria, S.: Conformal validity guarantees exist for any data distribution (and how to find them). In: Salakhutdinov, R., et al. (eds.) Proceedings of the 41st International Conference on Machine Learning, PMLR, vol. 235, pp. 41086–41118 (2024). https://proceedings.mlr.press/v235/prinster24a.html
15. Tibshirani, R.J., Foygel Barber, R., Candes, E., Ramdas, A.: Conformal prediction under covariate shift. In: Advances in Neural Information Processing Systems. vol. 32. Curran Associates, Inc. (2019), https://proceedings.neurips.cc/paper/2019/hash/8fb21ee7a2207526da55a679f0332de2-Abstract.html
16. Vovk, V., Gammerman, A., Shafer, G.: Algorithmic Learning in a Random World. Springer, New York (2005). https://doi.org/10.1007/978-3-031-06649-8
17. Vrao, S.: Daily climate time series data. https://www.kaggle.com/datasets/sumanthvrao/daily-climate-time-series-data (2017)
18. Wu, J., Hu, D., Bao, Y., Xia, S.T., Zou, C.: Error-quantified Conformal Inference for Time Series. In: The Thirteenth International Conference on Learning Representations (2025). https://openreview.net/forum?id=RD9q5vEe1Q
19. Xu, C., Xie, Y.: Sequential predictive conformal inference for time series. In: Proceedings of the 40th International Conference on Machine Learning. pp. 38707–38727. PMLR (Jul 2023), iSSN: 2640–3498
20. Zaffran, M., Feron, O., Goude, Y., Josse, J., Dieuleveut, A.: Adaptive conformal predictions for time series. In: Proceedings of the 39th International Conference on Machine Learning, pp. 25834–25866. PMLR (Jun 2022), iSSN: 2640–3498

Hidden Rhythms: an Embedding Framework for Downstream Tasks Validated on ECG Data

Simone Bartucci[1,2,3], Edoardo De Rose[1(✉)], Francesca Filice[1], Francesco Calimeri[1,3], and Simona Perri[1,3]

[1] Department of Mathematics and Computer Science, University of Calabria, Via Pietro Bucci, Rende, Italy
edoardo.derose@unical.it

[2] Department of Computer, Control and Management Engineering, Sapienza University of Rome, 00185 Rome, Italy

[3] DLVSystem Srl, Viale della Resistenza 19/C, 87036 Rende, Italy

Abstract. Foundation models (FMs) are large-scale deep neural networks trained on vast and diverse datasets, capable of learning transferable, domain-agnostic representations that enhance performance across a wide range of downstream tasks. These models have attracted significant attention across multiple fields, potentially reshaping standard paradigms of model design. However, adapting FMs to specific tasks typically requires computationally intensive fine-tuning and large labeled datasets, which can be significant limiting factors, especially in resource-constrained settings. In this work, we explore an alternative strategy: leveraging pre-trained FM embeddings (also called vector embeddings) as inputs to downstream supervised models. By utilizing these rich, general-purpose representations, the approach retains the expressive power of FMs while significantly reducing both computational costs and data requirements. We present a general framework, namely **CURE-FM** *(Context-aware Use of data REpresentations with Foundation Models)*, designed to extract embeddings from self-supervised FMs trained on raw data, and to leverage downstream models for generic tasks. We present an application of CURE-FM relying on raw time series data; in particular, the application is geared towards binary classification tasks over multi-lead electrocardiogram (ECG) signals. We report a comprehensive evaluation, including ablation studies on FM and classifier architectures, structural and explainability analyses of the embeddings, and a comparison between our approach and common fine-tuned based approaches, with the aim of investigating how different architecture and approaches affect performance and generalizability. Experimental results show that embedding-based approaches can provide a scalable, robust, and efficient solution for downstream tasks, and that **CURE-FM** holds significant promise for advancing ECG analysis.

Keywords: Foundation Models · Vector Embeddings · Electrocardiogram (ECG) Analysis

P. Bruno et al. (Eds.): HC_AIxIA_HYDRA 2025, CCIS 2830, pp. 218–230, 2026.
https://doi.org/10.1007/978-3-032-16708-8_18

1 Introduction

In recent years, artificial intelligence (AI) has seen rapid advances in Foundation Models (FMs), particularly in computer vision, natural language processing, and their intersection [8]. FMs are a major milestone in AI thanks to their ability to learn general, reusable representations from vast unlabeled data [8,13]. Their strong generalization makes them well-suited for complex domains like medicine, where data variability is high and accuracy is critical [13]. By distilling complex relationships into meaningful representations, FMs can reveal clinically relevant patterns often missed by traditional methods [28]. A key application of foundation models in medicine is the analysis of Electrocardiograms (ECGs) [26]: a low-cost, non-invasive tool widely used to detect and monitor cardiovascular diseases [13,24]. Standard 12-lead ECGs capture the heart's electrical activity from multiple viewpoints, providing rich diagnostic information but also increasing interpretation complexity and inter-observer variability [4,6]. Traditionally, ECG analysis relied on rule-based approaches and handcrafted features extracted through signal processing methods such as Fourier and wavelet transforms [10,11,14]. While traditional approaches have aided clinical ECG interpretation, they are sensitive to noise, lack robustness across patient populations, and struggle with atypical cases [6,15]. Crucially, they often miss non-linear and temporal patterns in ECG signals, limiting diagnostic precision [4,6]. Despite its importance, ECG interpretation remains complex and error-prone: misinterpretations are common, with studies reporting error rates exceeding 50% in certain arrhythmias [4,20]. The process is also time-consuming, especially critical in emergencies. Foundation models offer a promising path forward by enhancing signal analysis, reducing complexity, and improving diagnostic accuracy [13].
In this work, we propose **CURE-FM** *(Context-aware Use of data REpresentations with Foundation Models)* a general framework designed to harness the potential of FMs for advanced data analysis (see Fig. 1), along with a specific application to ECG binary classification task. One of the main points of interest of this framework lies in the use of pre-trained FMs, whose advantages are thoroughly discussed in Sect. 2.2, to extract robust, general-purpose latent space representations from raw general data. These representations are then employed for downstream tasks, particularly in scenarios involving small datasets, which are common in real-world applications. The core contributions of this study can be summarized as follows:

- We design and present **CURE-FM**, a general framework that researchers and clinicians can reuse as a pipeline for any downstream task (e.g., anomaly detection, segmentation, forecasting).
- We ground **CURE-FM** and apply it to a real-world scenario, i.e., classification tasks based on multi-lead ECG signals.
- We perform and report about a thorough evaluation of such workflow across several key dimensions:
  - An ablation study involving several foundation models and downstream model architectures applied to the extracted embeddings.

- An in-depth analysis of the embedding structures.
- A comparison between our approach and commonly used approaches in the literature, based on fine-tuning techniques.

Results show that the proposed framework can offer a viable solution for general data analysis, with potential applications across different domains and the possibility to outperform fine-tuning approaches.

The remainder of this paper is structured as follows. Section 2 introduces the key concepts of foundation models and embedding-based strategies, and provides an overview of related works in the context of ECG signal classification. Section 3 details our proposed framework for evaluating combinations of foundation models and downstream classifiers, including its mathematical formulation and operational pipeline.Section 4 presents the experimental results obtained reporting comparative performance analyses among multiple scenarios. Section 5 concludes the paper by summarizing the key findings and suggesting potential directions for future work.

2 Background and Related Works

Among the most compelling aspects of FMs is their versatility: they can serve as powerful tools for multiple downstream tasks without the need for task-specific architectures. In the context of biomedical data processing, where data is complex, high-dimensional, and often scarce, this flexibility is particularly valuable. This section introduces the fundamental concepts behind FMs and highlights the role of embedded-based approaches as efficient alternatives to traditional fine-tuning strategies.

2.1 Foundation Models and Vector Embeddings

Foundation models, often trained via self-supervised learning techniques, are capable of acquiring a broad and generalizable understanding of input data. This inherent versatility allows them to perform a wide variety of downstream tasks, such as classification, anomaly detection, and segmentation, without requiring task-specific architectures or training from scratch. Their scalability and adaptability make them a cornerstone in the advancement of modern AI systems [8]. Foundation models, typically trained with self-supervised learning, acquire broad and generalizable representations that enable a range of downstream tasks—such as classification, anomaly detection, and segmentation—without needing task-specific architectures [8]. Their scalability and adaptability make them central to modern AI systems. Traditionally, these models are adapted via fine-tuning on smaller, labeled datasets [21], but this approach is computationally intensive, requires substantial annotated data, and risks overfitting or reduced generalizability, especially in data-limited or clinical settings [9,18]. A promising alternative is to leverage the embeddings produced by foundation models for new tasks. These embeddings are compact, lower-dimensional representations that capture

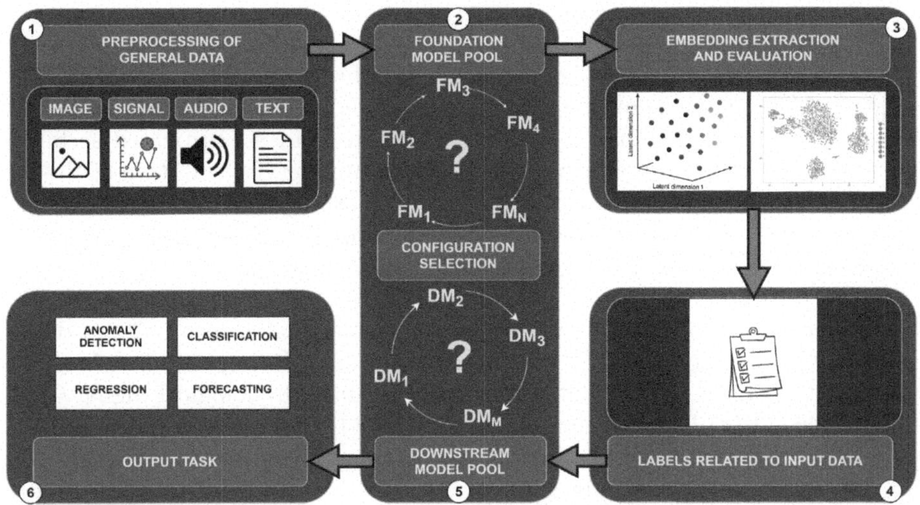

Fig. 1. Schematic representation of CURE-FM: *Frozen Embedding* workflow for systematic comparison of Foundation and Downstream Model combinations on downstream tasks.

the essential semantic and structural properties of the input data, learned during the initial pre-training phase [5,22]; their use in place of original data significantly reduces the need for computation resources and data storage, accelerates model deployment, and facilitates knowledge transfer across tasks [30].
Embedding-based approaches are particularly useful in medical/healthcare domains and other real world scenarios, where limited computational resources or unbalanced datasets are common challenges. In the context of medical signal analysis, such as ECG, embeddings can be used to transform multi-lead time series into clinically informative vector representations. This transformation not only improves the automation of diagnostic tasks, but can also help at enhancing interpretability by revealing latent patterns that would otherwise remain hidden when using conventional signal processing techniques [23]. In the latent space defined by these embeddings, patients with similar cardiovascular profiles tend to form coherent clusters, enabling improved stratification and more personalized treatment strategies [7]. Embedded representations also offer potential benefits for medical data analysis, such as contributing to anonymization by encoding raw clinical signals (e.g., ECGs) into abstract vector spaces that obscure direct identifiers [2,27]. While not guaranteeing full privacy, this approach can reduce re-identification risks when combined with other safeguards. Additionally, embeddings enable high-quality feature extraction without extensive compute or large labeled datasets, helping democratize AI development for less-resourced institutions and supporting fairness by providing more uniform features.

2.2 State of the Art of ECG Classifiers

The field of ECG analysis has witnessed significant advancements with the integration of deep learning techniques, transitioning from traditional models, such as Convolutional Neural Networks (CNN), to more sophisticated architectures, like FMs. In the following, we provides an overview of state-of-the-art methods, considering both conventional deep learning approaches and recent advancements. This progression can be seen through the various studies that first explored CNNs for ECG classification. Acharya et al. (2017) trained two CNNs to classify ECGs as normal or coronary artery disease, achieving 95% and 95.1% accuracy with 2 and 5 s segments [1]. Similarly, Zhu et al. (2020) developed a CNN model to classify cardiac arrhythmias, achieving a median F1 score of 0.84 with a 12-lead ECG dataset from the China Physiological Signal Challenge (CPSC 2018) [31]. Ribeiro et al. (2020) published a 12-lead ECG dataset with over 2 million labeled exams from the Telehealth Network of Minas Gerais (TNMG) as part of the study Clinical Outcomes in Digital Electrocardiography (CODE). They developed a ResNet model adapted for unidimensional ECG signals, with over 6 million parameters, to classify six abnormalities, achieving an average F1 score above 80% [19]. Vasconcellos et al. (2023) proposed the use of Siamese CNN trained on the open-source St Petersburg INCART 12-lead Arrhythmia dataset for classifying heartbeats from 12-lead ECGs, achieving an accuracy of 95% [25]. Yao et al. (2018) proposed a Time-Incremental CNN for the automatic detection of arrhythmias, overcoming the limitations of traditional CNN models that require fixed-length inputs, achieving an accuracy of 77.3% [29].

In recent years, the use of foundation models (FMs) has emerged as a versatile solution for clinical applications, overcoming many limitations of CNNs by supporting multiple tasks and integrating diverse data types [8]. For example, HuBERT-ECG—a FM pre-trained on 9.1 million ECGs—can be adapted to various downstream tasks, including disease diagnosis and risk prediction, and achieved AUCs above 90% for most cardiovascular conditions and 93.4% for two-year mortality prediction [3]. Similarly, ECG-FM, trained on 2.5 million samples, demonstrated robust performance across clinical tasks such as ECG label prediction and cardiac biomarker assessment, providing rich embeddings and strong generalizability for real-world medical applications [16].

3 Methodology

In the following we present **CURE-FM**, our general-purpose framework for identifying the best combination of FMs and *Downstream models* (DMs) for a selected task. We also introduce a case study to assess the potential of our framework in a medical context with time series data: a specific application for ECG signal classification.

3.1 Embedding Extraction

Let us consider a generic dataset consisting of n instances $\mathcal{X} = \{X_i\}_{i=1}^{n}$ where each input $X_i \in \mathbb{R}^D$ has dimension D. A FM is employed to project this data into a lower-dimensional latent embedding space:

$$Z_i = FM(X_i) \quad \text{with} \quad Z_i \in \mathbb{R}^d, \quad d \ll D, \quad Z = \bigcup_{i=1}^{n_{\text{samples}}} Z_i$$

where Z_i represents the embedding vector of the input data X_i mapped into the latent space, that captures its fundamental patterns and characteristics.
Three distinct embedding strategies can be defined as follows [12]:

- **Frozen Embeddings**: The FM parameters weights remain unchanged after the pre-training phase without further modification. Embeddings are directly used for downstream tasks.
- **Few-shot Embeddings**: A limited number of labeled examples are used to slightly fine-tune the foundational model parameters to adapt embeddings to specific tasks. This approach is particularly relevant in scenarios where data collection is impractical, such as in highly specialized fields or in the detection of rare events.
- **Fully Fine-tuned Embeddings**: The foundational model is extensively fine-tuned with substantial labeled data, optimizing embeddings specifically for a downstream task.

3.2 The CURE-FM Framework

Based on the *Frozen Embedding* strategy [12], we introduce **CURE-FM**, a general-purpose framework designed for the systematic evaluation of embeddings extracted from raw data and their performance in downstream tasks. The overall structure is depicted in Fig. 1; if we start from N FMs and M (untrained) DMs, we can schematically describe it as follows.

1. **Preprocessing:** the considered input data need to be preprocessed. This phase is configured and tuned depending on the specific use case and the specific requirements of each selected FM.
2. **Foundation model pool:** here, each FM_k is fed with the properly preprocessed data, for every $k \in \{0, \ldots, \text{N}\}$.
3. **Embedding Extraction**: each FM_k produces the k-th latent space Z^k of the considered dataset.
4. **Input label:** the input labels, combined with the embedded representation, are used to train the DMs to be employed in the next step.
5. **Downstream model pool:** each selected DM in the pool is fed with all vector embeddings and corresponding labels, in order to be trained for the final downstream task. More precisely, we train $DM^j(Z^k)$, for all $j \in \{0, \ldots, \text{M}\}$ and $k \in \{0, \ldots, \text{N}\}$, thus obtaining $N \times M$ trained models.

6. **Task output:** all the considered $N \times M$ trained DMs are tested, and the evaluation results are returned for each possible combination on a unique test set. This ensures a fair comparison across models and foundation embeddings under consistent conditions, over any task of choice.

3.3 Frozen Embedding Vs Few-Shot Embedding Vs Fully Fine-Tuned Embedding

Referring to Sect. 3.1 and 3.2, an experimental setting is designed for comparing the performance of our proposal based on a *Frozen Embedding* approach for FMs coupled with trained DMs against the more commonly used strategies *Few-shot Embedding* and *Fully Fine-tuned Embedding.* In particular, previously frozen FMs are fine-tuned on varying portions of the considered dataset and specialized for downstream tasks. In the case of the *Few-shot Embedding*, a portion of the benchmark dataset is considered, while in the case of *Fully Fine-tuned Embedding*, the entire dataset is taken into account. This comparison aims to determine which of the three approaches offers the best balance of performance and Training Time, thereby identifying the most suitable strategy for practical applications.

3.4 Case Study: ECG Binary Classification Task

In the following, we present a specific application of our framework, based on time series data and tailored for ECG analysis, in which the primary objective is to evaluate different combinations of FMs and DMs for binary classification tasks using a benchmark dataset. In the **preprocessing** step, raw ECG time series are prepared for input into the selected FMs, described in detail in Sect. 4.1, subsequently in the **embedding extraction** phase, the goal is to capture the relevant information of the ECG signals that can be used for classification. The **downstream model pool** consists of several classifiers, as presented in Sect. 4.1, trained with the aim of identifying the $FM^k + DM^j$ combination, i.e. in this case the couple *FM+classifier* that delivers the best performance. Each classifier DM^j is trained using the embedding representation Z^k and the chosen label, as follows:

$$\hat{y}^{j,k} = DM^j(Z^k)$$

where $\hat{y}^{j,k}$ represents the set of the predicted labels for each *FM+Classifier*.
In the **output task** step, performance is assessed using a unique test set. Proper key performance metrics are considered, as discussed in detail in Sect. 4.2, in order to ensure a fair and consistent comparison of models and foundation embeddings.

4 Experimental Setting

Building upon the methodology introduced in the previous section, we designed a structured experimental protocol to systematically evaluate the effectiveness of **CURE-FM** on ECG data. All experiments were conducted under controlled conditions to ensure comparability and reproducibility. In the following, we illustrate the experimental settings.

4.1 Dataset and Chosen Architectures

We employ the publicly available **CODE-15%** cohort [4,19], a stratified, literature-standard subsample of the full CODE database collected by TNMG (2010–2016) across 811 municipalities in Minas Gerais, Brazil. To ensure demographic equity, ECG exams from each one-year age bin (16–85 years) are uniformly sampled, yielding an age-balanced set of roughly **300,000 patients** unique first-recording tracings annotated with seven clinical labels. Importantly, this stratified subsampling directly addresses potential age-related bias, promoting fairness by preventing over-representation of any single demographic cohort [4,19]. Our evaluation focuses on the **Normal ECG class**, chosen for its minimal missing data and its role as a broad, healthy-tracing benchmark to verify if the models were capable to learn general ECG patterns. The selected foundation models for this study are *ECG-FM* [16], *HuBERT-ECG Small, HuBERT-ECG Base, and HuBERT-ECG Large* [3]; the choice was influenced by several factors. First, we only considered open-source FMs, in order to make our study accessible to a broad research community. This also mirrors the intention to rely on widely available dataset sources and architectures, that others can easily use and replicate. We selected *ECG-FM*, which outperformed several other FMs in the original study [17], for its robust contrastive-loss-based training and ability to capture discriminative ECG representations. In parallel, we chose *HuBERT-ECG* for its BERT-like architecture and innovative training that combines contrastive loss with clustering to enhance feature separation in the latent space. *HuBERT-ECG* is available in three parameter sizes, enabling us to investigate the impact of model scale—frozen or fine-tuned—on ECG classification performance.This allows us to explore the trade-offs between a frozen model and a fine-tuned model. Thanks to these variability, we can assess the impact of model parameter variability on the performance of the ECG classification task.
To complement the selected foundation models, we create a pool of downstream classifiers by chosing *XGBoost (XGB), Random Forest (RF), and Multi-Layer Perceptron (MLP)*, with the goal of introducing architectural diversity in the evaluation phase. This selection allows us to test the extracted embeddings under different learning assumptions: from tree-based ensemble methods, which are often effective with limited data (XGB and RF), to a neural model (MLP), which can exploit more complex, non-linear representations.

4.2 Workflow Unfolding

All experiments initially rely on frozen embeddings described in Sect. 3.2 based on the chosen FMs reported in Sect. 4.1. Two aggregation strategies are applied to summarize the token-level outputs into a fixed-size representation: *Last Token (LT)* and *Max Average Pooling (MAX)*. These strategies are selected to balance

Table 1. Performance comparison across embedding strategies, models, and dataset portions used related to MAX pooling strategy on **Normal ECG** label. All reported values have the same error of ±0.01, not shown in the table for simplicity.

Scenario	Foundation Model	Classifier	F1 score			AUROC			Training Time (seconds)		
			Dataset Portion			Dataset Portion			Dataset Portion		
			10%	20%	100%	10%	20%	100%	10%	20%	100%
Frozen	ECG-FM	XGB	0.76	0.77	0.80	0.80	0.82	0.87	3.73×10^2	5.63×10^2	2.30×10^3
		MLP	0.76	0.77	0.80	0.80	0.80	0.87	2.85×10^2	2.99×10^2	2.04×10^3
		RF	**0.77**	**0.78**	**0.88**	**0.82**	**0.85**	**0.96**	1.68×10^2	2.53×10^2	3.40×10^3
	HuBERT-ECG Small	XGB	0.73	0.72	0.73	0.76	0.76	0.77	5.43×10^2	6.99×10^2	9.55×10^2
		MLP	0.73	0.73	0.75	0.76	0.76	0.78	2.36×10^2	3.49×10^2	7.62×10^2
		RF	0.71	0.71	0.72	0.74	0.74	0.76	2.25×10^1	5.11×10^1	9.30×10^2
	HuBERT-ECG Base	XGB	0.69	0.70	0.71	0.72	0.74	0.75	1.72×10^2	3.06×10^2	1.03×10^3
		MLP	0.71	0.72	0.74	0.73	0.74	0.76	7.53×10^1	3.29×10^2	8.50×10^3
		RF	0.69	0.70	0.70	0.72	0.72	0.73	6.11×10^1	1.49×10^2	3.81×10^3
	HuBERT-ECG Large	XGB	0.70	0.71	0.72	0.75	0.75	0.77	3.14×10^2	5.47×10^2	1.06×10^3
		MLP	0.73	0.74	0.74	0.74	0.76	0.78	1.07×10^2	4.75×10^2	5.15×10^3
		RF	0.70	0.70	0.71	0.73	0.73	0.75	6.47×10^1	1.22×10^2	1.30×10^3
Few-shot/ Fully-Fine-tuned	ECG-FM		0.53	0.58	0.56	0.54	0.60	0.61	9.25×10^3	1.80×10^4	1.17×10^5
	HuBERT-ECG Small		0.60	0.61	0.71	0.60	0.62	0.74	6.13×10^2	1.56×10^3	6.43×10^3
	HuBERT-ECG Base		0.70	0.72	0.74	0.68	0.73	0.76	1.78×10^3	2.99×10^3	6.55×10^3
	HuBERT-ECG Large		0.72	0.72	0.74	0.73	0.74	0.77	2.77×10^3	3.46×10^3	1.98×10^4

simplicity and expressiveness, and are applied consistently across all models and classifiers. To optimize performance, each classifier is trained on the extracted embeddings using a grid-based hyperparameter search, validated through a 5-fold cross-validation procedure. Model performance is assessed on a held-out test set using three key metrics: **F1 score**, **AUROC**, and **Training Time**. We emphasize that, for a fair comparison focused solely on the advantages and disadvantages of the selected training strategies, the Training Time metric does not include the pre-processing time required for each specific Foundation Model selected. To complement the frozen embedding experiments, we explore two alternative training approaches: *Few-shot Embedding* where FMs are fine-tuned on 10% and 20% of the training data to simulate low data conditions, and *Fully fine-tuned Embedding*, which uses the entire dataset. The same 10% and 20% subsets are also used to train all the *FM-classifier* couples in the *Frozen Embedding* scenario, ensuring a fair comparison across methods. This analysis aims at quantifying the benefits of task-specific adaptation and assess whether the performance improvements justify the additional training cost.

4.3 Reproducibility

In the light of what discussed above, the reproducibility of our results is ensured by the use of open-source architectures and datasets, thus promoting transparency and allowing easy replicability.

In the *Frozen Embedding* scenario, all experiments rely on an extensive hyperparameter search, with optimal settings identified via grid search and k-fold cross-validation, ensuring robust and split-independent results. For the *Few-shot* and *Fully Fine-tuned* scenarios, hyperparameters are aligned with those reported in the original FM publications to ensure fairness and reproducibility.

To maintain consistency, all experiments are conducted with the same experimental setup and hardware configurations. Specifically, all fine-tuning, embedding extraction, and classifier training tasks are carried out using the same number of processors and GPUs. This setup reasonably ensures that any performance variations observed are due to the models themselves and not external factors.

The framework was developed using PyTorch (v2.6.0). For training, a high-performance computing node with the following specifications was used: two Tesla V100-PCIE-16GB GPUs, Intel® Xeon® Gold 5118 CPU (2.30GHz), and 512GB of RAM.

5 Results

In the "Frozen Embedding" scenario, Table 1 summarizes the performance on the **Normal ECG** class when using Max Pooling, which we found to be the top-performing aggregation strategy. This table reports F1 score, AUROC and Training Time for each *FM+classifier* pair, with all values (and their standard deviations) averaged over our 5-fold cross-validation. In the case where 100% of the dataset is used, the combination *ECG-FM+RF* outperforms all other configurations by a large margin, achieving an F1 score of 0.88 ± 0.01 and an AUROC of 0.96 ± 0.01, while maintaining training times comparable to XGB and significantly lower than those of MLP.
When analyzing the reduced dataset scenarios (10% and 20%), all classifiers paired with *ECG-FM* yield nearly identical F1 scores within the experimental error range. However, a closer look at AUROC values reveals that RF achieves slightly superior scores, 0.82 ± 0.01 for 10%, 0.85 ± 0.01 for 20%, compared to MLP and XGB, while still maintaining significantly shorter training times than MLP and comparable ones to XGB. Moreover, while increasing the dataset portion is justified for *ECG-FM* configurations, thanks to improved performance and comparable Training Times, this trend does not hold for any *HuBERT-ECG* configuration. For the latter, larger dataset sizes lead to longer training times without corresponding performance gains, making their use disadvantageous. Collectively, across all three evaluation metrics, the *ECG-FM* paired with *RF* delivers the best results in the Frozen Embedding configuration.

In the *Few-Shot* and *Fully* Fine-Tuned configurations, *ECG-FM* yields the lowest F1 and AUROC scores, but demanding the longest Training Time. On the other hand, *HuBERT-ECG* variants deliver better accuracy values related to lower Training Times.

Even under identical training-set proportions, the Frozen *ECG-FM + RF* pipeline delivers superior F1 and AUROC metrics compared to both adaptive strategies. Finally, the resilience of the frozen method is underscored by its ability to outperform all fine-tuned counterparts, including those trained on 100% of the data, even when is trained on only 10% of the dataset. These observations collectively demonstrate that, for the **Normal ECG** classification task, freezing pretrained embeddings yields a far more efficient and robust solution than adapting the entire model to the target domain.

6 Conclusion

We introduced **CURE-FM**, a general, modular framework that leverages pretrained foundation models (FMs) to extract latent representations from raw data and to drive downstream tasks. In a clinical case study on 12-lead ECG binary classification, FM embeddings delivered consistently strong performance with limited labels, and the framework clearly identified combinations that best trade off accuracy, robustness, and training speed. Compared with fine-tuning pipelines, CURE-FM achieved competitive or better accuracy at substantially lower computational cost and time, making it well-suited to resource-constrained settings. The framework is versatile, scalable, and adaptable beyond classification to tasks such as anomaly detection, segmentation, and forecasting. As future work, we will extend the evaluation to additional datasets and employ manifold visualizations (e.g., UMAP) to probe the geometry, separability, and stability of the learned embeddings.

Acknowledgments. This work has been carried out while **Simone Bartucci** was enrolled in the Italian National Doctorate on Artificial Intelligence run by Sapienza University of Rome in collaboration with **Università della Calabria**.

Disclosure of Interests. The authors declare that they have **no competing interests** relevant to the content of this article.

References

1. Acharya, U.R., Fujita, H., Lih, O.S., Adam, M., Tan, J.H., Chua, C.K.: Automated detection of coronary artery disease using different durations of ecg segments with convolutional neural network. Knowl.-Based Syst. **132**, 62–71 (2017)
2. Alves, V., et al..: Anonymization through substitution: words vs sentences. In: Proceedings of the Fifth Workshop on Privacy in Natural Language Processing, pp. 85–90 (2024)
3. Coppola, E., Savardi, M., Massussi, M., Adamo, M., Metra, M., Signoroni, A.: Hubert-ECG: a self-supervised foundation model for broad and scalable cardiac applications. medRxiv, pp. 2024–11 (2024)
4. van Dam, P.M., Boonstra, M., Locati, E.T., Loh, P.: The relation of 12 lead ECG to the cardiac anatomy: the normal cineecg. J. Electrocardiol. **69**, 67–74 (2021)
5. Darrin, M., Formont, P., Ben Ayed, I., Cheung, J.C.K., Piantanida, P.: When is an embedder more promising than another? (2024)
6. Fu, G., et al.: Cardiogpt: an ECG interpretation generation model. IEEE Access (2024)

7. Grossmann, N., Gröller, E., Waldner, M.: Concept splatters: exploration of latent spaces based on human interpretable concepts. Comput. Graph. **105**, 73–84 (2022)
8. Han, Y., Liu, X., Zhang, X., Ding, C.: Foundation models in electrocardiogram: a review. arXiv preprint arXiv:2410.19877 (2024)
9. Hsu, C.Y., et al.: Badtv: Unveiling backdoor threats in third-party task vectors. arXiv preprint arXiv:2501.02373 (2025)
10. Karel, J.M.: A wavelet approach to cardiac signal processing for low-power hardware applications (2009)
11. Kheirati Roonizi, A., Sassi, R.: ECG signal decomposition using Fourier analysis. EURASIP J. Adv. Signal Process. **2024**(1), 79 (2024)
12. Lee, S.A., Lee, J., Chiang, J.N.: Feet: A framework for evaluating embedding techniques. arXiv preprint arXiv:2411.01322 (2024)
13. Li, J., et al.: An electrocardiogram foundation model built on over 10 million recordings with external evaluation across multiple domains. arXiv preprint arXiv:2410.04133 (2024)
14. Luo, S., Johnston, P.: A review of electrocardiogram filtering. J. Electrocardiol. **43**(6), 486–496 (2010)
15. Mancia, G., et al.: 2023 ESH guidelines for the management of arterial hypertension the task force for the management of arterial hypertension of the european society of hypertension: Endorsed by the international society of hypertension (ish) and the european renal association (era). J. Hypertens. **41**(12), 1874–2071 (2023)
16. McKeen, K., Oliva, L., Masood, S., Toma, A., Rubin, B., Wang, B.: ECG-FM: An open electrocardiogram foundation model. arXiv preprint arXiv:2408.05178 (2024)
17. Oh, J., Chung, H., Kwon, J.m., Hong, D.g., Choi, E.: Lead-agnostic self-supervised learning for local and global representations of electrocardiogram. In: Conference on Health, Inference, and Learning, pp. 338–353. PMLR (2022)
18. Qin, S., Zhang, M.: Boosting generalization of fine-tuning bert for fake news detection. Inform. Process. Manage. **61**(4), 103745 (2024)
19. Ribeiro, A.H., et al.: Automatic diagnosis of the 12-lead ECG using a deep neural network. Nat. Commun. **11**(1), 1760 (2020)
20. Shaik, A., et al.: Erroneous electrocardiographic interpretations and its clinical implications. J. Cardiovasc. Electrophysiol. **34**(7), 1515–1522 (2023)
21. Song, J., Jang, J.H., Lee, B.T., Hong, D., Kwon, J.m., Jo, Y.Y.: Foundation models for ECG: Leveraging hybrid self-supervised learning for advanced cardiac diagnostics. arXiv preprint arXiv:2407.07110 (2024)
22. Tao, C., et al.: LLMs are also effective embedding models: An in-depth overview. arXiv preprint arXiv:2412.12591 (2024)
23. Tatyana, A.: Multi-way data representation: A comprehensive survey on tensor decomposition in machine learning
24. Vaid, A., et al.: A foundational vision transformer improves diagnostic performance for electrocardiograms. NPJ Digital Med. **6**(1), 108 (2023)
25. Vasconcellos, M.E., et al.: Siamese convolutional neural network for heartbeat classification using limited 12-lead ECG datasets. IEEE Access **11**, 5365–5376 (2023)
26. Wan, Z., Yu, Q., Mao, J., Duan, W., Ding, C.: Openecg: Benchmarking ECG foundation models with public 1.2 million records. arXiv preprint arXiv:2503.00711 (2025)
27. Willett, W., Jansen, Y., Dragicevic, P.: Embedded data representations. IEEE Trans. Visual Comput. Graph. **23**(1), 461–470 (2016)
28. Yang, W., Liu, M., Wang, Z., Liu, S.: Foundation models meet visualizations: challenges and opportunities. Comput. Visual Media **10**(3), 399–424 (2024)

29. Yao, Q., Fan, X., Cai, Y., Wang, R., Yin, L., Li, Y.: Time-incremental convolutional neural network for arrhythmia detection in varied-length electrocardiogram. In: 2018 IEEE 16th International Conference on Dependable, Autonomic and Secure Computing, 16th International Conference on Pervasive Intelligence and Computing, 4th International Conference on Big Data Intelligence and Computing and Cyber Science and Technology Congress (DASC/PiCom/DataCom/CyberSciTech), pp. 754–761. IEEE (2018)
30. Zhao, X., et al.: Embedding in recommender systems: a survey. arXiv preprint arXiv:2310.18608 (2023)
31. Zhu, H., et al.: Automatic multilabel electrocardiogram diagnosis of heart rhythm or conduction abnormalities with deep learning: a cohort study. Lancet Digital Health **2**(7), e348–e357 (2020)

Generating Patient Cohorts from Electronic Health Records Using Two-Step Retrieval-Augmented Text-to-SQL Generation

Angelo Ziletti(✉) and Leonardo D'Ambrosi

Bayer AG, Leverkusen, Germany
{angelo.ziletti,leonardo.dambrosi}@bayer.com

Abstract. Clinical cohort definition is crucial for patient recruitment and observational studies, yet translating inclusion/exclusion criteria into SQL queries remains challenging and manual. We present an automated system utilizing large language models that combines criteria parsing, two-level retrieval augmented generation with specialized knowledge bases, medical concept standardization, and SQL generation to retrieve patient cohorts with patient funnels. The top-performing configuration achieves 0.75 F1-score in cohort identification on EHR data, effectively capturing complex temporal and logical relationships. These results demonstrate the feasibility of automated cohort generation for epidemiological research.

Keywords: Text-to-SQL · Large Language Models · Electronic Health Records · Cohort Generation · Retrieval-Augmented Generation

1 Introduction

Electronic Health Records (EHR) have become essential resources for clinical research, serving as a foundational component across multiple healthcare applications. In clinical trials, accurate cohort identification directly impacts patient recruitment success, study validity, timeline adherence, and cost management [29]. For observational studies and epidemiological research, well-defined cohorts enable researchers to investigate disease patterns, treatment effectiveness, and health outcomes across specific patient populations, informing critical healthcare decisions from drug development to regulatory submissions [3, 32].

Problem Statement. Converting clinical inclusion/exclusion criteria into accurate database queries requires addressing multiple technical challenges simultaneously: (1) mapping natural language criteria to precise computational logic while leveraging medical domain knowledge, (2) preserving complex temporal and logical relationships across multiple criteria, (3) mapping diverse medical concepts to standardized codes, (4) generating queries that conform to established data models, (5) returning patient-level identifiers with associated index dates to enable subsequent time-anchored analyses.

P. Bruno et al. (Eds.): HC_AIxIA_HYDRA 2025, CCIS 2830, pp. 231–242, 2026.
https://doi.org/10.1007/978-3-032-16708-8_19

Contributions. This paper presents an approach for automatically generating patient cohorts from EHRs. Our main contributions are:

- A manually curated dataset of inclusion/exclusion criteria paired with SQL queries that conform to the Observational Medical Outcomes Partnership Common Data Model (OMOP-CDM) [19].
- A two-level retrieval-augmented generation (RAG) framework that substantially outperforms simple prompting across all tested models, demonstrating robust performance in translating complex clinical criteria into executable SQL queries.
- Open-source release of dataset, source code, and prompt configurations[1].

The system has been deployed and is currently being evaluated at Bayer by epidemiologists and data analysts.

2 Knowledge Base Generation

We create two complementary knowledge bases (KBs) for our retrieval-augmented approach: *EpiAskKB* and *EpiCohoKB*. Table 1 provides detailed statistics of both knowledge bases, highlighting their complementary nature and complexity.

EpiAskKB consists of 115 question-SQL pairs that capture typical analytical questions in observational studies, extending and refining the dataset from Ziletti and D'Ambrosi [42] to better reflect common epidemiological research questions.

EpiCohoKB contains inclusion/exclusion criteria for observational studies, which we create through structured language model prompting. The generation integrates three key elements: (1) a prompt specifying OMOP CDM vocabulary usage and structural constraints for cohort criteria, (2) standard guidelines for study criteria (including temporal relationships, assessment windows, and observable time definitions) [34], and (3) real observational study protocols from the European Medicines Agency (EMA) catalog [7] (89 samples) as exemplars for in-context learning. This ensures both structural rigor and clinical authenticity.

EpiCohoKB covers diverse therapeutic areas and study types, including drug safety analyses, comparative effectiveness research, and healthcare utilization studies, creating a comprehensive benchmark for clinical criteria translation. We generate an initial set of SQL queries through large language model (LLM) prompting, manually review and validate them for Snowflake SQL compatibility, resulting in 108 samples. Data scientists with extensive expertise in epidemiological research and SQL query development for observational studies curated and validated both knowledge bases, ensuring both technical accuracy and clinical relevance of the final dataset.

3 Methods

Our approach translates clinical cohort definitions into executable SQL queries through a multi-stage pipeline (Fig. 1). First, we use an LLM (Claude 3.5 Sonnet) to parse input criteria into a semi-structured format, explicitly identifying inclusion criteria, exclusion

[1] https://github.com/Bayer-Group/epi-cohort-text2sql-ecai2025.

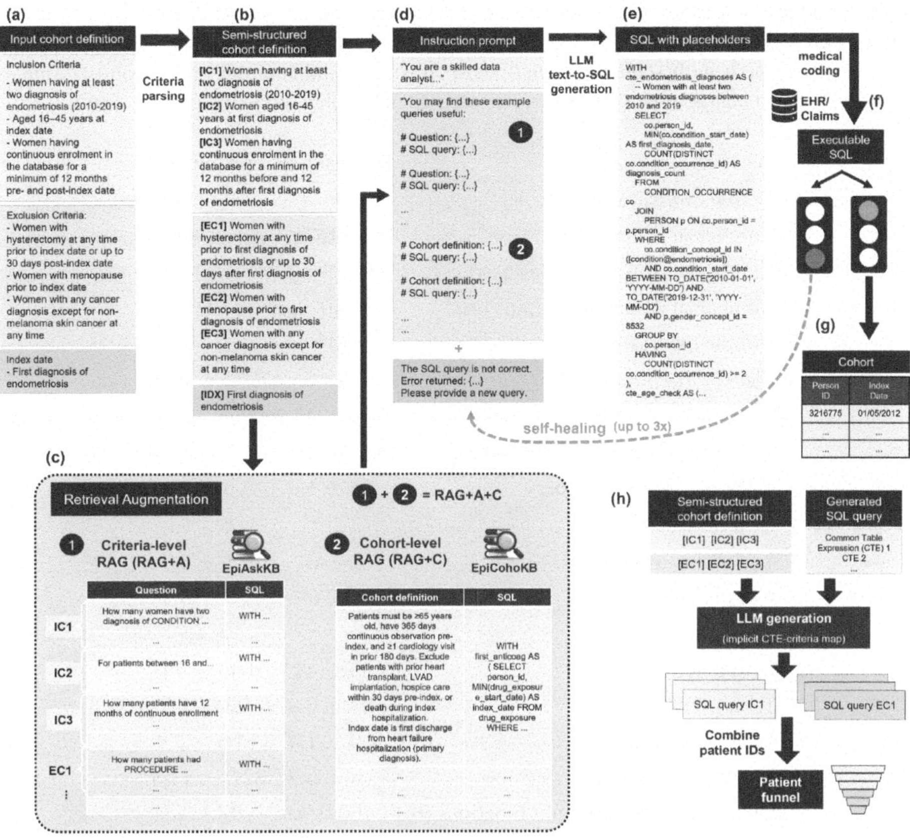

Fig. 1. (a-g) From inclusion/exclusion criteria in natural language to patient cohorts using electronic health record databases: end-to-end workflow. (h) Query decomposition and patient funnel generation through LLM-based processing.

criteria, and index date definition. We opted for this approach over passing raw text directly to the final generation model for two primary reasons. First, this decomposition allows our system to apply RAG strategies at a more granular level (e.g., per-criterion retrieval in RAG+A and RAG+A+C). Second, it simplifies the complex task for the final SQL-generating LLM, allowing it to focus solely on translating structured logic into code, which we found empirically to reduce errors related to missed or incorrectly combined criteria. We then compile an instruction prompt incorporating domain knowledge about OMOP CDM and SQL query construction, forming our baseline zero-shot (ZS) approach. We implement three retrieval augmentation strategies:

1. Criteria-level RAG (RAG + A) retrieves top-5 similar question-SQL pairs from EpiAskKB per criterion;

Table 1. Detailed statistics of the EpiAskKB and EpiCohoKB datasets. Global Statistics represent dataset-wide totals. Text Characteristics, Criteria Complexity, and SQL Complexity show averages per sample with standard deviations. Percentages indicate the proportion of samples with the specified characteristic. N/A denotes metrics not applicable to the dataset type.

Statistic	EpiAskKB	EpiCohoKB
Global Statistics		
Number of samples	115	108
Number of different tables used	13	12
Number of different columns used	40	32
Unique medical concepts	139	374
Text Characteristics		
Question/criteria length [chars]	82.2 ± 37.2	436.5 ± 82.1
Question/criteria length [words]	15.7 ± 7.6	76.3 ± 17.3
Medical entities per query	1.5 ± 1.0	8.0 ± 2.3
Criteria Complexity		
# of inclusion criteria	N/A	4.1 ± 0.7
# of exclusion criteria	N/A	3.7 ± 0.9
SQL Complexity		
SQL length [chars]	803 ± 475	3043 ± 741
Tables referenced	2.3 ± 0.8	5.3 ± 1.2
Joins per query	1.9 ± 1.4	14.6 ± 5.8
Logical conditions	5.8 ± 5.9	32.2 ± 11.4
Queries with aggregation functions (%)	100.0 %	98.1 %
Queries with date/time operations (%)	78.3 %	100.0 %
Queries with subqueries (%)	84.3 %	100.0 %
Samples with temporal constraints (%)	52.2%	100.0%

2. Cohort-level RAG (RAG + C) retrieves top-5 similar cohort definitions from EpiCohoKB;
3. Combined RAG (RAG + A + C) performs both criteria-level and cohort-level retrieval.

This modular design enables query pattern reuse at different granularities - individual criteria can be composed into complex cohort definitions while preserving temporal relationships. The augmented prompt is passed to the LLM to generate SQL with placeholder entities (e.g., [condition@hypertension]). This approach disentangles the query logic generation from the subsequent medical coding step where placeholders are mapped to specific concept IDs [42]. The system implements a self-healing mechanism, which attempts to fix non-executable queries by feeding compiler errors back to the LLM for up to three iterations [24]. The output is a cohort table with patient IDs and index dates.

To enhance interpretability for clinical users and enable criteria refinement, our system implements a patient funnel calculation pipeline (Fig. 1h). While the primary output of our system is the final patient cohort (a list of patient IDs and index dates), the funnel provides a transparent, step-by-step view of cohort attrition by quantifying the remaining patient count as each rule is applied. For example, a user can see that an initial pool of 10 000 patients is reduced to 8 000 after meeting an age requirement, and further reduced to 5 000 after excluding those with a recent medication. This breakdown allows researchers to validate the logic of individual criteria and identify if a specific rule is unexpectedly strict or lenient. To implement this, the LLM generates separate SQL queries for each criterion. These are executed independently and combined sequentially using set operations (set intersections for inclusion criteria and set differences for exclusion criteria), tracking the remaining patient count at each stage.

4 Evaluation

4.1 Experimental Setup

We evaluated several state-of-the-art LLMs: Claude 3.5 Sonnet (hereafter *Claude*) [1], Gemini 2.0 Flash (*Gemini*) [10], LLAMA 3.1 70B [11], and GPT-4o [20]. We also include reasoning models: o1 [21] and DeepSeek R1 (*deepseek*) [12]. All experiments were conducted in February 2025. We used a temperature of 0.0 for all models; top_p was set to 0.9 for LLAMA 3.1 70B and the provider's default for all other models. Due to computational cost constraints, we adopted a two-stage evaluation strategy for o1, DeepSeek R1, and LLAMA 3.1 70B, testing them only in the zero-shot (ZS) setting and with our best-performing RAG + A + C configuration to establish a performance baseline and measure the gains from our optimal augmentation strategy. Input prompts to LLMs range from 1 000 to 3 000 tokens depending on the RAG strategy. The total end-to-end time for the full pipeline, including all generation steps and subsequent query executions on Snowflake, was typically 2 to 6 min, confirming its viability for near-interactive analysis.

Our pipeline employs a two-stage approach to handle medical entities. For the RAG step, we use entity masking to improve the relevance of retrieved examples [42]. By replacing specific terms with generic labels (e.g., endometriosis → CONDITION), the system focuses on retrieving examples with similar analytical structures, rather than just similar medical concepts. This retrieval is powered by the BGE-LARGE-EN-V1.5 embedding model [39]. For the subsequent SQL generation, we instruct the LLM to use placeholders (e.g., condition@hypertension). This strategy decouples generating logical SQL from the specialized task of medical coding [15,23,40,41]. These placeholders are then resolved through a dedicated medical entity normalization process [42], which maps the natural language entity to a standardized OMOP Concept ID. This step is crucial for preventing the LLM from hallucinating invalid concept IDs and ensures the final query is both executable and accurate. This normalization also uses the BGE-LARGE-EN-V1.5 embeddings, with an additional verification layer from GPT-4o to ensure high fidelity [42].

The evaluation framework distinguishes between two key components: (1) the evaluation dataset consisting of inclusion/exclusion criteria paired with reference SQL queries, and (2) the healthcare database where these queries are executed. For the evaluation dataset, we use the 108 inclusion/exclusion criteria from EpiCohoKB described in Sect. 2, employing a leave-one-out approach to prevent data leakage during retrieval. For the database component, we execute both generated and reference SQL queries on Optum's de-identified Clinformatics® Data Mart Database (a major US claims database) converted to OMOP CDM to retrieve actual patient cohorts. Our methodology is compatible with any OMOP-formatted database, including the OMOP network (over 2.1 billion patient records worldwide [28]) and the freely available DE-SynPUF synthetic dataset [30]. For successful queries, we computed patient-level metrics (F1, precision, recall) and normalized cohort size differences based on matching patients, with temporal alignment assessed through exact matches and within a $\pm$ 30-day window. Failed queries (invalid SQL or empty results) contribute zero scores to the final cross-sample averages.

4.2 Experimental Results

Results are shown in Table 2, and outlined below.

Generated Queries have High Syntactic Validity.

Most models show high SQL compilation rates with RAG augmentation, while also improving data retrieval success. The retrieved data rate increases substantially with RAG.

RAG Strongly Improves Zero-Shot Performance.

The combined RAG strategy (RAG + A + C) substantially outperforms ZS across all models. RAG + A + C significantly improves patient cohort identification across all metrics. Precision increases (Claude: $\uparrow$14.6pp, Gemini $\uparrow$33.3pp, GPT-4o $\uparrow$29.6pp), while maintaining high recall (>70%). Similar patterns emerge in temporal alignment. The balanced improvement in precision and recall suggests that RAG helps models better understand both inclusion and exclusion criteria.

Complementary RAG Strategies Enhance Performance.

Cohort-level examples (RAG + C) are particularly effective. When compared to criteria-level RAG (RAG + A), cohort-level examples lead to substantially higher F1 scores. The combination of both strategies (RAG + A + C) further improves performance for most models, suggesting complementary benefits from both example types. Interestingly, GPT-4o shows slightly decreased performance with RAG + A + C compared to RAG + C ($\downarrow$6.4pp), indicating that longer input contexts may impact its generation capabilities.

Table 2. Performance evaluation of text-to-SQL generation for patient cohort identification. *Valid SQL* indicates syntactically correct queries, *Retrieved* indicates queries that successfully retrieved patient data. Patient-level metrics evaluate cohort membership accuracy, while date-level metrics assess the temporal alignment of cohort index dates. Higher values are better, all values in percentage. Bold indicates best results, underlined shows second best.

Model name	Settings	General metrics		Patient-level metrics				Date-level metrics	
		Valid SQL	Retrieved	F1	Prec.	Recall	Size sim.	Date overlap	Within 30d
Claude 3.5 Sonnet	ZS	**100.0**	78.1	57.8	61.0	63.1	62.8	75.9	74.9
Claude 3.5 Sonnet	RAG+A	99.0	82.6	58.4	59.5	68.6	62.6	80.8	77.5
Claude 3.5 Sonnet	RAG+C	99.0	91.4	69.5	72.0	74.7	74.5	88.2	87.4
Claude 3.5 Sonnet	RAG+A+C	99.0	**93.3**	72.8	75.6	79.0	77.6	**91.7**	**90.5**
Gemini 2.0 Flash	ZS	96.2	55.2	42.4	43.3	44.5	46.6	51.7	50.9
Gemini 2.0 Flash	RAG+A	99.0	62.9	41.6	42.1	48.6	46.0	58.7	58.4
Gemini 2.0 Flash	RAG+C	99.0	89.5	68.0	68.9	75.2	73.5	85.4	84.6
Gemini 2.0 Flash	RAG+A+C	99.0	91.3	**75.4**	**76.6**	**79.7**	**79.8**	89.1	89.1
GPT-4o	ZS	84.8	61.0	35.4	38.1	39.7	42.1	52.9	52.5
GPT-4o	RAG+A	86.7	50.5	31.7	32.8	34.7	37.4	44.9	44.6
GPT-4o	RAG+C	97.1	91.4	72.1	73.1	76.8	77.7	87.0	87.9
GPT-4o	RAG+A+C	98.1	84.8	65.7	67.7	71.1	70.5	80.9	82.3
o1	ZS	9.5	5.7	4.3	5.2	4.2	4.5	5.4	5.0
o1	RAG+A+C	78.1	73.3	60.0	62.0	62.2	63.0	71.5	70.0
DeepSeek R1	ZS	35.2	28.6	22.2	22.6	23.1	23.6	25.9	24.8
DeepSeek R1	RAG+A+C	36.2	31.4	23.6	25.0	25.4	25.4	29.6	30.2
LLAMA 3.1 70B	ZS	37.1	17.1	8.5	9.6	9.0	11.0	16.2	14.5
LLAMA 3.1 70B	RAG+A+C	79.1	69.5	47.0	51.2	52.0	52.7	66.6	65.3

Claude and Gemini Emerge as Top Performers.

Claude and Gemini achieve comparable performance when augmented with RAG+A+C. Claude exhibits the strongest ZS performance, while Gemini shows excellent in-context learning capabilities (↑33.3pp from ZS to RAG + A + C). Reasoning-focused models (o1, DeepSeek R1) struggle with SQL formatting despite their analytical capabilities.

To evaluate the patient funnel creation, for the best performing model (Claude RAG + A + C), we measure a 90% normalized cohort size similarity compared to the single-query approach, validating the funnel decomposition strategy.

Error Analysis.

To identify key areas for future improvement, we conduct a qualitative error analysis on the incorrect queries generated by our best-performing configuration (Claude 3.5 Sonnet with RAG+A+C).

The most significant challenges relate to the interpretation of complex temporal logic, a cornerstone of cohort study design. A frequent issue is the model's difficulty in correctly anchoring inclusion or exclusion criteria to the patient-specific index date. For instance, when defining a lookback window to identify new users of a drug, a query might incorrectly include the index date itself (e.g., using `BETWEEN DATEADD(day, -365, index_date) AND index_date`). This subtle discrepancy in boundary logic causes the index prescription to be found in the prior history, erroneously excluding every valid patient. Another common temporal challenge is atemporal exclusion; for a criterion to exclude patients with a diagnosis *before* the index date, the model generates logic to exclude patients with that diagnosis at *any time* in their record, incorrectly removing those who develop the condition after the index event.

Other significant error patterns also emerge. We observe challenges in understanding the specific conventions of the OMOP-CDM schema. For example, a query for "psychiatric evaluation" might incorrectly search the `VISIT_OCCURRENCE` table instead of the correct `PROCEDURE_OCCURRENCE` table. Similarly, a query for "mental health visits" often omits the required join from the `VISIT_OCCURRENCE` table to the `PROVIDER` table to filter by specialty. We also identify errors in complex query construction. A key example involves suboptimal sequences of operations, such as applying a date-range filter before an aggregation intended to find a patient's first-ever event. This leads to the model identifying the first event *within the specified window*, rather than the true *first-ever event* for that patient, thereby misidentifying the index date. Finally, some errors stem from a less nuanced interpretation of clinical concepts, such as translating "chronic use" into a check for any single prescription in the `DRUG_EXPOSURE` table instead of the more appropriate logic of identifying a long-term drug era in the `DRUG_ERA` table.

Collectively, these findings indicate that the primary opportunities for advancement lie not in improving syntactic SQL generation, but in enhancing the model's reasoning about the complex temporal relationships, data model conventions, and clinical semantics.

5 Related Work

Cohort Generation from EHR Data.

Rule-based systems can achieve high precision but require substantial expert curation [2, 13, 18, 25]. While early work combined rules and machine learning [37], recent approaches leverage LLMs: for OMOP-CDM clinical trial queries [22], for structured criteria extraction [16], for cross-schema templated queries [6], for phenotyping [36], and for eligibility criteria structuring [35]. Several EHR text-to-SQL datasets exist [14, 26, 31, 33, 42], though none maps observational study criteria to OMOP-SQL. Ziletti and D'Ambrosi [42] previously introduced RAG-enhanced epidemiological text-to-SQL for question answering. This work extends that approach to the more complex task of cohort generation, which requires preserving temporal relationships, handling logical combinations of criteria, and generating patient-level identifiers with index dates. As evidenced by the statistics in Table 1, cohort generation involves significantly more complex queries with more joins, logical conditions, and temporal constraints compared to analytical questions. Our innovations include two-level retrieval augmentation, patient funnel generation, and comprehensive evaluation of patient-level precision and recall with temporal alignment.

Text-to-SQL with in-Context Learning.

Recent work shows LLMs excel at text-to-SQL tasks when enhanced with in-context learning [27], particularly through optimized example selection [8, 17], query decomposition [24], diverse demonstrations [4,5], ensemble approaches [9], and chain-of-thought prompting [38].

6 Conclusions

This work shows that LLMs with RAG can effectively identify patient cohorts from EHR data. The pipeline combines medical concept standardization, criteria parsing, and two-level retrieval to handle complex temporal relationships, while the patient funnel provides interpretable intermediate metrics. Future applications to clinical trial recruitment could help bridge the gap between observational and interventional research.

7 Limitations

Our work has several limitations. The modest size of our dataset may not capture the full complexity and variety of real-world observational studies. The current system lacks formal uncertainty estimates for its predictions, making it difficult to identify cases where human review is particularly important. Additionally, the accuracy of intermediate preprocessing steps like semi-structured parsing and entity normalization was not separately evaluated, which would be required to fully characterize the pipeline's robustness. Although the patient funnel offers valuable transparency into the cohort attrition process, the generated SQL itself can be difficult to interpret for users unfamiliar with the language. This difficulty may limit the ability of clinical researchers to fully validate the query's underlying logic. The current methodology relies on OMOP-CDM, and although it could be in principle adapted to other data models through in-context learning, this was not tested.

References

1. Anthropic AI: Model card for claude 3 models. https://docs.anthropic.com/en/docs/resources/model-card (2024). Accessed Feb 15 2024
2. Banda, J.M., Halpern, Y., Sontag, D., Shah, N.H.: Electronic phenotyping with APHRODITE and the Observational Health Sciences and Informatics (OHDSI) data network. AMIA Joint Summits Transl. Sci. Proc. **2017**, 48–57 (2017)
3. Casey, J.A., Schwartz, B.S., Stewart, W.F., Adler, N.E.: Using electronic health records for population health research: a review of methods and applications. Ann. Rev. Public Health 37(Volume 37, 2016), 61–81 (2016). https://doi.org/10.1146/annurev-publhealth-032315-021353, https://www.annualreviews.org/content/journals/10.1146/annurev-publhealth-032315-021353
4. Chang, S., Fosler-Lussier, E.: How to prompt LLMs for text-to-SQL: a study in zero-shot, single-domain, and cross-domain settings (2023)

5. Chang, S., Fosler-Lussier, E.: Selective demonstrations for cross-domain text-to-SQL. In: Bouamor, H., Pino, J., Bali, K. (eds.) Findings of the Association for Computational Linguistics: EMNLP 2023, pp. 14174–14189. Association for Computational Linguistics, Singapore (Dec 2023). https://doi.org/10.18653/v1/2023.findings-emnlp.944, https://aclanthology.org/2023.findings-emnlp.944
6. Dobbins, N.J., et al.: Leafai: query generator for clinical cohort discovery rivaling a human programmer. J. Am. Med. Inform. Assoc. **30**(12), 1954–1964 (08 2023). https://doi.org/10.1093/jamia/ocad149
7. EMA: HMA-EMA catalogues of real-world data sources and studies (2024). https://catalogues.ema.europa.eu/. Accessed 21 Feb 2026 11:56:56
8. Gao, D., Wang, H., Li, Y., Sun, X., Qian, Y., Ding, B., Zhou, J.: Text-to-SQL empowered by large language models: a benchmark evaluation (2023)
9. Gao, Y., et al.: A preview of xiyan-SQL: a multi-generator ensemble framework for text-to-SQL (2025). https://arxiv.org/abs/2411.08599
10. Gemini Team: Gemini: A family of highly capable multimodal models. Tech. rep., Google (12 2023). https://storage.googleapis.com/deepmind-media/gemini_1_report.pdf. Accessed Feb 15 2024
11. Grattafiori, A., et al.: The llama 3 herd of models (2024). https://arxiv.org/abs/2407.21783
12. Guo, D., et al.: Deepseek-r1: Incentivizing reasoning capability in LLMs via reinforcement learning (2025). https://arxiv.org/abs/2501.12948
13. Hripcsak, G., et al.: Facilitating phenotype transfer using a common data model. J. Biomed. Inform. **96**, 103253 (2019). https://doi.org/10.1016/j.jbi.2019.103253, https://www.sciencedirect.com/science/article/pii/S1532046419301728
14. Lee, G., et al.: EHRSQL: A practical text-to-SQL benchmark for electronic health records. In: Koyejo, S., Mohamed, S., Agarwal, A., Belgrave, D., Cho, K., Oh, A. (eds.) Advances in Neural Information Processing Systems. vol. 35, pp. 15589–15601. Curran Associates, Inc. (2022)
15. Limsopatham, N., Collier, N.: Normalising medical concepts in social media texts by learning semantic representation. In: Erk, K., Smith, N.A. (eds.) Proceedings of the 54th Annual Meeting of the Association for Computational Linguistics (Volume 1: Long Papers), pp. 1014–1023. Association for Computational Linguistics, Berlin, Germany (Aug 2016). https://doi.org/10.18653/v1/P16-1096, https://aclanthology.org/P16-1096
16. Melnichenko, O.: Designing multi-step cohort creation flow for biomedical datasets. Microsoft Technical Community Blog (2023). https://techcommunity.microsoft.com/blog/healthcareandlifesciencesblog/designing-multi-step-cohort-creation-flow-for-biomedical-datasets/3964454
17. Nan, L., et al.: Enhancing text-to-SQL capabilities of large language models: a study on prompt design strategies. In: Bouamor, H., Pino, J., Bali, K. (eds.) Findings of the Association for Computational Linguistics: EMNLP 2023, pp. 14935–14956. Association for Computational Linguistics, Singapore (Dec 2023). https://doi.org/10.18653/v1/2023.findings-emnlp.996, https://aclanthology.org/2023.findings-emnlp.996
18. OHDSI Collaborative: The book of OHDSI. In: The Book of OHDSI, chap. 10. Observational Health Data Sciences and Informatics (2021). http://book.ohdsi.org
19. OMOP-CDM: OMOP CDM common data model. https://ohdsi.github.io/CommonDataModel/ (2023). Accessed Jan 23 2024
20. OpenAI: Gpt-4 technical report (2023)
21. OpenAI: Learning to reason with LLMs (September 2024). https://openai.com/index/learning-to-reason-with-llms/. Accessed Sept 2024
22. Park, J., et al.: Criteria2query 3.0: Leveraging generative large language models for clinical trial eligibility query generation. J. Biomed. Inform. **154**, 104649

(2024). https://doi.org/10.1016/j.jbi.2024.104649, https://www.sciencedirect.com/science/article/pii/S1532046424000674

23. Portelli, B., Scaboro, S., Santus, E., Sedghamiz, H., Chersoni, E., Serra, G.: Generalizing over long tail concepts for medical term normalization. In: Goldberg, Y., Kozareva, Z., Zhang, Y. (eds.) Proceedings of the 2022 Conference on Empirical Methods in Natural Language Processing, pp. 8580–8591. Association for Computational Linguistics, Abu Dhabi, United Arab Emirates (Dec 2022). https://doi.org/10.18653/v1/2022.emnlp-main.588, https://aclanthology.org/2022.emnlp-main.588
24. Pourreza, M., Rafiei, D.: DIN-SQL: decomposed in-context learning of text-to-SQL with self-correction. In: Thirty-seventh Conference on Neural Information Processing Systems (2023).https://openreview.net/forum?id=p53QDxSIc5
25. Privitera, S., Hartenstein, A.: Phenex: Automatic phenotype extractor. https://github.com/Bayer-Group/PhenEx (2024). Accessed 21 Feb 2026 11:56:56
26. Raghavan, P., Liang, J.J., Mahajan, D., Chandra, R., Szolovits, P.: emrKBQA: a clinical knowledge-base question answering dataset. In: Demner-Fushman, D., Cohen, K.B., Ananiadou, S., Tsujii, J. (eds.) Proceedings of the 20th Workshop on Biomedical Language Processing, pp. 64–73. Association for Computational Linguistics, Online (Jun 2021). https://doi.org/10.18653/v1/2021.bionlp-1.7, https://aclanthology.org/2021.bionlp-1.7
27. Rajkumar, N., Li, R., Bahdanau, D.: Evaluating the text-to-SQL capabilities of large language models. ArXiv abs/2204.00498 (2022). https://api.semanticscholar.org/CorpusID:247922681
28. Reich, C., et al.: OHDSI Standardized Vocabularies–a large-scale centralized reference ontology for international data harmonization. J. Am. Med. Inform. Assoc. ocad247 (01 2024). https://doi.org/10.1093/jamia/ocad247, https://doi.org/10.1093/jamia/ocad247
29. Sherman, R.E., et al.: Real-world evidence – what is it and what can it tell us? N. Engl. J. Med. **375**(23), 2293–2297 (2016). https://doi.org/10.1056/NEJMsb1609216, https://www.nejm.org/doi/full/10.1056/NEJMsb1609216
30. SynPUF: Medicare claims synthetic public use files (synpufs). https://www.cms.gov/data-research/statistics-trends-and-reports/medicare-claims-synthetic-public-use-files (2010). Accessed 23 Jan 2024
31. Tarbell, R., Choo, K.K.R., Dietrich, G., Rios, A.: Towards understanding the generalization of medical text-to-SQL models and datasets. AMIA ... Annual Symposium proceedings. AMIA Symposium 2023, 669–678 (2023). https://api.semanticscholar.org/CorpusID:257687830
32. U.S. FDA: Real-world data: Assessing electronic health records and medical claims data to support regulatory decision-making for drug and biological products. Guidance for Industry FDA-2020-D-2307, U.S. Food and Drug Administration (July 2024). https://www.fda.gov/regulatory-information/search-fda-guidance-documents/real-world-data-assessing-electronic-health-records-and-medical-claims-data-support-regulatory, final Level 1 Guidance
33. Wang, P., Shi, T., Reddy, C.K.: Text-to-SQL generation for question answering on electronic medical records. In: Proceedings of The Web Conference 2020, pp. 350–361. WWW '20, Association for Computing Machinery, New York, NY, USA (2020). https://doi.org/10.1145/3366423.3380120
34. Wang, S.V., et al.: Start-RWE: structured template for planning and reporting on the implementation of real world evidence studies. BMJ 372 (2021). https://doi.org/10.1136/bmj.m4856, https://www.bmj.com/content/372/bmj.m4856
35. Wong, C., et al.: Scaling clinical trial matching using large language models: a case study in oncology. In: Deshpande, K., Fiterau, M., Joshi, S., Lipton, Z., Ranganath, R., Urteaga, I.,

Yeung, S. (eds.) Proceedings of the 8th Machine Learning for Healthcare Conference. Proceedings of Machine Learning Research, vol. 219, pp. 846–862. PMLR (11–12 Aug 2023). https://proceedings.mlr.press/v219/wong23a.html

36. Yan, C., et al.: Large language models facilitate the generation of electronic health record phenotyping algorithms. J. Am. Med. Inform. Assoc. **31**(9), 1994–2001 (04 2024). https://doi.org/10.1093/jamia/ocae072, https://doi.org/10.1093/jamia/ocae072
37. Yuan, C., et al.: Criteria2Query: a natural language interface to clinical databases for cohort definition. J. Am Med. Inform. Assoc. **26**(4), 294–305 (02 2019). https://doi.org/10.1093/jamia/ocy178
38. Zhang, H., Cao, R., Chen, L., Xu, H., Yu, K.: ACT-SQL: In-context learning for text-to-SQL with automatically-generated chain-of-thought. In: Bouamor, H., Pino, J., Bali, K. (eds.) Findings of the Association for Computational Linguistics: EMNLP 2023, pp. 3501–3532. Association for Computational Linguistics, Singapore (Dec 2023). https://doi.org/10.18653/v1/2023.findings-emnlp.227, https://aclanthology.org/2023.findings-emnlp.227
39. Zhang, P., Xiao, S., Liu, Z., Dou, Z., Nie, J.Y.: Retrieve anything to augment large language models (2023)
40. Zhang, S., et al.: Knowledge-rich self-supervision for biomedical entity linking. In: Goldberg, Y., Kozareva, Z., Zhang, Y. (eds.) Findings of the Association for Computational Linguistics: EMNLP 2022, pp. 868–880. Association for Computational Linguistics, Abu Dhabi, United Arab Emirates (Dec 2022). https://doi.org/10.18653/v1/2022.findings-emnlp.61, https://aclanthology.org/2022.findings-emnlp.61
41. Ziletti, A., Akbik, A., Berns, C., Herold, T., Legler, M., Viell, M.: Medical coding with biomedical transformer ensembles and zero/few-shot learning. In: Loukina, A., Gangadharaiah, R., Min, B. (eds.) Proceedings of the 2022 Conference of the North American Chapter of the Association for Computational Linguistics: Human Language Technologies: Industry Track, pp. 176–187. Association for Computational Linguistics, Hybrid: Seattle, Washington + Online (Jul 2022). https://doi.org/10.18653/v1/2022.naacl-industry.21, https://aclanthology.org/2022.naacl-industry.21
42. Ziletti, A., D'Ambrosi, L.: Retrieval augmented text-to-SQL generation for epidemiological question answering using electronic health records. In: Naumann, T., Ben Abacha, A., Bethard, S., Roberts, K., Bitterman, D. (eds.) Proceedings of the 6th Clinical Natural Language Processing Workshop, pp. 47–53. Association for Computational Linguistics, Mexico City, Mexico (Jun 2024). https://doi.org/10.18653/v1/2024.clinicalnlp-1.4, https://aclanthology.org/2024.clinicalnlp-1.4

Which Metadata Matters? Evaluating Predictive Features for Environmental Time Series

Ann-Kathrin Dörr[1,2], Tina Schmidt[3], Jens Schoth[3], Ivana Kraiselburd[1], and Folker Meyer[1,2](✉)

[1] Institute for Artificial Intelligence in Medicine, University Hospital Essen, Department of Medicine, University of Duisburg-Essen, Essen, Germany
folker.meyer@uk-essen.de
[2] Department of Computer Science, University of Duisburg-Essen, Essen, Germany
[3] Emschergenossenschaft/Lippeverband, Kronprinzenstraße 24, 45128 Essen, Germany

Abstract. Forecasting complex, multivariate time series using machine learning presents significant challenges, particularly when dealing with high-dimensional biological data. One such application is the prediction of microbial community dynamics in wastewater treatment plants (WWTPs), which is directly relevant to public and environmental health. Previously, we addressed this problem by training different model architectures and comparing their performance. In this study, an attempt was made to enhance model performance by adding operational and environmental metadata, such as temperature, inflow rates, and nutrient levels. The parameters were incorporated into the time series, and their influence was systematically evaluated. The findings indicate that while metadata enhances predictive accuracy, the significance of individual features varies across WWTPs. Training a model on one dataset and retraining that model on site-specific data has been demonstrated to enhance performance, underscoring the necessity for adaptive, localized modeling strategies. The findings demonstrate the value of machine learning approaches for extracting predictive insights from complex, high-dimensional biological time series data in wastewater systems. The implementation of such a system as an additional wastewater monitoring technique has the potential to facilitate more timely public health decision-making in the future.

Keywords: Time series prediction · Wastewater · LSTM

1 Introduction

Machine learning, particularly deep learning for time series analysis, has demonstrated strong capabilities in modeling high-dimensional, temporally structured

Supplementary Information The online version contains supplementary material available at https://doi.org/10.1007/978-3-032-16708-8_20.

P. Bruno et al. (Eds.): HC_AIxIA_HYDRA 2025, CCIS 2830, pp. 243–253, 2026.
https://doi.org/10.1007/978-3-032-16708-8_20

data across domains. Architectures like Long Short-Term Memory (LSTM) models are especially effective at learning temporal dependencies and nonlinear dynamics in multivariate sequences [1]. These models are increasingly applied to real-world scenarios where distinguishing between baseline variability and significant deviation is essential [2].

One of the scenarios that this could be applied to is forecasting normality in microbial community fluctuations. There are already different approaches to use machine learning to forecast changes in microbial communities and link them to possible emerging diseases [3]. Due to the properties of microbial communities, including multivariability, interconnectedness, noise, and sparsity, LSTMs appear to be a suitable fit for modeling this type of data. Still, it requires additional research to refine such models [4].

A representative use case for such modeling is found in wastewater monitoring, where microbial community composition reflects a mixture of human and environmental inputs [5]. Using machine learning to explore wastewater microbial community shifts to define a normal baseline variability and detect outliers could be essential for building public health early warning systems. The integration of such an early warning system into a monitoring approach grounded in wastewater-based epidemiology (WBE) is a concept that merits further consideration. WBE incorporates the observation of chemical and biological markers in a sewage system to assess health and disease status in a population in a non-invasive way [6,7]. The process of measuring and tracking circulating pathogens in the population through wastewater monitoring has become a significant component in disease prevention and tracking, especially since the beginning of the COVID-19 pandemic [8].

Due to natural seasonal variability and the absence of a stable baseline microbial community, interpreting microbial signals in wastewater is particularly challenging [9–11]. As wastewater aggregates microbial input from diverse sources, distinguishing meaningful changes from expected variation requires robust, adaptive models [12]. Machine learning methods, especially when trained with relevant environmental and operational metadata, offer a scalable and data-driven solution to address these challenges, and can be extended to similar tasks in other ecological or public health contexts [13].

The current analysis is based on the findings of earlier studies that demonstrated the capability of LSTM models in the context of time series analysis and outlier detection within microbial communities [14,15]. It aims to investigate the impact of additional data and metadata on the model's performance and to identify the parameters that are beneficial to this type of analysis, helping to distinguish between outliers caused by external events or disease.

The present study employs 16S rRNA gene sequencing of wastewater data from a selection of WWTPs, with two located in Germany and two in the US. With this study, we aim to increase the predictive capabilities of LSTMs for forecasting microbial community composition and find issues and pitfalls when it comes to including additional metadata. A visual representation of the project's overview can be found in Fig. 1.

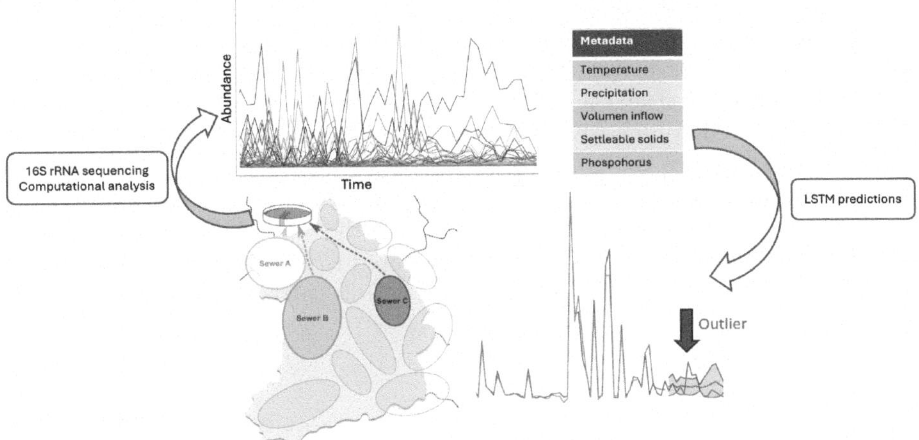

Fig. 1. Project overview, visualizing sampling point, input data, and model output. Bacterial abundances found in the WWTP over time and corresponding metadata are the input for the model, which then predicts future abundances with a 95% confidence interval.

2 Methods

2.1 Model Architectures

The model architecture selection was based on the findings of previous studies, which indicated that LSTM models are effective in predicting microbial community composition and traits in various environments, like beaches [14] and the human gut [2]. In a previous study, we found that LSTMs worked best for this kind of data in comparison to VARMA, Random Forests, and GRUs [4]. The focus of this study was to enhance the model that had been created previously, which contained 2048 LSTM cells in a single layer [4]. We used a ReLU activation function and the ADAM optimizer, both with their respective Keras default parameters. To allow for better generalization, we employed early stopping based on the model's loss with a waiting period of 10 epochs and dropout with a rate of 0.2. The input, consisting of the absolute abundance for the different bacterial genera, was generated from BIOM tables [16] resulting from the analysis of the samples. The model architecture was the same as used in Dörr *et al.* [4].

Prediction intervals were constructed from the distribution of model residuals. Specifically, residual quantiles were estimated to capture the variability of future observations. The lower and upper bounds were defined using the empirical quantiles of the residual distribution, respectively. The intervals were subsequently centered on the mean model prediction while preserving the observed asymmetry of the residual distribution, ensuring that the mean prediction always lies within the interval. This approach provides uncertainty bounds that reflect both prediction bias and heterogeneity in the data.

We split the continuous time series sequentially along the time axis: the first 70% of observations were used for training, the following 10% for validation, and the final 20% for testing. This preserves the temporal order of the data and avoids information leakage from the future into the past. The final model generates each prediction based on the preceding three time points. This design allows the model, once pre-trained, to be applied even to relatively short time series. The evaluation metrics employed for the assessment of prediction accuracy include the Mean Absolute Error (MAE), the Root Mean Squared Error (RMSE), and the Normalized Root Mean Squared Error (NRMSE). Code examples as well as input data can be found on GitHub (https://github.com/IKIM-Essen/Microbiome_TimeSeries).

2.2 Data

16S rRNA gene analysis involves the amplification and sequencing of one or more hypervariable regions of the 16S gene, which is specific to bacteria. The sequences are analyzed for differences and clustered based on similarity. These groups are then compared with reference sequences in a database to assign taxonomic labels, typically at the genus level. The number of different bacteria is determined by the number of clusters assigned to the taxonomic labels. For this project, 16S rRNA gene sequences from wastewater samples were obtained from two independent sources.

The sequences from the WWTPs in the USA were obtained from the publication of LaMartina *et al.* [10]. Samples were collected from two WWTPs in the Milwaukee area, namely Jones Island (JI) and South Shore (SH). The dataset provided supplementary metadata regarding environmental settings, including temperature, as well as wastewater-specific data, such as chemical parameters (see Table 1 for details). The samples were collected monthly over the course of several years.

The second dataset was created from over a year of weekly samples taken from the inlets of two WWTPs in Dinslaken, located in the Ruhr area in Germany. The WWTP in Dinslaken (KLDI) serves approximately 70,000 residents and two hospitals. It is equipped with a separate rainwater system. By contrast, the WWTP Emschermündung (KLEM) serves around 1.4 million residents and nine hospitals, including the University Hospital Essen. It treats both rainwater and human wastewater. For the KLDI, 138 samples were collected from March 2023 to December 2024, while 70 samples were obtained from April 2024 to December 2024 for KLEM. For both sampling sites, metadata similar to that collected for the Milwaukee samples has been gathered. Sequences for the samples from KLDI can be obtained from the European Nucleotide Archive under accession number PRJEB83882.

The sampling approach was based on the method described by Schmiege *et al.* [17], involving the collection of 2 L of untreated wastewater. Samples were stored at 4°C until processed. Aliquots of 200 mL were filtered using 0.45 μm pore-size electronegative filters (MF-Millipore). Nucleic acids were then extracted with the innuPREP AniPath DNA/RNA Kit using the InnuPure C16 touch system (Analytik Jena). Sequencing libraries were prepared following Illumina's 16S Metagenomic Sequencing Library Preparation protocol, using primers Bakt_341F and Bakt_805R targeting the V3–V4 region [18]. Sequencing was performed on an Illumina MiSeq platform with 2×250 V2 chemistry.

The resulting 16S rRNA gene sequences were analyzed with RiboSnake [19], a 16S rRNA gene sequence analysis pipeline based on Snakemake [20] and Qiime2 [21].

Additional metadata was included as supplementary columns in the model's input files. The metadata categories tested for impact on the model performance, as well as the subset utilized for training the model on all available wastewater data, are presented in Table 1. It is important to note that there are discrepancies in the manner in which the metadata was collected, and that missing values are present in the Milwaukee metadata. Columns of metadata with an excess of missing values were excluded from the training dataset of the models.

Table 1. Summary of available metadata from the two study sides. It was not possible to utilise the complete set of available metadata for the purposes of impact testing and training of the entire model, due to the absence of overlap between types and a significant number of missing values.

Metadata for KLDI & KLEM	Metadata for JI & SH	Used for impact evaluation	Used for complete training
Rainfall (l/m^2)	Precipitation (48h) (l/m^2)	Rainfall (l/m^2)	Rainfall/Precipitation (l/m^2)
Temperature (max) (°C)	Temperature (air) (°C)	Temperature (max) (°C)	Temperature (average) (°C)/ Temperature (air) (°C)
Temperature (min) (°C)	Temperature (sewer) (°C)	Temperature (min) (°C)	Volume inflow/ Flow (m^3/l)
Temperature (average) (°C)	Flow (per day) (m^3/l)	Temperature (average) (°C)	Settleable solids/ TSS (ml/l)
Volume inflow (m^3/d)	Ammonia (mg/l)	Volume inflow (m^3/d)	Phosphorus (mg/l)
pH (min)	BOD5 (mg/l)	pH (min)	
pH (max)	BOD5Total_Soluble (mg/l)	pH (max)	
Conductivity (min)	Cadmium (mg/l)	Conductivity (min)	
Conductivity (max)	Calcium (mg/l)	Conductivity (max)	
Temperature (inlet) (°C)	Chromium (mg/l)	Temperature (inlet) (°C)	
Settleable solids (ml/l)	Copper (mg/l)	Settleable solids (ml/l)	
Chemical Oxygen Demand (COD) (mg/l)	COD (mg/l)	COD (mg/l)	
Nitrogen (mg/l)	Iron (mg/l)	Nitrogen (mg/l)	
Phosphorus (mg/l)	Lead (mg/l)	Phosphorus (mg/l)	
Season	LowLevel_Mercury (ng/l)		
	Magnesium (mg/l)		
	Nickel (mg/l)		
	Nitrate/Nitrite (mg/l)		
	Phosphorus (mg/l)		
	TSS (total suspended solids) (ml/l)		
	TKN_Nitrogen (mg/l)		
	Zinc (mg/l)		

3 Results

To perform this analysis, 16S rRNA gene sequencing data was used to measure the abundances of the various bacterial genera present in wastewater samples. The complete list of genera used as input for the model was derived by combining all genera found in the different datasets. The genera not present across all datasets were included and assigned an abundance of zero, reflecting their biological absence in those samples. Although alternative imputation strategies may improve predictive performance, the choice of method remains a topic of scientific debate [22]. To avoid introducing assumptions or artifacts, we opted for the conservative approach of using zeros in this study. The initial tests were executed based on the KLDI dataset alone, as it is the longest time series with the densest sampling points and the least amount of missing values. This reduction in the initial training data has the effect of reducing the time required for the initial training and evaluation steps. The reduced amount of data may lead to overfitting, which should be tackled by training on further data as soon as the best-fitted parameter combinations are identified.

3.1 Metadata Impact on Prediction

To evaluate the impact of the various metadata types on the model's prediction accuracy, a comprehensive analysis of the model's performance was conducted, considering multiple combinations of the available metadata.

The parameters present in all four datasets used for final training were precipitation (l/m^2), average air temperature (°C), volume of inflow (m^3/day), total suspended solids (TSS, of which settleable solids are a part of) (ml/l), and concentration of phosphorus (mg/l).

As demonstrated in Table 2 (extended in Tables 5 and 6, Supplementary Material), the prediction accuracy exhibited significant variability, depending on the presence of metadata values. Models trained on the volume of inflow and precipitation demonstrated the best evaluation metrics.

Given the differing rainwater treatments in KLEM and KLDI, we examined whether precipitation affects the systems differently. As shown in Table 3, incorporating precipitation data improves both models, with a stronger impact on the KLEM-trained model.

As demonstrated in Fig. 2, the incorporation of metadata exerts an additional effect. The incorporation of additional metadata parameters into a model can indeed result in a reduction of overfitting, despite the absence of an increase in the accuracy of the predictions themselves.

Table 2. Evaluation metrics for the different metadata parameters, present in all datasets. The different parameters were added to the timeseries dataset from the KLDI separately as well as combined.

Metadata	Inflow vol	Temp	TSS	P total	Precipitation	5 combined parameters
MAE	19.24	27.26	34.84	27.25	17.80	17.81
MAE test	95.37	90.7	88.15	89	73.73	68.2
RMSE	347.17	450.94	527.06	470.2	309.41	315.11
RMSE test	890.27	842.12	824.46	811.19	1144.90	1101.55
NRMSE	0.37	0.52	0.63	0.52	0.41	0.44
NRMSE test	3.67	3.52	3.17	2.7	2.23	2.31

Table 3. A comparison of the evaluation metrics for models that have been trained on KLDI and KLEM data separately, with the addition of precipitation data, is presented here. The incorporation of precipitation leads to an enhancement in the model's performance across both datasets, with a marginally more pronounced effect in KLEM.

Evaluation Metrics	KLDI + Precipitation	KLDI only	KLEM + Precipitation	KLEM only
MAE	17.80	20.25	8.28	11.5
MAE test	73.73	98.47	81.14	114.51
RMSE	309.41	246.76	121.45	133.76
RMSE test	1144.90	1313.14	1142.37	1354.45
NRMSE	0.41	0.27	0.19	0.17
NRMSE test	2.23	2.07	4.51	4.03

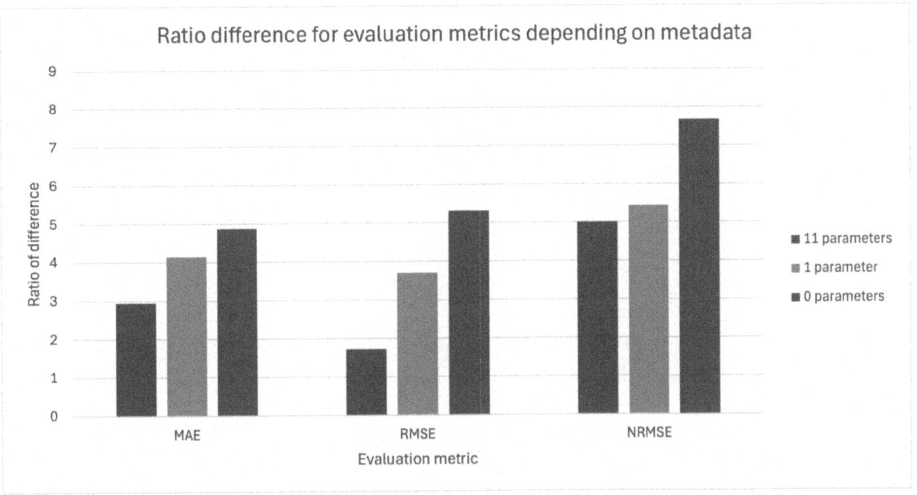

Fig. 2. Depicted are the differences between the evaluation metrics MAE, RMSE, and NRMSE for training and test sets, depending on the extent to which metadata categories are added to the model's prediction. The difference is depicted as a ratio between the values.

3.2 Retraining

To analyze possible reduction of overfitting by means of retraining, a model was initially trained on the KLDI dataset alone, with five metadata parameters that were present across all datasets. Subsequently, the resulting models were retrained using data from KLEM, JI, and SH. As illustrated in Table 4, the incorporation of additional datasets effectively mitigates the occurrence of overfitting, as evidenced by a reduction in the disparity between the evaluation metrics for the training and test sets.

The absence of overfitting in the model trained on the complete dataset is further supported by the progression of training and validation losses shown in

Table 4. The alterations in evaluation metrics can be attributed to the process of training and retraining the model on disparate datasets. The complete set of five overlapping metadata parameters was utilized to add to the model. Initially, the values are found to be suboptimal. However, as additional data is incorporated, the overfitting phenomenon is mitigated.

Evaluation metrics	DI	KLDI+KLEM	KLDI+KLEM+JI	KLDI+KLEM+JI+SH
MAE	17.81	44.98	32.23	26.29
MAE test	68.2	73.22	24.05	15.43
RMSE	315.11	498.93	336.21	251.65
RMSE test	1101.55	1090.77	265.85	123.11
NRMSE	0.44	1	1	1
NRMSE test	2.31	2.79	0.62	0.67

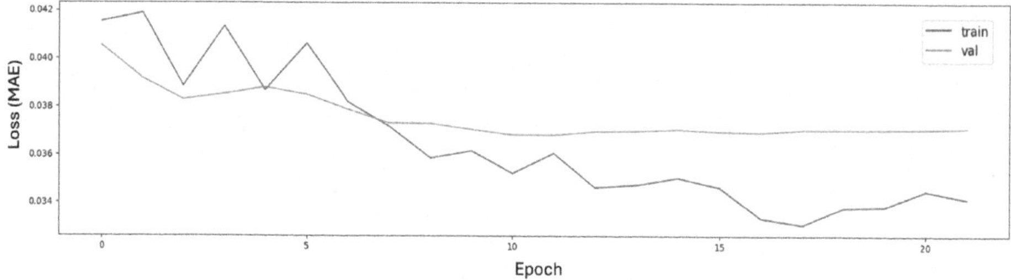

Fig. 3. The plot illustrates the model's loss values for the training and validation sets, which have been calculated based on the MAE. The loss function has been observed to decrease steadily, but from epoch 10 onwards, it has plateaued for the validation set.

Fig. 3. Both loss curves exhibit a consistent downward trend and remain in close proximity throughout the training process, indicating good generalization and stable model performance. However, the overall accuracy of predictions appears to be reduced when training is conducted on diverse datasets.

4 Conclusion

In this study, we examined the impact of distinct metadata values on the efficacy of LSTMs in predicting the composition of microbial communities in wastewater time series data. A number of parameters were analyzed, encompassing both general environmental information, such as temperature and precipitation, and more specific chemical properties, like phosphorus concentration. The parameters directly linked to the waterbody (precipitation, volume of inflow, chemical properties) had the greatest impact on the model's performance.

Incorporating precipitation data substantially improved model accuracy, with a stronger effect for the model trained solely on KLEM data. This aligns with the structural differences in KLDI, where rainwater is treated separately from other wastewater. Such context-dependent behavior suggests that the models adapt effectively to the structure and nuances of the input data and task. The observed feature-importance differences are thus meaningful, reflecting biologically plausible patterns rather than arbitrary variation.

Incorporating additional metadata reduced overfitting without requiring extra timepoints, as evidenced by the decreasing gap between training and test evaluation metrics with added metadata. Thus, even when additional timepoints are unavailable, appropriate metadata can enhance the model's generalization capability.

Retraining the LSTM on datasets from additional WWTPs further reduced overfitting compared to training on a single dataset. Combined with the benefits of additional metadata, this suggests that LSTM performance improves with longer, information-rich time series. However, the predictive value of metadata is context-dependent, and not all parameters enhance performance across environments. For short time series, selecting metadata optimally suited to the specific context is critical. In wastewater analysis, such parameters are often linked to the facility's inflow volume, driven by precipitation and total inflow.

Developing a model that predicts natural fluctuations in wastewater bacterial communities and detects outliers could be crucial for early warning systems. Such a system could enable timely detection of pathogen surges, providing valuable information for public health authorities to prevent outbreaks. Although further research is needed to automate outlier detection, extend prediction horizons, and explore alternative model architectures, this study offers valuable insights and promising results for future early warning system development.

Acknowledgments. We want to thank Prof. Christin Seifert for her advice and knowledge sharing.

Disclosure of Competing Interests. The authors have no competing interests to declare that are relevant to the content of this article. This work was supported in part by the WBEready consortium (grant no. ZMII2-2523COR10A-E), funded by the German Federal Ministry for Health (Bundesministerium für Gesundheit, BMG).

Code and Data Availability. Code for the models from Dörr et al. can be found on GitHub https://github.com/IKIM-Essen/Microbiome_TimeSeries. The data for KLDI is available under the accession number PRJEB83882.

References

1. Siami-Namini, S., Tavakoli, N., Namin, A. S. The performance of LSTM and biLSTM in forecasting time series. In: 2019505 IEEE International Conference on Big Data (Big Data), 3285–3292, (2019). https://doi.org/10.1109/BigData47090.2019.9005997
2. Baranwal, M., Clark, R.L., Thompson, J., Sun, Z., Hero, A.O., Venturelli, O.S. Recurrent neural networks enable design of multifunctional synthetic human gut microbiome dynamics. eLife, **11** e73870 (Jun 2022)
3. Sherwani, M.K., et al.: Multi-omics time-series analysis in microbiome research: a systematic review. bioRxiv 2025.07.03.659054; https://doi.org/10.1101/2025.07.03.659054
4. Dörr, A., Imangaliyev, S., Karadeniz, U., Schmidt, T., Meyer, F., Kraiselburd, I.: Distinguishing critical microbial community shifts from normal temporal variability in human and environmental ecosystems. Sci. Rep. **15**(1), 16934 (2025)
5. Hill, R., Stentiford, G.D., Walker, D.I., Baker-Austin, C., Ward, G., Maskrey, B.H., Von Aerle, R., Verner-Jeffreys, D., Peeler, E., Bass, D.: Realising a global one health disease surveillance approach: insights from wastewater and beyond. Nat. Commun. **15**(1), 5324 (2024)
6. Huizer, M., Ter Laak, T.L., De Voogt, P., Van Wezel, A.P.: Wastewater-based epidemiology for illicit drugs: A critical review on global data. Water Res. **207**, 117789 (2021)
7. Amin, V., Bowes, D.A., Halden, R.U.: Systematic scoping review evaluating the potential of wastewater-based epidemiology for monitoring cardiovascular disease and cancer. Sci. Total Environ. **858**, 160103 (2023)
8. Karthikeyan, S., et al.: Wastewater sequencing reveals early cryptic sars-cov-2 variant transmission. Nature **609**(7925), 101–108 (2022)
9. Guo, B., Liu, C., Gibson, C., Frigon, D.: Wastewater microbial community structure and functional traits change over short timescales. Sci. Total Environ. **662**, 779–785 (2019)
10. LaMartina, E.L., Mohaimani, A.A., Newton, R.J.: Urban wastewater bacterial communities assemble into seasonal steady states. Microbiome **9**(1), 116 (2021)
11. Liu, X., Nie, Y., Wu, X.-L.: Predicting microbial community compositions in wastewater treatment plants using artificial neural networks. Microbiome **11**(1), 93 (2023)
12. Becsei, Á., et al.: Time-series sewage metagenomics distinguishes seasonal, human-derived and environmental microbial communities potentially allowing source-attributed surveillance. Nature Commun. **15**(1), 7551 (Aug 2024)
13. Aßmann, E., et al.: Augmentation of wastewater-based epidemiology with machine learning to support global health surveillance. Nature Water (June 2025)
14. Jang, J., et al.: Prediction of antibiotic-resistance genes occurrence at a recreational beach with deep learning models. Water Res. **196**, 117001 (2021)
15. Karwowska, Z., Szczerbiak, P., Kosciolek, T.: Microbiome time series data reveal predictable patterns of change. bioRxiv (2023)
16. McDonald, D., et al.: The Biological Observation Matrix (BIOM) format or: how I learned to stop worrying and love the ome-ome. GigaScience, **1**(1), 2047–217X–1–7, (07 2012)
17. Schmiege, D., et al.: Analyzing community wastewater in sub-sewersheds for the small-scale detection of SARS-COV-2 variants in a german metropolitan area. Sci. Total Environ. **898**, 165458 (2023)

18. Klindworth, A., et al.: Evaluation of general 16S ribosomal RNA gene PCR primers for classical and next-generation sequencing-based diversity studies. Nucleic Acids Res. **41**(1), e1 (2012)
19. Dörr, A., et al.: RiboSnake – a user-friendly, robust, reproducible, multipurpose and documentation-extensive pipeline for 16S rRNA gene microbiome analysis. Gigabyte (2024)
20. Mölder, F., et al.: Sustainable data analysis with Snakemake [version 1; peer review: 1 approved, 1 approved with reservations]. F1000Research (2021)
21. Bolyen, E., et al.: Reproducible, interactive, scalable and extensible microbiome data science using qiime 2. Nature Biotechnol. **37**(8), 852–857 (Aug 2019)
22. Peleg, O., Borenstein, E.: Interpolation of microbiome composition in longitudinal data sets. mBio, 15, 9, (2024)

Causal Modeling and Data Reasoning

An Automatic Alignment Strategy for Medical Ontologies: the MedPix 2.0 Case Study

Luigi Colucci Cante[1], Mariangela Graziano[1], Irene Siragusa[2(✉)], Beniamino Di Martino[1], and Roberto Pirrone[2]

[1] Department of Engineering, University of Campania L. Vanvitelli, Aversa, Italy
{luigi.coluccicante,mariangela.graziano,beniamino.dimartino}@unicampania.it
[2] Department of Engineering, University of Palermo, Palermo, Italy
{irene.siragusa02,roberto.pirrone}@unipa.it

Abstract. In this paper, we present an automatic alignment strategy for the medical domain. Standard medical thesauri as the 11th Revision of the International Classification of Diseases (ICD-11) and a vocabulary of radiological terms (RadLex) are aligned with a multimodal medical data set (MedPix 2.0). The alignment process was conducted over their ontological representation and using Natural Language Processing techniques and Large Language Models to annotate both corpora. The obtained automatic pipeline ensures the terminology alignment between the terms in MedPix 2.0 and the standard terminology in ICD-11 and RadLex. Data and developed pipeline are available on https://github.com/CHILab1/MedOntoAlignment.

Keywords: Ontologies Alignment · Medical Ontologies · Large Language Models

1 Introduction

In recent years, the increasing availability of heterogeneous medical data has posed new challenges in terms of semantic integration and interoperability between clinical systems. In this context, the use of ontologies has established itself as an essential tool to represent medical knowledge in a structured and shared way. However, the coexistence of different standard terminology and the high complexity of multimodal data still make full semantic harmonization difficult.

In this paper, we propose an automatic alignment strategy for medical ontologies, in which **MedPix 2.0** [11], a multimodal data set of real clinical cases, was standardized according two medical thesauri, namely the **International Classification of Diseases 11th Revision (ICD-11)** [7] developed by the World Health Organization (WHO) and **RadLex**, a unified vocabulary to describe

L. Colucci Cante, M. Graziano, I. Siragusa—Equal contribution.

P. Bruno et al. (Eds.): HC_AIxIA_HYDRA 2025, CCIS 2830, pp. 257–269, 2026.
https://doi.org/10.1007/978-3-032-16708-8_21

radiological concepts [17]. ICD-11 and RadLex were selected as they are a well established and recognized medical source and are widely used in the hospital context by physicians. In addition, they provide a unique and standard form for concepts collected in the real clinical reports as in MedPix 2.0. To ensure proper alignment, an ontological representation of both MedPix 2.0 and ICD-11 has been built, while an existing ontological version of RadLex[1] was used. The proposed automatic alignment strategy involves the use of Natural Language Processing (NLP) techniques where Large Language Models (LLMs) are used as classifiers and evaluators of predicted annotations between MedPix 2.0 and both ICD-11, for body parts, disease, and sex information and RadLex for radiological terms involving the plane and the modality of a medical scan. The main contributions of this work can be summarized as follow:

1. An ontological representation of MedPix 2.0;
2. An ontological representation of ICD-11;
3. A LLM-based strategy for automatic annotation and matching of MedPix 2.0 entities with ICD-11 and RadLex ones.

This work is organized as follows: Sect. 2 illustrates the relevant contribution in the literature of existing ontologies in medical domain and their limitations. In Sect. 3 MedPix 2.0 and ICD-11 are described, while the process of building the corresponding ontologies and the alignment strategy proposed are illustrated in Sect. 4. An example of a possible use case over the obtained ontology after the alignment phase, is reported and discussed in Sect. 5, while concluding remarks are drawn in Sect. 6 respectively.

2 Related Works

Among the existing medical ontologies, the **Human Disease Ontology (DOID)** [18] is one of the most relevant one. It was developed to provide a standardized semantic representation of human diseases, facilitating the integration, analysis, and sharing of biomedical data. DOID was initially developed to address the need for a purpose-built ontology that covers the full spectrum of disease concepts annotated within biomedical repositories within an ontological framework that is extensible to meet community needs. The ontology uses *OWL (Ontology Web Language)* for formal representation and is structured according to the principles of the **Open Biomedical Ontologies (OBO) Foundry**[2]. Each disease is identified by a unique identifier and is annotated with synonyms, textual definitions, and possible cross-references to external resources. More in detail, DOID links to the main ontologies and classification systems used in biomedicine, so as to ensure a more complete and interoperable representation of diseases, integrating clinical, anatomical, genetic, and functional data. Examples are **UBERON** [14], an ontology describing anatomical structures, and **MIM**

[1] https://bioportal.bioontology.org/ontologies/RADLEX.
[2] https://obofoundry.org/.

(Online Mendelian Inheritance in Man) [1] and **Orphanet** [15], which collect information on hereditary and rare diseases.

In the clinical field, **Systematized Nomenclature of Medicine - Clinical Terms (SNOMED CT)** [5] and **Medical Subject Headings (MeSH)** [2] are worth mentioning. SNOMED CT is one of the most comprehensive and structured terminology systems for describing clinical data in a precise and uniform manner. It is designed to be used directly in electronic medical records, hospital software, health records and in all those contexts where a terminology standardization is required. Unlike other classifications, SNOMED CT is a complete clinical ontology: it represents concepts, relationships, and synonyms for each entry. MeSH, on the other hand, is the indexing system used by the *National Library of Medicine (NLM).* A particularly ambitious project is **MONDO** [23], an ontology that aims to unify all previously described sources, including DOID, Orphanet and other vocabularies, into a coherent and comprehensive structure. MONDO represents a decisive step towards semantic integration of disease knowledge, reducing ambiguities, and facilitating interoperability between different databases.
RadLex [17], on the other hand, is an ontology dedicated to radiology, developed by the Radiological Society of North America (RSNA) to standardize radiology vocabulary (such as examinations, techniques, structures, pathologies, etc.) and reduce ambiguity in reports and clinical data. Among the various standards and ontologies analyzed, we chose to adopt ICD-11 (Sect. 3.2) from WHO as the main reference for modeling diseases and body parts. Several factors motivate this choice: ICD-11 is currently the official international standard for the classification of diseases and health problems, developed to support systematic collection, analysis, and comparison of health data worldwide. Compared to previous versions, ICD-11 is designed to be natively digital and semantically richer, with an ontological structure that allows for a more precise and flexible representation of clinical concepts. In addition, ICD-11 incorporates both disease descriptions and anatomical topography, making it particularly suitable for use in the semantic modeling of medical knowledge. Therefore, adoption of ICD-11 allows us to ensure a high degree of interoperability with existing healthcare systems and, also, with the aforementioned international standardization initiatives. In addition, it is a widely used standard in the clinical context as a standardization source in the context of medical software, electronic health records, and decision support tools.

On this basis, we decide to use both ICD-11 and RadLex as standard and recognized medical sources to provide and alignment pipeline for MedPix 2.0 data set toward the two standards. ICD-11 is i) an international standard, ii) corresponds to the medical language of clinical cases, and is compatible with other standard medical resources; iii) it allows robust classification for searching, filtering, and navigating cases. In contrast, RadLex encodes the radiological terminology needed to standardize MedPix 2.0.

3 Data Set

3.1 MedPix 2.0

MedPix 2.0 [19] is a multimodal medical data set, derived from MedPix® [11], managed by the National Library of Medicine (NLM) of the National Institutes of Health (NIH). It collects real clinical cases annotated by doctors, which are used in the context of Continuing Medical Education (CME) of physicians, nurses, and healthcare students. MedPix 2.0 is a re-arranged version of MedPix, and includes both medical scans and textual content of the clinical cases, arranged in JSON files.

MedPix 2.0 consists of 2,550 medical scans grouped into 671 clinical cases, for which textual scan-level (*descriptions*) and clinical case information (*case-topic*) are reported. The case section reports information on the clinical case, while the topic section covers general information about the found disease. Both sections have a *title* field, which outlines a single annotated principal disease. This inherent structure of the data set, made it suitable for ontology modeling, leveraging the derivable abstractions such as for patient, clinical case, and medical scan.

MedPix 2.0 lacks standardization: annotated fields such as *Location*, which identifies the body part shown in a given scan, or *Disease*, which is reported in both *Case Title* and *Topic Title* fields, are not compliant with standard terminology, despite having been annotated by domain experts (doctors). This missing common terminology results in the collection of clinical cases labeled differently but referring to the same disease, e.g. `pancreatic ductal adenocarcinoma`, `pancreatic adenocarcinoma`, or its misspelled version `pancreatic adenocarinoma` appears different, but they commonly refer to the same disease `adenocarcinoma of pancreas`.

3.2 ICD-11

ICD-11 is the 11th revision of the International Classification of Diseases, which is an open-access resource developed by WHO. It can be seen as a taxonomy that collects diseases, disorders, and health conditions in a standard and structured manner, recognized and used by doctors and medical experts, representing a well-established standard in the medical domain.

ICD-11 contains over 55,000 diagnostic codes, organized into 28 chapters. Each chapter includes numerous categories and subcategories that allow a precise coding of clinical information. Each entry in the ICD-11 includes definitions eventually enriched with examples and cross-references with other chapters.

The first 26 chapters represent body systems, clinical conditions, or thematic areas such as mental disorders, nervous system diseases, etc. The other two chapters are transversal and complementary: Chap. 27 includes factors that influence the state of health or contact with health services, while Chap. 28 collects the *extension codes*, complementary external codes that enrich the information provided in previous chapters, such as a broad overview of the human anatomy. Each chapter is structured in a hierarchical manner, proceeding from broader categories to increasingly specific subcategories.

4 Methodology

The methodology used to build the ontological version of MedPix 2.0 and ICD-11 are reported in Subsect. 4.1 and Subsect. 4.2, while the proposed alignment annotation pipeline is described in Subsect. 4.3.

4.1 MedPix 2.0 Ontology Definition

Data on medical cases, scans, and patients were extracted from MedPix 2.0 and used to automatically populate an ontological representation of MedPix, through the API provided by the OWLReady2[3] module. A view of the ontology produced using the Protegè tool [20] is shown in Fig. 1.

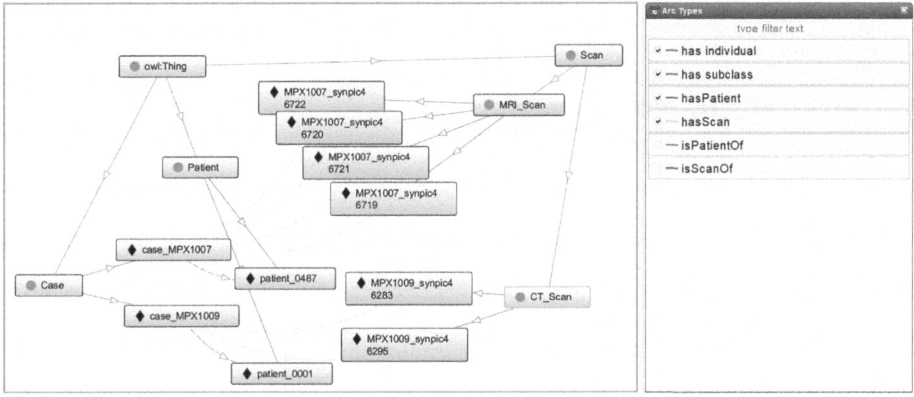

Fig. 1. MedPix 2.0 Ontology.

As can be seen from Fig. 1, all clinical cases in MedPix 2.0 were modeled as individuals of the class *Case*. Fields such as *title*, *exam*, *history*, *Findings* and *Case Diagnosis* and *Discussion* were modeled as textual data properties associated with the target cases. The scans were modeled as individuals of the classes *MRI_Scan* or *CT_Scan*, and associated with the respective clinical cases by the object property *hasScan* (edges in yellow). *caption* and *url* of the scans were modeled as data properties associated with the respective individuals. The *hasPatient* object property (edges in grey), associates the individuals of the class *Patient* with the clinical cases. Note that to properly address the purpose of this work, we modeled the data set and did not use automatic Knowledge Graph (KG) creation techniques. In addition, following this modeling, we ensure that each item has a suitable candidate over one of the standard ontology by design.

[3] https://owlready2.readthedocs.io/en/v0.47/.

4.2 ICD-11 Ontology Definition

Data from each chapter in ICD-11 for Mortality and Morbidity Statistics, in their last release from 2025-01, were downloaded via ICD-API access[4]. Obtained data have been then arranged according to the entity code from the foundational version of ICD-11. Furthermore, additional information such as description, included (synonyms) or excluded diseases, and the disease code used in clinical domains, were considered. The hierarchical structure of ICD-11 and the *classKind* field, which define if a given entity refers to a chapter, a block or a category, were also included. More specifically, only entities marked as categories have the clinical code and have been considered the leaf node of the taxonomy depicted in ICD-11. Figure 2 provides more details about the ontological modeling of ICD-11 obtained following its inherent structure.

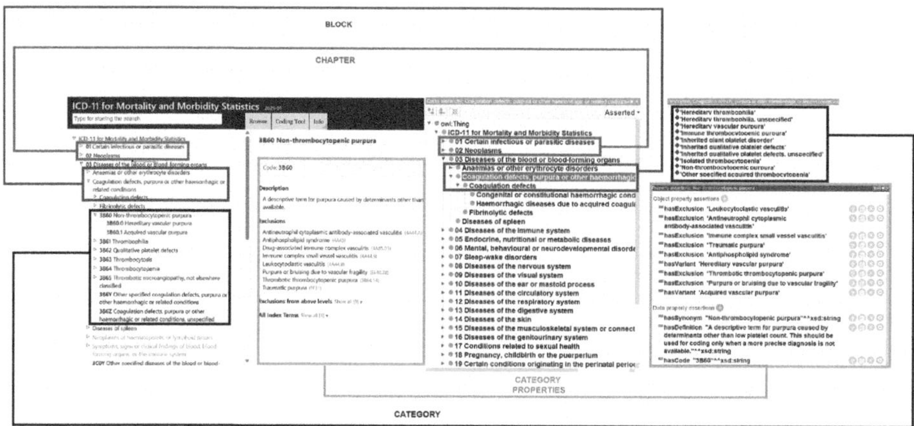

Fig. 2. ICD-11 Semantic Representation.

As can be seen in Fig. 2, all chapters and blocks of ICD-11 have been semantically represented as classes in the ontology: the blocks model the taxonomy of the various chapters, and individuals are associated with each of them, which correspond to the categories of ICD-11. Each individual is associated through data properties with the clinical code, a definition, and one or more synonyms. Through the object property *hasExclusion*, each individual, representing a disease, can be linked to other individuals to model explicit exclusion conditions between diseases. Furthermore, in ICD-11 each category can be further specialized into other subcategories, leading to a very complex taxonomic structure: these specializations have been modeled through the object property *hasVariant*.

[4] https://icd.who.int/icdapi.

4.3 Automatic Alignment Strategy

To properly define an alignment strategy, a connection between the built MedPix and ICD-11 Ontologies is needed. In particular, leaf entities in ICD-11 Ontology can be associated with *Location*, *Sex* and *Disease* fields in MedPix. Similarly to the alignment with MedPix and the Radlex ontology, the fields *Modality* and *Plane* are involved.

Traditional ontology alignment strategies leverage lexical information and ontologies structures [16,22]. In this study case, MedPix 2.0 is an ontological representation of a clinical corpus and terms in target fields lacks of standardization and these strategies cannot properly used when dealing with the peculiarities which are characteristic of the medical domain. For these reasons, an *ad hoc* alignment strategy based on LLMs in needed, coupled with simply exact-match strategies among target terms.

The proposed annotation and alignment strategy (Fig. 3) has the scope to provide to MedPix 2.0, a terminology compliant with ICD-11 and RadLex, leveraging NLP techniques and the use of LLMs for classification and evaluation purposes in the annotation process. Below, the alignment between MedPix and ICD-11 is reported, and alignment with RadLex follows the same principles.

As a first step, all the occurrences in MedPix 2.0 which found an exact correspondence in the ICD-11 entities, were directly associated, via an exact-match alignment. More in detail, exact matches were searched among the MedPix 2.0 fields and in the ICD-11 entity title or synonyms. For *Sex* field, all values found their exact match, excluding the case of missing values (3%), that have been set as to *Biological sex not specified* as in ICD-11 standard. On the contrary, *Disease* and *Location*, results much more challenging than for the number of matches found and their possible values, namely 25% and 12% exact matches have been found. This first step assured a preliminary correspondence for the target fields, but the simple usage of traditional alignment strategies is far from perfect, given the low obtained results in this phase.

To overcome this issue, the annotation pipeline was extended with an LLM-based alignment strategy. Based on the information recovered from ICD-11, a document was created for each entity following the template in Fig. 3. If additional information from ICD-11, such as entity definition or its synonyms, is available, it is included to the document. From the built documents, the corresponding embeddings are calculated via an LLM tailored for embedding extraction and retrieval. In particular, NV-Embed-v2 [8,12] was used as it was the most promising open-source model for retrieve capabilities in the medical domain as for the MTEB Leaderboard [13] in March 2025. The so-obtained embeddings are then stored in a FAISS Vector Database (VDB) [3]. Two different VDBs were built: one that collects all the diseases in ICD-11 (from Chap. 1 to Chap. 26) and one with the only section that collects the annotated body parts (subsection in Chap. 28). The created VDBs are queried with two *ad hoc* queries created, one for the disease and one for the body parts (Fig. 3). Queries were designed to provide as much information as possible to the LLM for an effective and coherent retrieve. The obtained output consists of a list of the entities in the VDB,

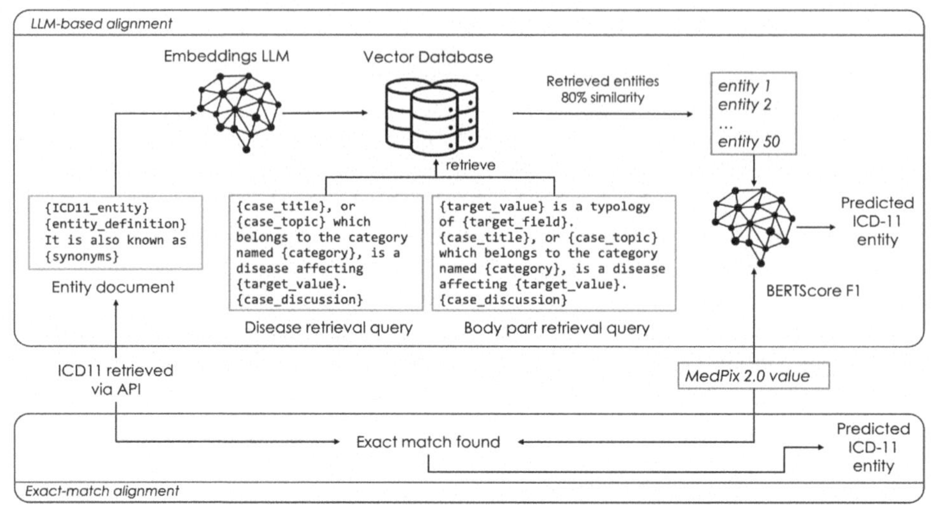

Fig. 3. Overview of the proposed alignment strategy for ICD-11 automatic annotation.

and only retrieved elements with a similarity score no less than the 80%[5] of the highest similarity score found, are considered for the subsequent phase.

The ICD-11 candidates obtained are then compared with the corresponding MedPix 2.0 labels for *Disease* and *Body part*. BERT F1 score metric [24] was selected for comparison and the ICD-11 entity achieving the highest score is selected as the annotated MedPix 2.0 values in ICD-11. BERTScore values have been calculated with BioSyn [21], a fine-tuned version of BioBERT [9] trained on biomedical data and disease synonym corpora [4].

Analogously, a simplified retrieval query[6] has been used for RadLex alignment over *Modality* and *Plane* fields. In this case, no exact matches have been found for the *Modality* field, while reaching the 96% for *Plane*. The proposed automatic alignment, involving the usage of LLMs and state of the art techniques in NLP field, allows a proper annotation of MedPix terms to the standard terminology according to the trustworthy, recognized, and standard medical resources (ICD-11 and RadLex), thus permitting an appropriate alignment of the three ontologies as in Fig. 4. Although obtained alignments result promising via a preliminary evaluation, a subsequent evaluation phase is required by domain experts.

After importing all three ontologies, alignment object property assertions are applied to link individuals from MedPix 2.0 with individuals defined in ICD-11 and RadLex. In particular, with the object property *hasDisease*, diseases in MedPix 2.0 are connected to the corresponding terms in ICD-11, and more complex queries, spreading both ontologies can be performed.

[5] this threshold was empirically found.

[6] *{target_value} is a typology of {target_field}.*

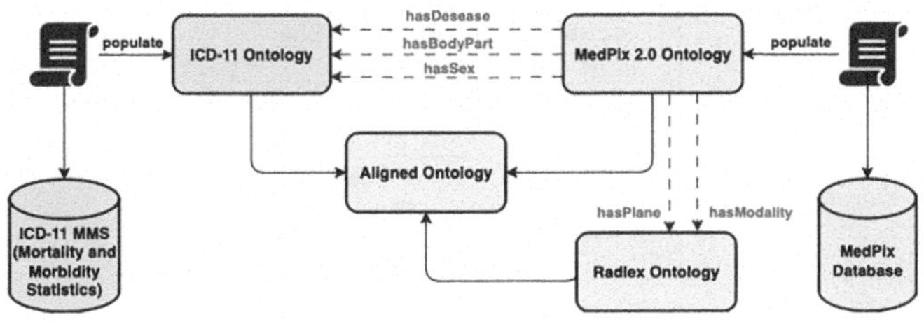

Fig. 4. Overview of the obtained ontology after the alignment annotations.

5 Application

The proposed semantic modeling of MedPix 2.0 and subsequent alignment, provides a number of advantages, one of which is the ability to use semantic technologies, such as **SPARQL** and **SWRL**, to query and infer via OWL ontologies [6]. With the SWRL rule (Fig. 7a) reported in Appendix, it is possible to leverage knowledge of Medpix 2.0's past history to associate one or more *disease categories* (classes of disease) with each *location category* (macro-body part) involving the knowledge from the two standard ontologies.

To do this, two steps are performed:

- SPARQL query (Fig. 6a) is used to retrieve the *location category* in ICD-11 associated with the location reported in the MedPix 2.0 scan.
- SPARQL query (Fig. 6b) is used to retrieve the *disease category* in ICD-11 associated with the disease diagnosed by doctors in aligned Medpix 2.0.

According to SWRL rule 7a : 1) if a clinical case *c* has at least one scan showing the body part *bp* involved; 2) then the Location Categories *lc* of ICD-11, to which *bp* belongs is found; 3) if the clinical case *c* has a diagnosed disease *d*; 4) then the disease category *dc* of ICD-11 to which *d* belongs is retrieved, and 5) an association *hasPossibleDisease* exists linking *lc* and *dc*.

The associations inferred with the SWRL Rule 7a are also used by SWRL Rule 7b to identify, given a new clinical case represented semantically, a list of possible diseases that can be diagnosed in the patient known the body part involved in the scans performed.

Each time a new clinical case is provided, the alignment described in Sect. 4 will be performed. Then, using the SWRL Rule 7b, the system automatically predicts a set of diagnosable diseases for the clinical case based on the *location category* identified from the medical scan in the clinical case, and on the object properties inferred by the SWRL Rule 7a that connect each location category to multiple disease categories.

To clarify the inference obtained with rule 7b, an example is illustrated in Fig. 5.

The diagram illustrates a clinical reasoning process supported by a semantic infrastructure based on OWL and SWRL rules.

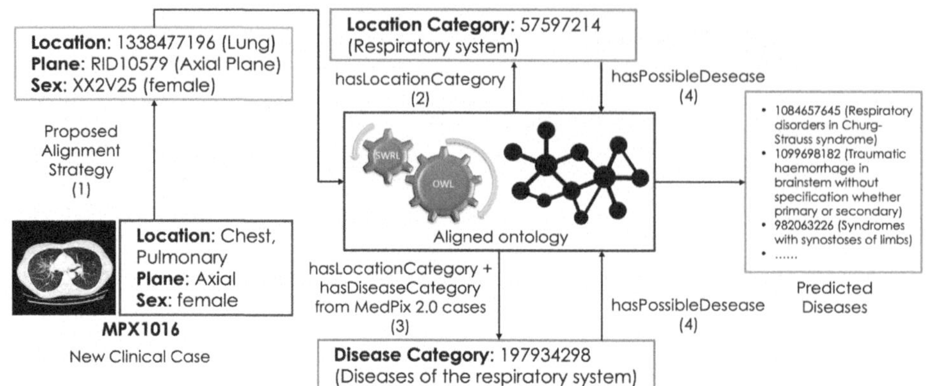

Fig. 5. Clinical reasoning process.

- A new clinical case (bottom left), described in simple terms as in the anatomical location (*thorax*, *lung*), the plane of the scan (*axial plane*) and the gender (*female*) is compared with the information already present in the knowledge base and aligned with a structured ontological representation that includes unique codes and semantic categories.
- The SWRL Rule 7a connects the specific location category (*Lung*) to its broader anatomical category, *Respiratory System*.
- Possible associated disease for each anatomical category are retrieved from all the cases contained in MedPix 2.0, thus simulating prior knowledge.
- The results obtained are combined in the SWRL Rule 7b, which enables the system to automatically deduce a list of diseases that might be relevant to the scenario.

This architecture illustrates how the combination of clinical ontologies, semantic rules, and structured medical databases can promote interoperability between different sources and facilitate more intelligent and customized clinical treatment.

The result of the proposed application can be seen as a first attempt towards an Ontology-Augmented Generation (OAG) approach. Following the proposed strategy, a list of candidate diseases (ICD-11 individuals) can be obtained. Then it can serve as an input to an LLM to generate a verbose diagnostic suggestion. The obtained answer will depend on the retrieved diseases following a semantic-based strategy, thus reducing the level of "hallucination" of the LLM at generation time, due to the first filtering. Furthermore, all candidate diseases are standardized according to ICD-11, each associated with a unique code recognized by numerous medical systems.

6 Conclusions and Future Works

In this work, we presented an ontology alignment strategy between two relevant ontological sources in the medical field, namely ICD-11, RadLex, and the multimodal data set MedPix 2.0. We proposed an automatic pipeline involving NLP techniques and usage of LLMs to obtain the desired annotation for a proper ontology alignment. The aim of this integration is to provide an automatic structured and semantic representation of clinical knowledge, useful both for educational purposes and for applications that support diagnosis, leveraging standard, recognized and trustworthy resources in the medical domain. We plan to use the results of this ontology alignment a basis for an Ontology-Augmented Generation (OAG) system, with the aim of developing a hybrid reasoning system, which combines the robustness of ontologies with the flexibility of LLMs and the Retrieval-Augmented Generation (RAG) approach [10]. On doing this, we aim to reduce risks of hallucinations in LLMs, in generating implausible diagnoses or not-entailed output. In addition, the usage of ontologies in the retrieval phase in a RAG approach can provide a more semantic meaningful and robust data sources for subsequent generation phase. We can therefore consider this medical ontology alignment strategy as a concrete step towards more transparent, interpretable, and clinically robust decision support systems, paving the way for new solutions at the intersection of artificial intelligence, ontologies, and medicine. Although a promising empirical and manual evaluation of the proposed terms alignments, the robustness of the presented alignment strategy can be enhanced by a more extensive evaluation leveraging both additional medical data sets and involving the validation of domain experts such as doctors and physicians. Overall, the proposed strategy attempts to obtain promising alignment results via exact matching strategies and the usage of semantic-oriented metrics as BERTScore.

Acknowledgments. This work is supported by the cup project B73C22000810001, project code ECS_00000022 "SAMOTHRACE" (Sicilian MicronanoTech Research And Innovation Center), and the cup project J73C24000070007, "CAESAR" (Cognitive evolution in Ai: Explainable and Self-Aware Robots through multimodal data processing). Annotation pipeline was built on the Leonardo supercomputer with the support of CINECA-Italian Super Computing Resource Allocation, class C project IscrC_DOC-VLM (HP10C64J82) and IscrC_DOCVLM2 (HP10C97VNN).

Disclosure of Interests. The authors have no competing interests to declare that are relevant to the content of this article.

A SPARQL Query and SWRL Rules

a. SPARQL Query to retrieve the "Location Category"

```
PREFIX rdf: <http://www.w3.org/22-rdf-syntax-ns#>
PREFIX owl: <http://www.w3.org/owl#>
PREFIX rdfs: <http://www.w3.org/rdf-schema#>
PREFIX xsd: <http://www.w3.org/XMLSchema#>
PREFIX medpix: <http://www.semanticweb.org/MedPix#>
PREFIX ontomedpix: <http://example.org/ontoMedPix.
    owl#>
PREFIX icd: <http://www.semanticweb.org/icd11#>

SELECT DISTINCT ?LocationCategory
WHERE {
  ?LocationCategory rdfs:subClassOf ?mid1.
  ?mid1 rdfs:subClassOf ?mid2.
  ?mid2 rdfs:subClassOf icd:1154280071.
  icd:NameLocation a ?class.
  ?class rdfs:subClassOf+ ?LocationCategory.
}
```

b. SPARQL Query to retrieve the "Disease Category"

```
PREFIX rdf: <http://www.w3.org/22-rdf-syntax-ns#>
PREFIX owl: <http://www.w3.org/owl#>
PREFIX rdfs: <http://www.w3.org/rdf-schema#>
PREFIX xsd: <http://www.w3.org/XMLSchema#>
PREFIX medpix: <http://www.semanticweb.org/MedPix#>
PREFIX ontomedpix: <http://example.org/ontoMedPix.
    owl#>
PREFIX icd: <http://www.semanticweb.org/icd11#>

SELECT DISTINCT ?DiseaseCategory
WHERE {
  icd:NameDisease a ?DiseaseCategory .
}
```

Fig. 6. SPARQL queries

a. SWRL Rule to infer all possible associations between Location Category and Disease Category

```
medpix:Case(?c),
medpix:Scan(?s),
medpix:hasScan(?c,?s),
ontomedpix:hasBodyPart(?s,?bp),
ontomedpix:hasLocationCategory(?bp,?lc),
ontomedpix:hasDisease(?c,?d),
ontomedpix:hasDiseaseCategory(?d,?dc) ->
hasPossibleDisease(?lc, ?dc)
```

b. SWRL Rule to infer a candidate disease pool given a body part

```
medpix:Case(?c),
medpix:Scan(?s),
medpix:hasScan(?c,?s),
ontomedpix:hasBodyPart(?s,?bp),
ontomedpix:hasLocationCategory(?bp,?lc),
rdfs:subPropertyOf(?p, ontomedpix:
    hasPossibleDisease),
rdfs:domain(?p,?lc),
rdfs:range(?p,?d),
ontomedpix:p(?lc,?dc),
rdf:type(?dc,?d) ->
ontomedpix:hasPossibleDisease(?c,?d)
```

Fig. 7. SWRL rules

References

1. Amberger, J.S., Hamosh, A.: Searching online mendelian inheritance in man (omim): a knowledgebase of human genes and genetic phenotypes. Curr. Protoc. Bioinform. **58**(1), 1–2 (2017)
2. Baumann, N.: How to use the medical subject headings (mesh). Int. J. Clin. Pract. **70**(2), 171–174 (2016). https://doi.org/10.1111/ijcp.12767
3. Douze, M., et al.: The Faiss library. Preprint arXiv:2401.08281 (2024)
4. Doğan, R.I., Leaman, R., Lu, Z.: NCBI disease corpus: a resource for disease name recognition and concept normalization. J. Biomed. Inform. 1–10 (2014)
5. El-Sappagh, S., Franda, F., Ali, F., Kwak, K.S.: Snomed CT standard ontology based on the ontology for general medical science. BMC Med. Inform. Decis. Mak. **18**, 1–19 (2018)

6. Essani, F.H., Rajput, Q.: Ontology based system for expert searching in academia using swrl and sparql. KIET J. Comput. Inform. Sci. **2**(1), 10–10 (2019)
7. ICD-11. https://icd.who.int/en/
8. Lee, C., et al.: Nv-embed: Improved techniques for training LLMs as generalist embedding models. Preprint arXiv:2405.17428 (2024)
9. Lee, J., et al.: BioBERT: a pre-trained biomedical language representation model for biomedical text mining. Bioinformatics 1234–1240 (2019)
10. Lewis, P., et al.: Retrieval-augmented generation for knowledge-intensive NLP Tasks. In: Advances in Neural Information Processing Systems (2020)
11. MedPix. https://medpix.nlm.nih.gov/home
12. Moreira, G.d.S.P., Osmulski, R., Xu, M., Ak, R., Schifferer, B., Oldridge, E.: Nv-retriever: Improving text embedding models with effective hard-negative mining. Preprint arXiv:2407.15831 (2024)
13. Muennighoff, N., Tazi, N., Magne, L., Reimers, N.: MTEB: Massive text embedding benchmark. In: Proceedings of the 17th Conference of the European Chapter of the Association for Computational Linguistics, pp. 2014–2037 (2023)
14. Mungall, C.J., Torniai, C., Gkoutos, G.V., Lewis, S.E., Haendel, M.A.: Uberon, an integrative multi-species anatomy ontology. Genome Biol. **13**(1), R5–R5 (2012)
15. Rath, A., Olry, A., Dhombres, F., Brandt, M.M., Urbero, B., Ayme, S.: Representation of rare diseases in health information systems: the orphanet approach to serve a wide range of end users. Hum. Mutat. **33**(5), 803–808 (2012). https://doi.org/10.1002/humu.22078
16. Romero, M.M., Naya, J.M.V., Loureiro, J.P., Ezquerra, N.: Ontology alignment techniques. In: Encyclopedia of Artificial Intelligence, pp. 1290–1295. IGI Global Scientific Publishing (2009)
17. Rubin, D.L.: Creating and curating a terminology for radiology: Ontology modeling and analysis. J. Digital Imaging **21**(4), 355–362 (2008). https://doi.org/10.1007/s10278-007-9073-0
18. Schriml, L.M., et al.: The human disease ontology 2022 update. Nucleic Acids Res. **50**(D1), D1255–D1261 (2022)
19. Siragusa, I., Contino, S., Ciura, M.L., Alicata, R., Pirrone, R.: Medpix 2.0: a comprehensive multimodal biomedical data set for advanced ai applications with retrieval augmented generation and knowledge graphs. Data Sci. Eng. 1–17 (2025)
20. Sivakumar, R., Arivoli, P.: Ontology visualization protégé tools-a review. Int. J. Adv. Inform. Technol. (IJAIT) Vol 1 (2011)
21. Sung, M., Jeon, H., Lee, J., Kang, J.: Biomedical entity representations with synonym marginalization. In: Proceedings of the 58th Annual Meeting of the Association for Computational Linguistics, pp. 3641–3650 (2020)
22. Taye, M.M., Alalwan, N.: Ontology alignment technique for improving semantic integration. SEMAPRO **2010**, 22 (2010)
23. Vasilevsky, N., et al.: Mondo disease ontology: harmonizing disease concepts across the world. In: CEUR Workshop Proceedings, CEUR-WS, vol. 2807 (2020)
24. Zhang, T., Kishore, V., Wu, F., Weinberger, K.Q., Artzi, Y.: BERTScore: evaluating Text Generation with BERT. Preprint arXiv:1904.09675 (2020)

Learning a Causal Model for Intracranial Pressure in Patients with Traumatic Brain Injury

Alessio Zanga[1,2(✉)], Francesca Graziano[2,3], Giuseppe Citerio[2,3], Paola Rebora[2], Stefania Galiberti[2], Shubhayu Bhattacharyay[4], David K. Menon[5], Ewout W. Steyerberg[6], and Fabio Stella[1]

[1] Models and Algorithms for Data and Text Mining Laboratory (MADLab), Department of Informatics, Systems and Communication (DISCo), University of Milano-Bicocca, Milan, Italy

[2] School of Medicine and Surgery, University of Milano-Bicocca, Monza, Italy
alessio.zanga@unimib.it

[3] Fondazione IRCCS San Gerardo dei Tintori, Monza, Italy

[4] Harvard Medical School, Boston, MA, USA

[5] University of Cambridge, Cambridge, UK

[6] University Medical Center Utrecht, Utrecht, The Netherlands

Abstract. Traumatic brain injury is a sequence of pathophysiological events that originates from an acute biomechanical insult. One of the major challenges physician face routinely in traumatic brain injury patients is the management of intracranial pressure. Elevated intracranial pressure may lead to herniation, causing injury through compression of brain tissue. Studying the underlying mechanism of intracranial pressure is crucial to develop personalized therapy planning. In this paper, we build a causal model from clinical experts knowledge and partially-observed event-based data to represent the trajectory of patients over time. We show how to derive insights on the effectiveness of multiple treatments allocations from the model parameters and evaluate the model against treatment policies reported in clinical guidelines.

Keywords: Traumatic brain injury · Intracranial pressure · Intensive care unit · Continuous time Bayesian network

1 Introduction

1.1 Traumatic Brain Injury and Intracranial Pressure Management

Traumatic brain injury (TBI) [1,2] is a sequence of pathophysiological events that begin with an acute biomechanical insult and evolve into prolonged secondary cascades. The heterogeneity of the occurring conditions, such as impact location, impact force (e.g. variations in acceleration), and injury type (e.g. closed versus penetrating), leads to a definition of TBI that is more akin to a spectrum of conditions, rather than a single condition.

P. Bruno et al. (Eds.): HC_AIxIA_HYDRA 2025, CCIS 2830, pp. 270–282, 2026.
https://doi.org/10.1007/978-3-032-16708-8_22

Patients that experience severe TBI are admitted to intensive care units (ICUs), where multiple factors are monitored in time. Intracranial pressure (ICP) [3] monitoring allows the identification of several life-threatening brain insults, such as severe traumatic brain injury, subarachnoid hemorrhage, and malignant stroke. Figure 1 depicts the ICP monitoring setup and different herniation subtypes, associated with elevated ICP, causing injury through compression of brain tissue or cerebral vessels.

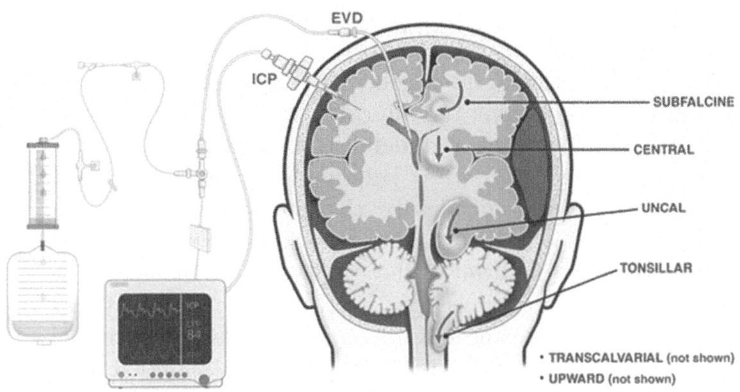

Fig. 1. Elevated intracranial pressure is associated with herniation of brain tissue is most cases. Different herniation subtypes are reported in red. (Color figure online)

However, the complex pathophysiological mechanism that leads to an increase in ICP in TBI patients is still under study. Existing guidelines [4] for TBI treatment advocate for an incremental approach to ICP management, where multiple treatments are cautiously administered with increasing intensity, until the desired ICP is reached. An aggregated level of intensity of ICP treatment management can be measured on the Therapy Intensity Level (TIL) [5] scale.

1.2 The CENTER-TBI Research Project

Traumatic brain injury is a wide spread public health problem, but patients characteristics and their care pathways in Europe are under-explored [6]. The *Collaborative European NeuroTrauma Effectiveness Research* (CENTER-TBI) [7] project is a European study which is specificially designed to better describe TBI as a disease in the European context and identify the most effective clinical decisions for managing it.

The CENTER-TBI project includes two cohorts: a multicentre clinical-based, longitudinal, observational cohort study, the *core study*, consisting in 4509 patients from 18 European countries between 2014 and 2017, with highly granular data ranging from clinical and outcome data; a population-based *registry*, consisting in 22782 patients with different information derived from basic administrative data. Patients were diagnosed TBI in less than 24 h after injury and assigned to three different strata: emergency room (ER), hospital ward admission and intensive care unit (ICU).

The outcome assessments were done at 6 months after injury, where the primary outcome measures global function using the Glasgow Outcome Scale-Extended (GOSE) [8]. Incomplete recovery at 6 months (GOSE < 8) was found in 1547 (84%) patients in the ICU stratum, calling for more research in personalized medicine and the identification of best practices to improve outcomes.

1.3 Leveraging Causal Artificial Intelligence

In the last few years, artificial intelligence (AI) applications to medicine showed promising results for explaining the interplay of multiple risk factors [9], acquiring insights on existing treatment guidelines [10], and more [11]. More recently, a novel branch of AI, named *Causal AI* [12], has been developed to take advantage of cause-effect relationships encoded by the data generating mechanism. When the mechanism is unknown, *causal discovery* [13] can be used to learn a *causal graph*, a graphical representation of these causal relationships.

Probabilistic graphical models (PGMs) [14] are a prominent class of AI models that are able to leverage causal graphs to enable causal inference [15], decision making [16] and uncertainty quantification [17]. In this context, continuous-time Bayesian networks (CTBNs) [18] are PGMs that have been specifically designed to learn the behaviour of complex systems from event-based data, with applications in cardiology [19], immunology [20] and personalized medicine [21].

However, constructing a CTBN from ICU data on TBI patients is not a trivial task: sparse, high-dimensional and uncertain data can hinder the quality of the resulting model, requiring prior knowledge elicitation.

In this context, our contributions are:

- the development of a CTBN, acting as the first causal model to study ICP management in TBI patients from partially-observed event-based data and clinical experts knowledge,
- the acquisition of insights on the interaction between multiple treatments and ICP changes derived from the inspection of the learned quantities,
- the draw out of current theoretical limitations that must be addressed to allow a meaningful extension of the model and layout the validation steps.

The reminder of this paper is organized as follows: Sect. 2 lists the few existing related works, Sect. 3 introduces the methodology framework, Sect. 4 layouts the experimental setup, Sect. 5 reports the results, Sect. 6 discusses the obtained results, finally Sect. 7 draws the conclusions.

2 Related Work

Recent AI applications on ICP management in TBI patients included in the CENTER-TBI project focused on predicting the TIL on a daily basis. Authors in [22] studied the variability in care pathways between centres by modelling the patient-level predictors of changes in ICP management leveraging recurrent neural networks, mapping a token-embedded time series representation to a prediction of the five-category TIL score. This work constitutes the first approach to dynamic prediction of future TIL in ICP-monitored TBI patients relying on more than two thousands variables. The rationale is that a more standardized management of ICP would also be more predictable, making the factors that drive day-to-day changes in TIL measurable on an individual level.

However, this approach relies on a high-dimensional black-box model that is not designed to discover and explain cause-effect relationships, resulting in associational findings that suffers from confounding bias [15]. Moreover, these methods rely on time discretisation, which fails to capture event-based relationships, making their ability to handle irregular patterns limited. These are frequent conditions in clinical practice, where precise timing is essential for meaningful decision-making. Recent Causal AI applications to personalized treatment and risk prediction for event-based data leverage CTBNs to integrate causal information from experts clinicians, dynamically adjusting transition intensities based on covariate effects [21].

3 Preliminaries

3.1 Continuous-Time Markov Processes

Variables in time are represented by trajectories.

Definition 1 (Trajectory).
Let $\mathbf{X}$ *be a random vector, a trajectory* $\sigma : \mathbb{R}^+ \rightarrow \mathcal{D}(\mathbf{X})$ *is a right-continuous, piece-wise constant, function that assigns a value to* $\mathbf{X}^t$ *for each time* $t \in \mathbb{R}^+$ *(Fig. 2).*

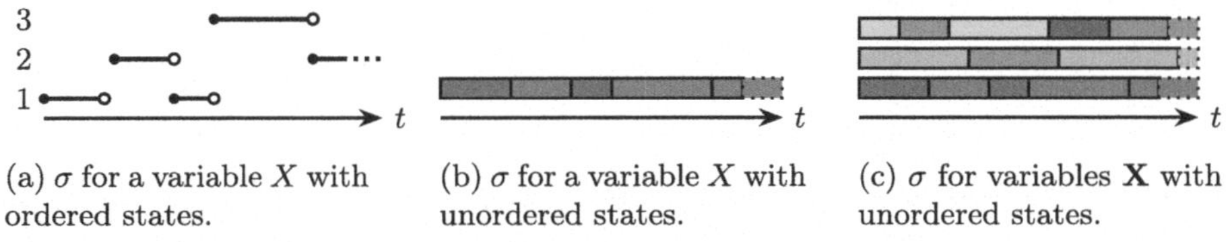

(a) σ for a variable X with ordered states. (b) σ for a variable X with unordered states. (c) σ for variables $\mathbf{X}$ with unordered states.

Fig. 2. Different trajectories with different variables $\mathbf{X}$.

To model the trajectories behaviour we can rely on a Markov process.

Definition 2 (Continuous-Time Markov Process).
A Continuous-Time Markov Process (CTMP) [23] is a stochastic process over $\mathbf{X}$ *defined by a tuple* $\langle P^0_{\mathbf{X}}, \mathbf{Q}_{\mathbf{X}} \rangle$*, where:*

- $P^0_{\mathbf{X}}$ *is an* initial distribution *that represents the probability distribution of the state of the process at time* $t = 0$*,*

- $\mathbf{Q}_\mathbf{X}$ *is an* intensity matrix *(IM) that describes the process at time* $t > 0$.

The IM $\mathbf{Q}_\mathbf{X}$ is a square matrix where:

- the *sojourn time* in state i follows an exponential distribution $\text{Exp}(q_i)$ with parameter $q_i = -q_{ii}$ and an *expected transition time* of $1/q_i$,
- the *probability of transitioning* from state i to state j follows a categorical distribution $\text{Cat}(\boldsymbol{\theta}_i)$ with parameters $\theta_{ij} = q_{ij}/q_i$ for $j \neq i$, zero otherwise.

Parameter Learning. Given a complete trajectory σ, we can estimate $\mathbf{Q}_\mathbf{X}$ from its sufficient statistics $\mathbf{N}_{ij}$ the number of transitions from state i to state j, and $\mathbf{T}_i$ the time spent in state i. Then we can specify a non-informative gamma prior Γ^0 with parameters α_{ij} and τ_{ij} to derive the posterior parameters:

$$\hat{q}_{ij} = \begin{cases} (\mathbf{N}_{ij} + \alpha_{ij}) \,/\, (\mathbf{T}_i + \tau_{ij}) & i \neq j \\ -\sum_{i \neq j} (\mathbf{N}_{ij} + \alpha_{ij}) \,/\, (\mathbf{T}_i + \tau_{ij}) & i = j \end{cases} \tag{1}$$

3.2 Continuous-Time Bayesian Networks

The size of $\mathbf{Q}_\mathbf{X}$ grows exponentially with the number of random variables in $\mathbf{X}$. To mitigate this issue, continuous-time Bayesian networks have been introduced.

Definition 3 (Continuous-Time Bayesian Network). *Let* $\mathbf{X}$ *be a random vector, a Continuous-Time Bayesian Network (CTBN) [18, 24] is stochastic process over* $\mathbf{X}$ *defined by a tuple* $\langle P^0_\mathbf{X}, \mathcal{G}, \mathbf{Q}_\mathbf{X} \rangle$, *where:*

- $P^0_\mathbf{X}$ *is an initial distribution,*
- $\mathcal{G}$ *is a directed graph* $(\mathbf{V}, \mathbf{E})$, *where each* $V_i \in \mathbf{V}$ *is mapped to a* $X_i \in \mathbf{X}$,
- $\mathbf{Q}_\mathbf{X}$ *is an IM factorized into multiple* conditional *intensity matrices (CIMs)* $\mathbf{Q}_{X_i|\boldsymbol{\Pi}_i}$ *according to the graph* $\mathcal{G}$:

$$\mathbf{Q}_\mathbf{X} = \sum_{X_i \in \mathbf{X}} \sum_{\boldsymbol{\Pi}_i \in \boldsymbol{\Pi}_i} \bigotimes_{X_j \in \mathbf{X}} \begin{cases} \mathbf{Q}_{X_i|\boldsymbol{\Pi}_i} & X_i = X_j \\ \boldsymbol{\Delta}_{X_j} & X_i \neq X_j \wedge X_j \in \boldsymbol{\Pi}_i \\ & X_i \neq X_j \wedge X_j \notin \boldsymbol{\Pi}_i \end{cases} \tag{2}$$

with $\otimes$ *the Kronecker product,* $\boldsymbol{\Pi}_i$ *the parents of* X_i *in* $\mathcal{G}$, $\boldsymbol{\Delta}_{X_j}$ *a squared matrix with one at* (j, j) *and zeros elsewhere, and* $\mathbf{I}$ *the identity matrix.*

Since $\mathcal{G}$ factorizes the state space according to Eq. (2), $\mathcal{G}$ is said to be a *structure* over $\mathbf{X}$. For this reason, CTBNs are also referred in the literature as *structured* (or *factorized*) CTMPs, which means that instead of modelling $\mathbf{Q}_\mathbf{X}$ we can use collection of CIMs as $\{\mathbf{Q}_{X_0|\boldsymbol{\Pi}_0}, \ldots, \mathbf{Q}_{X_{n-1}|\boldsymbol{\Pi}_{n-1}}\}$, reducing the asymptotic space complexity. The factorization of CIMs in CTBNs is analogous to the one of CPDs in BNs. See [25] on how to read a CIM.

Learning a CTBN means not only to estimate the parameters by computing the CIMs, but also to construct the structure that allows to factorize the state space, that is the space of all the possible combinations of states of the variables.

Parameter Learning. Estimating a CIM $\mathbf{Q}_{X_i|\mathbf{\Pi}_i}$ of a CTBN is essentially equivalent to estimating the IM $\mathbf{Q}$ of a CTMP: we can apply Eq. (1) to the *conditional* counts $\mathbf{N}_{ijk}$ and times $\mathbf{T}_{ij}$ along the conditioning axis.

So far the estimation of the sufficient statistics $\mathbf{N}_{ijk}$ and $\mathbf{T}_{ij}$ was performed from a *complete* trajectory σ, but it is unlikely to observe a variable continuously. See [25] on how to learn parameters from incomplete trajectories.

Structure Learning. While learning the parameters $\mathbf{Q}_{X_i|\mathbf{\Pi}_i}$ of a CTBN is a relatively simple task, learning its structure $\mathcal{G}$ is more complicated. In general, to estimate the graph $\mathcal{G}$ of a CTBN from a trajectory σ there are two approaches:

- the *score-based* [26] approach, which aims to find the graph that maximizes the penalized log-likelihood of the CTBN built on it,
- the *constraint-based* [27] approach, which starts from a complete graph and performs conditional independence testing iteratively, removing edges between independent variables, until no more edges can be removed.

4 Application to the CENTER-TBI Research Project

4.1 Data Selection

Patients Inclusion. Patients inclusion criteria were aligned to previous work on ICP monitoring in the CENTER-TBI project core study [22]:

- active ICP monitoring,
- age greater or equal than 16 years,
- admission to ICU and minimum ICU stay of at least 24 h,
- no withdrawal of life-sustaining therapies within minimum ICU stay.

Variables Selection. Table 1 reports the selected variables, along with a brief description. The selection was performed jointly with clinicians to collect the necessary information to study the impact of various treatments on ICP.

4.2 Data Preprocessing

Each patient is assigned a global unique patient identifier (GUPI), which is then filtered according to patients selection criteria. For each variable in Table 1 a query to the CENTER-TBI database is executed to retrieve the actual value of the variable and the associated datetime field, filtering by GUPI.

Value Encoding. Extracted values are checked against the CENTER-TBI data dictionary to ensure consistency, rejecting values that do not belong to the variables domain. Discretization is applied to the two continuous variables, `HVICP` and `TILMannitolDose`, according to intervals provided by clinicians. See [25] for the categorical levels of the selected variables.

Table 1. Variables selected from the CENTER-TBI database.

Variable	Description
`HVICP`	ICP measured twice hourly.
`HosComplEventHypocapnia`	Measures inadvertent hypocapnia, i.e. abnormally low CO2, defined as a PaCO2 $\leq$ 3.3 kPa.
`MarshallCTClassification`	A general CT grading scale, for outcome prediction.
`TILCSFDrainage`	Reflects if cerebrospinal fluid (CSF) drainage.
`TILFever`	Records whether there was treatment of fever $\geq$38°C or spontaneous temperature of 34.5 °C.
`TILHyperosmolarTherapy`	Records whether there was hyperosmolar therapy with mannitol up to 2 g/kg/24 h.
`TILHyperventilation`	Records whether there was mild hypocapnia for ICP control (PaCO2 4.6–5.3 kPa).
`TILMannitolDose`	Indicates the total dose of mannitol administered calculated over a 24-h period, if applicable.
`TILSedation`	Records whether there was sedation (low dose as required for mechanical ventilation).

Evidence Encoding. Once both values x_i and datetimes t_s are properly encoded, variables are concatenated together, sorted by datetime and grouped by GUPI. Each group represents the incomplete trajectory σ^- of a single patient. The conversion of σ^- to evidence $\mathbf{e}$ is a two step procedure:

1. Choosing the state x_i - In some cases, for a variable X_i at time t_s there are different states x_i reported in σ^-. This is probably due to some inconsistency in the data entry procedure. Since there is no evidence in favour of one state or the other, we encoded it as *uncertain evidence* [28], see [25].
2. Setting the end time t_e - The datetime t_s is the *start time* of the evidence, the point in time at which the value x_i of X_i was observed. It does not necessary coincide with the time at which X_i transitioned to x_i: this is generally unknown when the trajectory is incomplete. Several inference algorithms are designed to work with interval-like evidence, rather than point evidence, which means that an *end time* t_e must be provided. In this context we set $t_e = t_s + \epsilon$, with $\epsilon = 1$ minute. Note that the selected variables are observed hourly, or even less frequently.

The resulting $\mathbf{e}$ is a sequence of tuples (X_i, x_i, t_s, t_e) with the value x_i of X_i in the time interval $[t_s, t_e)$. Refer to [25] for prior knowledge encoding.

4.3 Experimental Layout

The core of the experimental section is described by Algorithm 1.

Algorithm 1 Pseudocode of the causal discovery procedure.

Input: An initial graph $\mathcal{G}^0$, the prior knowledge $\mathcal{K}$, the evidence $\mathbf{e}$, the maximum SEM iterations n, the maximum EM iterations m.
Output: A CTBN $\mathcal{M}$.

```
 1: procedure SEM-IS-CTPC(G^0, K, e, n, m)
 2:     i ← 0                                  ▷ Initialize SEM counter.
 3:     M ← RAWE(G^0, e)                       ▷ Initialize M arbitrarily.
 4:     repeat
 5:         j ← 0                              ▷ Initialize EM counter.
 6:         M' ← M
 7:         repeat
 8:             M'' ← M'
 9:             D+ ← IS(M', e)                 ▷ Sample completed trajectories.
10:             M' ← BE(G', D+)                ▷ Update current EM solution.
11:             j ← j + 1
12:         until ||M'' − M'|| < ε ∨ j ≥ m
13:         M ← CTPC(G^0, D+, K)               ▷ Update current SEM solution.
14:         i ← i + 1
15:     until ||M' − M|| < ε ∨ i ≥ n
16:     return M                               ▷ Return current SEM solution.
```

Here are the key lines:

- Line 3 - The initial model was fitted with a *raw estimator* (RAWE) that naïvely fills the incomplete trajectory by backward propagating the observed values. The rationale is that many of the variables in Table 1 are computed as hourly or daily aggregates, therefore an initial rough approximation could be done by merging consecutive evidence in the same state.
- Line 7–12 - The inner Expectation-Maximization (EM) [29] cycle estimates the expected sufficient statistics by completing the trajectories using importance sampling (IS) [28] and fitting the model using a Bayesian estimator (BE) [29] with a non-informative prior from Eq. (1), see [25].
- Line 4–15 - The outer Structural Expectation-Maximization (SEM) cycle builds upon the completed trajectories and the prior knowledge to learn a new structure to use as input for the next EM iteration. The CTPC [27] algorithm was chosen due to its recovery capabilities, see [25].

The convergence criterion checks for differences between the previous and the current model, up to a maximum of 100 iterations for both EM and SEM.

5 Results

Since the sampling step is performed using a random number generator, the execution of Algorithm 1 is repeated 30 times and the results are aggregated following a model averaging strategy. The resulting model is reported in Fig. 3.

With 8 categorical parents and a total of 1728 parents combinations, the ICP CIM is high-dimensional, which makes it difficult to inspect the actual

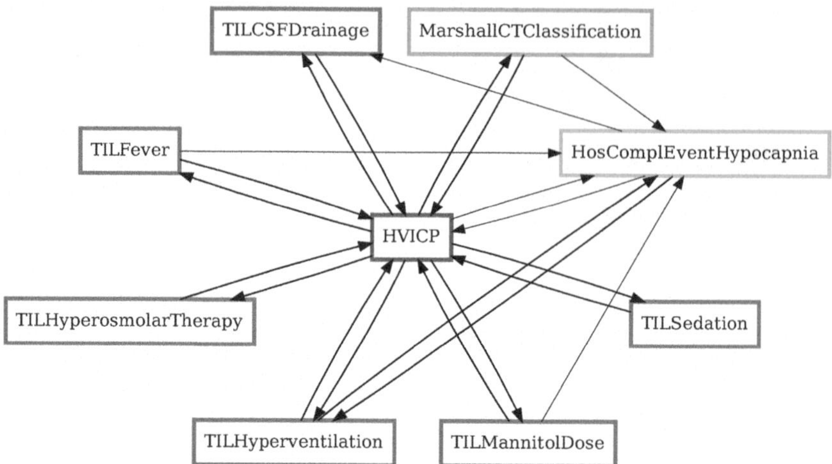

Fig. 3. Structure of the CTBN of the interactions between treatments and ICP. Variables related to treatments are in red, imaging in green, vitals in orange, and hourly values of ICP in blue. (Color figure online)

learned parameters. To filter out non-informative combinations the amount of information contained in each IM can be measured using the Kullback-Leibler divergence $D(P \,||\, Q)$ and its symmetrized Jeffreys divergence $J(P \,||\, Q)$:

$$D(P \,||\, Q) = \sum P \log \frac{P}{Q} \tag{3}$$

$$J(P \,||\, Q) = \frac{1}{2} D(P \,||\, Q) + \frac{1}{2} D(Q \,||\, P) \tag{4}$$

so that each IM in the CIM $\mathbf{Q}_{\mathtt{ICP}|\boldsymbol{\Pi}_{\mathtt{ICP}}}$ can be compared to the non-informative prior Γ^0 used in Equation (1) via Equation (4) as:

$$J\left(\Gamma^0 \,||\, \exp\left(\mathbf{Q}_{\mathtt{ICP}|\boldsymbol{\Pi}_{\mathtt{ICP}}} \cdot \varepsilon\right)\right) \qquad \forall \boldsymbol{\Pi}_{\mathtt{ICP}} \in \boldsymbol{\Pi}_{\mathtt{ICP}} \tag{5}$$

with exp the matrix exponentiation, mapping each $\mathbf{Q}_{\mathtt{ICP}|\boldsymbol{\Pi}_{\mathtt{ICP}}}$ to its instantaneous transition probability.

The IM with the highest Jeffreys divergence is reported in Fig. 4, the other top three can be found in [25].

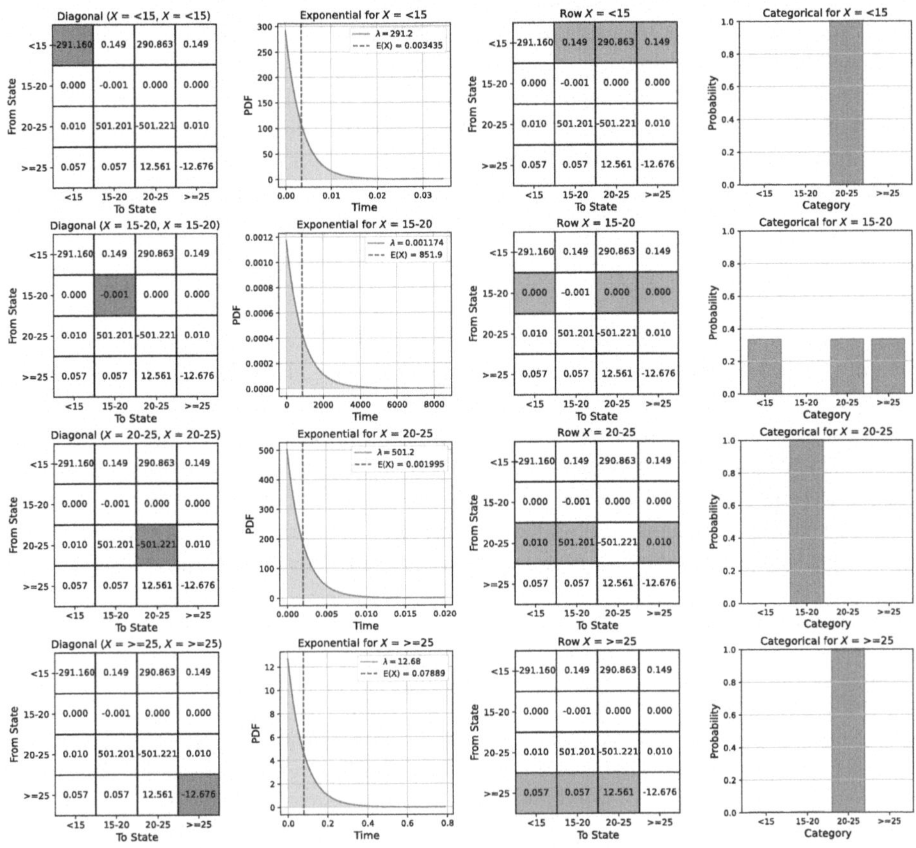

Fig. 4. ICP parameters for a patient with a Marshall CT classification of 5, treated with CFS drainage and daily cumulative mannitol dose between 0–2 g.

6 Discussion

The learned model structure in Fig. 3 is mostly derived from the prior knowledge provided by clinical experts, with the only exception being the hypocapnia variable, acting as an hub. This can be explained by the fact that it is a complication caused by therapeutic hyperventilation when ICP remains high despite osmotic therapies. While hypocapnia initially reduces ICP by constricting blood vessels, it also reduces blood flow to the brain, which can lead to further injury. The model structure captures this trade-off between short-term ICP control and long-term cerebral perfusion.

The learned parameter in Fig. 4 are associated to a patient with a severe TBI (Marshall CT 5), treated with CSF drainage and low-dose mannitol. Here the ICP does not stabilize at values below 15 mmHg, instead it rapidly rebounds in the 20–25 mmHg range. Excursions above 25 mmHg do occur but they are short-lived, usually resolving downward into the 20–25 mmHg range, rather than to normal ranges. No observations are present for the 15–20 mmHg range. This suggests that the combination of therapies is effective at preventing catastrophic and sustained intracranial hypertension, but is insufficient to reach a physiological ICP baseline. The overall picture is one of partial control rather than normalization, consistent with the severity of the injury.

A detailed discussion on the limitations of this work can be found in [25].

7 Conclusion

One of the major challenges physician face routinely in traumatic brain injury patients is the management of intracranial pressure. In this paper, we built a causal model to study the underlying mechanism of intracranial pressure, which is crucial to develop personalized therapy planning. To do so we leveraged clinical experts knowledge and partially-observed event-based data representing the trajectory of patients over time. We showed how to derive insights on the effectiveness of multiple treatments allocations from the model parameters and evaluated the model against treatment policies reported in clinical guidelines.

Acknowledgments. Zanga, Citerio, Galimberti and Stella are funded by the Project 2022-NAZ-0036, European Union, CUP H53D23001810006. Citerio, Rebora and Galimberti participated in the manuscript preparation as part of their involvement in the MUR under the grant "Dipartimenti di Eccellenza 2023-2027". Rebora was partially funded by the European Union - Next Generation EU - NRRP M6C2 - Investment 2.1 Enhancement and strengthening of biomedical research in the NHS project PNRR-MAD-2022-12376033. Stella was partially supported by the MUR under the grant "Dipartimenti di Eccellenza 2023-2027" of the Department of Informatics, Systems and Communication of the University of Milano-Bicocca, Milan, Italy, and by the National Plan for NRRP Complementary Investments (Project n. PNC0000003 - AdvaNced Technologies for Human-centrEd Medicine (ANTHEM)).

References

1. Robba, C., et al.: Traumatic brain injury management in the intensive care unit: standard of care and knowledge gaps. Intens. Care Med. **51** (2025). https://doi.org/10.1007/s00134-025-07967-1
2. Maas, A.I.R., et al.: Traumatic brain injury: progress and challenges in prevention, clinical care, and research. Lancet Neurol. **21**(11) (2022). https://doi.org/10.1016/S1474-4422(22)00309-X
3. Hawryluk, G.W.J., et al.: Intracranial pressure: current perspectives on physiology and monitoring. Intens. Care Med. **48** (2022). https://doi.org/10.1007/s00134-022-06786-y
4. Hawryluk, G.W.J., et al.: A management algorithm for patients with intracranial pressure monitoring: the Seattle International Severe Traumatic Brain Injury Consensus Conference (SIBICC). Intens. Care Med. **45**(12) (2019). https://doi.org/10.1007/S00134-019-05805-9

5. Zuercher, P., et al.: Reliability and validity of the therapy intensity level scale: analysis of clinimetric properties of a novel approach to assess management of intracranial pressure in traumatic brain injury. J. Neurotrauma **33**(19) (2016). https://doi.org/10.1089/neu.2015.4266
6. Maas, A.I.R., et al.: Collaborative European NeuroTrauma effectiveness research in traumatic brain injury (CENTER-TBI). Neurosurgery **76**(1) (2015). https://doi.org/10.1227/NEU.0000000000000575
7. Steyerberg, E.W., et al.: Case-mix, care pathways, and outcomes in patients with traumatic brain injury in CENTER-TBI: a European prospective, multicentre, longitudinal, cohort study. Lancet Neurol. **18**(10) (2019). https://doi.org/10.1016/S1474-4422(19)30232-7
8. Wilson, L., et al.: A manual for the glasgow outcome scale-extended interview. J. Neurotrauma **38**(17) (2021). https://doi.org/10.1089/neu.2020.7527
9. Scutari, M., et al.: Causal networks of infodemiological data: modelling dermatitis (2025). https://doi.org/10.1007/978-3-031-95838-0_39
10. Bernasconi, A., et al.: A causal network model to estimate the cardiotoxic effect of oncological treatments in young breast cancer survivors. Progr. Artif. Intell. (2024). https://doi.org/10.1007/s13748-024-00348-7
11. Liu, P.-R., et al.: Application of artificial intelligence in medicine: an overview. Curr. Med. Sci. **41**(6) (2021). https://doi.org/10.1007/s11596-021-2474-3
12. Sanchez, P., et al.: Causal machine learning for healthcare and precision medicine. Roy. Soc. Open Sci. **9**(8) (2022). https://doi.org/10.1098/rsos.220638
13. Zanga, A., et al.: A survey on causal discovery: theory and practice. Int. J. Approx. Reason. **151** (2022). https://doi.org/10.1016/j.ijar.2022.09.004
14. Koller, D., et al.: Probabilistic Graphical Models: Principles and Techniques. The MIT Press, USA (2009)
15. Geffner, H., et al. (eds.) Probabilistic and Causal Inference. ACM, New York, NY, USA (2022). https://doi.org/10.1145/3501714
16. Cavenaghi, E., et al.: Towards a causal decision-making framework for recommender systems. ACM Trans. Recomm. Syst. **2**(2) (2024). https://doi.org/10.1145/3629169
17. Hüllermeier, E., et al.: Aleatoric and epistemic uncertainty in machine learning: an introduction to concepts and methods. Mach. Learn. **110** (2021). https://doi.org/10.1007/s10994-021-05946-3
18. Nodelman, U., et al.: Continuous Time Bayesian Networks (2002)
19. Gatti, E., et al.: A continuous time Bayesian network model for cardiogenic heart failure. Flexible Serv. Manuf. J. **24**(4) (2012). https://doi.org/10.1007/s10696-011-9131-2
20. Acerbi, E., et al.: Continuous time Bayesian networks identify Prdm1 as a negative regulator of TH17 cell differentiation in humans. Sci. Rep. **6**(1) (2016). https://doi.org/10.1038/srep23128
21. Guillamet, G.H., et al.: CTBN-PH: A Continuous-Time Bayesian Network for Individualised Diagnostic Risk Prediction (2025). https://doi.org/10.2139/ssrn.5264449
22. Bhattacharyay, S., et al.: TILTomorrow today: dynamic factors predicting changes in intracranial pressure treatment intensity after traumatic brain injury. Sci. Rep. **15**(1) (2025). https://doi.org/10.1038/s41598-024-83862-x
23. Norris, J.R.: Cambridge University Press. Markov Chains (1997). https://doi.org/10.1017/CBO9780511810633
24. Shelton, C.R., et al.: Tutorial on structured continuous-time Markov processes. J. Artif. Intell. Res. **51** (2014). https://doi.org/10.1613/jair.4415

25. Zanga, A., et al.: Supplementary Material for: "Learning a Causal Model for Intracranial Pressure in Patients with Traumatic Brain Injury (2025). https://doi.org/10.5281/zenodo.17566334
26. Nodelman, U., et al.: Learning Continuous Time Bayesian Networks (2003)
27. Bregoli, A., et al.: A constraint-based algorithm for the structural learning of continuous-time Bayesian networks. Int. J. Approx. Reason. **138** (2021). https://doi.org/10.1016/j.ijar.2021.08.005
28. Sturlaugson, L., et al.: Uncertain and negative evidence in continuous time Bayesian networks". . Int. J. Approx. Reason. **70** (2016). https://doi.org/10.1016/j.ijar.2015.12.013
29. Nodelman, U., et al.: Expectation maximization and complex duration distributions for continuous time Bayesian networks. In: Proceedings of the 21st Conference on Uncertainty in Artificial Intelligence, UAI 2005 (2005)

Survival Hidden Markov Model

Alessandro Bregoli[1(✉)], Francesco Bellocchio[1], Luca Neri[1], and Fabio Stella[2,3,4]

[1] Fresenius Medical Care, Vaiano Cremasco, CR, Italy
a.bregoli1@campus.unimib.it,
{francesco.bellocchio,luca.neri}@freseniusmedicalcare.com
[2] University of Milano-Bicocca, Viale Sarca, 336, 20126 Milan, Italy
fabio.stella@unimib.it
[3] BReCHS – Bicocca Research Centre in Health Services, Milan, Italy
[4] Bicocca Bioinformatics Biostatistics and Bioimaging Centre - B4, University of Milano-Bicocca, Vedano al Lambro, MB, Italy

Abstract. Survival analysis is a statistical approach used to predict the time until the occurrence of a specific event. It has broad applications across various domains, including healthcare, manufacturing, and logistics. In this paper, we advance standard statistical approaches by introducing the Survival Hidden Markov Model (SHMM), which decouples the modeling of the failure event from the representation of the hidden state. This design choice enhances the model's interpretability and allows the latent states to capture underlying dynamics independently of the event occurrence. We evaluate SHMM by comparing its performance to state-of-the-art survival analysis methods, including the Cox proportional hazards model and Random Survival Forests, on synthetic data as well as on chronic kidney disease (CKD) single session data.

Keywords: Survival Analysis · Hidden Markov Models · Event Prediction

1 Introduction

Survival analysis is a statistical method for predicting the time until a specific event happens. It is used in many different fields, including healthcare [12,13], manufacturing [7], and logistics [1]. Because of its wide applicability, this topic is extensively researched in the literature.

Accordingly to [11], the models used in survival analysis can be discriminated in two main categories: *statistical methods*, which focus on modeling the survival curve, and *machine learning methods*, that focus on predicting the event of interest. Typical statistical methods for survival analysis include the Kaplan–Meier estimator [10] and the Cox proportional hazards model [5]. In contrast, machine learning approaches encompass both algorithms specifically designed for survival analysis, such as Random Survival Forests, and adaptations of classical machine learning techniques, including Naive Bayes and gradient boosting [11].

P. Bruno et al. (Eds.): HC_AIxIA_HYDRA 2025, CCIS 2830, pp. 283–295, 2026.
https://doi.org/10.1007/978-3-032-16708-8_23

The main contribution of this work is represented by the Survival Hidden Markov Model (SHMM), a new and original machine learning model that specializes the Hidden Markov Model framework to survival analysis.

The key idea of our approach is to decouple the modeling of the failure event from the representation of the hidden state, thereby enabling a more flexible and interpretable framework. The central idea is to treat the failure event as an observable emission generated by the Hidden Markov Model (HMM), rather than embedding it directly within the hidden state space. This separation allows the model to capture latent physiological dynamics independently, while still accounting for clinically significant outcomes such as vascular access failure.

We compare the performance of SHMM against state-of-the-art survival analysis methods, including the Cox proportional hazards model and Random Survival Forests, using synthetic data. Furthermore, to evaluate the real-world applicability of SHMM, we utilized the EUCLID dataset, a rich, real-world dataset of patients with chronic kidney disease (CKD) provided by Fresenius Medical Care. A major clinical concern for CKD patients undergoing hemodialysis is the failure of vascular access, most commonly an arteriovenous fistula, which is vital for effective treatment delivery [6]. We trained SHMM to predict the risk of fistula failure using only the data available to the dialysis machine during a single session. This approach enables seamless integration of the model into the dialysis machine itself, allowing for real-time risk assessment and timely alerts to medical staff, thereby supporting early intervention and potentially improving patient outcomes.

The rest of the paper is organized as follows: Sect. 2 introduces the core concepts of survival analysis and presents the HMM framework along with the associated notation. Section 3 describes the main contribution of this manuscript, i.e., the Survival Hidden Markov Model. Section 4 presents the results from both the synthetic data experiments and the chronic kidney disease (CKD) case study. Finally, Sect. 5 summarizes the main findings of the paper and outlines potential directions for future research.

2 Methods

In this section, we introduce and examine the core methodologies that support the manuscript's key contributions: survival analysis and hidden Markov models.

2.1 Survival Analysis

Many real-world phenomena involve estimating the expected time until a specific event occurs. For example, in the field of maintenance [1,7] , estimating the expected time until the next equipment failure is crucial for proactive planning and minimizing costly downtime. Similarly, in healthcare [14,18], forecasting disease progression and estimating the risk of death within a given time frame enables physicians to make more informed, timely, and effective treatment decisions.

This class of problems is extensively studied within the field of survival analysis [11], whose key concepts are survival function, lifetime distribution function, hazard function, and right-censored data, all of which we present below.

Let T be a random variable representing the survival time or time without events. Then, the *survival function* $S(\cdot)$, modelling the probability of surviving at least until time t, is defined as follows:

$$S(t) = P(T > t),\ 0 < t < \infty \tag{1}$$

The *lifetime distribution function* $F(\cdot)$, which is the complement of the survival function, represents the probability of the event occurring before a given time t, and it is defined as follows:

$$F(t) = P(T < t) = 1 - S(t),\ 0 < t < \infty \tag{2}$$

If it exists, the probability density function associated with the lifetime distribution describes the rate at which events occur per unit of time:

$$f(t) = \frac{dF(t)}{dt} = \frac{d(1 - S(t))}{dt} \tag{3}$$

The *hazard function*, which quantifies the instantaneous risk of an event occurring at time t for an individual, given that the individual has survived up to that time, is defined as follows:

$$h(t) = \lim_{\delta t \to 0} \frac{P(t \leq T < t + \delta t | T \geq t)}{\delta t} = \lim_{\delta t \to 0} \frac{P(t \leq T < t + \delta t)}{\delta t S(t)} = \frac{f(t)}{S(t)} \tag{4}$$

Also, the *cumulative hazard function* is strictly tied to the survival function as follows:

$$H(t) = \int h(t)dt = \int \frac{f(t)}{S(t)}dt = \int \frac{-S'(t)}{S(t)}dt = -logS(t) \tag{5}$$

According to [11], a defining feature of survival analysis is the potential presence of *right-censored data*, that is, instances where the event of interest is not observed for all individuals under study.

To estimate the survival function in presence of censored data, the most widely used method is the Kaplan–Meier estimator [10], a non-parametric approach defined as follows:

$$\hat{S}(t) = \prod_{j:t_j \geq t} \frac{n_j - d_j}{n_j} \tag{6}$$

where n_j denotes the number of individuals at risk of experiencing the event at time t, while d_j represents the number of individuals for whom the event actually occurs at that time.

The main limitation of the survival function as defined in (1) is that it does not account for any covariates; consequently, the probability of survival is assumed to be the same for all individuals, regardless of their specific characteristics. This assumption is both difficult to justify and to leverage in practice. As a result, various models have been developed to address this limitation, most notably the Cox proportional hazards model [5]. Moreover, when the objective of the analysis is to predict the likelihood of an event occurring within a specific time frame, the survival analysis problem can be reformulated as a binary classification task [13].

2.2 Hidden Markov Model

A HMM, as described by [4], is a statistical model used to represent processes that evolve over time. Like a standard Markov Chain, it satisfies the first-order Markov property. A defining feature of HMMs is that the underlying process generating the data is unobservable, or hidden. Instead, we observe emissions, observable variables whose states are directly influenced by the hidden states of the system.

To better illustrate the structure of a HMM, let $\mathbf{X}$ denote an unobservable discrete stochastic process, and $\mathbf{Y}$ the corresponding observable emission process. The pair $(\mathbf{X}, \mathbf{Y})$ constitutes an HMM if the following conditions are satisfied

- The process $\mathbf{X}$ satisfies the first-order Markov property, meaning that the future state depends only on the current state, and not on the sequence of past states. Formally, this condition can be expressed as follows:

$$P(X_t|X_{t-1}, \dots, X_0) = P(X_t|X_{t-1}) \tag{7}$$

- The state of the emission process Y_t depends solely on the current hidden state X_t. Formally, we have:

$$P(Y_t|X_t, X_0, \dots, X_n) = P(Y_t|X_t) \; \forall n \in \mathbb{N}^+ \tag{8}$$

where X_t and Y_t are the processes $\mathbf{X}$ and $\mathbf{Y}$ observed at time t. The structure of an HMM can be represented as a graph (Fig. 1).

In the standard formulation of HMMs, the hidden process $\mathbf{X}$ assumes values from a finite set of discrete states, while the emission process $\mathbf{Y}$ may take on either discrete or continuous values, depending on the application. For this type of HMM, the parameters required to specify the model are:

- $P(X_0)$; initial distribution (categorical).
- $P(X_t|X_{t-1})$; transition distribution (conditional categorical).
- $P(Y_t|X_t)$; emission distribution (conditional categorical/Gaussian).

A realization of the HMM is called *trajectory* and consists in a sequence of time indexed variables (Table 1).

Table 1. Example of trajectory for an HMM with a discrete hidden process **X** and a discrete emission process **Y**.

T	0	1	2	...	n
X	1	1	0	...	0
Y	0	2	1	...	0

Learning the parameters of a HMM involves estimating three probability distributions: the initial state distribution of **X**, the state transition distribution of **X**, and the emission distribution of **Y**.

The main difficulty to solve the parameters learning problem arises from the fact that the underlying process **X** is hidden and cannot be directly observed. The classical approach to addressing this type of problem is to employ the Expectation-Maximization (EM) algorithm. This method consists of two steps: in the *Expectation step* (E-step), the algorithm estimates the posterior distribution of the unobserved variables given the observed data; in the *maximization step* (M-step), it optimizes the model parameters based on the posterior distribution obtained in the E-step.

The task of parameter learning in HMMs has been extensively studied in the literature. In particular, Baum and colleagues [3] introduced the Baum–Welch algorithm, an adaptation of the EM algorithm that leverages the structure and conditional independencies inherent in HMMs

3 Survival Hidden Markov Model

In this section, we present our main contribution to the specialized literature. We begin by exploring the relationship between HMMs and survival analysis, and then introduce the core innovation of this work: the Survival Hidden Markov Model (SHMM). The application of HMMs is well established in the field of survival analysis. For instance, the authors of [9,15,17,19], employ the HMM

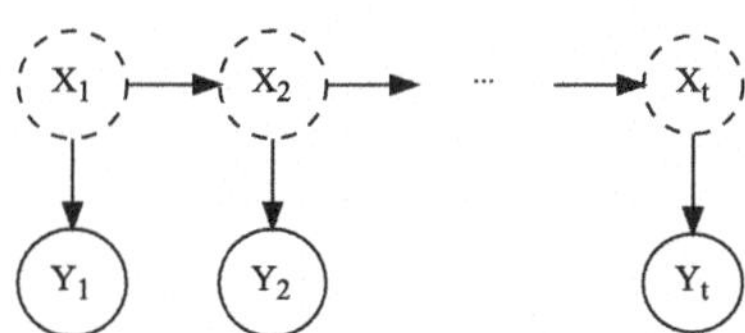

Fig. 1. Graphical representation of an HMM. The dashed nodes represent hidden process while the solid nodes represent the observable emission.

framework to model disease progression over time. Similarly, in industrial contexts, HMMs have been used for time-to-event prediction and reliability analysis, as demonstrated by [7,16]. A common underlying assumption in these studies is that the hidden variable not only captures the system's internal dynamics but also implicitly represents the occurrence of failure or the terminal stage of a disease.

In contrast to this approach, we propose decoupling the modeling of the failure event from the representation of the hidden state, allowing for a more flexible and interpretable framework. The key idea is to treat the failure event as an observable emission generated by the HMM, rather than embedding it directly within the hidden state space. Figure 2 illustrates the structure of a SHMM, in which the processes $\mathbf{X}$ and $\mathbf{Y}$ represent the hidden states and observable emissions, respectively, consistent with the classical HMM framework.

The SHMM extends the classical framework by introducing an additional observable process $\mathbf{S}$, where S_t is a discrete variable representing survival status at time t. To fully specify a SHMM, the following components are required:

- $P(X_0)$; initial distribution (categorical distribution over the states of $\mathbf{X}$).
- $P(X_t|X_{t-1})$; transition distribution (conditional categorical distribution over the states of $\mathbf{X}$).
- $P(Y_t|X_t)$; emission distribution. It is worthwhile to mention that no constraints are set on the form of this distribution.
- $P(S_t|X_t)$; conditional survival distribution (conditional categorical distribution with binary domain).

Given a trajectory in which only the realizations of $\mathbf{Y}$ and $\mathbf{S}$ are observed, the parameters of the SHMM can be estimated using the Baum–Welch algorithm [3].

3.1 Survival HMM and Survival Analysis

In this subsection, we reinterpret the SHMM within the framework of survival analysis. As a starting point, we introduce the concept of the survival function. By combining Eq. (1) with the Markov property described in Eq. (7), along with

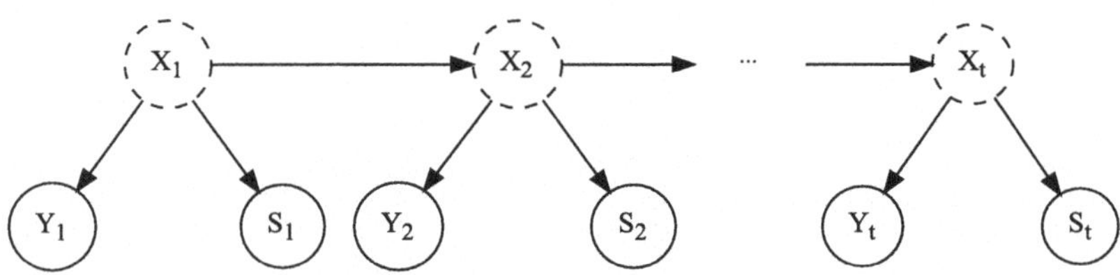

Fig. 2. Graphical representation of a Survival Hidden Markov Model.

the independence assumption of the emission process stated in Eq. (8), we derive the following expression:

$$\hat{S}(t) = P(S_0^s \ldots S_t^s) = P(S_0^s|X_0)P(X_0)\prod_{i=1}^{t} P(S_i^s|X_i)P(X_i|X_{i-1}) \tag{9}$$

where S_i^s indicates that the individual s is still alive at time i.

The hazard function (4), describes the instantaneous risk of death/failure at time t given that the individual survived until time t. Combining Eq. (4) with Eq. (7) and Eq. (8), we obtain:

$$h(t) = P(S_t^{ns}|S_{t-1}^s \ \ldots \ S_0^s) = P(S_t^{ns}|X_t) \tag{10}$$

where S_i^{ns} indicates that, at time i, the individual is no longer alive.

To incorporate the covariate Y into Eq. (9) and estimate the survival function from a single time point (similar to the approach used in Cox and Survival Random Forest models), we can modify the Eq. (9) as follows:

$$\hat{S}(t, Y_0) = P(S_0^s \ldots S_t^s|Y_0) = P(S_0^s|X_0)P(X_0|Y_0)\prod_{i=1}^{t} P(S_i^s|X_i)P(X_i|X_{i-1}) \tag{11}$$

where $P(X_0|Y_0)$ can be estimated starting from the emission probability $P(Y_t|X_t)$ and appling the Bayes theorem.

A distinctive feature of the SHMM is its ability to identify the underlying mechanism, represented by the sequence of hidden states, that leads to a failure. This is particularly valuable in scenarios where multiple failure mechanisms coexist, especially when they operate at different rates. Such capability is beneficial both operationally, by enabling targeted and effective interventions, and analytically, by helping to distinguish between failures that were potentially preventable and those that occurred suddenly and were unavoidable.

4 Numerical Experiments

In this section, we begin by evaluating the performance of the SHMM, the Cox proportional hazards model, and random survival forests on synthetic data. We then illustrate the practical application of the SHMM in predicting arteriovenous fistula failure during single-session dialysis.

4.1 Synthetic Data

In this subsection, we present a series of synthetic experiments aimed at evaluating the performance of our model and gaining insights into its behavior under idealized conditions. Additionally, we explore the distinctive features of the SHMM by comparing it with classical survival analysis methods, including the Cox proportional hazards model [5] and the random survival forest (RSF) [8].

Table 2. Concordance Index - Fully random SHMM.

	Generating Model	SHMM	Cox	RSF
Train Test	0.59(0.03)	0.59(0.03)	0.55(0.02)	0.57(0.02)
		0.58(0.03)	0.54(0.03)	0.53(0.02)

In the first experiment, we randomly generated 10 different SHMMs, each comprising 5 hidden states. The emission variable $\mathbf{Y}$ was modeled using a 5-dimensional Gaussian distribution. For each SHMM, we simulated 1,000 trajectories by sampling from the model until a failure event occurred. The hyperparameters used to generate each SHMM are as follows:

- $P(X_0)$; categorical distribution with 5 states randomly generated.
- $P(X_t|X_{t-1})$; conditional categorical distribution with 5 states randomly generated with the constraint that the probability of staying in the same state $P(X_t = x|X_{t-1} = x)$ is greater than 0.5.
- $P(S_t|X_t)$; conditional categorical distribution with 2 states randomly sampled.
- The mean of the conditional multivariate Gaussian distribution $P(Y_t|X_t)$ is a 5-dimensional vector, with each component independently sampled from a uniform range between –3 and 3.
- The covariance matrix of the conditional multivariate Gaussian $P(Y_t|X_t)$ is a symmetric matrix 5×5 where each element off-diagonal element can take values between –9 and 9 while the elements on the main diagonal can assume values between 0 and 9.

Since the RSF and Cox models are not designed to handle entire trajectories, we trained them independently at each time point. During the prediction phase, all models, including the SHMM, were tasked with providing survival estimates at each time point. The results of this experiment (Table 2) indicate that the SHMM slightly outperforms the other models, achieving performance levels comparable to those of the generative model.

In the second synthetic experiment, we aimed to simulate the progression of a disease. To achieve this, we ordered the hidden states from least to most severe, constrained transitions to allow only forward progression, and imposed a decreasing survival probability as the disease advanced. Based on these conditions, we randomly generated 10 SHMMs using the following hyperparameters and constraints:

- $P(X_0)$; categorical distribution with 5 states randomly generated.
- $P(X_t|X_{t-1})$; conditional categorical distribution with 5 states randomly generated with the constraint that the probability of staying the same state $P(X_t = x|X_{t-1} = x)$ is greater than 0.5 and when $x < k$ then $P(X_t = x|X_{t-1} = k) = 0$.
- $P(S_t|X_t)$; conditional categorical distribution with 2 states randomly generated with the constraint that $P(S_t = \text{survive}|X_t = x) < P(S_t = \text{survive}|X_t = y)\ \forall y < x$.

Table 3. Concordance Index - SHMM with triangular transition matrix.

	Generating Model	SHMM	Cox	RSF
Train Test	0.71(0.02)	0.71(0.03)	0.59(0.04)	0.57(0.05)
		0.71(0.04)	0.59(0.04)	0.55(0.05)

- The mean of the conditional multivariate Gaussian $P(Y_t|X_t)$ is 5-dimensional vector, with each component independently sampled from a uniform distribution over the interval $[0, 9]$.
- The covariance matrix of the conditional multivariate Gaussian $P(Y_t|X_t)$ is a symmetric matrix 5×5 where each element off-diagonal element can take values between -9 and 9 while the elements on the main diagonal can assume values between 0 and 9.

The results of this experiment are summarized in Table 3.

As in the previous experiment, the model trained on the synthetic data achieves performance comparable to that of the generative SHMM. However, in this scenario, the SHMM significantly outperforms both the Cox proportional hazards model and the RSF.

4.2 Single Session Arteriovenous Fistula Failure

For patients with chronic kidney disease (CKD), renal replacement therapy (RRT) is a vital treatment. Hemodialysis is one of the most commonly used forms of RRT, and it requires well-functioning vascular access (VA) for administration. Accordingly, to [6], arteriovenous fistula (AVF) is one of the most common VA, especially in Europe. As a result, considerable efforts have been dedicated to ensuring the survival and long-term patency of arteriovenous fistulas (AVFs) [13]. The most common complication of an AVF that can lead to a failure are [6]: *Stenosis* - a reduction of the vascular lumen that determine an insufficient blodflow, *Thrombosis* - formation of a thrombus in the AVF reducing the bloodflow, *Infection* - presence of pathogen in the area of the AVF.

In this subsection, we evaluate the performance of the SHMM in estimating the risk of AVF failure, and compare it against two established methods: Random Survival Forests (RSF) and the Cox proportional hazards model.

All models rely solely on data collected from the dialysis machine during a single treatment session. This represents a relevant use case, as such a model could be directly integrated into dialysis equipment to provide real-time alerts to medical staff. Nevertheless the goal is to develop a single session model, the dataset used for this work is a subset of the Nephrocare European Clinical Database (EuCliD) [2]. We include all adult patients in Portugal who underwent dialysis between January 1, 2023, and January 31, 2024. During this period, a total of 523,061 dialysis sessions were recorded across 1,581 unique patients. Among these, 945 patients experienced at least one AVF failure, resulting in 1,581 documented AVF failure events.

A failure event was defined as the occurrence of any of the following: identification of a stenosis, identification of a thrombosis, a required change in vascular access, or the need for vascular surgery. The variables recorded by the dialysis machines at 15-min intervals and available for analysis are:

- *Arterial pressure*: blood pressure entering the machine (negative value).
- *Venous pressure*: blood pressure put back into circulation (positive value).
- *Clearance*: urea removal rate.

We enriched the dataset with two additional features derived from expert knowledge. The first feature is:

$$\textit{Sum pressure} = \textit{Arterial pressure} + \textit{Venous pressure}$$

The rationale behind this feature is that, in a well-functioning fistula, pressure values may fluctuate; however, their sum is expected to remain close to zero. The second feature we used is defined as follows:

$$\textit{Clearance-Reference ratio} = \frac{\textit{Clearance}}{\textit{Reference Clearance}}$$

This feature assesses how closely the observed clearance aligns with the reference clearance value. Starting from the raw variables and engineered features, we constructed the dataset used to train our models. Since our objective was not to capture the temporal dynamics of the variables throughout the dialysis session, we chose to summarize each variable by its median value per session. Furthermore, we included only a carefully selected subset of variables and features in the final dataset. Specifically, we included only the following variables and features: *Arterial pressure, Venous pressure, Sum pressure, Clearance, Clearance-Reference clearance ratio.* The final variable to be introduced is the target variable. In this study, our objective is to estimate the risk of fistula failure. Accordingly, for each dialysis session, we associated the data with the occurrence of the next failure event, if one was recorded.

The hyperparameters values used in this experiment were as follows: for the RSF, we employed 50 trees with a maximum depth of 6; for the SHMM, we used 15 hidden states. Model performance was evaluated using 3-fold cross-validation, and the results are summarized in Table 4.

Table 4. Concordance Index - 3-Fold cross validation - Fresenius dataset.

Fold	Split	SHMM	Cox	RSF
0	Train	0.67	0.68	0.69
	Test	0.68	0.68	0.69
1	Train	0.67	0.68	0.69
	Test	0.67	0.68	0.69
2	Train	0.67	0.68	0.70
	Test	0.67	0.67	0.68

From a purely predictive standpoint, all three models performed comparably, although the RSF showed a slight advantage.

However, as noted in [6], AVF failure can occur due to different underlying mechanisms. While stenosis typically reflects a progressive deterioration of vascular access, thrombosis is often a sudden and acute event. Motivated by this distinction, we further examined the parameters learned by the SHMM to gain deeper insights into its ability to differentiate between these failure types. We began by analyzing the conditional survival distribution shown in Fig. 3, which revealed that hidden states 3 and 13 are associated with the highest probability of failure. Next, we examined the transition probabilities in Fig. 4 for these two states. We found that patients in state 3 tend to remain in that state with a high probability (0.95), whereas patients in state 13 are much more likely to transition to other states, with a self-transition probability of only 0.14. This

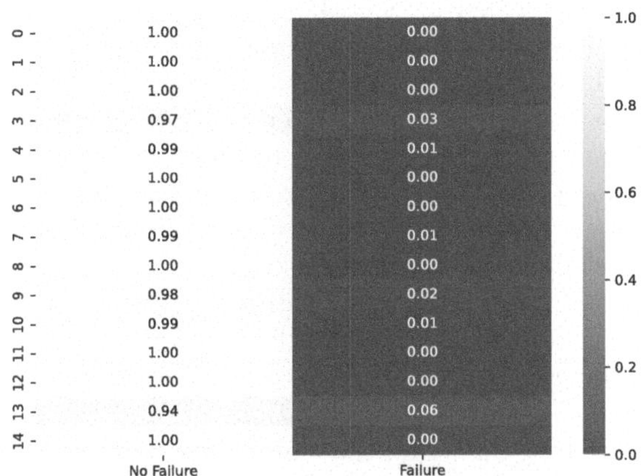

Fig. 3. Conditional survival distribution learned by SHMM on Fresenius data.

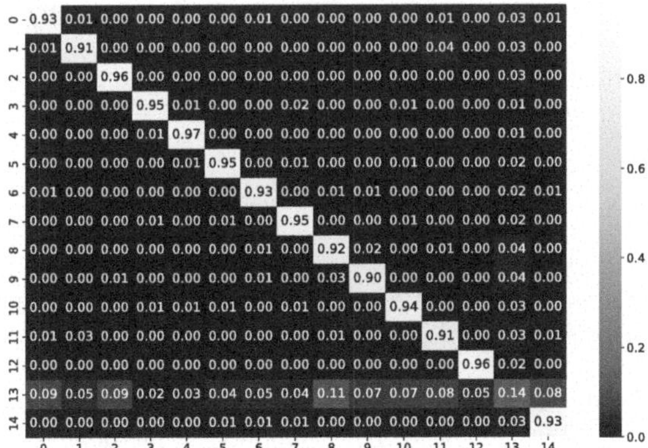

Fig. 4. Transition distribution learned by SHMM on Fresenius data. Each cell is the probability of transitioning from state i at time t to state j at $t+1$.

suggests that the SHMM is capturing at least two distinct failure mechanisms. State 3 appears to represent the terminal phase of a predictable failure, such as stenosis, characterized by gradual deterioration. In contrast, the high volatility of state 13 indicates that it may be used by the model to explain abrupt events like thrombosis.

5 Conclusions and Future Work

Survival analysis is a well established field focused on predicting the time until the occurrence of a specific event. In this study, we introduce a new and original formulation of the survival problem in which the data available during training differs from that available at prediction time. Specifically, while the training phase benefits from longitudinal data capturing the evolution of the process over time, the prediction phase is limited to a single time point. This setup reflects the clinical scenario described in Sect. 4.2, where the model is trained using a patient's historical dialysis data but must generate predictions based solely on information from the current session. Experimental results demonstrate that the SHMM performs competitively compared to classical approaches such as the Cox proportional hazards model and the Random Survival Forest. Moreover, the SHMM offers interpretability by uncovering latent mechanisms leading to failure—an advantage that becomes particularly valuable when combined with expert clinical knowledge.

This work can be extended in several directions. First, the model could be enriched with expert knowledge by introducing constraints on the transition probabilities, thereby guiding the learning process toward clinically meaningful patterns. Additionally, alternative distributions beyond the multivariate Gaussian could be explored for modeling the emission process, potentially improving the SHHM's flexibility and robustness in capturing complex data characteristics.

Acknowledgements. FS has been partially supported by the MUR under the grant "Dipartimenti di Eccellenza 2023-2027" of DISCo of the University of Milano-Bicocca, and by the National Plan for NRRP Complementary Investments (Project n. PNC0000003 - AdvaNced Technologies for Human-centrEd Medicine (ANTHEM)).

References

1. de Almeida Costa, M., de Azevedo Peixoto Braga, J.P., Ramos Andrade, A.: A data-driven maintenance policy for railway wheelset based on survival analysis and markov decision process. Qual. Reliab. Eng. Int. **37**(1), 176–198 (2020). https://doi.org/10.1002/qre.2729
2. Amato, C., Carioni, C., Kirchgessner, J., Marcelli, D., Mitteregger, A., Moscardo, V., Orlandini, G., Gatti, E., Steil, H.: Euclid® – a medical registry. Methods Inf. Med. **43**(01), 83–88 (2004)
3. Baum, L.E., et al.: An inequality and associated maximization technique in statistical estimation for probabilistic functions of Markov processes. Inequalities **3**(1), 1–8 (1972)

4. Bishop, C.M., Nasrabadi, N.M.: Pattern recognition and machine learning, vol. 4. Springer (2006)
5. Cox, D.R.: Regression models and life-tables. J. Royal Statis. Soc. Series B (Methodol.) **34**(2), 187–220 (1972). http://www.jstor.org/stable/2985181
6. Fazendeiro Matos, J., et al.: Vascular Access, Cannulation and Care. EDTNA (2015)
7. Gámiz, M.L., Limnios, N., Segovia-García, M.d.C.: Hidden markov models in reliability and maintenance. Eur. J. Oper. Res. **304**(3), 1242–1255 (2023). https://doi.org/10.1016/j.ejor.2022.05.006
8. Ishwaran, H., Kogalur, U.B., Blackstone, E.H., Lauer, M.S.: Random survival forests. Ann. Appl. Statis. **2**(3) (2008)
9. Jackson, C.H., Sharples, L.D., Thompson, S.G., Duffy, S.W., Couto, E.: Multistate Markov models for disease progression with classification error. J. Royal Statist. Soc.: Series D (Statis) **52**(2), 193–209 (2003). https://doi.org/10.1111/1467-9884.00351
10. Kaplan, E.L., Meier, P.: Nonparametric estimation from incomplete observations. J. Am. Stat. Assoc. **53**(282), 457–481 (1958). https://doi.org/10.1080/01621459.1958.10501452
11. Kartsonaki, C.: Survival analysis. Diagn. Histopathol. **22**(7), 263–270 (2016). https://doi.org/10.1016/j.mpdhp.2016.06.005
12. Lin, R.H., Lin, C.S., Chuang, C.L., Kujabi, B.K., Chen, Y.C.: Breast cancer survival analysis model. Appl. Sci. **12**(4), 1971 (2022)
13. Peralta, R., et al.: Development and validation of a machine learning model predicting arteriovenous fistula failure in a large network of dialysis clinics. Int. J. Environ. Res. Publ. Health **18**(23), 12355 (2021)
14. Rai, S., Mishra, P., Ghoshal, U.C.: Survival analysis: a primer for the clinician scientists. Indian J. Gastroenterol. **40**(5), 541–549 (2022). https://doi.org/10.1007/s12664-021-01232-1
15. Sukkar, R., Katz, E., Zhang, Y., Raunig, D., Wyman, B.T.: Disease progression modeling using hidden markov models. In: 2012 Annual International Conference of the IEEE Engineering in Medicine and Biology Society. pp. 2845–2848. IEEE (2012). https://doi.org/10.1109/embc.2012.6346556
16. Vrignat, P., Avila, M., Duculty, F., Kratz, F.: Failure event prediction using hidden markov model approaches. IEEE Trans. Reliab. **64**(3), 1038–1048 (2015). https://doi.org/10.1109/tr.2015.2423191
17. Wang, X., Sontag, D., Wang, F.: Unsupervised learning of disease progression models. In: Proceedings of the 20th ACM SIGKDD international conference on Knowledge discovery and data mining. KDD '14, ACM (2014)
18. Xu, Z., et al.: Risk-aware survival time prediction from whole slide pathological images. Sci. Rep. **12**, 21948 (2022). https://doi.org/10.1038/s41598-022-26096-z
19. Zhou, X., Kang, K., Kwok, T., Song, X.: Joint hidden markov model for longitudinal and time-to-event data with latent variables. Multivar. Behav. Res. **57**(2–3), 441–457 (2021). https://doi.org/10.1080/00273171.2020.1865864

An Approach Leveraging Deep Learning and Stream Reasoning for Dynamic Task Assignments Balancing Productivity and Well Being

Luca Laboccetta[1(✉)], Francesco Calimeri[1], Davide Iacopino[2], Salvatore Iiritano[2], Marta Maria[2], Simona Perri[1], Massimiliano Ruffolo[2], and Giorgio Terracina[1]

[1] University of Calabria, Rende 87036, Italy
luca.laboccetta@unical.it
[2] Revelis S.r.l., Rende 87036, Italy

Abstract. Employee well-being is an increasingly crucial factor for sustainability and efficiency in modern industry, especially within the context of Industry 5.0, which places humans at the center of production processes. This article presents some innovative aspects of the InCoP platform, which is part of a more general project developed under the NRRP MUR initiative FAIR (Future AI Research): Green-aware AI, and integrates Stream Reasoning (SR) and Machine Learning (ML). In particular, we focus on the real-time monitoring of operators' psychophysical well-being and optimization of task assignment in a real industrial bakery environment. Here, an Assignment Module integrates results from ML-based models, used to predict stress, with the deductive capabilities of the SR engine, used to dynamically reassign operators to departments and suggest breaks in cases of persistent or dangerous stress levels. The goal is to minimize worker stress and prevent overload, while maintaining adherence to the production plan. Notably, the dynamic assignment module is fully integrated within the InCoP platform and leverages also sensors data coming from smartwatches and environmental monitoring devices which are fed into the system through Kafka, Elasticsearch, and MongoDB based technologies.

1 Introduction

The contemporary manufacturing sector is undergoing a profound transformation, driven by the principles of Industry 4.0 and progressively advancing towards Industry 5.0. This evolution positions human well-being, sustainability, and human-centric methodologies at the very core of industrial processes, thereby elevating the health and psychophysical state of employees to a critical determinant of operational efficiency and sustained long-term success. This paradigm shift necessitates the development of sophisticated technological solutions capable of real-time monitoring and adaptive management of human factors. A fundamental aspect of this capability involves the precise assessment and proactive

P. Bruno et al. (Eds.): HC_AIxIA_HYDRA 2025, CCIS 2830, pp. 296–307, 2026.
https://doi.org/10.1007/978-3-032-16708-8_25

prediction of critical human conditions, such as employee stress levels, to facilitate timely interventions and optimize resource allocation.

This work presents some ongoing work on the design and development of a platform, named InCoP (Industry 5.0 Collaborative Platform), which is part of the activities funded by the NRRP MUR initiative FAIR (Future AI Research). The general goal of InCoP is to establish a versatile and scalable technological platform capable of supporting the widespread implementation of Industry 5.0 principles across diverse industrial sectors.

Our aim is to address the issue of dynamically assigning tasks to achieve sustainable production in a real bakery setting. This is an integral component of the broader InCoP platform. To address this complex challenge, our methodology uniquely integrates two pivotal domains of Artificial Intelligence, namely Machine Learning and declarative Stream Reasoning. Machine Learning (ML) techniques, particularly Deep Learning (DL) models such as Recurrent Neural Networks (RNNs) including Gated Recurrent Units (GRU) and Long Short-Term Memory (LSTM) [14], are employed for discerning subtle patterns within physiological data and for forecasting future human states, such as stress levels. This predictive capability is then synergistically combined with Stream Reasoning (SR) [11]. Addressing the complexities inherent in the dynamic, and frequently voluminous, nature of data streams has been a key focus in recent years. This effort has led to the proliferation of various Stream Reasoning (SR) approaches [1–6,8,12,13,15,16,18–21], notably within the spheres of Data Stream Management Systems (DSMS), Complex Event Processing (CEP), Semantic Web, and Knowledge Representation and Reasoning (KRR).

While task assignment is typically addressed using classical numerical optimization paradigms or with workflow management tools, in our context SR has proven to be an effective approach for handling the complexities of real-time data analysis and deductive inference over continuous, high-volume data streams. Its ability to apply logical reasoning to extract meaningful insights from an incessant flow of heterogeneous and dynamic data is exceptionally relevant in domains like Smart Cities, the Internet of Things (IoT), and Healthcare, where timely and accurate decision-making is paramount.

The specific Stream Reasoning framework utilized in this project for the dynamic assignment of tasks is known as *DP*-sr [9,16], whose main features are: *(i)* disjunctive logic programming, allowing to address non-determinism in logic programs, *(ii)* the integration of external sources of computation, enabling imperative programming capabilities into the deductive realm, and *(iii)* inertial event generators, i.e. complex events with stream-controlled lifespan. These ingredients proved to be effective in the development of the application at hand.

2 General InCop Architecture

The InCoP platform is built upon a sophisticated Internet of Everything (IoE) infrastructure, designed to optimize work organization by balancing productivity and the psycho-physical well-being of operators. The overall architecture,

illustrated in Fig. 1, depicts a continuous, dynamic data flow that underpins the system's adaptive capabilities.
Operators are equipped with smartwatches that continuously monitor a range of biometric parameters, including their estimated stress level, blood pressure, heart rate, blood oxygen level, and body temperature. Complementing this, Airgloss environmental sensors are strategically deployed across critical production departments (production, ovens, packaging) to provide real-time measurements of environmental conditions such as temperature and humidity. These heterogeneous data streams are reliably transmitted via dedicated gateways to a centralized Kafka-based messaging system, which acts as the primary data ingestion point.
From Kafka, a specialized Ingester component processes the raw data, structuring and storing it efficiently within an Elasticsearch database. This structured data in Elasticsearch is the analytical backbone for various system modules. The architectural design prioritizes maximum efficiency and responsiveness, enabling the system to make informed decisions dynamically based on prevailing conditions.

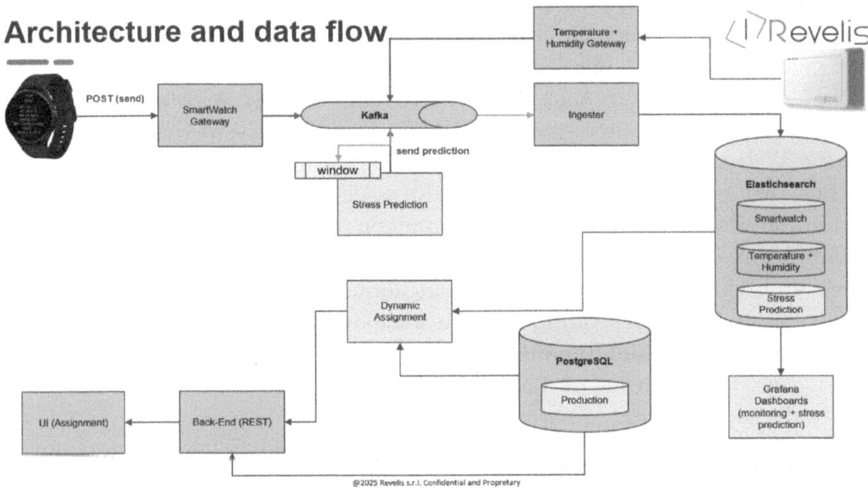

Fig. 1. General Architecture.

2.1 Interaction Between Deep Learning and Stream Reasoning

A pivotal aspect is the iterative interaction between its Deep Learning-based predictive component and its Stream Reasoning-based decision-making core. This synergy enables proactive well-being management and dynamic operational adjustments.

The Stress Prediction module, continuously monitors the Kafka queue to acquire the latest biometric measurements from operators. This algorithm, leveraging a specially trained Machine Learning model (implemented in Python using Tensorflow and Keras), processes these biometric data to forecast future stress level trends for each operator. These stress predictions are then fed back into the Kafka queue and subsequently stored in a dedicated Elasticsearch index, creating a historical record of anticipated stress levels vital for proactive strategies. This predictive output becomes a critical input for the Dynamic Assignment module, which is powered by the *DP*-sr Stream Reasoning engine. The *DP*-sr logic program then consumes this stream of predicted stress data, combining it with other essential contextual information such as operators' weekly shift rotations and the daily production schedule. The core function of *DP*-sr is to dynamically process this integrated data to infer optimal task assignments or to trigger "Pause" states for operators. This continuous feedback loop—where Deep Learning provides anticipatory insights (stress predictions) which are then processed by Stream Reasoning for adaptive, logical task management—is central to the system's ability to optimize workload distribution while safeguarding operator health and productivity. The resultant assignment decisions are stored back into MongoDB and exposed via a REST API for visualization on Grafana dashboards, enabling production managers to monitor real and expected stress levels and to facilitate timely interventions.

3 Stream Reasoning Based Solution for Dynamic Assignment

In this section, we focus on the Dynamic Assignment module. This module features a logic program that, in turn, is processed by the *DP*-sr system; it is designed to process real-time operator data and environmental conditions, integrating outputs from the Deep Learning stress prediction module to make informed staffing decisions. The program operates on a continuous stream of information, dynamically adapting assignments based on inferred stress levels and predefined operational constraints.

In order to allow readers unfamiliar with *DP*-sr to easily follow our proposal, we first provide some background on *DP*-sr architecture and language, and then present our solution.

3.1 The DP-sr Stream Reasoning System

The DP-sr system [10] is an innovative ASP-based stream reasoner designed to efficiently tackle the challenges of real-time inference over dynamic data streams. Its core functionality relies on a tight integration between a custom Java application built on Apache Flink and an ASP system.

System Architecture and Workflow. The architecture of DP-sr is based on a continuous collaboration between three main modules: the Execution Manager, the Stream Manager, and the Subprogram Manager, all leveraging Flink APIs.

The system workflow consists of two main phases:

- Configuration Phase: The Execution Manager receives an input DP-sr program. It then splits this program into subprograms based on predicate dependencies introduced by streaming atoms. An evaluation order among these subprograms is established to build the Flink dataflow graph. Each subprogram is also "flattened" into a standard ASP program. This information, along with the dataflow graph, is passed to the Stream Manager and Subprogram Manager. The Subprogram Manager instantiates Reasoner instances for each subprogram, which will handle the incremental evaluation.
- Execution Phase: The Stream Manager connects to the data source and continuously consumes the input stream, feeding its elements into the Flink dataflow graph. For each subprogram, the Stream Manager executes Flink operators to compute the semantics of streaming literals. The results are forwarded to the Subprogram Manager, which translates them into ground standard ASP literals. These are then fed to the dedicated reasoner instance for incremental evaluation of the flattened subprogram. The new derivations are sent back to the Stream Manager, which updates the overall output and proceeds with the next subprogram. This iterative process forms the output stream at each time point. The system is designed to manage backpressure, ensuring no data loss and correctness of output.

Input Language and Constructs. The input language of DP-sr is an extension of ASP-Core-2 [7] enriched with constructs for reasoning over data streams.

- Stream and Events: A stream is fundamentally a sequence of sets of ground predicate atoms, where each set is associated with a specific time point. An event is an information true at a specific time point, represented as a predicate atom.
- Streaming Literals: These allow evaluation of formulas on an input stream. A streaming literal comprises a predicate atom, an operator, and a lookup set (a set of time points for evaluation). Supported operators include `always`, `at least`, `at most`, and `count`, which check the persistence or count occurrences of an event within the specified time points.
- `@now` Construct: This special term allows explicit reasoning about time points within rule bodies. At each evaluation time point t, `@now` takes t as its value, enabling dynamic temporal conditions and derivations. It can be numeric (seconds, minutes, hours) or textual (datetime format).
- Inertial Event Generator: An *inertial event* is a complex event with stream-controlled lifespan; in particular, it is defined by means of a special construct called *inertial event generator*. [17]
- Rule Types: DP-sr supports normal rules (similar to classical ASP rules), trigger rules (evaluated with a user-specified frequency), and temporary rules

(whose inferred atoms are considered true only at the current time point and then forgotten).
- Safety and Stratification: The language also adheres to concepts of safe rules and program stratification, which guide the evaluation process and ensure consistency.

3.2 The Proposed Solution

In what follows, we present our solution by explicitly illustrating various fragments of the program in separate sections, to ease the presentation.

Input and Base Facts. At first, static facts about the operational environment and deriving basic operator information must be defined.

```
1 area("NEW_WAREHOUSE").
2 department("PRODUCTION").
3 department("PACKAGING").
4 department("OVENS").
5 operator(X) :- stressOperator(X, _).
6 operatorStressLevel(X, Y) :- stressOperator(X, Stress),
      stressOperatorPred(X,StressPred),&compute_stress(Stress
      ,StressPred; Y).
```

These rules define available areas and departments. `operator(X)` is derived for any operator for whom stress data `stress_operator(X)` is available. Crucially, `operator_stress_level(X,Y)` categorizes the operator's stress into qualitative levels (‘‘LOW",‘‘MEDIUM",‘‘HIGH") based on raw stress measurements and their predicted values `stress_pred` using an external atom `&compute_stress`. This external atom bridges the sub-symbolic output of the Deep Learning model with the symbolic reasoning of *DP*-sr.

Stream Population and Stress Persistence. This section uses *DP*-sr **#generate** construct to maintain “inertial" facts related to persistent stress levels. The **#generate** construct defines facts that, once derived, remain true until explicitly deactivated by a contradicting condition or a timer expiration.

```
1 #generate(medium_stress_threshold(O);operatorStressLevel(O,"
      MEDIUM"):operatorStressLevel(O,"LOW")).
2 #generate(critical_stress_threshold(O);operatorStressLevel(O
      ,"HIGH"):operatorStressLevel(O,"MEDIUM")|
      operatorStressLevel(O,"LOW")).
```

The predicate `medium_stress_threshold` is generated if an operator reaches a ‘‘MEDIUM" stress level, persisting until their level drops to ‘‘LOW" . Similarly, `critical_stress_threshold` is generated for ‘‘HIGH" stress, persisting until the level becomes ‘‘MEDIUM" or ‘‘LOW". These rules convert transient measurements into persistent states, which are essential for decision-making.

Operator Pause Management. The system explicitly manages operator pauses based on critical stress levels.

```
1 activate_generator(O):-critical_stress_threshold(O) always
      in [20],operator(O) at least 4 in [20].
2
3 #generate(pause(O,stress_threshold);activate_generator(O):
      operatorStressLevel(O,"MEDIUM")|operatorStressLevel(O,"
      LOW")).
```

The `activate_generator(O)` atom becomes true if an operator `O` has been in a critical stress state always within the last 20 time units (meaning 4 consecutive measurements, as data is received every 5 minutes), and has been actively monitored for at least 4 time units within that window. This logic enables the system to detect persistent high stress which, according to the system's rules, triggers a pause. The **#generate** rule then activates a pause for the operator that will persist until the operator's stress level drops to "`MEDIUM`" or "`LOW`".

Shift Assignment and Constraints. This section defines the core assignment problem and enforces fundamental operational constraints.

```
1 shift(A, D) :- area(A), department(D).
2
3 assigned(O, D, A) | not_assigned(O, D, A) :- operator(O),
      shift(A, D).
4
5 covered(A, D) :- assigned(_, D, A), shift(A, D).
6
7 :- shift(A, D), not covered(A, D).
8
9 :- assigned(O, D1, A), assigned(O, D2, A), D1 != D2.
10
11 :- assigned(O, _, _), pause(O, _).
12
13 assigned_operators_count(O,C):-#count { O : assigned(O, _,
      _) } = C,operator(O).
14
15 unassigned_operator(O):-#count { O : assigned(O, _, _) } =
      0,operator(O).
16
17 :-unassigned_operator(O),not pause(O,stress_threshold).
```

The predicate `shift` defines all possible area and department shifts. The disjunctive rule `assigned(O, R, A) | not_assigned(O, R, A)` guesses whether an operator is assigned to a specific shift. *DP*-sr extended language supports such non-deterministic rules for robust solution finding. Hard constraints ensure that: every shift is covered, all non-paused operators are assigned to exactly only one shift, operators in pause are not assigned.

Capacity Constraints. Operational limits on department capacity are enforced through integrity constraints and weak constraints for flexibility.

```
1 :- shift(A, D),covered(A,D),#count { O : assigned(O, D, A)
      } > 3.
2
3 :~shift(A, D),covered(A,D),#count { O : assigned(O, "
      PACKAGING",A) } !=2.[10@1]
```

The first rule ensures no more than 3 operators are assigned to any single shift. The second rule is a weak constraint indicating a preference (with weight 10 and level 1) for exactly 2 operators in the "PACKAGING" department, allowing for solutions that deviate if necessary but penalizing them[1].

Shift Balancing Across Departments. To optimize workload distribution, the program includes rules to balance the number of operators across different departments.

```
1  department_operator_count(D, A, C) :- #count { O : assigned
       (O, D, A) }=C,department(D),area(A).
2  total_operators_assigned(Tot) :- #count{O: assigned(O,_,_)}
       = Tot.
3  minimum_target(TMin) :- total_operators_assigned(Tot), TMin
       = Tot / 3 .
4  maximum_target(TMax) :- total_operators_assigned(Tot), TMax
       = (Tot / 3 ) + 1.
5  target_difference(D, Diff) :- department_operator_count(D,
       _, Count),
6                                 minimum_target(TMin),
7                                 maximum_target(TMax),
8                                 Count < TMin, Diff = TMin -
       Count.
9  target_difference(D, Diff) :- department_operator_count(D,
       _, Count),
10                                minimum_target(TMin),
11                                maximum_target(TMax),
12                                Count > TMax, Diff = Count -
       TMax.
13 :~ target_difference(D, Diff). [20@2]
```

These rules calculate the total number of assigned operators and define minimum and maximum target ranges (e.g., 1/3 of total operators) for each department, `target_difference` computes the deviation from these targets. The weak constraint at line 13 with a high weight (20) penalizes solutions where departments significantly deviate from their ideal operator counts, promoting balanced distribution.

[1] These specifications have been provided by the company, based on departments and operational requirements.

Stress-Driven Reassignment and Swap Constraints. This critical block implements the dynamic reassignment logic based on operator stress, leveraging the categorized stress levels.

```
1 operator_stress_integer(O,SInt):-stressOperator(O,Stress),&
      return_stress_int(Stress; SInt).
2 total_department_stress(D,A,S) :- S = #sum{ Stress,O :
      assigned(O, D, _), operator_stress_integer(O, Stress)
      }, department(D),area(A).
3 average_department_stress(D, A, M) :-
      total_department_stress(D, A, S),
      department_operator_count(D, A, C), C > 0, M = S / C.
4 maximum_stress(Max) :- Max = #max { M :
      average_department_stress(D, A, M) }.
5 most_stressed_department(D,A) :- maximum_stress(Max),
      average_department_stress(D,A,Max).
6
7 activate_swap_constraint(O):-medium_stress_threshold(O)
      always in [20],operator(O) at least 4 in [20],not
      activate_swap_constraint(O) in {5,10,15}.
8 :~assigned(O,D,A),most_stressed_department(D,A),
      activate_swap_constraint(O),operator(O) at least 4 in
      [20].[10@3,O]
9
10 :~assigned(O,D,A),activate_swap_constraint(O),operator(O)
      at least 4 in [20],previous_assignment(O,D,A).[10@3,O]
```

The predicate `operator_stress_integer(O)` converts raw stress values into integers by relying on the `$return_stress_int` external atom, and rules number 4 and 5 compute departmental stress metrics. The maximum average stress within any department is then identified by `maximum_stress` and linked to the specific `most_stressed_department`. The `activate_swap_constraint(O)` rule activates a constraint for an operator `O` if they have persistently been in a medium stress state, are active, and this swap condition hasn't been recently triggered (e.g., in the last 5, 10, or 15 time units). The two subsequent weak constraints (both with weight 10 and level 3):

- Penalize assigning an operator `O` to the most stressed department if the swap constraint is true. This mechanism forces the reassignment of medium-stressed operators to less stressful departments.
- Penalize assigning an operator `O` to the same department of the previous assignment if a swap constraint is active, ensuring that a detected need for reassignment results in a move to a different department.

Minimizing Reassignments. To ensure stability and minimize disruptions, the program includes a weak constraint that penalizes unnecessary reassignments.

```
1 :~previous_assignment(O,D,A),assigned(O,D1,A),D1!=D. [10@2,
    0]
```

This weak constraint (with weight 10 and level 2) penalizes any change in assignment (D1!=D) for an operator from their previous assignment, favoring solutions that maintain existing assignments unless critical conditions necessitate a change.

4 Conclusion and Future Work

We presented some preliminary results on the ongoing design, development and testing of the InCoP platform. In particular, we focused on the dynamic task assignment, developed for a real bakery towards sustainable production. Preliminary analyses show the practical feasibility and tangible benefits of using a mixture of ML and SR approaches to address operator stress and dynamic task assignment. The actual implementation and some preliminary tests show that the proposed approach is promising to enhance employee well-being and operational efficiency.

As future work is concerned, we plan to conduct a series of experiments designed to systematically quantify the relationship between operator stress levels and production output. The primary objective is to measure productivity as a function of stress variation, specifically by adjusting intervention thresholds within our dynamic assignment module. A key experimental variable will be k, representing the number of consecutive high-stress measurements required to trigger an operator's pause. We hypothesize that by decreasing k, the average operator stress will likely reduce due to more frequent interventions, but this might concurrently lead to a decrease in overall productivity. Conversely, an excessively large k would allow stress to escalate significantly before intervention. Productivity will be defined as the time necessary for a department to reach its designated production target, while average stress will serve as another key parameter. Through the systematic variation of k, we aim to identify the optimal balance point where operator well-being is effectively managed without excessively compromising production efficiency. These experiments are crucial for fine-tuning the system's adaptive capabilities and establishing empirical evidence for the optimal trade-off in human-centric manufacturing.

Acknowledgment. We acknowledge financial support from: PNRR MUR project PE0000013-FAIR. Francesco Calimeri is member of the Gruppo Nazionale Calcolo Scientifico-Istituto Nazionale di Alta Matematica (GNCS-INdAM).

Declaration on Generative AI. The author(s) confirm that no Generative AI tools were used in the creation of this article.

References

1. Anicic, D., Fodor, P., Rudolph, S., Stojanovic, N.: EP-SPARQL: a unified language for event processing and stream reasoning. In: Srinivasan, S., Ramamritham, K., Kumar, A., Ravindra, M.P., Bertino, E., Kumar, R. (eds.) Proceedings of the 20th International Conference on World Wide Web, WWW 2011, Hyderabad, March 28 - April 1, 2011, pp. 635–644. ACM (2011). https://doi.org/10.1145/1963405.1963495
2. Barbieri, D.F., Braga, D., Ceri, S., Valle, E.D., Grossniklaus, M.: C-SPARQL: a continuous query language for RDF data streams. Int. J. Semantic Comput. **4**(1), 3–25 (2010). https://doi.org/10.1142/S1793351X10000936
3. Bazoobandi, H.R., Beck, H., Urbani, J.: Expressive stream reasoning with laser. In: d'Amato, C., et al., (eds.) The Semantic Web - ISWC 2017 - 16th International Semantic Web Conference, Vienna, Austria, October 21-25, 2017, Proceedings, Part I. Lecture Notes in Computer Science, vol. 10587, pp. 87–103. Springer (2017). https://doi.org/10.1007/978-3-319-68288-4_6
4. Beck, H., Dao-Tran, M., Eiter, T.: LARS: a logic-based framework for analytic reasoning over streams. Artif. Intell. **261**, 16–70 (2018). https://doi.org/10.1016/J.ARTINT.2018.04.003
5. Beck, H., Eiter, T., Folie, C.: Ticker: a system for incremental asp-based stream reasoning. Theory Pract. Log. Program. **17**(5–6), 744–763 (2017). https://doi.org/10.1017/S1471068417000370
6. Calbimonte, J., Corcho, Ó., Gray, A.J.G.: Enabling ontology-based access to streaming data sources. In: Patel-Schneider, P.F., Pan, Y., Hitzler, P., Mika, P., Zhang, L., Pan, J.Z., Horrocks, I., Glimm, B. (eds.) The Semantic Web - ISWC 2010 - 9th International Semantic Web Conference, ISWC 2010, Shanghai, November 7-11, 2010, Revised Selected Papers, Part I. Lecture Notes in Computer Science, vol. 6496, pp. 96–111. Springer (2010). https://doi.org/10.1007/978-3-642-17746-0_7
7. Calimeri, F., et al.: Asp-core-2 input language format. Theory Pract. Log. Program. **20**(2), 294–309 (2020)
8. Calimeri, F., Manna, M., Mastria, E., Morelli, M.C., Perri, S., Zangari, J.: I-DLV-SR: a stream reasoning system based on I-DLV. Theory Pract. Log. Program. **21**(5), 610–628 (2021). https://doi.org/10.1017/S147106842100034X
9. Calimeri, F., Mastria, E., Perri, S.: DP-SR: a purely declarative programming framework for stream reasoning (2024). https://sites.google.com/unical.it/dp-sr
10. Calimeri, F., Mastria, E., Perri, S., Zangari, J.: The stream reasoning system I-DLV-SR: enhancements and applications in smart cities. In: Governatori, G., Turhan, A. (eds.) Rules and Reasoning - 6th International Joint Conference on Rules and Reasoning, RuleML+RR 2022, Berlin, Germany, September 26-28, 2022, Proceedings. Lecture Notes in Computer Science, vol. 13752, pp. 38–53. Springer (2022). https://doi.org/10.1007/978-3-031-21541-4_3
11. Dell'Aglio, D., Valle, E.D., van Harmelen, F., Bernstein, A.: Stream reasoning: a survey and outlook. Data Sci. **1**(1–2), 59–83 (2017). https://doi.org/10.3233/DS-170006
12. Do, T.M., Loke, S.W., Liu, F.: Answer set programming for stream reasoning. In: Butz, C.J., Lingras, P. (eds.) Advances in Artificial Intelligence - 24th Canadian Conference on Artificial Intelligence, Canadian AI 2011, St. John's, Canada, May 25-27, 2011. Proceedings. Lecture Notes in Computer Science, vol. 6657, pp. 104–109. Springer (2011). https://doi.org/10.1007/978-3-642-21043-3_13

13. Gebser, M., Grote, T., Kaminski, R., Schaub, T.: Reactive answer set programming. In: Delgrande, J.P., Faber, W. (eds.) Logic Programming and Nonmonotonic Reasoning - 11th International Conference, LPNMR 2011, Vancouver, Canada, May 16-19, 2011. Proceedings. Lecture Notes in Computer Science, vol. 6645, pp. 54–66. Springer (2011). https://doi.org/10.1007/978-3-642-20895-9_7
14. Hochreiter, S., Schmidhuber, J.: Long short-term memory. Neural Comput. **9**(8), 1735–1780 (1997). https://doi.org/10.1162/neco.1997.9.8.1735
15. Hoeksema, J., Kotoulas, S.: High-performance distributed stream reasoning using s4. In: Ordring Workshop at ISWC (2011)
16. Laboccetta, L., Mastria, E., Calimeri, F., Leone, N., Perri, S., Terracina, G.: Towards effective asp-based stream reasoning: Facilitate the reasoning over patterns of events. In: PPDP, pp. 18:1–18:12. ACM (2024)
17. Laboccetta, L., Mastria, E., Calimeri, F., Leone, N., Perri, S., Terracina, G.: Towards effective asp-based stream reasoning: facilitate the reasoning over patterns of events. In: Proceedings of the 26th International Symposium on Principles and Practice of Declarative Programming. PPDP '24, Association for Computing Machinery, New York (2024). https://doi.org/10.1145/3678232.3678248
18. Mileo, A., Abdelrahman, A., Policarpio, S., Hauswirth, M.: Streamrule: a non-monotonic stream reasoning system for the semantic web. In: Faber, W., Lembo, D. (eds.) Web Reasoning and Rule Systems - 7th International Conference, RR 2013, Mannheim, July 27-29, 2013. Proceedings. Lecture Notes in Computer Science, vol. 7994, pp. 247–252. Springer (2013). https://doi.org/10.1007/978-3-642-39666-3_23
19. Pham, T., Ali, M.I., Mileo, A.: C-ASP: continuous asp-based reasoning over RDF streams. In: Balduccini, M., Lierler, Y., Woltran, S. (eds.) Logic Programming and Nonmonotonic Reasoning - 15th International Conference, LPNMR 2019, Philadelphia, June 3-7, 2019, Proceedings. Lecture Notes in Computer Science, vol. 11481, pp. 45–50. Springer (2019). https://doi.org/10.1007/978-3-030-20528-7_4
20. Phuoc, D.L., Dao-Tran, M., Parreira, J.X., Hauswirth, M.: A native and adaptive approach for unified processing of linked streams and linked data. In: Aroyo, L., et al., (eds.) The Semantic Web - ISWC 2011 - 10th International Semantic Web Conference, Bonn, Germany, October 23-27, 2011, Proceedings, Part I. Lecture Notes in Computer Science, vol. 7031, pp. 370–388. Springer (2011). https://doi.org/10.1007/978-3-642-25073-6_24
21. Ren, X., Curé, O., Naacke, H., Xiao, G.: Bigsr: real-time expressive RDF stream reasoning on modern big data platforms. In: Abe, N., et al., (eds.) IEEE International Conference on Big Data (IEEE BigData 2018), Seattle, December 10-13, 2018, pp. 811–820. IEEE (2018). https://doi.org/10.1109/BIGDATA.2018.8621947

Machine Learning and Statistical Insights Into Hospital Stay Durations: The Italian Healthcare Administrative Data Case

Marina Andrić(✉) and Mauro Dragoni

Fondazione Bruno Kessler, Trento, Italy
{mandric,dragoni}@fbk.eu

Abstract. Length of hospital stay (LoS) is a key metric for healthcare quality and hospital resource management. This study investigates factors influencing LoS within the Italian healthcare system, using patient-level hospitalization records from standardized hospital discharge forms (Schede di Dimissione Ospedaliera, SDO) for the population served by a local health authority in Piedmont. The dataset included 37,526 patients across 66 facilities over four years. We analyzed patient characteristics, comorbidities, admission details, and hospital-specific factors. Significant associations were observed with age group, comorbidity burden, admission type, and month of admission. Machine learning models, CatBoost and Random Forest, were used to predict LoS, with CatBoost achieving the highest validation R^2 of 0.49. Historical LoS and procedure were the most influential predictors. As diagnosis and procedure information is recorded at discharge, the models are intended for retrospective analysis rather than real-time prediction at admission. The results demonstrate the potential of administrative SDO data for understanding LoS patterns and supporting hospital planning.

Keywords: Healthcare research · Length of hospital stay · Machine learning

1 Introduction

Length of stay (LoS) is an important indicator of the use of medical services that is used to assess the efficiency of hospital management, patient quality of care, and functional performance [10]. Shorter LoS has been associated with decreased risks of infections, improvements in treatment outcomes, reduced medical costs, and increased hospital bed turnover [5,18].

LoS varies even among patients with the same condition or undergoing the same type of intervention due to a complex interplay of individual characteristics, differences in medical practices across facilities [2], and external influences like seasonal trends and public health crises. Understanding LoS requires accounting for these complexities.

To investigate these factors, this study utilized administrative healthcare records from the Local Health Authority of Alba and Bra (Azienda Sanitaria

P. Bruno et al. (Eds.): HC_AIxIA_HYDRA 2025, CCIS 2830, pp. 308–320, 2026.
https://doi.org/10.1007/978-3-032-16708-8_26

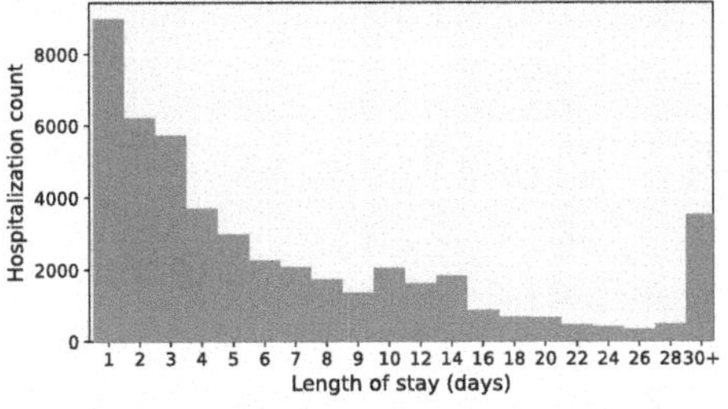

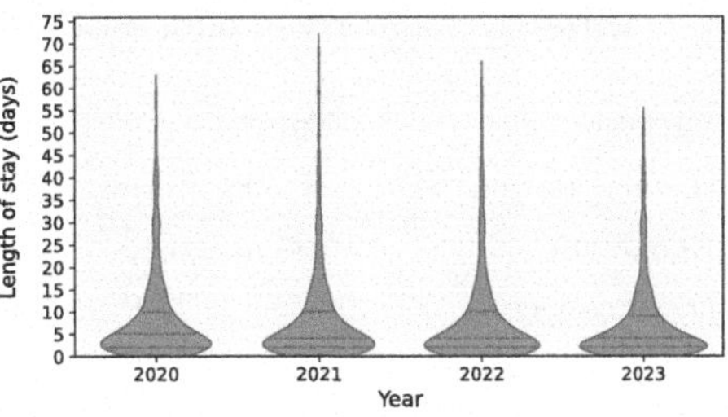

Fig. 1. Distribution of length of stay in days overall (left) and for specific years (right). In the violin plots, observations above the 98th percentile have been excluded for clarity, while black horizontal bars denote the 25th, 50th (median), and 75th percentiles.

Locale di Alba e Bra, ASL CN2) in Piedmont, Italy, made available through the TrustAlert research project,[1] an Italian initiative aimed at developing early-warning, monitoring, and forecasting tools for public health agencies. Spanning four years (2020–2023) and encompassing 37,526 unique patients, 55,684 hospitalizations, and 66 healthcare facilities, the dataset provides a comprehensive view of patient- and hospital-related factors. This enabled a systematic exploration of factors associated with LoS, providing preliminary evidence that may inform future analyses and decision-support efforts in hospital management.

Our methodology (Sect. 2) began with selecting relevant patient records (Sect. 2.1) and transforming them into a structured dataset of patient, admission, and hospital features (Sect. 2.2). These features formed the basis of two analyses: (1) a statistical analysis examining their relationship with LoS (Sect. 2.3) and (2) a predictive modeling approach using machine learning—Random Forest and CatBoost regression models—with different encoding techniques, including pretrained embeddings for diagnosis and procedure codes (Sect. 2.4).

Our results (Sect. 3) revealed significant statistical correlations between LoS and selected features (Sect. 3.1) and demonstrated strong predictive performance, with CatBoost consistently outperforming Random Forest and all features contributing to model accuracy (Sect. 3.2). The study's conclusions (Sect. 5) offer valuable insights for future LoS analysis and prediction.

2 Methodology

2.1 Data

The dataset originates from the administrative healthcare flows of the Local Health Authority of Alba and Bra (ASL CN2) and includes healthcare events for residents of the municipalities within its jurisdiction. Record linkage across multiple administrative sources was carried out by Innovo Srl, which pseudonymized patient identifiers (e.g., encrypted fiscal codes) to enable the connection of healthcare events while preserving anonymity.

[1] https://www.trustalert.it/.

Table 1. Summary of data set characteristics (example data is artificial).

Variable	Value	Example
Hashed patient ID	37,526 unique patients	JL(&LFURP(!2
Age group	20 categories	35–39
Diagnosis code	3,689 ICD-9 unique codes	724.2 - Lumbago
Procedure code	1,645 ICD-9 unique codes	88.93 - MRI of the Spinal Canal
Facility	66 unique values	Az. Ospedal. S. Croce E Carle
Department	52 unique values	Neurology
Hospitalization type	Surgical, medical, ordinary	Medical
Admission date	01/01/2020 – 31/12/2023	22/07/2021
Discharge date	01/01/2020 – 31/12/2023	25/07/2021

Table 2. Facilities and % samples by cat.

Category	#	%
General/teaching hospitals	13	16.4
Specialized hospitals	6	5.8
Private clinics and rehab. centers	21	13.4
Local/community hospitals	19	62.6
Geriatric/long-term care facilities	2	0.7
Religious or charitable facilities	2	0.9
Rehab. centers and research inst.	3	0.3

Table 3. Yearly LoS statistics.

Year	#	%	Median	Std	IQR	Min	Max
2020	10,147	17.0	5	20.80	2–11	1	362
2021	15,142	25.4	5	23.67	2–11	1	360
2022	16,674	27.9	4	22.74	2–10	1	357
2023	17,721	29.7	4	16.17	2–9	1	328
all	59,684	100	4	20.94	2–10	1	362

We analyzed inpatient hospitalization records from January 2020 to December 2023, extracted from the administrative healthcare sources of ASL CN2. These records originate from the Hospital Discharge Records (Scheda di Dimissione Ospedaliera – SDO), the standardized form used nationwide in Italy to document all inpatient stays. The extracted dataset encompasses 66 healthcare facilities spanning multiple categories: local and community hospitals (62.6%), general and teaching hospitals (16.4%), private clinics and rehabilitation centers (13.4%), and smaller shares from specialized, geriatric, religious, and research institutions. The majority of hospitalizations are concentrated in a limited number of departments, out of a total of 52, specifically General Medicine (8,200), General Surgery (7,000), Orthopedics and Traumatology (6,700), Obstetrics and Gynecology (6,400), Physical Medicine and Rehabilitation (4,600), Cardiology (4,000), Urology (3,600), and Neonatology (3,600), which together account for approximately 75% of all inpatient stays. Although the majority of hospitalizations occurred within ASL CN2 facilities, the dataset also includes events involving ASL CN2 residents treated in hospitals outside its jurisdiction. Table 1 summarizes dataset characteristics, while Table 2 details facility categories.

The dataset includes 59,684 hospitalizations ($\geq$ 1 day) involving 37,526 patients. Admission and discharge dates enabled LoS calculation, while de-identified patient IDs allowed hospitalization history reconstruction. Each record

Table 4. Description of features used in the analysis.

Variable	Description
Age group	Age category as a four-year interval (e.g., 0 for newborns, 1–4, up to 90+).
# of comorbidities	Count of unique comorbid conditions based on patient's past diagnoses.
Comorbidity index	Elixhauser comorbidity index.
Diagnosis	Main diagnosis associated with the hospitalization.
Procedure	Main medical procedure performed during hospitalization.
Admission type	Hospitalization type: day hospital (medical/surgical) or standard inpatient.
Admission month	Month when the hospitalization occurred.
Patient volume	Adjusted hospitalizations for a diagnosis in the past three months.
Historical LoS	Average LoS for a diagnosis and hospital over the past three months.

contained age group, hospitalization type, main diagnosis, main procedure, hospital, and department. Diagnoses and interventions were coded according to the 9th revision of the International Classification of Diseases (ICD-9-CM), including the ICD-9 Procedure Coding System (PCS).

Figure 1 illustrates the distribution of the length of stay. The right panel shows the distribution of the length of stay separately for each year. In terms of hospitalization share, 2020 accounts for 17% of sample, while 2021, 2022, and 2023 contribute approximately 25%, 28% and 30% percent, respectively. Table 3 shows key statistics for each year. Notably, for each following year, the plot shows broader section around the median, meaning higher concentration around the typical values. The years 2020 and 2021 exhibit larger interquartile ranges (IQRs) compared to 2022 and 2023, suggesting greater variability and unpredictability in the LoS during those earlier years. These patterns likely reflect the impact of the COVID-19 pandemic. In 2020 and 2021, hospitals faced significant strain, leading to a reduction in non-COVID hospitalizations [19]. However, by 2022 and 2023, healthcare systems began to recover, resulting in more consistent hospitalization patterns.

2.2 Features

In this study, we examined features broadly classified into three categories: patient-related, admission-related, and hospital-related (see Table 4). While previous research has explored these feature categories in LoS prediction (see [10, 20] and references therein), existing studies often emphasize patient- and admission-related features, with less attention given to the role of hospital-related features and their temporal trends.

We transformed the raw hospitalization dataset into a structured feature set. For each entry in the original dataset, a corresponding record was created in the feature dataset. In some cases, the data were used directly, while in others, we applied transformations that incorporated historical records, as detailed below. This feature set was then analyzed for its relationship with LoS using statistical and predictive methods.

Patient Features. The patient's age group was taken directly from the hospitalization record and was represented as a categorical variable based on four-year intervals, starting with *0* (newborns), followed by *1–4*, *5–9*, and so on, up to *90+*. We computed the number of comorbidities and the Elixhauser comorbidity index [9], which quantify a patient's overall health, and have been previously associated with LoS [15]. These calculations were based on the patient's diagnosis history, which we constructed by extracting unique ICD-9 codes for prior diagnoses of a patient using admission dates to establish time ordering. We leveraged Python's comorbidity (`comorbiPy`) library[2] to calculate comorbidity measures.

Admission Features. Diagnosis and procedure are clearly important features that influence care complexity and, consequently, the LoS. We explored different representations for diagnoses and procedures to determine their suitability for our analysis. We used 100-dimensional diagnosis embeddings from Kane et al. [14] based on the BioGPT large language model [16], and 300-dimensional procedure embeddings from Choi et al. [8], trained with a neural language model. Since the diagnosis embeddings were originally designed for ICD-10 codes, we mapped ICD-9 codes to ICD-10 using the General Equivalence Mappings in Python's `icdmappings` library[3]. We also tested one-hot and target encoding as alternative representations in preliminary experiments to identify the effective approach. Furthermore, we included month and type of admission to capture seasonal trends and variations in hospital practices.

Hospital Features. Previous studies suggest that higher-volume hospitals may have more experience, specialized expertise, and established care protocols [3, 13]. It is therefore plausible that hospital volume influences LoS. We modeled the hospital patient volume feature as the number of patients admitted to the hospital with a specific diagnosis over the past three months, normalized by the total number of observation days. To account for LoS variations across hospitals, we introduced a feature reflecting the average past hospitalization duration for each hospital, department, and diagnosis. For a given hospitalization record, we identified prior hospitalizations within the past three months that shared the same hospital, department, and diagnosis. Based on these historical records, we computed the observed mean LoS. To mitigate data scarcity, we also calculated a global mean LoS for related diagnoses using the `drgpy` library, which groups diagnoses into Diagnosis Related Groups (MS-DRG) based on hospital resource usage [7]. Finally, a smoothed mean was obtained by combining the observed and global means using a Bayesian approach with a smoothing parameter of five.

2.3 Statistical Analysis

The statistical analysis explored features influencing LoS from multiple angles. Since diagnosis and procedure are known to be strong predictors of LoS [20], they

[2] https://comorbidipy.readthedocs.io/en/latest/.
[3] https://pypi.org/project/icd-mappings/.

were excluded from our statistical analysis to focus on broader, less explored hospital-, admission-, and patient-related factors.

Using the feature set outlined in Sect. 2.2, the number of comorbidities and comorbidity index were discretized into categories [1], while other categorical variables (age group, admission type, and admission month) were used directly. Because some patients experienced multiple hospitalizations, we aggregated the data at the patient level to satisfy the independence assumption. Specifically, for each patient we computed the median length of stay and assigned a dominant category for each grouping variable (i.e., the most frequent value observed for that patient). The relationship between each of these variables and LoS was then assessed using the Kruskal-Wallis test [6], which is robust to non-normal distributions and suitable for comparing LoS across independent groups. Additionally, LoS variability within each category was summarized by the median, interquartile range, and standard deviation. To examine the relationships between patient volume, historical LoS, and LoS, we employed mixed-effects linear models with LoS as the outcome variable. Separate models were estimated using patient volume and historical LoS as independent variables, incorporating diagnosis as a random effect. To account for potential temporal variations, we explored interaction terms to assess how these relationships change over time. Statistical significance was assessed at a 0.05 significance level to identify meaningful associations. The results are presented in Sect. 3.1.

2.4 Predictive Modeling

Machine Learning Models. We employed machine learning models to assess the predictive power of the considered features (see Table 4). Due to likely complex, non-linear relationship between features and LoS, we framed the task as a non-linear regression problem and employed two robust tree-based models: Random Forest and CatBoost [17]. Random Forest uses multiple decision trees to reduce overfitting and achieve model generalization. On the other hand, CatBoost is specifically optimized for categorical data and often outperforms other gradient boosting algorithms in structured data sets, particularly when dealing with large numbers of categorical features [17]. Both models efficiently handle large, diverse datasets and have been shown to outperform other regression models in predicting LoS [11]. Interestingly, the models exhibited different sensitivities to how categorical features were represented. CatBoost performed best when diagnosis and procedure features were used as categorical variables, likely because of its built-in target encoding, which encodes each category based on the mean value of the target variable for that category. In contrast, Random Forest showed weaker performance when categorical features were used directly or one-hot encoded but performed best when represented as embeddings. In our results (Sect. 3.2), we present only the best-performing configurations: embeddings for Random Forest and categorical variables for CatBoost.

Validation Approach. Given the potential seasonal trends exhibited by LoS, we split data into training, validation and test sets on a per-year basis to assess the models' capability to capture these variations. To assess the impact of additional historical data on model performance, we designed two *split scenarios*. In the first, machine learning models were trained on hospitalization records from 2021, validated on 2022 records, and tested on 2023 records. In the second, the training set was expanded to include records from both 2020 and 2021, while the validation and test sets remained the same (2022 and 2023, respectively). This comparison enabled us to evaluate whether incorporating additional historical data from further in the past improves model performance. For hyperparameter tuning, we conducted a grid search to evaluate various hyperparameter combinations and determine the best configuration for each model.

Evaluation Metrics. To evaluate the quality of fit, we used adjusted R^2 and mean absolute error (MAE). We assessed these metrics for both the training and validation sets. Adjusted R^2 measures the proportion of variance explained by the model. Because it accounts for the number of predictors, it is more suitable than standard R^2 when comparing models with different feature sets [12]. A consistently high adjusted R^2 value across the training and validation sets suggests that the model captures a significant portion of variability without overfitting. On the other side, MAE offers a straightforward measure of prediction accuracy by averaging the absolute differences between predicted and actual values. To evaluate the generalizability of the models on the test sets, in addition to MAE we used also root mean squared error (RMSE), which in contrast to MAE, penalizes large errors more heavily due to squaring [4].

3 Results

3.1 Statistical Analysis

Tables 5 and 6 summarize the descriptive statistics for the analyzed features, including patient-related variables (age group, number of comorbidities, and Elixhauser comorbidity index) and admission-related variables (month and type of admission).

The largest patient cohort, aged 70–84 years, made up about 28% of all cases. The youngest group (0–14 years) had a narrow IQR (1–4 days), indicating short, predictable stays. Young adults (15–24 years) showed the highest LoS variability, with a standard deviation of 30 days, while the oldest patients (90+) had the most predictable stays, with a standard deviation of around 10 days.

Around 90% of hospitalizations involved patients with no comorbidities, with a median LoS of 4 days. The presence of comorbidities doubled the median LoS to 8 days, with no significant change across 1, 2, or 3+ comorbidities. A higher Elixhauser index was associated with significantly longer and more variable stays.

Hospital admissions peaked in October–November and dropped sharply in December. January and February had the highest LoS variability, while October, November, and December showed the lowest variability.

Ordinary admissions, making up 80% of cases, had a median LoS of 5 days. Surgical cases had the shortest and most predictable stays (median: 1 day), while medical cases had the longest and most variable stays.

Table 5. Patient statistics for different variables across all inpatient admissions. All analyzed variables showed a statistically significant relationship with LoS ($p < 0.001$)

Variable	Type	Number	%	Length of stay (days)				
				Median	Std	IQR	Min	Max
Age group	0	3,215	5.39	3	4.50	2–4	1	158
	1–4	2,215	3.71	3	7.67	2–4	1	108
	5–9	898	1.50	2	22.41	1–4	1	349
	10–14	599	1.00	2	25.11	1–4	1	357
	15–19	927	1.55	3	29.55	1–6	1	316
	20–24	1,183	1.98	3	31.24	1–6	1	352
	25–29	1,824	3.06	3	22.25	2–5	1	343
	30–34	2,646	4.43	3	13.08	2–4	1	351
	35–39	2,485	4.16	3	20.71	2–5	1	348
	40–44	1,976	3.31	3	22.14	1–6	1	355
	45–49	2,510	4.21	3	26.02	1–9	1	342
	50–54	3,184	5.33	3	29.75	1–9	1	352
	55–59	4,092	6.86	4	21.55	1–11	1	338
	60–64	4,374	7.33	4	24.11	2–11	1	339
	65–69	4,793	8.03	5	19.97	2–12	1	322
	70–74	5,558	9.31	6	22.71	2–14	1	362
	75–79	5,734	9.61	7	18.50	3–14	1	359
	80–84	5,566	9.33	8	19.79	4–15	1	362
	85–89	3,893	6.52	9	17.69	5–16	1	350
	90+	2,012	3.37	9	10.41	5–15	1	118
Number of comorbidities	0	53,533	89.69	4	19.50	2–9	1	362
	1	5,578	9.35	8	30.88	3–17	1	338
	2	552	0.92	8	18.23	4–17	1	198
	3+	21	0.04	8	8.89	4–19	1	31
Elixhauser comorbidity index	Low (,2]	54,542	91.38	4	19.47	2–10	1	362
	Moderate [3,5]	629	1.05	8	14.79	3–15	1	191
	High [6,10]	3,165	5.30	7	35.86	2–17	1	338
	Very High [11,)	1,348	2.26	9	27.07	4–18	1	323

Age group, number of comorbidities, comorbidity index, admission type, and month all showed a statistically significant relationship with LoS ($p < 0.001$).

The mixed-effects model results indicated that in 2020, higher patient volume was associated with shorter LoS, but this relationship weakened or reversed in the following years, 2021, 2022, and 2023, with higher volume leading to longer LoS over time. Additionally, the influence of past hospitalization durations on

Table 6. Admission-related statistics across all inpatient admissions. All analyzed features showed a statistically significant relationship with LoS ($p < 0.001$)

Variable	Type	Number	%	Length of stay (days)				
				Median	Std	IQR	Min	Max
Month of admission	January	4,641	7.78	5	44.62	2–13	1	362
	February	4,617	7.74	4	26.07	2–10	1	323
	March	5,175	8.67	4	23.04	2–11	1	294
	April	4,381	7.34	5	20.60	2–12	1	267
	May	5,076	8.50	5	18.93	2–11	1	232
	June	5,079	8.51	4	17.41	2–10	1	198
	July	5,329	8.93	4	18.77	2–11	1	180
	August	4,509	7.55	5	16.08	2–11	1	146
	September	5,270	8.83	4	13.35	2–10	1	112
	October	5,900	9.89	4	12.24	2–10	1	90
	November	5,600	9.38	4	9.03	2–10	1	58
	December	4,107	6.88	3	4.79	2–7	1	30
Type of admission	Surgical	8,090	13.55	1	11.82	1–1	1	253
	Medical	3,777	6.33	7	58.92	2–35	1	362
	Ordinary	47,817	80.12	5	14.34	3–11	1	359

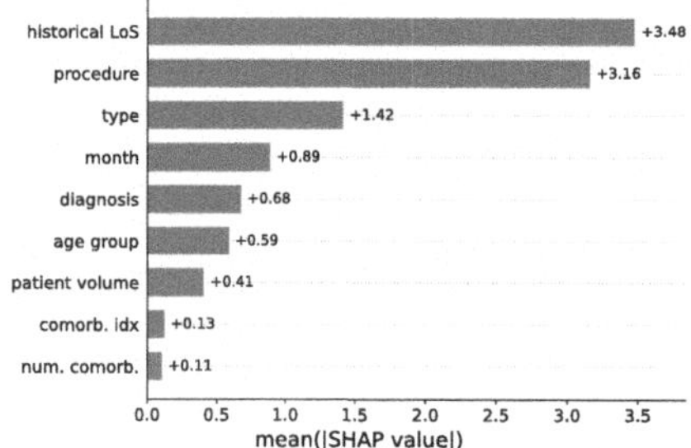

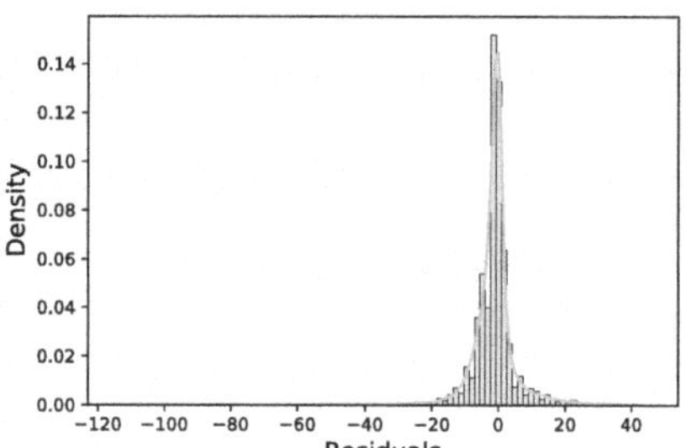

Fig. 2. SHAP feature importance bar plot (Left) and residuals distribution histogram (Right) for the CatBoost model trained on 2021 data with all features. Outliers below the 2nd and above the 98th percentile were removed from the histogram for clarity.

current LoS has grown stronger in recent years. These trends were supported by statistically significant interaction terms at the 0.05 level.

3.2 LoS Prediction Performance

We conducted experiments with six distinct feature sets to assess their impact on model performance. Starting with patient characteristics and diagnosis, we incrementally added procedure, admission type, month, patient volume, and

Table 7. Performance of regression models on training, validation, and test datasets across two evaluation splits. Acronyms: RF – Random Forest, CB – CatBoost. Metrics: MAE – Mean Absolute Error, R^2 – R-squared, RMSE – Root Mean Squared Error.

R#	Model	Train: 2021, Val: 2022, Test: 2023						Train: 2020–21, Val: 2022, Test: 2023					
		Train		Validation		Test		Train		Validation		Test	
		MAE	R^2	MAE	R^2	MAE	RMSE	MAE	R^2	MAE	R^2	MAE	RMSE
Patient features + diagnosis													
1	RF	8.40	0.29	8.62	0.21	7.71	14.74	8.26	0.28	8.50	0.22	7.62	14.71
2	CB	7.37	0.26	7.64	0.16	6.82	15.40	7.17	0.26	7.34	0.19	6.41	14.70
+ procedure													
3	RF	7.79	0.33	8.12	0.19	7.25	14.26	7.67	0.31	7.91	0.20	7.07	14.11
4	CB	6.79	0.34	7.02	0.23	6.28	14.59	6.78	0.33	6.72	0.27	5.89	13.92
+ type													
5	RF	7.77	0.35	8.06	0.22	7.24	14.12	7.63	0.34	7.85	0.24	7.07	13.95
6	CB	6.58	0.43	6.94	0.34	6.09	13.98	6.33	0.44	6.73	0.36	5.90	13.76
+ month													
7	RF	7.75	0.36	8.08	0.22	7.27	14.18	7.65	0.33	7.89	0.23	7.10	14.00
8	CB	6.40	0.48	6.90	0.38	6.17	14.06	6.17	0.51	6.68	0.42	5.86	13.34
+ patient volume													
9	RF	7.77	0.35	8.07	0.22	7.26	14.13	7.65	0.32	7.88	0.23	7.07	13.97
10	CB	5.93	0.55	6.74	0.39	6.03	13.69	6.20	0.51	6.64	0.43	5.88	13.13
+ historical LoS													
11	RF	7.58	0.39	7.83	0.26	6.99	13.58	7.52	0.36	7.71	0.27	6.88	13.49
12	CB	5.66	0.60	6.04	0.49	4.88	11.44	5.73	0.57	6.01	0.49	4.91	11.62

historical LoS, evaluating models across two split scenarios. Results for Random Forest and CatBoost are shown in Table 7.

Overall, CatBoost consistently outperformed Random Forest across all metrics, feature combinations, and evaluation scenarios. For the CatBoost models, the best configuration consisted of a maximum of 128 one-hot splits, a tree depth of 10, 5000 boosting iterations, an L2 regularization coefficient of 3, a learning rate of 0.05, a random seed of 42, and a random strength of 1.

Further analysis of CatBoost revealed that adding the procedure feature alongside patient characteristics and diagnosis improved performance, as reflected by reduced validation and test MAE/RMSE and increased R^2 (rows 2 and 4). Incorporating admission type significantly boosted validation R^2 from 0.23 to 0.34 (rows 4 and 6), while validation MAE remained stable. Test results supported this improvement, with RMSE decreasing from 14.59 to 13.89 in the first evaluation split and from 13.92 to 13.76 in the second. Adding admission month had the most impact in the two-year split scenario, where validation R^2 rose from 0.36 to 0.42, and test RMSE dropped from 13.76 to 13.34 (rows 6 and 8). This suggests that a larger dataset helps the model capture seasonal trends more effectively. The inclusion of patient volume led to further performance gains (rows 8 and 10). Finally, historical LoS provided the greatest improvement (rows

10 and 12). However, training on both 2020 and 2021 data did not outperform using 2021 alone on the 2023 test set, likely due to shifts in patterns from 2020 making the model less representative (see Sect. 3.1).

Figure 2 illustrates the SHAP feature importance bar plot (Left) and residuals distribution histogram (Right) for the best-performing CatBoost model (trained on 2021 data with all features). Historical length of stay and procedure were the most influential features, which is consistent with expectations, as both are strong predictors of a patient's length of stay. On the other hand, the number of comorbidities and the Elixhauser comorbidity index show minimal impact, which is expected due to the highly skewed distribution of these values in our dataset. The residuals exhibit an approximately normal distribution, indicating that the model is well-fitted with random, unbiased errors. The distribution is centered around zero, which suggests there is no significant bias in the predictions.

4 Discussion

In our dataset, diagnoses are recorded at hospital discharge, reflecting information primarily used for administrative and reimbursement purposes rather than detailed clinical assessment. This has two main implications. First, discharge diagnoses may not fully capture the patient's condition at admission, particularly in cases with complications or comorbidities that develop during hospitalization. Second, predictive models based on these diagnoses cannot be applied in real time at admission, since the final discharge diagnosis is inherently unknown at that stage.

A further limitation is that model evaluation was performed at the aggregate level, without stratifying by patient subgroups. Consequently, systematic differences in predictive accuracy across specific subpopulations cannot be ruled out. Future work will involve subgroup-level analyses to assess model robustness and identify potential biases.

Finally, the mapping from ICD-9 to ICD-10 codes is not always one-to-one, which may introduce some inaccuracy in the analysis employing ICD-10-based embeddings for diagnoses.

5 Conclusions

Understanding hospital length of stay is crucial for optimizing resource management and improving patient care. By identifying the key factors influencing LoS, hospitals can better anticipate inpatient demand and allocate resources efficiently.

In this study, we examined patient-, admission-, and hospital-related features for LoS prediction. CatBoost consistently outperformed Random Forest, with model performance improving as additional features were incorporated. Historical LoS emerged as the most influential predictor. Interestingly, while higher patient volume in 2020 was associated with shorter LoS, this trend reversed from

2021 onward, suggesting that increasing patient loads may have strained hospital capacity over time.

With all features included, CatBoost achieved a validation R^2 of 0.49, indicating moderate predictive power and demonstrating the potential of machine learning approaches to capture complex relationships in administrative healthcare data. Additionally, target encoding for diagnosis and procedures outperformed previously published embeddings.

While these models provide useful insights into factors associated with LoS, predictions cannot currently be applied at admission, and subgroup-level performance remains to be evaluated. Future work should include subgroup-level analyses and explore integration with task-specific embeddings from large language models to improve robustness and generalizability.

References

1. Austin, S.R., Wong, Y.N., Uzzo, R.G., Beck, J.R., Egleston, B.L.: Why summary comorbidity measures such as the charlson comorbidity index and elixhauser score work. Medical Care **53**(9) (2015)
2. Baek, H., Cho, M., Kim, S., Hwang, H., Song, M., Yoo, S.: Analysis of length of hospital stay using electronic health records: a statistical and data mining approach. PLOS ONE (2018)
3. Birkmeyer, J.D., et al.: Hospital volume and surgical mortality in the united states. NEJM **346**(15), 1128–1137 (2002)
4. Bishop, C.M.: Pattern Recognition and Machine Learning. ISS, Springer, New York (2006). https://doi.org/10.1007/978-0-387-45528-0_9
5. Bueno, H.: Trends in length of stay and short-term outcomes among medicare patients hospitalized for heart failure, 1993–2006. JAMA **303**(21), 2141 (2010)
6. Carter, E.M., Potts, H.W.: Predicting length of stay from an electronic patient record system: a primary total knee replacement example. BMC Med. Inform. Decis. Mak. **14**(1) (2014)
7. Centers for Medicare and Medicaid Services: Design and development of the Diagnosis Related Group (DRG) (2025), Accessed 21 Feb 2026
8. Choi, Y., Chiu, C.Y.I., Sontag, D.: Learning low-dimensional representations of medical concepts. AMIA Summits Translational Sci. Proc. **2016**, 41 (2016)
9. Elixhauser, A., Steiner, C., Harris, D.R., Coffey, R.M.: Comorbidity measures for use with administrative data. Med. Care **36**(1), 8–27 (1998)
10. Gokhale, S., et al.: Hospital length of stay prediction tools for all hospital admissions and general medicine populations: systematic review and meta-analysis. Front. Med. **10** (2023)
11. Jain, R., Singh, M., Rao, A.R., Garg, R.: Predicting hospital length of stay using machine learning on a large open health dataset. BMC Heal. Serv. Res. **24**(1) (2024)
12. James, G., Witten, D., Hastie, T., Tibshirani, R.: An introduction to statistical learning: with applications in R. Springer (2013)
13. Kahn, J.M., Goss, C.H., Heagerty, P.J., Kramer, A.A., O'Brien, C.R., Rubenfeld, G.D.: Hospital volume and the outcomes of mechanical ventilation. NEJM **355**(1), 41–50 (2006)

14. Kane, M.J., King, C., Esserman, D., Latham, N.K., Greene, E.J., Ganz, D.A.: A compressed large language model embedding dataset of ICD 10 CM descriptions. medRxiv (2023)
15. Liu, J., Larson, E., Hessels, A., Cohen, B., Zachariah, P., Caplan, D., Shang, J.: Comparison of measures to predict mortality and length of stay in hospitalized patients. Nurs. Res. **68**(3), 200–209 (2019)
16. Luo, R., et al.: BioGPT: generative pre-trained transformer for biomedical text generation and mining. Brief, Bioinform (2022)
17. Prokhorenkova, L., Gusev, G., Vorobev, A., Dorogush, A.V., Gulin, A.: CatBoost: unbiased boosting with categorical features. In: NIPS. vol. 31 (2018)
18. Rotter, T., et al.: Clinical pathways: effects on professional practice, patient outcomes, length of stay and hospital costs. Cochrane Database Syst. Rev. (2010)
19. Santi, L., et al.: Non-covid-19 patients in times of pandemic: Emergency department visits, hospitalizations and cause-specific mortality in northern italy. PLoS ONE **16**(3), e0248995 (2021)
20. Stone, K., Zwiggelaar, R., Jones, P., Mac Parthaláin, N.: A systematic review of the prediction of hospital length of stay: towards a unified framework. PLOS Digital Heal. **1**(4) (2022)

Patient management

Depth Sensor Based AI-Services for Nursing Homes

Rinu Elizabeth Paul(✉), Lucas Deichsel, and Tanja Schultz

Cognitive Systems Lab (CSL), University of Bremen, Bremen, Germany
{rinueliz,luc_dei,tanja.schultz}@uni-bremen.de

Abstract. Falls are a frequent and critical event among older adults, often leading to severe consequences such as injuries, loss of independence, fear of walking, and even death. Therefore, it is essential to detect and prevent them. AI services in homes and nursing facilities enable early fall detection and timely support. Another major concern in nursing homes and clinics is the frequency of bed-exit attempts by residents or patients who cannot stand independently. These individuals often overlook their limitations and attempt to get out of bed alone, increasing the risk of falling. Our approach focuses on bed-exit detection to notify caregivers in real time, potentially preventing these incidents. We present a system that uses depth video to detect falls and bed-exit attempts among older adults. A configuration interface is developed to provide seamless access to fall and bed-exit detection functionalities and their results. The interface is compatible with various operating systems and optimized for both CPU and GPU versions, making it suitable for home and nursing facility applications. Our system achieves 68% accuracy and a 69% F1-score for fall detection, and 82% accuracy and an 88% F1-score for bed-exit detection. Room occupancy detection, which determines whether an older adult is present in the room, achieved 92% accuracy and an 89% F1-score. This work demonstrates significant potential to enhance services that improve assisted living environments.

Keywords: Fall detection · Bed-exit detection · Room occupancy detection · Depth video · Elderly care · Smart healthcare · Computer vision · Assisted living · Interface · Real-time monitoring · AI for accessibility

1 Introduction

Falls in older adults can occur for various reasons, including medication side effects, balance problems, and mobility disorders [14,21,30]. They also happen when older adults walk to the toilet, stumble over obstacles or carpets, or forget to call for assistance before getting up. The annual fall rate for adults over 65 is 30%, increases with age, and half of those affected fall more than once per

R. E. Paul and L. Deichsel—These authors contributed equally to this work.

P. Bruno et al. (Eds.): HC_AIxIA_HYDRA 2025, CCIS 2830, pp. 323–335, 2026.
https://doi.org/10.1007/978-3-032-16708-8_27

year [18]. Falls can cause injuries, increase the need for walking aids, trigger a fear of falling again, and may even result in death [3,28]. About 10% of falls cause serious injuries [24]. They also place both mental and physical stress on caregivers [12,20,29]. The most urgent detection cases involve residents falling in their rooms without being found, such as during the night. Another critical case is when a resident gets up after a fall—either on their own or with help from friends or relatives—and forgets to notify the caregiver [17]. In such situations, serious or even fatal injuries may go unnoticed, leading to severe consequences. Therefore, detecting falls and notifying caregivers is crucial to ensure timely assistance. Falls also frequently occur when older adults leave their beds without support. Some residents face a temporary or permanent risk of falling while getting out of bed. Temporary risk factors include recent surgery or medication, while permanent factors include balance issues when transitioning from lying to standing. Bed-exit detection is essential, as many falls happen during this activity, often due to a loss of balance. Timely caregiver intervention can prevent such incidents. In these cases, attempting to get out of bed without help can lead to falls. Thus, detecting bed exits and notifying caregivers can help prevent such accidents.

AI services in healthcare are a growing research focus. Here, we focus on camera and sensor-based monitoring for fall and bed-exit detection, and a few prior studies in this field are as follows. The work in [10] studied 5–10 independent older adults in their homes, collecting data using infrared motion, light, temperature, and humidity sensors, along with weekly telehealth and monthly in-person nurse visits over six months. AI algorithms were trained to detect falls, sleep disturbances, and chronic conditions. The study in [32] used a simulated dataset with motion and wearable sensors over nine years, modeling individual homes to detect abnormalities such as falls. The smart home study in [4] involved 30 older adults over three years, logging daily patterns using infrared and contact sensors to predict next-day activity and detect anomalies. In [23], air quality, infrared motion, temperature, and humidity sensors were used along with wearable devices monitoring heart rate, blood pressure, and respiration. Their system detected falls and health anomalies with over 90% accuracy. The real-time system in [33] used an RGB video-based human activity recognition model to detect falls, chest pain, and staggering. In [5], a pressure-sensitive mattress in hospital wards detected bed exits and prevented 88% of related falls by notifying staff via smartphones.

While most studies focus on fall detection, only a few address bed-exit detection in smart homes with AI services. Our focus is on nursing homes, which house many older adults across multiple rooms—a setting rarely explored in existing research. Instead of relying on wearable sensors—which are uncomfortable, easy to forget, and often impractical—or privacy-sensitive RGB and RGB+depth sensors, we used a depth sensor–only setup. We also developed a configuration interface to improve the AI service system. This paper presents two AI services designed to support care in nursing homes: fall detection, which identifies when a fall occurs, and bed-exit detection, which detects attempts to leave the bed and helps prevent falls. Both services use depth images as input, offering partial privacy protection. We used privacy-aware depth sensors, where individuals can only be identified by their gait. In addition, we developed room occupancy detection to determine whether a resident is present in the room. The configuration interface combines these services, allowing users to start the system and check results. We created different versions of the interface for different environments—for example, a CPU version for individual homes and a GPU version that can support multiple rooms in a nursing home.

2 AI Pipeline

The AI pipeline is shown in Fig. 1. AI services include fall, bed exit, and room occupancy detection in nursing homes with multiple rooms at any given time, utilizing depth sensors. The pipeline comprises feature extraction models and AI service models that identify falls, bed exits, and room occupancy, all integrated through a configuration interface to form an end-to-end system. In this study, we evaluated each model and the configuration interface with the full pipeline. Depth images were continuously transferred to the processor. When the interface was started, the pretrained feature extraction model began extracting skeleton joint features from the depth images. Models for room occupancy detection (OD), fall detection (FD), and bed-exit detection (BD) were executed sequentially, and the results were stored in a file. This file was used to record all detected events. The feature extraction, OD, FD, and BD models were trained and tested separately and were integrated into the interface.

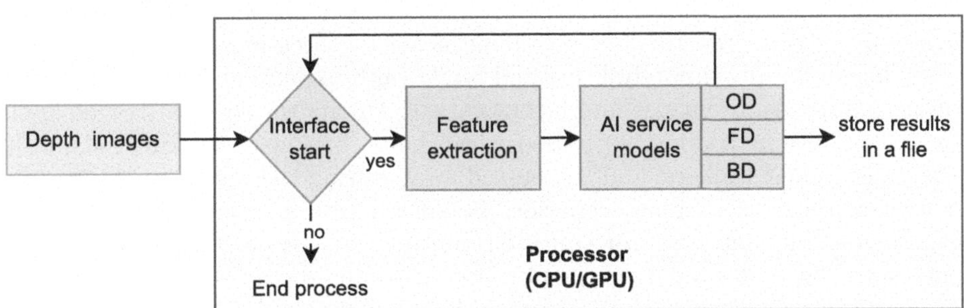

Fig. 1. AI pipeline; the interface is executed in the processor using depth images. AI service models denote OD: occupancy detection, FD: fall detection, and BD: Bed-exit detection.

In the following sections, we describe the devices used, the training process, and the parameterization of the feature extraction and AI service models (OD, FD, and BD). Before training the models, we introduce the dataset used for training and evaluation.

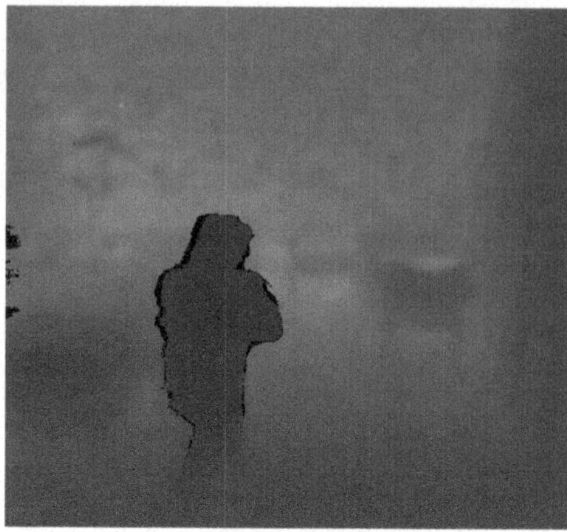

Fig. 2. Reference depth image showing a person in a resident room.

2.1 Dataset

We collected depth images from nursing facilities using wall-mounted depth sensors; one sensor per room [25]. The depth images, such as those shown in Fig. 2, included headers with the date, time, and IP address of the sensor. Each image had a resolution of 640 × 480 pixels, was recorded at 10 frames per second (fps), and stored in a 16-bit depth map format. The data was collected after ethical approval from the German Society of Nursing Science. Our dataset comprises 58,037 h of depth data from 45 residents (average per month: 3,627 h; standard deviation: 1,327 h), recorded over 27 months across three nursing homes. While sensor height (approximately 2 m) and angle (approximately 20°) were consistent across rooms, room size and layout varied. Among the residents (aged ≥ 60 years), 8% were bedridden, 20% used wheelchairs, 38% used walking aids, 30% were independent walkers, and 3% passed away during the study. In this paper, we focused on single-person scenarios, as older adults typically reside alone in their rooms. The depth sensor captured multiple images per second, creating a continuous video stream. Each pixel represented the distance from the sensor. The depth images, such as those shown in Fig. 2, included headers with the date, time, and IP address of the sensor. Each image had a resolution of 640 × 480 pixels, was recorded at 10 frames per second (fps), and stored in a 16-bit depth map format.

2.2 Metrics

We used the following metrics to evaluate the performance of the skeleton extraction model. The Percentage of Correct Keypoints (PCK) measures the percentage of joints within a certain distance (typically 15cm) [34]. This metric ranges from 0–100%, with higher values indicating better performance.

$$PCK = \frac{100}{N} \sum_{i=1}^{N} \begin{cases} 1, & \text{if } \|K_i - J_i\|_2 < 15\,cm \\ 0, & \text{else} \end{cases} \tag{1}$$

For occupancy, fall, and bed-exit detection, we used accuracy, precision, recall, and F1 score. Precision, recall, and F1 score are especially valuable when evaluating models on imbalanced datasets. True Positive (TP), True Negative (TN), False Positive (FP), and False Negative (FN).

$$\text{Precision} = \frac{TP}{TP + FP} \tag{2}$$

$$\text{Recall} = \frac{TP}{TP + FN} \tag{3}$$

$$\text{F1 Score} = 2 \cdot \frac{\text{Precision} \cdot \text{Recall}}{\text{Precision} + \text{Recall}} \tag{4}$$

Cohen's Kappa (κ) is a statistical measure used to evaluate the interrater agreement for activity annotations. Unlike simple percent agreement, it takes into account the agreement occurring by chance. P_o is the observed agreement between raters (i.e., the proportion of times the raters agree), and P_e is the expected agreement by chance, calculated based on the marginal probabilities of each category.

$$\kappa = \frac{P_o - P_e}{1 - P_e} \tag{5}$$

Annotation: We used the Computer Vision Annotation Tool (CVAT) [6] to annotate skeletons and activities. Fifteen skeleton joints and several activities were annotated in the depth videos. To ensure consistency among annotators, we provided proper training and evaluation. We achieved interrater reliability with an average PCK score above 85% for skeleton annotations and an average Kappa score of 90% for activity annotations. Activities labeled for the fall detection model included 'fall' and 'controlled fall'. Controlled falls were performed by staff to augment the dataset. For bed-exit detection, we used the activity 'sit in bed', which indicated a person sitting on the bed edge with legs down. This posture was considered a precursor to a bed exit; thus, detecting it could alert caregivers. Other annotated activities included 'walk', 'stand', 'sit in chair', 'stand to sit', and 'sit to stand'.

2.3 Feature Extraction: Skeleton Extraction Model

Pose estimation involves extracting human structural features from images. Common approaches include skeleton extraction [22], silhouette extraction [8], and Center of Mass (CoM) estimation [7]. In this study, we used skeleton extraction to obtain joint features from depth images. Well-known skeleton extraction models include ResNet [31], OpenPose [11], and PopNet [13], typically trained on ground truth data from intrusive Motion Capture (MoCap) systems. In our previous studies [15,16], we evaluated these models on lab-collected depth data and found ResNet performed best. For feature extraction in this work, we used the ResNet model [31], trained separately using the L1 norm as proposed by Sun et al.

2.4 Occupied Room Detection Model

Although the primary focus was fall and bed-exit detection, we also developed an occupied room detection feature to determine whether the room was occupied. This is useful when residents should not leave the room unaccompanied. Previous studies have used depth or infrared sensors [2] and environmental sensors [19] (e.g., CO_2, temperature) for occupancy detection. In contrast, we used only a depth sensor. Unoccupied frames appeared when residents left for meals or group activities. We applied frame subtraction to identify contours, using contour size and count as features. As presented in our previous work [25], we determined room occupancy by detecting changes across consecutive frames using absolute frame subtraction. Specifically, each frame was subtracted from the next 15 consecutive frames, and the resulting heatmaps were analyzed to identify contours—regions of significant pixel change. Two features were extracted: the number of contours and the size of the largest contour. Ideally, the largest contour corresponded to the shape of a human figure. We used Decision Tree (DT) and K-Nearest Neighbor (KNN) classifiers for room occupancy detection.

2.5 Fall Detection Model

Most fall detection studies used RGB cameras [27], RGB+depth sensors [26], or accelerometers [1]. We used depth-only sensors to preserve residents' privacy. A fall occurs when a person drops to the ground, often from a chair, bed, or while standing. Our dataset included controlled falls, where trained staff safely simulated a fall for data augmentation. In total, we collected 25 falls across both hard and controlled categories. The skeleton joint coordinates extracted from the feature extraction model were converted into global 3D coordinates using camera intrinsics (focal length, camera height, and tilt). Fall detection was based on the vertical position of the neck joint in global coordinates. A threshold was selected from the training set; data points were classified as 'fall' if the neck's vertical position dropped below this threshold. The optimal threshold was determined by iteratively evaluating multiple values on the training set.

2.6 Bed-Exit Detection Model

Prior work [5] used zone-based depth sensors specific to bed height and position, while another study [9] employed mattress pressure sensors. We developed an activity recognition model to detect bed exits. The labels used for human activity recognition included 'sit in bed', 'sit in chair', 'walk with walker', 'walk', 'stand', 'stand to sit', 'sit to stand', and 'stand with walker'. We used an LSTM-based model to classify these activities. The activity 'sit in bed'—defined as a person sitting at the edge of the bed with legs down—was labeled as a bed-exit. The model was trained for multi-class detection across the eight activities. After classification, activities labeled as 'sit in bed' were considered bed-exits, and all others as non-bed-exits.

3 Configuration Interface

The configuration interface was developed to integrate and execute all models for the AI service system. It manages input and output of depth data, preprocesses input for each model, runs the models, generates a CSV output file, maintains logs, and removes temporary files after post-processing. During real-time, the input file is updated with the latest frames. Both CPU-based and GPU-based versions of the interface were developed to accommodate different use cases, such as single-person monitoring at home or multi-person monitoring in nursing homes.

3.1 CPU-Based Interface

The CPU-based interface is suitable for continuous home monitoring, where a single depth sensor is sufficient. The graphical configuration interface was implemented in Python using the Kivy framework. As shown in Fig. 3, the application provides editable fields to specify input and output folders, along with a 'Process' button to initiate execution. The steps include reading the binary depth file, detecting room occupancy, extracting skeletons, identifying falls and bed exits, and managing temporary files. Real-time status updates are displayed at the bottom of the interface. Final results are saved as a CSV file for long-term use. All steps and errors are recorded in logs for debugging. To simplify deployment, the complete AI package was converted into a standalone executable using PyInstaller, which includes all required Python modules and trained model weights, allowing the system to run without additional installations.

3.2 GPU-Based Interface

The GPU-based interface is designed for nursing homes and clinics with multiple sensors. In this setup, sensor data is streamed to a central GPU where processing is executed. GPU acceleration and parallel processing across multiple GPU cores are utilized. Unlike the graphical interface used in the CPU version, this version employs a Command Line Interface (CLI), which is more suitable for centralized systems. The interface reads data from a continuously updated input file and processes frames in batches. Logs track progress and errors, with each sensor assigned a corresponding output file updated in real time. This version was also packaged as a standalone executable using PyInstaller, designed for deployment on Linux systems with CUDA support.

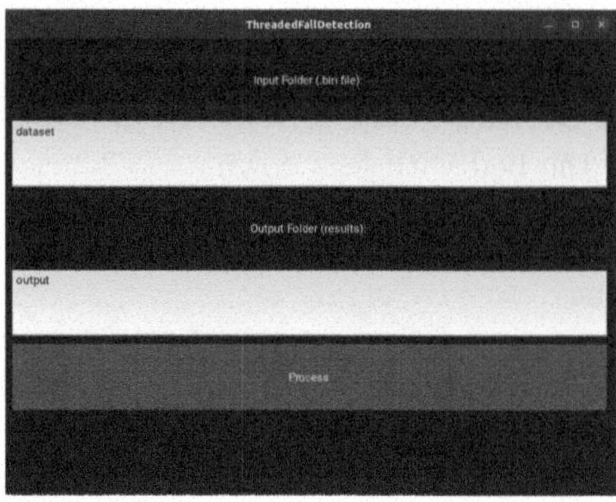

Fig. 3. AI Application graphical configuration interface and process flow.

4 Results and Discussion

4.1 Evaluation of Occupied Room Detection

The occupied room detection model developed in our previous paper [25] was used in this pipeline. We used 17 h of non-occupied data and 11 h of occupied data. The entire dataset was split into training, validation, and test sets using an 80:10:10 ratio, ensuring a balanced distribution of occupied and non-occupied data in each set. The training set was used to train the models, the validation set to optimize parameters, and the test set to evaluate model accuracy. Due to the low visibility of distant beds, a resident lying still was sometimes classified as unoccupied. We achieved 92% accuracy with Decision Trees (DT), 85% with K-Nearest Neighbors (KNN), and 73% for the baseline. The best-performing DT model was selected for use in this pipeline. The majority-class baseline accuracy was 61% when always predicting the dominant class. Table 1 shows the classification results using DT.

4.2 Evaluation of Skeleton Extraction

We used 11 h of annotated depth data from occupied rooms, split into training, validation, and test sets using the same split as in Sect. 4.1. All data included occupants. We used the Percentage of Correct Keypoints (PCK) (see Sect. 2.2) and L1 accuracy as evaluation metrics. L1 loss was used for accuracy, and PCK was defined as the percentage of joint predictions within 15 centimeters of the ground truth. Feature extraction and AI service models were implemented in PyTorch, using the Stochastic Gradient Descent (SGD) optimizer with a momentum of 0.9. We achieved a PCK of 69% and an L1 accuracy of 74%.

4.3 Evaluation of Fall Detection

Table 1 shows performance on the test set, with the detection threshold fixed using the training set. Fall and bed-exit detection data were taken from the skeleton extraction test set. The dataset duration was 90 min (70 min non-fall, 20 min fall), split 80:20 into training and test sets. The binary classification task was to detect fall vs. no-fall. A fall was detected when the neck position fell below the threshold defined during training. The test set accuracy was 68%. The baseline accuracy was 78% when always predicting non-fall.

4.4 Evaluation of Bed-Exit Detection

The dataset included 60 min of data, with 20 min corresponding to the 'sit in bed' activity. We used the same split as in Sect. 4.1. We evaluated different temporal windows and found that a six-frame window with a two-frame overlap gave the best results, compared to 12-frame and 18-frame windows with six-frame overlaps. A smaller window length was preferred to detect critical events more promptly. The frame rate was six frames per second. We achieved 82% accuracy in binary classification (bed-exit or not). The baseline accuracy was 67% when always predicting non-bed-exit. Table 1 shows the classification results for binary classification for bed-exit and others.

Table 1. Model performance for detection tasks (per-class metrics) in %.

Task	Class	Accuracy	Precision	Recall	F1 score
Occupancy detection	Unoccupied	95	78	95	86
(baseline accuracy: 61%)	Occupied	88	97	87	91
Fall detection	No fall	73	74	66	69
(baseline accuracy: 78%)	Fall	63	71	62	67
Bed-Exit detection	No bed-exit	74	80	86	83
(baseline accuracy: 67%)	Bed-exit (sit in bed)	90	89	96	92

4.5 Assessment of Configuration Interface

Once the executable file was created on Linux or Windows OS, it could run standalone on the respective system. A settings file was also developed with various parameters (e.g., input/output folder paths, core count) to suit specific environments such as homes and nursing homes. These parameters could be edited according to the environment and machine specifications at each location. There were slight differences between the CPU and GPU versions. Here, we compare CPU and GPU usage and interface latency (Table 2). The output of this interface was a file containing all recorded events.

CPU: The CPU version of the GUI was tested with one sensor input. The executable was generated for both Linux and Windows using PyInstaller on the respective OS. All reported values are from the Linux executable. The machine used had the following specifications: architecture x86_64, 64-bit CPU op-mode, Intel(R) Core(TM) i5-6600 CPU @ 3.30 GHz, with four cores. For a 10-second file (six frames per second), memory usage was 300 MB, and latency was 55 s.

GPU: The GPU experiments used an Nvidia GeForce RTX 2000 with CUDA version 12.4, 12 GB of available memory, and 16 cores. Processing one second of data from a single sensor consumed approximately 700 MB of memory with a latency of one second. Up to eight sensors could be processed in parallel without increasing latency, due to memory availability. For streaming sensors, either ten frames or the maximum number of available frames (if any were lost during transfer from the camera to the GPU over the internet) were processed. After processing, frames were deleted, and new frames continued to be processed. To reduce processing time, direct memory mapping was used for loading and deleting frames.

Table 2. Latency and resource usage for inference.

version	avg inference time	processor utilization	fps	sensor count
CPU	55 s	85%	6–10	1
GPU	0.07 s	35%	6–10	1
GPU	1 s	95%	6–10	6

4.6 Discussion

Our study demonstrated the feasibility of using depth images for occupancy detection, fall detection, and bed-exit detection by extracting skeletons in a natural environment. The models were trained and tested for single-person scenarios, as falls and bed exits typically occur when the older adult is alone in the room. Since skeleton extraction performance is critical to all other models, its extracted features were reused across the detection models. However, our skeleton extraction achieved only 69% PCK accuracy, primarily due to the lack of accurate ground truth data, such as motion capture (MoCap) used in related works like PopNet [13], which reported 95% PCK accuracy. Instead, we relied on manual annotations from depth images, a time-consuming and challenging process.

Only five true falls occurred in the entire dataset. Three were used in the training set along with 17 controlled falls, while two true falls and three controlled falls were included in the test set. The bed-exit detection model faced limitations due to a limited number of 'sit in bed' samples, which were affected by distant beds and occlusions. Additionally, 'sit in bed' also describes scenarios where a patient sits at the edge of the bed to eat or converse with another resident or nurse. Therefore, the bed-exit detection system could be enhanced by incorporating time and context constraints, making it active only during nighttime to early morning and for residents at higher risk of bed exit. Compared to previous studies in fall and bed-exit detection, our models achieved competitive accuracy while using fewer sensors and modest computational resources. The pipeline incorporated three detection modules: room occupancy, fall, and bed-exit detection. This enabled identification of whether a resident was in the room, if a fall occurred, or if a bed-exit attempt was made. Integrating multiple detection modules within a single pipeline enhances applicability in healthcare settings where multi-event monitoring is essential. Additional modules, such as activity recognition or sleep monitoring, could further improve insights into the daily routines of older adults.

The CPU version of the pipeline accumulated delays during continuous operation, resulting in latency of up to several weeks, rendering it impractical for real-time use. To mitigate this, we executed the CPU version at regular one-minute intervals. However, this approach reduced the continuity of monitoring and resulted in suboptimal latency for critical events like falls. The GPU version offered two main advantages: (1) the ability to process multiple sensors in parallel, and (2) reduced latency, enabling real-time or near-real-time processing. In our implementation, memory constraints limited the number of sensors to six per GPU. By using GPUs with more memory or multiple GPUs, the number of supported sensors could be increased. With the current setup, we were able to run up to 12 sensors using two GPUs with 12 GB of memory each.

5 Conclusion and Future Work

In this paper, we presented AI services for 24/7 monitoring developed for older adults in nursing homes, utilizing privacy-protecting depth sensors mounted on the walls of individual rooms. The AI services we focused on include fall detection, bed-exit detection, and room occupancy monitoring. Key joints were extracted from depth images using a skeleton extraction model, and these features were used to detect falls and bed exits. The fall detection model achieved 68% accuracy, the bed-exit model 82%, and the room occupancy model 92%. These models were integrated into a configuration interface for deployment in real-world scenarios. Both CPU and GPU versions of the interface were developed. The CPU-based interface is well-suited for individual rooms due to its minimal hardware requirements. In contrast, the GPU-based solution is ideal for monitoring multiple rooms, such as in nursing homes with several residents. Our GPU-based system can monitor up to six rooms simultaneously without delays in results. This work lays the foundation for real-time, privacy-preserving monitoring systems that address fall risks in nursing homes while reducing caregiver burden. Unlike prior efforts focused on individual homes or simulated data, our system is designed for scalable deployment in multi-room care facilities.

The AI service supports up to six rooms. We aim to cut memory use without hurting performance. The skeleton extraction model uses the most memory, while the fall, bed exit, and occupancy detection models are light. Logging and event storage use moderate memory and can be optimized. Current models handle single-person rooms, matching our dataset. Detecting falls and bed exits was the first focus since they are vital even for one resident. The next step is handling multi-bed rooms with two or three residents. The system can send real-time alerts to caregivers' smartphones during critical events. New services, such as activity recognition and mobility tests, could be added in common areas. The setup should allow these services to run only when needed. We also plan to automate event and activity records to help caregivers with care planning. Over time, reports can reveal fall risks, support clinical decisions, and guide interventions. To support shared rooms, we will train models on multi-person datasets.

Acknowledgments. The research reported in this paper was supported by the German Ministry of Health (BMG) as part of the research project ETAP – Evaluation of semi-automated care processes in long-term care using AI-based movement monitoring (etap-projekt.de/). We sincerely thank the staff and residents of AWO Karlsruhe GmbH, Stift Tilbeck GmbH Havixbeck, and Ss. Fabian und Sebastian Rosendahl for their invaluable support during data collection. We acknowledge ChatGPT, an AI language model developed by OpenAI, for its assistance in editing this paper.

References

1. Al Nahian, M.J., et al.: Towards an accelerometer-based elderly fall detection system using cross-disciplinary time series features. IEEE Access **9**, 39413– (2021)
2. Billah, M.F.R.M., et al.: BLE can see: a reinforcement learning approach for RF-based indoor occupancy detection. In: Proc. 20th Int. Conf. Inf. Process. Sensor Netw, pp. 132–147 (2021)
3. Blumenberg, P., et al.: Expertenstandard sturzprophylaxe in der pflege. DNQP (2013)
4. Cejudo, A., et al.: Smart home-assisted anomaly detection system for older adults: a deep learning approach with a comprehensive set of daily activities. Med. Biol. Eng. Comp, pp. 1–15 (2025)
5. Cheung, J.C.W., et al.: Night-time monitoring system (eNightLog) for elderly wandering behavior. Sensors **21**(3), 704 (2021)
6. CVAT.ai Corporation: computer vision annotation tool (CVAT)
7. Dubois, A., et al.: A gait analysis method based on a depth camera for fall prevention. In: 2014 36th Annual Int. Conf. IEEE Eng. Med. Biol. Soc, pp. 4515–4518 (2014)
8. Dutta, A., et al.: Poise: pose guided human silhouette extraction under occlusions. In: Proc. of the IEEE/CVF Winter Conf. on Applications of Comp. Vis, pp. 6153–6163 (2024)
9. Fernández-Bermejo Ruiz, J., et al.: Bedtime monitoring for fall detection and prevention in older adults. Int. J. Environ. Res. Public Health **19**(12), 7139 (2022)
10. Fritz, R.L., et al.: A nurse-driven method for developing artificial intelligence in "smart" homes for aging-in-place. Nurs. Outlook **67**(2), 140–153 (2019)
11. Gama, F., et al.: Automatic infant 2D pose estimation from videos: comparing seven deep neural network methods. arXiv:2406.17382 (2024)

12. Gruss, V., et al.: Job stress among nursing home certified nursing assistants: comparison of empowered and nonempowered work environments. Alzheimer's Care Today **5**(3), 207–216 (2004)
13. Guo, Y., et al.: Pop-net: pose over parts network for multi-person 3D pose estimation from a depth image. In: Proc. of the IEEE/CVF Winter Conf. on Applications of Comp. Vis, pp. 1240–1249 (2022)
14. Görres, S.: Sturzprävention im Fokus, pp. 11–13 (2018)
15. Hartmann, Y., et al.: Gait parameter estimation from a single privacy preserving depth sensor. In: Proc. 17th Int. Joint Conf. on Biomedical Eng. Systems and Technologies - BIOSIGNALS, pp. 637–645 (2024)
16. Hartmann, Y., et al.: Gait parameter estimation from a single depth sensor. J. of Smart Cities and Soc. **4**(1), 35–61 (2025)
17. Hoffman, G.J., et al.: Underreporting of fall injuries of older adults: implications for wellness visit fall risk screening. J. Am. Geriatr. Soc. **66**(6), 1195 (2018)
18. Kaeding, T.: Stürze im alter. Sportwissenschaft **39**(1), 45–51 (2009)
19. Kampezidou, S.I., et al.: Real-time occupancy detection with physics-informed pattern-recognition machines based on limited CO2 and temperature sensors. Energy Buildings **242**, 110863 (2021)
20. Krankenkasse, T.: Gesundheitsreport. pflegefall pflegebranche? so geht's deutschlands pflegekräften (2019)
21. Li, Y., et al.: Risk factors for falls among community-dwelling older adults: a systematic review and meta-analysis. Front. Med. **9**, 1019094 (2023)
22. Mejia-Trujillo, J.D., et al.: Kinect^{TM} and Intel Realsense^{TM} D435 comparison: a preliminary study for motion analysis. In: 2019 IEEE Int. Conf. on E-health Networking, Application & Services (HealthCom), pp. 1–4 (2019)
23. Naseer, F., et al.: Integrating generative adversarial networks with IoT for adaptive AI-powered personalized elderly care in smart homes. Front. Artifi. Intell. **8**, 1520592 (2025)
24. Nevitt, M.C., et al.: Risk factors for injurious falls: a prospective study. J. Gerontol. **46**(5), M164–M170 (1991)
25. Paul, R.E., et al.: Longitudinal data acquisition for AI services in long-term care facilities for older adults. In: Proc. of the 18th Int. Joint Conf. on Biomedical Eng. Systems and Technologies - Scale-IT-up, p. 1099 (2025)
26. Planinc, R., et al.: Introducing the use of depth data for fall detection. Personal Ubiquitous Comput. **17**, 1063–1072 (2013)
27. Ramirez, H., et al.: Fall detection and activity recognition using human skeleton features. IEEE Access **9**, 33532–33542 (2021)
28. Saß, A.C., et al.: Sturzunfälle in deutschland (2016)
29. Scheel, J., et al.: Krankenhausaufenthalte verringern und besser gestalten. Geriatrie-Report **15**, 32–38 (2020)
30. Strutz, N., et al.: Predictors of falling events in nursing homes: a cross-sectional study in germany. HeilberufeSCIENCE **11**, 44–51 (2020)
31. Sun, X., et al.: Compositional human pose regression. In: Proc. of the IEEE Int. Conf. on Comp. Vis, pp. 2602–2611 (2017)
32. Tanaka, K., et al.: Long-term detection system for six kinds of abnormal behavior of the elderly living alone. arXiv:2411.13153 (2024)
33. Wang, Y., et al.: A real-time human action recognition model for assisted living. arXiv:2503.18957 (2025)
34. Zheng, C., et al.: Deep learning-based human pose estimation: a survey (2022)

A Hybrid Inductive-Deductive Approach for Resource-Efficient Suicide Risk Detection in Counseling Conversations

Ron Franco[1], Avi Segal[1(✉)], and Kobi Gal[1,2]

[1] Ben-Gurion University of the Negev, Beer-Sheva, Israel
ronfr@post.bgu.ac.il, avisegal@gmail.com
[2] The University of Edinburgh, Edinburgh, UK

Abstract. The growing reliance on online platforms for mental health support underscores the need for accurate, real-time suicide risk detection. Most existing datasets utilized in training AI models for suicide risk detection consist of conversation level training examples, missing critical turning points within interactions. Research is especially limited in low-resource languages like Hebrew, restricting broader applicability. We propose a hybrid inductive-deductive framework for crisis hotline chats: an inductive component uses large language models to generate message-level pseudo-labels, distilled into a compact classifier for resource-constrained settings; a deductive component links predictions to a clinically curated taxonomy of risk factors. Experiments on real-world data from a national support service show that pseudo-labeling with curriculum learning improves performance over strong baselines. Our results highlight the promise of combining inductive and deductive strategies for resource-efficient, clinically meaningful AI in suicide prevention.

Keywords: AI in Mental Health · Model Distillation · Inductive and Deductive Reasoning

1 Introduction

The rapid development of large language models (LLMs) is reshaping modern life, enabling advances in knowledge access, productivity, and natural language processing applications [3]. Mental healthcare is no exception: diagnostic and therapeutic practices often rely on text-based interactions, where recent LLM progress suggests potential for supporting such tasks [10,24]. This trend parallels the growing reliance on online platforms for mental health support, where digital interventions and online communities increasingly complement traditional care pathway [4,17,22].

A promising use of LLMs in this domain is real-time detection of General Suicidal Risk (GSR) or its absence (NoSR) during conversations. These models can support human responders by flagging high-risk cases early, improving response times and outcomes [6]. Such systems could also expand the capacity of emotional support centers by reducing time spent on false alarms. Importantly, concise risk-score outputs place less cognitive load on operators, allowing

P. Bruno et al. (Eds.): HC_AIxIA_HYDRA 2025, CCIS 2830, pp. 336–351, 2026.
https://doi.org/10.1007/978-3-032-16708-8_28

each to handle more conversations. However, to the best of our knowledge, no lightweight Hebrew-specific model currently exists for binary real-time suicide risk detection under resource constraints.

Several challenges compound this problem. Hebrew remains underrepresented in the LLM landscape compared to high-resource languages. Volunteer-based organizations also lack the infrastructure needed for deploying very large models, and data privacy concerns limit the use of cloud-hosted models. Purely inductive, transformer-based architectures further struggle to provide deductive explanations for the mental health indicators underlying predictions. Most critically, the real-time nature of the task contrasts with existing datasets, which label entire conversations rather than turning points within them. Constructing a dedicated real-time dataset would require costly manual annotation.

To address these challenges, we propose a semi-supervised, distillation-based framework. Multilingual LLMs automatically generate pseudo-labels at the message level, enabling the transfer of their broad linguistic abilities into a compact, domain-specific classifier deployable in real time. We deconstruct annotated conversations into message-level units to make training feasible on previously unavailable real-time data. Beyond this inductive step, we also perform a complementary deductive analysis to test whether predictions align with known symptom indicators from mental health research.

We demonstrate our methodology by using LLaMA 3.3 70B Instruct [5] to pseudo-label anonymized conversations from a leading online mental health support organization, and fine-tune AlephBERT [21] for binary classification on this dataset. We further explore combining human-labeled and LLM-labeled data to balance quality and coverage. Complementing the inductive stage, we conduct a deductive analysis of predictions against a 48-category taxonomy of mental health symptoms, using a similarity-based model to provide interpretable symptom profiles. We report the resulting performance, an ablation study, and future directions.

2 Related Work

Our work relates to three main strands of prior research: (1) AI for mental health risk detection, (2) knowledge distillation and semi-supervised labeling in low-resource settings, and (3) approaches for explainability in mental health AI.

A large body of research has examined NLP methods for suicide risk detection and related tasks. Bialer et al. [1] introduced SI-BERT, a domain-adapted language model for Hebrew, leveraging lexicons to improve suicide ideation detection. Building on this, Izmaylov et al. [13] combined psychological theory with pretraining to develop SR-BERT. More recently, Grimland et al. [9] integrated machine learning with theory-driven psychological risk factors in real-time crisis hotline chats, highlighting the predictive role of hopelessness and thwarted belongingness. Large-scale reviews emphasize the growing role of AI in suicide prevention [8], while decision-tree analyses highlight structural and social factors in suicide risk assessment [7]. Our work differs by employing pseudo-labeling at the *message level*, enabling real-time detection within conversations, rather than relying solely on conversation-level signals or post-hoc labeling.

Knowledge distillation (KD) and semi-supervised learning are central to building efficient NLP models in low-resource settings. Kim and Rush [16] introduced sequence-level knowledge distillation for neural machine translation, showing that smaller student models can approximate large teacher models while retaining translation quality. Sanh et al. [19] and Jiao et al. [14] demonstrated how KD can produce smaller BERT variants with minimal performance loss. In mental health contexts, real-world deployment often faces data scarcity. Recent surveys underscore the importance of semi-supervised labeling techniques, including pseudo-labeling and back-translation, especially relevant for applications where annotated data are expensive to obtain [25]. Our approach adapts KD and pseudo-labeling specifically to Hebrew suicide prevention, a highly low-resource setting, showing how compact classifiers can still be clinically meaningful.

Explainability and interpretability are central concerns in clinical AI. Huang et al. [12] provided a systematic review of interpretability techniques in healthcare NLP. Bittar et al. [2] highlighted the limitations of applying general-purpose sentiment lexicons to suicide risk detection in electronic health records, motivating the need for domain-specific, theory-driven resources. Joyce et al. [15] proposed the TIFU framework (Transparency and Interpretability for Understandability) for mental health AI, while Grimland et al. [9] explicitly integrated psychological factors into a BERT-based model to open the "black box" of suicide risk prediction. Collectively, these works emphasize both technical and clinical motivations for interpretable AI. Our work contributes by coupling inductive pseudo-labeling with deductive, taxonomy-based symptom labeling, thus balancing performance with clinically grounded interpretability.

3 Methodology

3.1 Preliminaries

We first review the data resources and models used in this study.

The Models. Two models were employed. The first, *AlephBERT*, is a compact Hebrew-specific model used as the fine-tuning base. It has a memory footprint of $\sim$ 500 MB, supports 512 tokens, and we denote it as AlephBERT. When composed with a binary classification head, it is denoted $\text{AlephBERT}_{\text{cls}}$. This efficient model enables real-time inference on CPUs, making it suitable for cost-sensitive organizations.

The second, *Llama 3.3 70B-Instruct*, served as the teacher model in our distillation pipeline. We used its 4-bit quantized version ($\sim$ 32 GB memory, 8192 tokens), denoted Llama.

We define Train as the operation that trains $\text{AlephBERT}_{\text{cls}}$ using PyTorch with `batch_size` = 16, `learning_rate` = 2e-5, and AdamW optimizer.

The Data. The dataset was provided by Sahar[1], a leading online mental-health support service in Israel. It contains 30,234 anonymized Hebrew conversations, each a sequence of messages exchanged between a help-seeker and a volunteer. Conversations are annotated with binary labels assigned by volunteers: 5506 positive (high-risk, GSR) and 24,728 negative (NoSR). The data was split with ratio 80:20 into training and test sets.

We also received a smaller human-labeled dataset of 109 individual messages with risk labels, used only for evaluation.

Formally, the conversation dataset is

$$\mathcal{C} = \{c_1, \ldots, c_{30234}\},$$

where each c_i is defined as a sequence $(m_1, \ldots, m_{k_i})$ of k_i messages. And the Train and Test splits are denoted as $\mathcal{C}_{\text{train}}$ and $\mathcal{C}_{\text{test}}$. The smaller message-level dataset is denoted

$$\mathcal{H} = \{h_1, \ldots, h_{109}\}.$$

The Taxonomy. We were also provided with a taxonomy of mental health symptoms curated by psychology researchers collaborating with the organization. It defines 48 categories of suicidal symptoms in help-seekers' text messages, divided into 24 male-specific and 24 female-specific symptoms. The partitioning of symptoms into binary genders arises from the gendered structure of the Hebrew language; no additional gender categories were defined. Each category includes a name, a description, and a set of illustrative example sentences.

Formally, the taxonomy is

$$\text{Tax} = (N, D, \mathcal{E}),$$

where $N = (n_1, \ldots, n_{48})$ are symptom names, $D = (d_1, \ldots, d_{48})$ their descriptions, and $\mathcal{E} = (E_1, \ldots, E_{48})$ the corresponding sets of examples. For each $1 \leq i \leq 48$, E_i is a list of sentences of varying size, i.e., $|E_i|$ differs across categories.

The taxonomy plays a deductive role: while inductive training on pseudo-labeled data yields generalizable patterns, the taxonomy provides a clinically grounded basis to analyze and explain predictions.

All data used in this research is obtained through informed consent and this research is approved with the Institutional Review Board (IRB) protocols of the participating organizations.

3.2 Inductive Model Training

The inductive component is trained in two phases: The first is *pseudo-labeling* by LLM. The second is *progressive curriculum learning* [23], a complementary strategy that integrates pseudo-labeled data with the original human-labeled conversations.

[1] https://sahar.org.il/about-us/.

Pseudo-Labeling. We hypothesize that training data labeled only at the full-conversation level is insufficient for real-time suicide risk detection. Augmenting it with machine-labeled segments, specifically, individual help-seeker messages-may be essential to capture risk as it emerges.

To this end, we selected a subset of 11,506 conversations from $\mathcal{C}$ (6000 NoSR chosen randomly and uniformly, and 5506 GSR, comprising all conversations expressing GSR within $\mathcal{C}$). From each conversation, we extracted only the help-seeker messages and processed them individually using LLAMA. Each message was passed through the model with a fixed prompt (Appendix item A), instructing LLAMA to respond with a single token, either *Yes* or *No*, indicating whether the message exhibits signs of suicidal risk. By constraining both the format and output space, we obtained consistent binary pseudo-labels across all messages.

This process (see Fig. 1a) yields a new pseudo-labeled message dataset, denoted by $\mathcal{M}$. We define $\mathcal{M}_{\text{train}}$ and $\mathcal{M}_{\text{test}}$ as the subsets of $\mathcal{M}$ derived from $\mathcal{C}_{\text{train}}$ and $\mathcal{C}_{\text{test}}$, respectively. The subsequent phase presents a methodology of combining both $\mathcal{C}_{\text{train}}$ and $\mathcal{M}_{\text{train}}$ in the training process.

Progressive Curriculum Learning. This method fine-tunes ALEPHBERT$_{\text{cls}}$ on both $\mathcal{M}_{\text{train}}$ and $\mathcal{C}_{\text{train}}$, aiming to unify the strengths of both data sources without significantly degrading performance on either domain.

The training is structured progressively, transitioning from simpler to more complex examples [23]. Initially, the model is trained mainly on $\mathcal{M}_{\text{train}}$ (isolated messages). Over time, $\mathcal{C}_{\text{train}}$ (context-rich conversations) is introduced with increasing frequency, while a smaller proportion of simpler examples is retained throughout to reinforce foundational behavior (Fig. 1b).

This progression is governed by a curriculum *plan*, a sequence of weights determining the sampling proportions of each dataset at every epoch:

$$\mathcal{P} = [(w_1, w'_1), (w_2, w'_2), \ldots, (w_n, w'_n)],$$

where $w_1, ..., w_n$ form a monotonic decreasing sequence and $w'_1, ..., w'_n$ a monotonic increasing sequence, with n the number of epochs. For epoch i, subsets are drawn from $\mathcal{M}_i \subseteq \mathcal{M}_{\text{train}}$ and $\mathcal{C}_i \subseteq \mathcal{C}_{\text{train}}$ in proportions w_i and w'_i, giving $\mathcal{D}_i = \mathcal{M}_i \cup \mathcal{C}_i$. For algorithmic form, see:

Algorithm 1. PROGRESSIVECURRICULUMLEARNING

Input:
$\mathcal{M}_{\text{train}}, \mathcal{C}_{\text{train}}, \mathcal{P}$, ALEPHBERT$_{\text{cls}}$

1: **for** $(w_i, w'_i) \in \mathcal{P}$ **do**
2: $\quad \mathcal{M}_i \leftarrow \text{sample}(\mathcal{M}_{\text{train}}, \text{frac} = w_i)$
3: $\quad \mathcal{C}_i \leftarrow \text{sample}(\mathcal{C}_{\text{train}}, \text{frac} = w'_i)$
4: $\quad \mathcal{D}_i \leftarrow \mathcal{M}_i \cup \mathcal{C}_i$
5: $\quad$ Train(ALEPHBERT$_{\text{cls}}$, $\mathcal{D}_i$)
6: **end for**

In our specific implementation, we use the following curriculum plan:

i	0	1	2	3	4	5
$\mathcal{P}[i]$	(0.9, 0.1)	(0.8, 0.2)	(0.65, 0.3)	(0.1, 0.7)	(0.05, 0.9)	(0.025, 0.95)

constructed based on empirical results.

Conceptually, using $\mathcal{M}_{\text{train}}$ constitutes a form of knowledge distillation: a large, general-purpose model (LLAMA) transfers knowledge to the smaller, ALEPHBERT$_{\text{cls}}$ model, enabling deployment in resource-constrained environments.

We denote the model obtained by this method as IND, which serves as the inductive component in this paper.

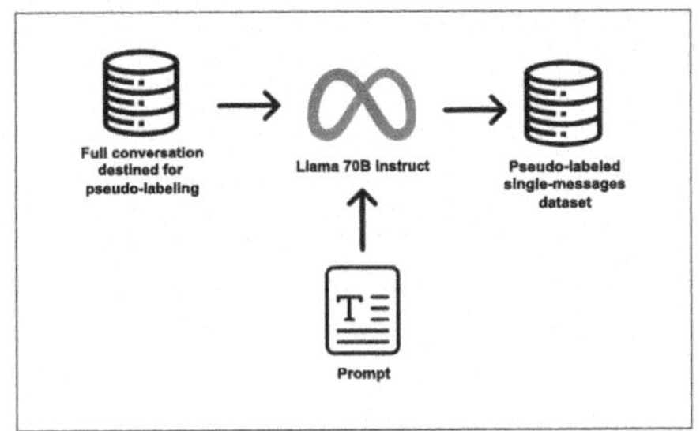

(a) Prompting Pipeline

(b) Inductive Model's Training Process

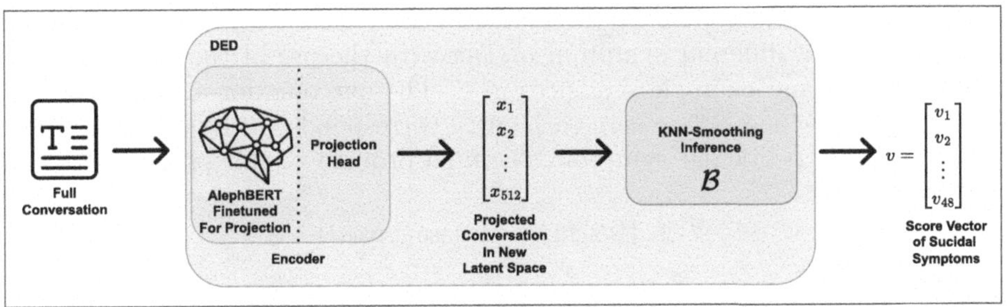

(c) Deductive Model (DED) Inference Methodology

Fig. 1. (a) Pseudo-labeling pipeline for single messages. (b) Progressive curriculum learning strategy, producing model IND. (c) Complete architecture of DED. The input is a full conversation, which is projected into the learned latent space $\mathbb{R}^{512}$. This embedding is passed through a KNN-smoothing inference (over projections of conversations from $\mathcal{T}_{\text{train}}$), producing a final score vector $v \in [0, 1]^{48}$.

3.3 Deductive Model Training

To complement the inductive model, which provides a high-level GSR score, we introduce a deductive model that leverages Tax to generate a resource-efficient, clinically informed score for each of the 48 suicidal symptoms.

Training proceeds in two phases: (1) *Symptom pseudo-labeling*, where LLAMA evaluates each conversation in the training set for the presence of every symptom in Tax, producing a clinically informed dataset in which each conversation is represented by a 48-dimensional symptom vector. (2) Fine-tuning ALEPHBERT with a contrastive learning objective to learn latent representations of conversations emphasizing symptom-level similarity.

Inference on a new conversation applies a KNN-smoothing [18] inspired method, producing a 48-dimensional score vector that estimates symptom presence based on proximity in the latent space. This vector offers clinically grounded explanations of the 48 possible symptoms.

Like the inductive model, this approach performs model distillation: LLAMA first generates the annotated dataset, and the smaller ALEPHBERT student model is fine-tuned, yielding a fast, resource-efficient, Hebrew-specific model. The inference procedure allows a single forward pass to output the full 48-dimensional prediction vector.

Symptom Pseudo-Labeling. In this phase, we randomly sampled 1000 conversations from $\mathcal{C}_{\text{train}}$, maintaining balance between GSR and NoSR by including 500 conversations labeled as GSR (chosen randomly) and 500 as NoSR (chosen randomly). We denote this subset as T. Since Tax includes 24 gender-specific symptoms per gender, it is note-worthy that 667 conversations are authored by females and 327 by males (6 unknowns).

Similar to the method in the inductive training, for each conversation $c \in T$, we prompt (Appendix item B) LLAMA 48 times, where each prompt queries the presence of a different symptom in Tax with the use of the corresponding definition in D and example sentences in $\mathcal{E}$. The outcome for a conversation c is a binary vector $v \in \mathbb{B}^{48}$, where each entry corresponds to the presence (1) or absence (0) of a particular symptom. the final product of this phase is denoted as

$$\mathcal{T} = \{(c_1, v_1), ..., (c_{1000}, v_{1000})\}$$

Contrastive Learning. After procuring $\mathcal{T}$, we finetuned ALEPHBERT on a projection task, mapping conversations into a latent space where conversations with similar symptom vectors are close and dissimilar ones are farther apart.

We split $\mathcal{T}$ into $\mathcal{T}_{\text{train}}$ and $\mathcal{T}_{\text{test}}$ (80:20). And computed the similarity matrix $\mathbf{Sim} = \mathbf{A}^\top \mathbf{A}$, where $\mathbf{A} = \left[\frac{v_1}{\|v_1\|_2} \mid \frac{v_2}{\|v_2\|_2} \mid \cdots \mid \frac{v_{800}}{\|v_{800}\|_2} \right]$ such that each v_i is a symptom vector of conversation c_i where $(c_i, v_i) \in \mathcal{T}_{\text{train}}$.

For each epoch, we sample n conversation pairs (c_i, c_j). If $\mathbf{Sim}_{i,j} >$ `threshold` (for a predetermined `threshold`; in our case 0.7, set empirically), we assign *similar* (1); otherwise *dissimilar* (0). This yields a new dataset of n labeled pairs per epoch, used to finetune ALEPHBERT with Contrastive Loss.

The choice of similarity-based contrastive learning is motivated by the small size of $\mathcal{T}$ and the high cost of enlarging it. Pairwise sampling generates up to $1000^2 - 1000$ unique training examples. The per-epoch approach enables fresh datasets at each round. The resulting model is denoted ENCODER : $\mathbb{N}^{512} \rightarrow \mathbb{R}^{512}$.

KNN-Smoothing Inference Methodology. After projecting conversations into a similarity-preserving latent space, we evaluate a score vector predicting the expression level of each of the 48 symptoms. To this end, $\mathcal{T}_{\text{train}}$ is encoded into the latent space, yielding anchor points with symptom vectors:

$$\mathcal{B} = (e_1, \dots, e_{800}) = (\textsc{Encoder}(c_1), \dots, \textsc{Encoder}(c_{800})).$$

For a new conversation c, we compute $e = \textsc{Encoder}(c)$ and retrieve its k nearest neighbors from $\mathcal{B}$ via Euclidean distance ($k = 100$, selected empirically from $\{5, 15, 25, 50, 75, 100\}$). Let $\mathcal{N}_k(e)$ denote their indices. Each neighbor e_j receives a weight

$$w_j = \frac{\frac{1}{\|e - e_j\|_2 + \varepsilon}}{\sum_{j' \in \mathcal{N}_k(e)} \frac{1}{\|e - e_{j'}\|_2 + \varepsilon}},$$

with $\varepsilon > 0$ ensuring numerical stability.

The score vector is the weighted average of neighbors' symptom vectors:

$$v = \sum_{j \in \mathcal{N}_k(e)} w_j \, v_j.$$

The model mapping a conversation c to $e = \textsc{Encoder}(c)$ and outputting v via the above inference procedure (Fig. 1c) is denoted DED, serving as the deductive component of our framework.

4 Experiments

4.1 Ablation Studies

We conducted three ablations to evaluate the inductive training framework. The first is a naive baseline trained only on conversation-level data:

$$\textsc{Naive} \leftarrow \text{Train}(\textsc{AlephBERT}_{\text{cls}}, \mathcal{C}_{\text{train}}),$$

removing all pseudo-labeling to test whether conversation-level supervision suffices.

The second uses only single messages from $\mathcal{M}_{\text{train}}$:

$$\textsc{SingMess} \leftarrow \text{Train}(\textsc{AlephBERT}_{\text{cls}}, \mathcal{M}_{\text{train}}),$$

thereby ablating the joint training bridge between messages and conversations.

The third removes progressive curriculum. We first train on $\mathcal{M}_{\text{train}}$ and then train on $\mathcal{C}_{\text{train}}$:

$$\textsc{AlephBERT}'_{\text{cls}} \leftarrow \text{Train}(\textsc{AlephBERT}_{\text{cls}}, \mathcal{M}_{\text{train}}),$$

$$\textsc{StageWise} \leftarrow \text{Train}(\textsc{AlephBERT}'_{\text{cls}}, \mathcal{C}_{\text{train}}).$$

This stage-wise scheme tests whether progressive blending is needed to prevent catastrophic forgetting.

4.2 Deductive-Inductive Relation Experiment

We further examined the relationship between DED and IND. For each conversation $c_i \in \mathcal{C}_{\text{test}}$, we compute:

$$p_i = \text{IND}(c_i) \in \mathbb{B}, \qquad v_i = \text{DED}(c_i) \in [0,1]^{48}.$$

The vector v_i is then discretized with a threshold of 0.5, producing $v_i' \in \mathbb{B}^{48}$. IND's predictions induce a partition:

$$Pos = \{c_i : p_i = 1\}, \qquad Neg = \{c_i : p_i = 0\}.$$

For each symptom $s = N[k]$, for $k \in \{1, \ldots, 48\}$, we define

$$Pos^{(s)} = \{c_i : c_i \in Pos \wedge v_i'[k] = 1\}, \qquad Neg^{(s)} = \{c_i : c_i \in Neg \wedge v_i'[k] = 1\}.$$

In words, $Pos^{(s)}$ corresponds to conversations where IND predicts GSR and DED predicts symptom s, while $Neg^{(s)}$ corresponds to conversations where IND predicts NoSR but DED predicts s. Comparing $|Pos^{(s)}|$ and $|Neg^{(s)}|$ highlights which symptoms differ most between GSR and NoSR, providing insight into how the deductive symptom reasoning aligns with the inductive GSR predictions.

5 Results

We present the performance of IND and DED, along with analyses of $\mathcal{M}$ and $\mathcal{T}$. Additionally, we report the results of the Deductive–Inductive Relation experiment, illustrating the interaction between IND and DED.

5.1 Datasets

The pseudo-labeled single-message dataset $\mathcal{M}$ contains 409,286 entries, 10.64% of which were labeled as positive by LLAMA (indicating GSR). Among messages originating from GSR conversations, 15.57% were labeled positive, compared to 5.66% for those derived from NoSR conversations.

Meanwhile, $\mathcal{T}$ comprises 1,000 conversations, each associated with a 48-dimensional binary symptom vector. Figure 2 presents its distribution, geometric structure, and symptom-level disparities. The results exhibit bias toward female-associated symptoms, consistent with the gender imbalance among help-seekers in $\mathcal{T}$.

5.2 Model Performance

Table 1 reports the performance of IND, the ablation models, and LLAMA. For each model, an additional row shows the average over $\mathcal{M}_{\text{test}}$ and $\mathcal{C}_{\text{test}}$, referred to as *"Averaged Results"* (AR). Figure 3 presents the ROC, Precision–Recall (PR), and calibration curves of all ablation models as well as IND. The deductive model DED achieved $F1 = 0.69$ and $BCE = 0.18$ on $\mathcal{T}_{\text{test}}$. Here, the F1 score was computed by rounding each entry in the predicted score vectors (`threshold`=0.5) and comparing them element-wise to the corresponding entries in the corresponding vectors from $\mathcal{T}_{\text{test}}$.

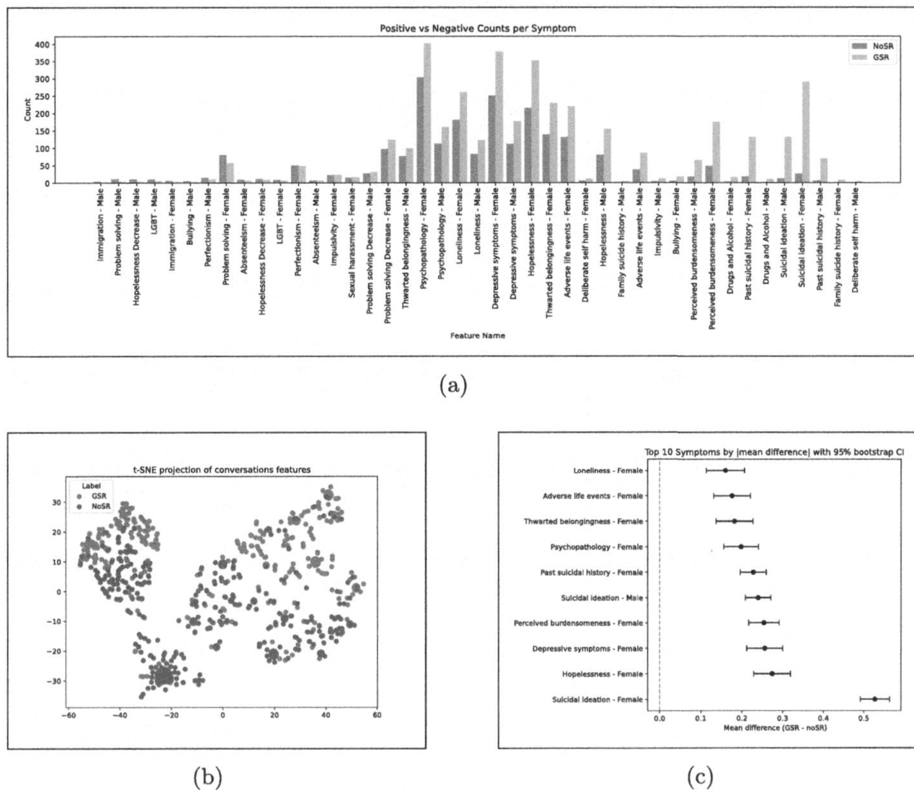

Fig. 2. Analysis of the symptom-based dataset $\mathcal{T}$. (a) Distribution of conversations per symptom (x-axis), stratified by GSR/NoSR. (b) t-SNE projection of 48-d feature vectors (`perplexity` = 15), showing a separation pattern. (c) Top 10 symptoms by mean difference between GSR and NoSR (bootstrapped, 100k resamples, 95% CI).

5.3 Inductive-Deductive Relation

We examined correspondence between IND predictions and DED symptom signals. For each $s \in N$, we computed $|Pos^{(s)}|$ and $|Neg^{(s)}|$, the counts of conversations predicted by IND as GSR or NoSR in which DED identified symptom s, with standard deviations reported in Table 2.

To highlight discriminative symptoms, we ranked s by $|Pos^{(s)}| - |Neg^{(s)}|$, exposing markers most associated with GSR and linking conversation-level decisions to symptom-level predictions.

6 Discussion and Conclusions

The empirical results highlight several key observations. The AR of IND improves over NAIVE in all measured metrics, with notable gains in recall

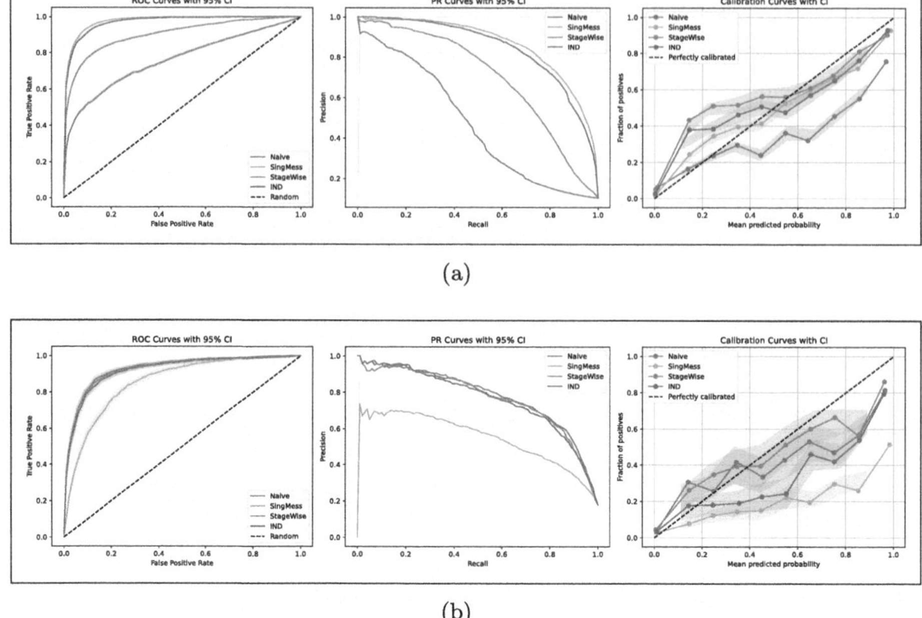

Fig. 3. ROC, Precision–Recall (PR), and calibration curves evaluated for IND and the three ablation models, with 95% confidence intervals estimated via bootstrapping over 1000 resamples. Calibration was performed using 10 bins. (a) Evaluation on $\mathcal{M}_{\text{test}}$. (b) Evaluation on $\mathcal{C}_{\text{test}}$.

(+18.7%) and F_2 (+17.7%), suggesting that integrating single-message and full-conversation training enhances generalization across granularities. This claim is further supported by the curves presented in Fig. 3, as models that underperform on a specific dataset are consistently those that were not exposed to or reinforced with that dataset. Some ablation variants of AR surpassed IND in recall (+3.3%) or precision (+4.8%) but underperformed on all other metrics. Although the Average Results measurement may favor IND, it captures the notion that performance on both $\mathcal{C}_{\text{test}}$ and $\mathcal{M}_{\text{test}}$ is essential for robust real-time GSR detection. Moreover, IND outperformed LLAMA across all metrics when evaluated on $\mathcal{H}$, indicating successful knowledge distillation likely aided by the Hebrew-specific ALEPHBERT$_{\text{cls}}$, which confers a linguistic advantage over the general-purpose multilingual LLAMA. This claim should be interpreted with caution due to the limited size of $\mathcal{H}$, which constrains the statistical strength of the findings.

The deductive model DED adds further insight. the deductive-inductive relation experiment (Table 2) aligns closely with the independent analysis of $\mathcal{T}$ (Fig. 2c). Suicidal ideation in females consistently emerged as the strongest GSR indicator across analyses. Eight of the top ten indicators overlapped, consistent with a methodologically independent study [9] reporting five overlapping symp-

Table 1. Performance of IND, LLAMA, and the ablation studies. Here, MCC and BS denote the Matthews Correlation Coefficient and Brier Score, respectively. Rows labeled as AR report the mean of the corresponding cells in $\mathcal{M}_{test}$ and $\mathcal{C}_{test}$ for the same model. Boldfaced cells indicate the highest score among the AR rows.

Model	Test Set	Accuracy	Precision	Recall	F1	F2	AUC-ROC	MCC	BS
NAIVE	$\mathcal{M}_{test}$	0.911	0.622	0.368	0.462	0.401	0.760	0.434	0.078
NAIVE	$\mathcal{C}_{test}$	0.897	0.706	0.738	0.722	0.731	0.924	0.659	0.082
NAIVE	$\mathcal{H}$	0.606	0.882	0.435	0.583	0.484	0.846	0.348	0.335
NAIVE	AR	0.904	0.664	0.553	0.592	0.566	0.842	0.546	0.080
SINGMESS	$\mathcal{M}_{test}$	0.956	0.827	0.726	0.774	0.744	0.976	0.751	0.034
SINGMESS	$\mathcal{C}_{test}$	0.757	0.413	0.820	0.550	0.685	0.854	0.452	0.195
SINGMESS	$\mathcal{H}$	0.761	0.922	0.681	0.783	0.719	0.908	0.561	0.195
SINGMESS	AR	0.857	0.62	**0.773**	0.661	0.715	0.915	0.601	0.114
STAGEWISE	$\mathcal{M}_{test}$	0.934	0.827	0.461	0.592	0.506	0.902	0.587	0.058
STAGEWISE	$\mathcal{C}_{test}$	0.899	0.730	0.702	0.716	0.707	0.923	0.654	0.081
STAGEWISE	$\mathcal{H}$	0.752	0.957	0.638	0.765	0.684	0.898	0.574	0.232
STAGEWISE	AR	0.917	**0.779**	0.582	0.654	0.607	0.913	0.620	0.069
IND	$\mathcal{M}_{test}$	0.952	0.823	0.683	0.746	0.707	0.970	0.724	0.039
IND	$\mathcal{C}_{test}$	0.881	0.638	0.797	0.709	0.759	0.921	0.642	0.092
IND	$\mathcal{H}$	0.789	0.911	0.739	0.816	0.768	0.910	0.592	0.185
IND	AR	**0.917**	0.731	0.74	**0.728**	**0.733**	**0.946**	**0.683**	**0.065**
LLAMA	$\mathcal{H}$	0.789	0.893	0.725	0.800	0.753	–	–	–

Table 2. Top DED-Identified Symptoms Ranked by Mean Difference Between GSR and NoSR (IND Predictions)

Symptom	Mean Pos	Mean Neg	Std Pos	Std Neg	Mean Diff	t-value	p-value
Suicidal ideation - Female	0.472	0.206	0.499	0.404	0.266	18.074	1.466e-67
Perceived burdensomeness - Female	0.346	0.168	0.476	0.374	0.179	12.766	7.377e-36
Adverse life events - Female	0.599	0.426	0.490	0.495	0.173	11.476	1.152e-29
Thwarted belongingness - Female	0.631	0.524	0.483	0.499	0.107	7.127	1.368e-12
Loneliness - Female	0.686	0.613	0.464	0.487	0.073	5.067	4.359e-07
Hopelessness - Female	0.798	0.745	0.401	0.436	0.053	4.245	2.273e-05
Depressive symptoms - Female	0.955	0.909	0.206	0.288	0.047	6.702	2.432e-11
Problem solving Decrease - Female	0.178	0.135	0.382	0.342	0.042	3.669	2.502e-04
Hopelessness - Male	0.175	0.147	0.380	0.354	0.028	2.406	1.623e-02
Psychopathology - Female	0.964	0.939	0.186	0.239	0.025	4.098	4.286e-05

toms. Convergence across models of independent nature - an inductive classifier trained on examples, a deductive symptom-similarity model, pseudo-labels from a general-purpose LLM, and an external study - suggests these signals are stable, clinically meaningful markers of GSR. Nevertheless, differences in ranking and relative importance remain, warranting further examination.

Despite these promising findings, several limitations should be acknowledged. The reliance on LLAMA for pseudo-labeling $\mathcal{M}$ and $\mathcal{T}$ introduces a dependency on the classification quality of a generative model, which may not match human annotators. While symptom-level pseudo-labeling arguably leverages LLM strengths in textual pattern recognition and comparison (due to the use of $\mathcal{E}$), the validity of message-level labels is more tenuous. The robustness of IND is also called into question, as the model was trained solely on data originating from the organization, without exposure to out-of-domain samples. In addition, as shown in Fig. 3b, IND exhibits degraded calibration performance in the conversation classification task. Moreover, not all symptoms were equally represented: as shown in Fig. 2a, some were severely underrepresented in $\mathcal{T}$, and five symptoms were not expressed at all. Whether this reflects genuine clinical distribution, limited coverage in the source corpus, or systematic misclassification by LLAMA remains unclear. Furthermore, although IND, DED, and external findings partially overlap, discrepancies persist in both symptom presence and the relative weight assigned to each. These divergences underscore the necessity of validation using carefully annotated human datasets.

Beyond technical limitations, deploying AI for suicide prevention raises governance and ethical considerations. Our framework is intended only as a decision-support tool, with human responders maintaining responsibility for all interventions. Safeguards such as confidence calibration [26], explainable symptom profiles [20], and human-in-the-loop oversight [11] are critical to prevent over-reliance on automated predictions. Misuse mitigation also requires clear governance: deployment should be limited to accredited organizations with training protocols, ethical review, and data protection measures in place. Addressing these risks will be essential for ensuring that efficiency gains do not come at the expense of safety, fairness, or trustworthiness.

In conclusion, the contributions of this study are multi-dimensional. From a resource perspective, the pseudo-labeled datasets $\mathcal{M}$ and $\mathcal{T}$ provide valuable assets, while IND and DED offer complementary strengths: real-time GSR detection and interpretable symptom-level explanations. These efficiencies support deployment in resource-constrained settings. Methodologically, we present a generalizable framework that decomposes data into fine-grained units, applies LLM-based pseudo-labeling, and recombines them into a curriculum integrating granular and holistic views. Convergence between inductive and deductive findings aligns with external clinical theories, providing preliminary validation. Using pseudo-labeled data from LLAMA, we demonstrate the potential of LLMs to augment domain-specific models. Future work includes extending pseudo-labeling to additional conversational entities, performing a more detailed error analysis to better understand sources of misclassification, evaluating IND for potential gender-related biases in $\mathcal{T}$ to ensure robustness across demographic groups, and exploring ensembles of IND and DED to further enhance predictive performance and clinical interpretability.

Conflict of Interest. The authors declare that they have no conflict of interest.

Appendix

(A) Prompt for labeling single messages

<s>[INST] «SYS» You are a helpful assistant that evaluates text for suicide risk factors and responds only with "Yes" or "No". «/SYS»
Does the following text show signs of any of the following risk factors?
Text: "..."
Risk factors to consider:
1. Suicidal intent (explicit or implicit mentions of wanting to die or end one's life)
2. Hopelessness or extreme despair (statements like "there's no way out" or "nothing will ever get better")
3. Social withdrawal or isolation (mentioning feeling alone, abandoned, or disconnected)
4. Self-harm or past suicidal behavior (references to cutting, previous attempts, or self-inflicted harm)
5. Giving away possessions or saying goodbye (indicating preparation for suicide)
6. Expressing a burden mentality ("Everyone would be better off without me")
7. Extreme guilt or self-hatred (statements like "I am worthless" or "I deserve to suffer")
8. Sudden calmness after distress (which might indicate a decision to act)
9. Lack of future-oriented thinking ("I won't be here much longer" or "It doesn't matter anymore")
10. Expressions of unbearable emotional pain ("I can't take this anymore" or "The pain is too much")
Please respond only with a single word: Yes or No: [/INST]

(B) Prompt For Symptoms Pseudo-labeling

<s>[INST] «SYS» You are a helpful assistant that classifies text into a given category.
You must respond with exactly one word: "Yes" or "No".
The text comes from a conversation between two people, and only one participant's messages are shown.
«/SYS»
A text is define to show signs of "{feature}" if: {defintion}
Does the following Hebrew text show signs of "{feature}"?
Text:
{text} Here are some example sentences that might appear in conversations with "{feature}" signs:
{example_block}
Answer with only "Yes" or "No". [/INST]</s>\n

(A) the prompt used in curating labels for single-messages, in line three instead of "..." we inserted the message (B) The prompt used in curating the 48-dimensional vector of symptoms for conversations in T. For every symptom $i \in \{1, ..., 48\}$ {feature}, {definition}, {example_block} are replaced with $N[i], D[i], \mathcal{E}[i]$ respectively while {text} is replaced with the conversation itself.

References

1. Bialer, A., Izmaylov, D., Segal, A., Tsur, O., Levi-Belz, Y., Gal, K.: Detecting suicide risk in online counseling services: a study in a low-resource language. arXiv preprint arXiv:2209.04830 (2022)
2. Bittar, A., Velupillai, S., Roberts, A., Dutta, R.: Using general-purpose sentiment lexicons for suicide risk assessment in electronic health records: corpus-based analysis. JMIR Med. Inform. **9**(4), e22397 (2021)
3. Chiarello, F., Giordano, V., Spada, I., Barandoni, S., Fantoni, G.: Future applications of generative large language models: a data-driven case study on chatgpt. Technovation **133**, 103002 (2024)
4. Coelho, J., Pécune, F., Micoulaud-Franchi, J.A., Bioulac, B., Philip, P.: Promoting mental health in the age of new digital tools: balancing challenges and opportunities of social media, chatbots, and wearables. Front. Digit. Heal. **7**, 1560580 (2025)
5. Dubey, A., et al.: The llama 3 herd of models. arXiv e-prints pp. arXiv–2407 (2024)
6. Ehtemam, H., et al.: Role of machine learning algorithms in suicide risk prediction: a systematic review-meta analysis of clinical studies. BMC Med. Inform. Decis. Mak. **24**(1), 138 (2024)
7. Fulginiti, A., Segal, A., Wilson, J., Hill, C., Tambe, M., Castro, C., Rice, E.: Getting to the root of the problem: a decision-tree analysis for suicide risk among young people experiencing homelessness. J. Soc. Soc. Work Res. **13**(2), 327–350 (2022)
8. Gaur, V., Maggu, G., Bairwa, K., Chaudhury, S., Dhamija, S., Ali, T.: Artificial intelligence in suicide prevention: utilizing deep learning approach for early detection. Ind. Psychiatry J. **33**(2), 226–233 (2024)

9. Grimland, M., et al.: Predicting suicide risk in real-time crisis hotline chats integrating machine learning with psychological factors: exploring the black box. Suicide Life-Threatening Behav. **54**(3), 416–424 (2024)
10. Guo, Z., Lai, A., Thygesen, J.H., Farrington, J., Keen, T., Li, K., et al.: Large language models for mental health applications: systematic review. JMIR Mental Heal. **11**(1), e57400 (2024)
11. Holzinger, A., Zatloukal, K., Müller, H.: Is human oversight to ai systems still possible? (2025)
12. Huang, G., Li, Y., Jameel, S., Long, Y., Papanastasiou, G.: From explainable to interpretable deep learning for natural language processing in healthcare: How far from reality? Comput. Struct. Biotechnol. J. **24**, 362–373 (2024)
13. Izmaylov, D., Bialer, A., Segal, A., Grimland, M., Levi-Belz, Y., Gal, K.: Combining psychological theory with language models for suicide risk detection. In: Findings of the Association for Computational Linguistics: EACL 2023, pp. 2430–2438 (2023)
14. Jiao, X., et al.: Tinybert: distilling Bert for natural language understanding. In: Findings of the Association for Computational Linguistics: EMNLP 2020, pp. 4163–4174 (2020)
15. Joyce, D.W., Kormilitzin, A., Smith, K.A., Cipriani, A.: Explainable artificial intelligence for mental health through transparency and interpretability for understandability. NPJ Digital Med. **6**(6) (2023)
16. Kim, Y., Rush, A.M.: Sequence-level knowledge distillation. In: Proceedings of EMNLP (2016)
17. Löchner, J., Carlbring, P., Schuller, B., Torous, J., Sander, L.B.: Digital interventions in mental health: an overview and future perspectives. Internet Interv. **40**, 100824 (2025)
18. Matabuena, M., Vidal, J.C., Padilla, O.H.M., Onnela, J.P.: KNN algorithm for conditional mean and variance estimation with automated uncertainty quantification and variable selection. arXiv preprint arXiv:2402.01635 (2024)
19. Sanh, V., Debut, L., Chaumond, J., Wolf, T.: Distilbert, a distilled version of Bert: smaller, faster, cheaper and lighter. arXiv preprint arXiv:1910.01108 (2019)
20. Saraswat, D., et al.: Explainable AI for healthcare 5.0: opportunities and challenges. IEEE Access **10**, 84486–84517 (2022)
21. Seker, A., Bandel, E., Bareket, D., Brusilovsky, I., Greenfeld, R., Tsarfaty, R.: Alephbert: language model pre-training and evaluation from sub-word to sentence level. In: Proceedings of the 60th Annual Meeting of the Association for Computational Linguistics (vol. 1: Long Papers), pp. 46–56 (2022)
22. Srivastava, A., Gupta, T., Cerezo, A., Lord, S.P., Akhtar, M.S., Chakraborty, T.: Critical behavioral traits foster peer engagement in online mental health communities. PLoS ONE **20**(1), e0316906 (2025)
23. Wang, X., Chen, Y., Zhu, W.: A survey on curriculum learning. IEEE Trans. Pattern Anal. Mach. Intell. **44**(9), 4555–4576 (2021)
24. Xu, X., et al.: Mental-LLM: leveraging large language models for mental health prediction via online text data. In: Proceedings of the ACM on Interactive, Mobile, Wearable and Ubiquitous Technologies, vol. 8, no. 1, pp. 1–32 (2024)
25. Yang, X., Song, Z., King, I., Xu, Z.: A survey on deep semi-supervised learning. IEEE Trans. Knowl. Data Eng. **35**(9), 8934–8954 (2022)
26. Zhang, Y., Liao, Q.V., Bellamy, R.K.: Effect of confidence and explanation on accuracy and trust calibration in ai-assisted decision making. In: Proceedings of the 2020 Conference on Fairness, Accountability, and Transparency, pp. 295–305 (2020)

Triage Discrimination: Myth or Reality?

Justin Armanini[1,4](✉) and Fabio Stella[1,2,3]

[1] University of Milano-Bicocca, Viale Sarca. 336, 20126 Milan, Italy
j.armanini@campus.unimib.it, fabio.stella@unimib.it
[2] BReCHS – Bicocca Research Centre in Health Services, Milan, Italy
[3] Bicocca Bioinformatics Biostatistics and Bioimaging Centre - B4, University of Milano-Bicocca, Vedano al Lambro, MB, Italy
[4] Department of Epidemiology and Data Science, Fondazione IRCCS Istituto Nazionale dei Tumori, Via Giacomo Venezian 1, 20133 Milan, Italy

Abstract. Discrimination, understood as the unjust or prejudicial treatment of individuals based on characteristics such as age, gender, race, or disability, is a deeply contested issue and a significant challenge for contemporary society. This paper examines potential instances of discrimination within the healthcare sector, with particular focus on the triage process. We employ causal networks and causal mediation analysis to answer two key questions: (1) Does triage decision-making exhibit disparity based on demographic factors such as race, gender, or age? (2) If such disparities are identified, to what extent can they be attributed to clinically relevant factors rather than to demographic characteristics? The results reveal demographic disparities in triage assignments for age, gender, and race. However, causal mediation analysis shows that gender and race disparities are entirely explained by clinical mediators. In contrast, age exhibits a direct effect on acuity scores beyond its influence on vital signs, though this may reflect clinically appropriate age-based triage protocols rather than unjustified discrimination. These findings highlight the importance of causal analysis in distinguishing between statistical disparities and actual discrimination in healthcare settings.

Keywords: Causal Networks · Mediation Analysis · Triage · Discrimination

1 Introduction

Triage is the process of sorting patients in an emergency department according to the severity of their injuries and their need for care and monitoring. This process is fundamental in healthcare, as it determines how quickly emergency providers can attend to patients. Essentially, triage is an optimisation problem aimed at minimizing the use of hospital resources while ensuring appropriate

---

Supplementary Information The online version contains supplementary material available at https://doi.org/10.1007/978-3-032-16708-8_29.

P. Bruno et al. (Eds.): HC_AIxIA_HYDRA 2025, CCIS 2830, pp. 352–365, 2026.
https://doi.org/10.1007/978-3-032-16708-8_29

care for patients. Providing inadequate care can lead to poorer health outcomes, which can have a significant impact on a country's healthcare system, incurring economic and social costs.

When a patient arrives at the Emergency Department (ED), they undergo a brief evaluation by a nurse according to a specific protocol. During this evaluation, *vital signs* are recorded, and the patient is assigned an *acuity* score reflecting the urgency of their medical needs. The most common protocol is the Emergency Severity Index (ESI) [3], recommended by the Emergency Nurses Association and the American College of Emergency Physicians. The ESI has five acuity levels, with an ESI of 1 indicating the most acute condition and an ESI of 5 the least acute. This scoring system determines where a patient will be evaluated, for example, in a designated high-acuity or stabilisation bed, how quickly they will be admitted, and how long they will wait for evaluation and definitive care [1]. By design, the ESI and the triage process rely on the subjective assessments made by the nurse about a patient's illness severity, whether the patient is facing an immediate life threat and their expected resource needs in the emergency department (ED). The only objective data used in this evaluation are vital signs, which may be subjectively interpreted in nuanced cases. The triage decisions of emergency nurses can be influenced by numerous cognitive biases, including confirmation and anchoring biases, premature closure, risk tolerance, satisficing, the framing effect, and blind obedience. These biases can be even heightened by factors like cognitive stress or pressure to improve ED throughput for better patient care [1,10], and may contribute to well-documented disparities in medical care. The literature demonstrates that in the United States, factors such as race, sex, and language impact the quality of care. For instance, Black and Hispanic patients are often subjected to longer wait times and offered less intensive treatment, highlighting a pattern of systemic inequity in emergency services [6]. Such discrimination can cause delayed diagnosis, inadequate pain management, increased mortality rates among affected populations, and perpetuation of health disparities that undermine both individual patient outcomes and public health equity [7]. Beyond the immediate clinical impact, discrimination in healthcare settings erodes trust in medical institutions and violates fundamental principles of medical ethics and social justice. In the existing literature, discrimination in triage has been assessed through statistical analysis, primarily using odds ratios.

Inspired by the Simpson's Paradox in COVID-19 [5], which demonstrated that incorrect conclusions can be drawn without a causal understanding of the underlying mechanisms, this work studies discrimination in triage through the lens of causality [8], to answer the following questions:

- RQ1: Is there discrimination in triage based on demographics such as race, gender, and age?
- RQ2: If discrimination exists, what underlying mechanisms drive such disparities? Is there any justifiable discrimination based on clinical factors?

To answer the above research questions we take a causal perspective. Indeed, it is well known that observational data alone is in general not enough to draw reliable conclusions and to make effective decisions. A causal perspective is crucial for gathering information about the data generation process and avoiding erroneous, unsound and even paradoxical conclusions. When randomized controlled trials are unfeasible or unethical, as in the case of triage, the causal inference framework provides the appropriate methodology for conducting causal investigations using observational data.

In this work, we show that traditional statistical analysis fails to unveil the underlying mechanisms behind observed patterns, while causal inference can help resolve statistical paradoxes and provide deeper insights into the true relationships between the quantities of interest. To the best of our knowledge, this is the first application of causal analysis to better understand demographic discrimination in triage, offering a novel methodological approach to addressing this critical healthcare equity issue.

The rest of the paper is organized as follows; Sect. 2 presents a brief overview of the scientific literature on racial and gender discrimination in healthcare. Definitions and notation about causal networks and inference are given in Sect. 3. The case study on triage is presented and developed in Sect. 4. Conclusions and further directions are described in Sect. 5. Additional methodological information and results are available in the Supplementary Material.

2 Related Work

There is a growing body of evidence in the healthcare literature on the existence of racial and gender discrimination in clinical triage in the United States. However, this consensus is largely built on descriptive statistical approaches that may not adequately account for the clinical complexity of triage decisions, raising concerns about the validity of the conclusions. The most significant and pervasive limitation of this body of work is the risk of uncontrolled confounding from omitted clinical variables. Several key studies compute odds ratios adjusted for patient demographics, but fail to incorporate detailed clinical data. For example, [1] observed that Black patients were more likely to be triaged to a dedicated fast-track area (rather than the main ED), and less likely to be given a high acuity score by controlling for sex, ED arrival time, insurance type, age, chief complaint and vital signs, but only using a coarse binary classification ('any abnormal vital signs versus none'), which misses to capture critical patient-level variability. A similar approach was taken by [11], who matched patients based on the presence of abnormal vital signs, not the values themselves. Other works are further weakened by the complete absence of clinical status variables, as in [10], which makes its conclusions about the drivers of disparity affecting Black and Hispanic adults unreliable. Even a multi-site study [7] that adjusted for ED operational factors, such as ED wait time, time of day, and day of week (used as proxies for ED saturation level), did not account for specific clinical indicators, a critical omission when evaluating triage acuity. Beyond clinical confounding factors, other methodological limitations challenge the findings. [1] used the patient encounter as the unit of analysis, without accounting for within-patient correlations when individuals visit an emergency department multiple times. The generalizability of findings is also limited in some cases by the use of site-specific, resource-based triage to acuity pods rather than the ESI [10] or by data sourced from a single site [1,10,11]. A more robust methodological approach is provided by [13], which concluded that Black and Hispanic patients were assigned less urgent ESI scores than White patients, and this effect was higher for males. This work controlled for both some patients' vitals (heart rate, respiratory rate, and patient-reported pain score), and nurses' information (gender, age, and number of years of experience) to try to model nurses' potential bias. However, it included only a subset of the vital signs measured during triage. It also accounted for patients with multiple visits by employing linear cross-classified, random-effects models. To conclude, while evidence points towards disparities in clinical triage, its methodological robustness varies significantly.

3 Preliminaries

In this work, we leverage on causal networks and causal inference to investigate potential discrimination in medical triage by answering to RQ1 and RQ2. Therefore, this section is devoted to give the main definitions and notation needed to describe our contributions.

3.1 Basic Definitions

Definition 1 (Bayesian Network). *A Bayesian Network is a type of probabilistic graphical model represented as a pair $\langle G, P(X, \Theta)\rangle$, where:*

- *$G = \langle V, E\rangle$ is a Direct Acyclic Graph (DAG);*
- *$P(X, \Theta)$ is a global probability distribution over a vector X of random variables, with parameters Θ, such that each node $V_i \in V$ is associated with a random variable $X_i \in X$.*

We will use the terms "nodes" and "variables" interchangeably from now on. The edges in the graph define relationships between any two nodes X_i and X_j:

- If a directed edge $X_i \rightarrow X_j$ exists, X_i is a *parent* of X_j, and X_j is a *child* of X_i. The set of parents of X_j is denoted $\text{Pa}(X_j)$;
- If a directed path exists from X_i to X_j, X_i is an *ancestor* of X_j, and X_j is a *descendant* of X_i. Given $G = \langle V, E\rangle$, a directed path is a sequence of distinct vertices $X = (X_1, X_2, \ldots, X_k)$ such that for each $i = 1, 2, \ldots, k-1$, there exists an edge $(X_i, X_{i+1}) \in E$.

The structure of the DAG G encodes conditional independence relationships among the random variables $X_i \in X$, allowing to factorize the joint distribution as a product of local conditional probabilities for each variable given its parents:

$$P(X, \Theta) = \prod_{i=1}^{n} P(X_i | \text{Pa}(X_i), \theta_{X_i})$$

Making the *Causal Edge Assumption*, i.e., *every parent is a direct cause of all its children*, allows us to move from BNs to causal networks.

Definition 2 (Causal Network). *A Causal Network is a Bayesian Network where the edges of G are interpreted as direct causal relationships.*

In a causal network, each directed edge $X_i \to X_j \in E$ represents a cause-effect relationship, where X_i is said to be a cause (or treatment) of X_j, whereas X_j is an effect (or outcome) of X_i. The structure of a causal graph allows to determine statistical independence using a graphical criterion known as *d-separation*. This concept is fundamental to understanding how information and association flow through the network.

Definition 3 (d-separation). *A path p is said to be blocked by a set of nodes S if and only if:*

1. *p contains a chain of nodes* $(A \to B \to C)$ *or a fork* $(A \leftarrow B \to C)$ *such that the middle node B is in S (i.e., is conditioned on),*
2. *or p contains a collider* $(A \to B \leftarrow C)$ *such that the collision node B is not in S, and no descendant of B is in S.*

If S blocks every path between two nodes X and Y, then X and Y are d-separated conditional on S, and thus are independent conditional on S. d-separation implies conditional independence thanks to the *Markov assumption.*

Another relevant concept is that of *information flow* which helps in understanding the mechanisms through which causes transmit their influence to produce effects through the network paths. The structure of a causal graph dictates how both statistical and causal associations propagate through the system. Causal association flows along directed causal paths from causes to effects. Statistical association, however, can propagate through any connecting path, including non-causal paths that create spurious correlations (confounding). The principle of d-separation determines when paths are blocked, thereby preventing the flow of both types of association.

3.2 Learning Causal Networks from Data

A Bayesian Network is learned by combining domain knowledge and data. When domain knowledge is partial or unavailable, specific algorithms allow to retrieve a network from observational data. The discussion of the different algorithms in the literature is beyond the scope of this work. However, constructing a causal network from observational data involves two main stages:

$$\underbrace{P(G, \Theta \mid D)}_{\text{Learning}} = \underbrace{P(G \mid D)}_{\text{Structure learning}} \cdot \underbrace{P(\Theta \mid G, D)}_{\text{Parameter learning}}$$

- *Structure Learning* (or *Causal Discovery*); The process of learning the DAG $G = \langle X, E \rangle$ from a dataset $D = \{\mathbf{x}^{(1)}, \mathbf{x}^{(2)}, \ldots, \mathbf{x}^{(N)}\}$ with $\mathbf{x}^{(i)} \in \mathbb{R}^M$, where each $\mathbf{x}^{(i)} = (x_1^{(i)}, x_2^{(i)}, \ldots, x_M^{(i)})$ is an instance of the random vector $X = \{X_1, X_2, \ldots, X_M\}$. The goal is to infer the edge set E such that the d-separation properties in G correspond to the conditional independencies observed in the data (an assumption known as *Faithfulness*). Typically, when working with observational data alone, the best we can hope is to determine a Markov equivalence class of graphs. In such cases, input from domain experts can help identify a unique DAG.
- *Parameter Learning*; Once the structure G is known, this stage involves estimating the parameters Θ of the conditional probability distributions, which quantify the strength of the causal relationships defined by the graph's edges. Specifically, for each variable X_i in the graph, we estimate the parameters θ_{X_i} of its local conditional distribution $P(X_i \mid \text{Pa}(X_i); \theta_{X_i})$.

3.3 Causal Mediation Analysis

To answer RQ2, we leverage causal mediation analysis [9] which decomposes the total causal effect of a treatment variable on an outcome into its constituent paths, thus allowing to understand the mechanisms through which causal association flows.

Definition 4 (Mediator). *A mediator is a variable that lies on a causal path between a treatment and an outcome.*

A mediator explains how the treatment influences the outcome, also blocking the causal flow between the treatment and the outcome.

In a causal network, mediators determine two types of effects:

- *Direct Effect*; The causal association from a treatment T to an outcome Y that does not pass through any intermediate variables. This corresponds to the direct edge $T \to Y$.
- *Indirect Effect*: The causal association from T to Y that is transmitted through one or more mediator variables. For a single mediator M, this corresponds to the path $T \to M \to Y$.

In the most elementary case a single mediator is present, while more complex scenarios can involve multiple mediators operating in parallel or series (Supplementary Material Fig. S1). Mediation analysis provides the tools to estimate both direct and indirect effects, thereby providing a detailed understanding of the causal mechanisms involved [9]. To discuss the causal queries provided by mediation analysis, we first need to introduce the key concepts of intervention and counterfactual.

- *Intervention*; An *intervention* refers to an external manipulation of a variable, setting it to a specific value regardless of its natural causes. This is denoted using the *do*-operator and represents the hypothetical scenario in which variable X is forcibly set to x ($do(X = x)$). This notation distinguishes causal effects from mere statistical associations: conditioning on a variable narrows the focus to the subset of cases in which the variable takes a specific value, without changing anything. In distributional terms, $P(Y = y|X = x)$ stands for the population distribution of Y among individuals whose X value is x; $P(Y = y|do(X = x))$ stands for the population distribution of Y if *everyone* in the population had their X value fixed at x [8].
- *Counterfactual*; A *counterfactual* describes a *hypothetical* alternative outcome that would have occurred under a different treatment, contrary to what actually happened. It is typically expressed using the notation $Y_{(X=x)}$, which means "the value that Y would have taken if X had been x". The probability $P(Y_{(X=x')} \mid X = x)$ represents the probability of Y if X had taken the value x' given that we observed it took the value x. Counterfactuals enable questions like "*What would the outcome have been if the treatment had been different?*" and play a central role in causal reasoning.

In the case of a binary treatment with a single mediator, causal mediation analysis defines the following causal queries:

- *Total Causal Effect (TCE)*; The overall causal association, flowing through all directed paths between T and Y:

$$TCE_{0\to1} = \mathbb{E}[Y|do(T = 1)] - \mathbb{E}[Y|do(T = 0)]$$

- *Controlled Direct Effect (CDE)*; The effect of changing treatment T from 0 to 1, while fixing the mediator M at a value x.

$$CDE_{0\to1}(x) = \mathbb{E}[Y \mid do(T = 1, M = x)] - \mathbb{E}[Y \mid do(T = 0, M = x)]$$

- *Natural Direct Effect (NIE)*; The effect of changing treatment T from 0 to 1 while letting the mediator M behave as it would under no treatment ($M_{(T=0)}$). This isolates the direct effect because the indirect effect is blocked by the counterfactual mediator $M_{(T=0)}$.

$$NDE_{0\to1} = \mathbb{E}[Y_{M(T=0)} \mid T = 1] - \mathbb{E}[Y \mid T = 0]$$

- *Natural Indirect Effect (NIE)*; The effect of changing the mediator M from what it would be under treatment 0 to what it would be under treatment 1 ($M(T = 1)$), while keeping treatment constant ($T = 0$). This isolates the indirect effect because the direct effect does not actually occur due to the non-treatment.

$$NIE_{0\to1} = \mathbb{E}[Y_{M(T=1)} \mid T = 0] - \mathbb{E}[Y \mid T = 0]$$

4 Triage Mediation and Confounding

4.1 Dataset

We used the MIMIC-IV-ED (v2.2) dataset [4] for our experiments. The study population is derived from the Beth Israel Deaconess Medical Center, a tertiary academic medical center in Boston, with data spanning from 2011 to 2019.

We selected the following variables for analysis: *subject_id*, *stay_id*, gender, race, age, the Emergency Severity Index score (*acuity*), and vital signs, which include temperature, heart rate, respiratory rate, oxygen saturation, systolic blood pressure, diastolic blood pressure, and pain level. Furthermore, we applied some exclusion criteria and then discretized continuous variables according to common strategies adopted in the clinical literature [2]. The final cohort was composed of 160,883 data units. We reported the details in Supplementary Material Section S.2.

4.2 Learning the Causal Network

The problem of learning the structure of the causal network was tackled by leveraging on domain knowledge, which has been translated into a black-list, i.e., by specifying those edges that can not be included in the causal network. The *bnlearn* package [12] has been used to specify the following black-list:

- *Root nodes*: demographics (*age*, *race*, *gender*) cannot point to each other;
- *Leaf node*: *acuity*;
- *Clinical variables*: cannot point to demographics.

We opted for a score-based causal discovery, thus Tabu search has been used to optimize the Akaike Information Criterion (AIC):

$$AIC = -2\ln(\hat{L}) + 2k$$

$$\hat{L} = L(\hat{E}|D) \quad \hat{E} = \arg max_E L(E|D).$$

where E stands for the set of included edges, D represents the available data, $\hat{L}$ is the optimal value of the likelihood function measuring the fitness of the model given the data, and k is the number of estimated parameters, acting as a penalty term for models with high parameter complexity.

The triage causal network (Fig. 1) has been obtained repeating the structural learning procedure 100 times with varying seeds, by using the *bnlearn* package [12], and by retaining edges which occurred at least 80% of the times. Parameter learning has been carried out by computing the expected values of the Bayesian posterior distributions, using a uniform prior to accommodate unobserved variable configurations in the data.

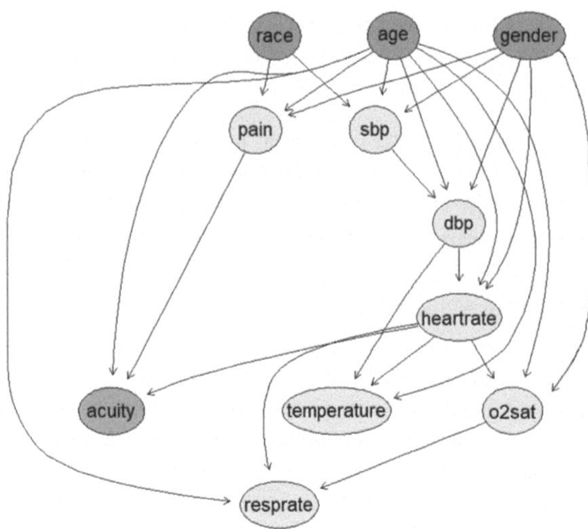

Fig. 1. The triage causal network.

4.3 Mediation Analysis

In our triage case study, we employed causal inference and mediation analysis to investigate disparities linked to demographic attributes. As these characteristics are immutable, their "effect" is not interventional; rather, it quantifies the statistical disparity in outcomes between different groups. We use mediation analysis to decompose this total disparity and determine the extent to which it is associated directly with a demographic factor versus being mediated by clinical variables. This framework rests on the assumptions of causal sufficiency (no unmeasured confounders) and positivity.

Does Discrimination Occur in Triage? In the algorithmic fairness literature, discrimination is defined as the causal influence from a protected attribute, such as age, gender, or race, towards an outcome through paths deemed unfair in specific contexts [5]. For our analysis, we adopted a broader, neutral definition of a *disparity*: any causal association flowing from a demographic attribute to the acuity score.

Our first research question (RQ1) therefore translates to: "*Does a causal association exist between age, gender, or race and the assigned acuity score?*"

The answer is *yes*. Our triage DAG demonstrates that all three demographic attributes are causally linked to the acuity score through multiple paths. For example, paths run from demographics through clinical mediators like *heartrate*, *pain*, *sbp*, and *dbp*, to acuity. Age also has a direct path to acuity. According to d-separation, the chain structure of these paths are naturally open when no variables are conditioned on (i.e., $S = \emptyset$), thereby establishing a causal association. To measure the strength of these associations, we calculated the Total

Causal Effect (TCE) which quantifies the average change in the acuity score when comparing a “treatment” group to a “control” group. Since all treatment nodes are root nodes, there are no backdoor paths to block between treatment and outcome. Therefore, identification tells us the causal estimands (Sect. 3.3) coincide with the statistical estimands. In our setting, recall that a higher acuity score number corresponds to a lower clinical urgency. It follows that a positive TCE means the treatment group is assigned higher scores (lower urgency) than the control group. Symmetrically, a negative TCE means the treatment group is assigned lower scores (higher urgency) than the control group.

For *age* as treatment, the disparity is significant (Fig. 2a). The group’s sorting by average TCE reflects a natural ordering: the older the individuals are, the lower acuity score they are assigned (higher urgency). Comparing the youngest group (‘16–24’) to the oldest (‘85+’), there is a TCE of −0.53, indicating a substantially higher urgency assignment for the elderly. For *gender* the effect is smaller (Supplementary Material Fig. S6). Males receive a slightly lower acuity score (−0.01) on average than females, suggesting marginally higher urgency. For *race*, we observed small but notable differences (Fig. 2b). ‘Hispanic or Latino’ and ‘Black or African American’ groups tended to receive higher acuity scores (between +0.01 and +0.04, lower urgency) compared to other groups, a finding consistent with previous studies [6,13].

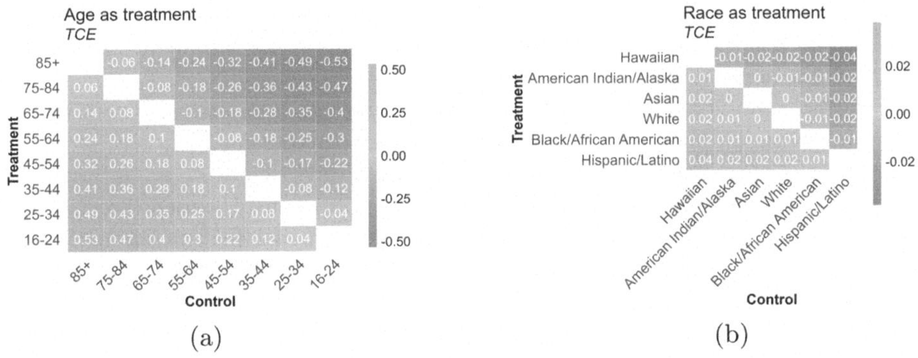

Fig. 2. Groups are sorted by their average TCE as a treatment over the remaining groups as a control. (a) Age, (b) Race.

Having established that demographic disparities exist, the crucial next step is to understand their underlying mechanisms. Are these effects driven directly by demographics in a way that might be unfair, or are they explained by differences in patients’ clinical conditions? This leads us to our second research question.

Why Does Discrimination Occur in Triage? To investigate the mechanisms driving the observed demographic disparities, we employ causal mediation analysis, which allows us to decompose the total causal effect into:

- A direct effect, which we term *potentially unfair disparity*[1]; representing a causal association from a demographic variable to the acuity score that bypasses the measured clinical variables;
- An indirect effect, which we term *clinically explained disparity*, representing a causal association mediated through those same clinical variables.

This framework allows us to address whether there is actually some form of discrimination, or whether the observed disparities are entirely explained by patients' clinical presentations. RQ2 can be thereby rephrased as: "*Is disparity in triage totally unfair?*". The answer is *no*. We quantified the magnitude of potentially unfair and clinically explained disparities through NDE and NIE, respectively. To identify the two effects, we verified the `Assumption Set B (sequential ignorability)` and used `eq. 14a, 14b` from [9] as statistical estimands. The interpretation of positive and negative NDE and NIE is similar to that provided for TCE.

Our analysis indicates that the nature of these disparities varies significantly across demographic groups. For *gender* and *race*, the disparities are entirely indirect and clinically explained. The causal model shows no direct path from these attributes to the *acuity* score, while d-separation confirms that indirect paths are open, establishing an indirect causal association. These indirect paths would be blocked by the set of mediator clinical variables. Quantitatively, the NDE is zero (Supplementary Material, Fig. S9, S10), meaning the entire TCE is channeled through the NIE. In practical terms, this suggests that two individuals of different *gender* or *race* but with identical clinical measurements would be assigned the same *acuity* score.

For *age*, however, the disparity is driven primarily by a strong direct effect. The causal model shows a direct path from *age* to the *acuity* score, while d-separation confirms that it is open, establishing a direct causal association. The NDE (Fig. 3a) accounts for the majority of the total causal association (TCE), indicating that *age* influences the *acuity* score beyond its effect on the measured vital signs. While our framework labels this direct effect 'potentially unfair', it likely reflects clinically appropriate considerations. Triage protocols such as the ESI often use age-dependent thresholds for vital signs [3], and we hypothesize that nurses may use a patient's age as a heuristic for estimating physiological reserve or the risk of unobserved comorbidities.

In summary, our findings indicate that demographic disparity exists in triage acuity assignments, a conclusion that aligns with previous literature. However, the mechanisms behind these disparities differ by demographic group. *Age* was found to have a direct effect on acuity assignments, introducing a potential for bias. We hypothesize this may be clinically motivated, as nurses might adjust their assessment based on age-dependent vital sign thresholds or use age as a proxy for unobserved comorbidities. In contrast, the disparities related to *gender* and *race* are indirect. Our causal analysis reveals a causal association where these demographic factors are associated with the patient's clinical condition, and it

[1] This reflects the concept of discrimination in algorithmic fairness.

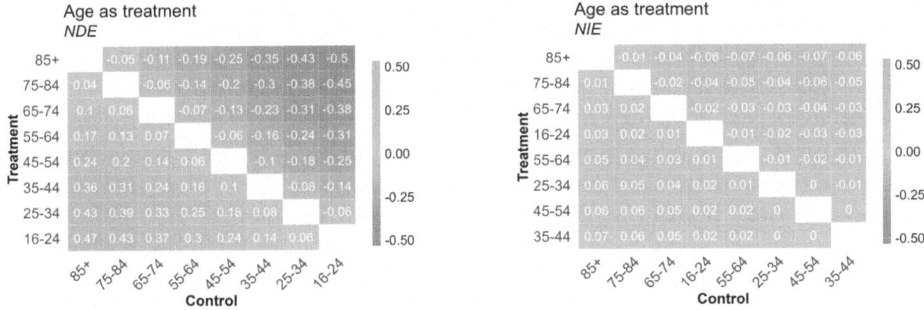

Fig. 3. Age groups are sorted by their average effect as a treatment over the remaining groups as a control.

is the clinical condition itself that primarily drives the acuity score. Therefore, the statistical association between gender/race and the triage decision is mediated by the patient's presenting medical state, rather than these demographics directly influencing the nurse's assignment. In conclusion, our results indicate discrimination based solely on age, as the term is defined and understood in the literature. To strengthen our findings, we reproduced commonly used statistical methods from prior work on our data (Sect. 2; Supplementary Material Section S.4). The results confirmed the disparities observed for RQ1. However, whereas our approach disentangled mechanisms and recognised clinical justification, the compared approaches could not, thereby risking interpretation as demographic discrimination.

5 Conclusions and Future Works

This study demonstrates how causal reasoning enhances understanding of triage discrimination by modeling the data generation mechanism. To our knowledge, this is the first work to move beyond traditional statistical methods, which identified but could not explain disparities.

In response to (RQ1), our analysis confirmed demographic disparities in triage in the MIMIC-IV-ED dataset. However, through causal mediation analysis (RQ2), we found that gender and race contribute to clinically explained disparity, while age exerts a potentially unfair disparity that may be clinically justified by established, age-based triage protocols.

Our study has some limitations to acknowledge. The causal sufficiency assumption is strong but reasonable, given we assumed access to all information available to nurses in triage. Positivity is discussed in Supplementary Material Section S.3.1. There may be unobserved factors, such as socio-economic proxies, which might explain causal relationships between demographics and clinical status without altering our conclusions. The causal model incorporates relationships well-supported by established physiological and clinical evidence. For example, we validated the influence of gender on pain perception, shaped by biological and psychosocial factors; the relationship between blood pressure and heart rate, regulated by arterial baroreflex; and the impact of age on increasing systolic blood pressure due to arterial stiffness. State-dependent cardio-respiratory coupling between heart rate and respiratory rate was also verified. While these are some of the pathways grounded in existing literature, other learned relationships are more nuanced and would benefit from further review by a physician. Lastly, single-center data limits the generalizability of our findings.

Future research should refine variable discretization by age to investigate our hypothesis regarding its potentially unfair direct effect. Exploring joint effects and interactions between demographic factors is another promising direction. Our findings suggest interventions should be tailored to specific mechanisms driving each disparity type. For gender and race, attention should focus on upstream factors contributing to differential clinical presentations across demographic groups.

Acknowledgements. This work has been partially supported by the MUR under the grant "Dipartimenti di Eccellenza 2023–2027" of the DISCo, University of Milano-Bicocca, and by the National Plan for NRRP Complementary Investments (Project n. PNC0000003 - AdvaNced Technologies for Human-centrEd Medicine (ANTHEM)). The PhD fellowship of JA is funded by the IRCCS National Cancer Institute Foundation.

References

1. Boley, S., et al.: Investigating racial disparities within an emergency department rapid-triage system. Am. J. Emergency Med. **60**, 65–72 (2022). https://doi.org/10.1016/j.ajem.2022.07.030. https://www.sciencedirect.com/science/article/pii/S0735675722004685
2. Candel, B., et al.: The association between vital signs and clinical outcomes in emergency department patients of different age categories. Emergency Med. J. **39**, emermed–2020 (2022). https://doi.org/10.1136/emermed-2020-210628
3. Emergency Nurses Association: Emergency Severity Index Handbook, 5th edn. (2023). https://californiaena.org/wp-content/uploads/2023/05/ESI-Handbook-5th-Edition-3-2023.pdf. Accessed 30 July 2025
4. Johnson, A., Bulgarelli, L., Pollard, T., Celi, L.A., Mark, R., Horng, S.: Mimic-iv-ed (version 2.2) (2023). https://doi.org/10.13026/5ntk-km72. https://doi.org/10.13026/5ntk-km72, rRID:SCR_007345
5. von Kugelgen, J., Gresele, L., Scholkopf, B.: Simpson's paradox in COVID-19 case fatality rates: a mediation analysis of Age-Related causal effects. IEEE Trans. Artif. Intell. **2**(1), 18–27 (2021)
6. Lu, F.Q., Hanchate, A.D., Paasche-Orlow, M.K.: Racial/ethnic disparities in emergency department wait times in the united states, 2013–2017. Am. J. Emergency Med. **47**, 138–144 (2021). https://doi.org/10.1016/j.ajem.2021.03.051. https://www.sciencedirect.com/science/article/pii/S0735675721002369
7. Patel, M., et al.: Patient sex, racial and ethnic disparities in emergency department triage: a multi-site retrospective study. Am. J. Emergency Med. **76** (2023). https://doi.org/10.1016/j.ajem.2023.11.008

8. Pearl, J., Glymour, M., Jewell, N.: Causal Inference in Statistics: A Primer. Wiley (2016). https://books.google.it/books?id=L3G-CgAAQBAJ
9. Pearl, J.: Interpretation and identification of causal mediation. Psychol. Methods **19**(4), 459 (2014)
10. Peitzman, C., Tartak, J., Samuels-Kalow, M., Raja, A., Konstantopoulos, W.: Racial differences in triage for emergency department patients with subjective chief complaints. Western J. Emergency Med. **24** (2023). https://doi.org/10.5811/WESTJEM.59044
11. Schrader, C.D., Lewis, L.M.: Racial disparity in emergency department triage. J. Emergency Med. **44**(2), 511–518 (2013). https://doi.org/10.1016/j.jemermed.2012.05.010. https://www.sciencedirect.com/science/article/pii/S0736467912006518
12. Scutari, M.: Learning Bayesian networks with the bnlearn R package. J. Stat. Softw. **35**(3), 1–22 (2010). https://doi.org/10.18637/jss.v035.i03
13. Vigil, J.M., et al.: Ethnic disparities in emergency severity index scores among U.S. veteran's affairs emergency department patients. PLoS One **10**(5), e0126792 (2015)

Neuro-symbolic and Multi-modal Learning

Expert-Guided POMDP Learning for Data-Efficient Modeling in Healthcare

Marco Locatelli[1(✉)], Arjen Hommersom[2], Roberto Clemens Cerioli[1], Daniela Besozzi[1,3,4], and Fabio Stella[1,3,4]

[1] Department of Informatics, Systems and Communication, University of Milano-Bicocca, Milan, Italy
m.locatelli60@campus.unimib.it
[2] Department of Computer Science, Open University, P.O. Box 2960, 6401DL Heerlen, The Netherlands
[3] Bicocca Bioinformatics Biostatistics and Bioimaging Centre - B4, University of Milano-Bicocca, Vedano al Lambro, MB, Italy
[4] BReCHS – Bicocca Research Centre in Health Services, University of Milano-Bicocca, Milan, Italy

Abstract. Learning the parameters of Partially Observable Markov Decision Processes (POMDPs) from limited data is a significant challenge. We introduce the Fuzzy-MAP EM algorithm, a novel approach that incorporates expert knowledge into the parameter estimation process by enriching the Expectation–Maximization (EM) framework with fuzzy pseudo-counts derived from an expert-defined fuzzy model. This integration naturally reformulates the problem as a Maximum A Posteriori (MAP) estimation, effectively guiding learning in environments with limited data. In synthetic medical simulations, our method consistently outperforms the standard EM algorithm under both low-data and high-noise conditions. Furthermore, a case study on Myasthenia Gravis illustrates the ability of the Fuzzy-MAP EM algorithm to recover a clinically coherent POMDP, demonstrating its potential as a practical tool for data-efficient modeling in healthcare.

1 Introduction

Sequential decision-making poses a critical challenge across numerous real-world domains, particularly in healthcare, where diagnostic and treatment decisions must be made over time in response to patients' dynamic conditions. This complexity is further amplified in the context of rare diseases, which are marked by small, heterogeneous patients populations, limited clinical data, and an incomplete understanding of underlying disease mechanisms.

Partially Observable Markov Decision Processes (POMDPs) provide a general framework for making sequential decisions in environments where the true state of the system is uncertain or hidden [2]. POMDPs maintain a probabilistic belief over latent states and use this information to inform decision-making. This

P. Bruno et al. (Eds.): HC_AIxIA_HYDRA 2025, CCIS 2830, pp. 369–383, 2026.
https://doi.org/10.1007/978-3-032-16708-8_30

enables policies to evolve over time by combining current observations with probabilistic estimates of disease progression, making POMDPs particularly well-suited for rare diseases, which are characterized by limited data availability and substantial uncertainty [8]. Despite their theoretical advantages, POMDPs face practical challenges: *i*) exact solution methods scale poorly with state and observation complexity, and *ii*) learning parameters under data paucity is difficult.

In this work a novel Fuzzy-MAP EM algorithm is designed to tackle the second challenge by integrating medical knowledge into a POMDP model. Our approach leverages expert knowledge of disease dynamics, encoded within a fuzzy modeling framework, to inform a Maximum A Posteriori (MAP) estimation algorithm. The fuzzy model generates *fuzzy pseudo-counts* that serve as informative priors, thereby regularizing parameter updates and enhancing the robustness of the estimation process. To the best of our knowledge, constructing a prior using fuzzy rules for the M-step of the EM algorithm represents a novel methodological contribution. Specifically, the central contributions of this study are:

- The introduction of the Fuzzy-MAP EM algorithm, a novel method for integrating expert knowledge into POMDP parameter estimation by augmenting the M-step of the EM algorithm with *fuzzy pseudo-counts*.
- A demonstration, via synthetic medical simulations, that the proposed approach consistently outperforms the standard EM algorithm, particularly in challenging low-data and high-noise environments.
- A validation of the algorithm's practical utility through a real-world case study on Myasthenia Gravis, a rare autoimmune disorder that impairs communication between nerves and muscles. This study demonstrates the possibility to learn a clinically coherent POMDP from expert knowledge alone.

This paper begins by reviewing the foundational concepts of POMDPs, the EM algorithm, and Takagi-Sugeno fuzzy models in Sect. 2. Section 3 introduces our novel Fuzzy-MAP EM algorithm, and describes how expert knowledge is integrated through *fuzzy pseudo-counts*. In Sect. 4, we evaluate the algorithm's performance in a simulated medical environment characterized by limited and noisy data. Section 5 presents a real-world case study focused on the management of Myasthenia Gravis, a rare autoimmune disease. Finally, Sect. 6 concludes the paper and outlines directions for future research.

2 Preliminaries

2.1 Partially Observable Markov Decision Processes

A Partially Observable Markov Decision Processes (POMDP) [2] is a mathematical framework for modeling an agent acting in a stochastic, partially observable environment.

A POMDP is formally defined as a tuple $\langle S, A, \Omega, T, O, R \rangle$, where:

- S is a finite set of hidden states.
- A is a finite set of actions.

- Ω is a continuous observation space, $\Omega \subseteq \mathbb{R}^d$. The vector of observations at time t is represented by $o_t \in \Omega$, where $o_{t,j}$ denotes the j-th component.
- $T(s,a,s') = P(s_{t+1} = s' \mid s_t = s, a_t = a)$ is the state transition probability function, which defines the probability of transitioning from state s to state s' after taking action a.
- $O(o \mid s) = p(o_t = o \mid s_t = s)$ is the observation probability density function, which defines the probability of observing o when the system is in state s.
- $R(s,a,s')$ is the reward function, which specifies the immediate reward for transitioning from s to s' via action a. While crucial for control, the reward function is not involved in the parameter learning problem addressed here.

2.2 Expectation-Maximization for POMDPs

The Expectation-Maximization (EM) algorithm [4] is an iterative algorithm for finding the maximum likelihood estimates of parameters in probabilistic models with latent variables. For POMPDs the latent variables are the unobserved state trajectories $s^{(i)}_{1:T_i}$, where (i) indexes a specific patient trajectory in the dataset and $1 : T_i$ denote the sequence of time steps for that trajectory. EM treats each full state sequence as missing data and marginalizes over it.

Given a dataset $\mathcal{D} = \{a^{(i)}_{1:T_i}, o^{(i)}_{1:T_i}\}_{i=1}^N$ consisting of N action-observation trajectories, the goal is to find the parameters θ that maximize the log-likelihood of the data:

$$\mathcal{L}(\theta) = \sum_{i=1}^{N} \log P(o^{(i)}_{i:T_i} \mid a^{(i)}_{i:T_i-1}; \theta). \tag{1}$$

The EM algorithm solves this problem by alternating between two steps:

E-Step (Expectation). Given the parameters estimate θ^k at the *k-th* EM iteration, this step computes the posterior probability of the latent sequences using the forward-backward algorithm [1]. In detail, the computed quantities are:

1. **State occupancy probability:** the probability of being in state s at time t: $\gamma_t(s) = P(s_t = s \mid o_{i:T_i}, a_{i:T_i-1}; \theta^k)$.
2. **State transition probability:** the joint probability of transitioning from state s to state s' at time t: $\xi_t(s,s') = P(s_t = s, s_{t+1} = s' \mid o_{i:T_i}, a_{i:T_i-1}; \theta^k)$.

M-Step (Maximization). This step updates the model parameters from θ^k to θ^{k+1} by maximizing the expected complete-data log-likelihood. This is obtained by using the probabilities values computed by the *E-step* as expected counts.

- **Transition model update:** $T^{k+1}(s,a,s') = \frac{\sum_{i=1}^{N}\sum_{t=1}^{T_i-1} \mathbb{I}(a_t^{(i)}=a)\xi_t(s,s')}{\sum_{i=1}^{N}\sum_{t=1}^{T_i-1} \mathbb{I}(a_t^{(i)}=a)\gamma_t(s)} = \frac{\hat{N}_T(s,a,s')}{\sum_{s''\in S}\hat{N}_T(s,a,s'')}$, where $\mathbb{I}(\cdot)$ is the indicator function.

- **Observation model update** (for a multivariate normal distribution):

$$\mu_s^{(k+1)} = \frac{\sum_{i=1}^{N} \sum_{t=1}^{T_i} \gamma_t^{(i)}(s) o_t^{(i)}}{\sum_{i=1}^{N} \sum_{t=1}^{T_i} \gamma_t^{(i)}(s)} = \frac{\hat{S}_O(s)}{\hat{N}_O(s)}$$

$$\Sigma_s^{(k+1)} = \frac{\sum_{i=1}^{N} \sum_{t=1}^{T_i} \gamma_t^{(i)}(s)(o_t^{(i)} - \mu_s^{(k+1)})(o_t^{(i)} - \mu_s^{(k+1)})^{\mathrm{T}}}{\sum_{i=1}^{N} \sum_{t=1}^{T_i} \gamma_t^{(i)}(s)}$$
$$= \frac{\hat{S}_{O,2}(s)}{\hat{N}_O(s)} - \mu_{s'}^{(k+1)} \mu_{s'}^{(k+1)\,\mathrm{T}}$$

2.3 Takagi-Sugeno Fuzzy Models

To integrate expert knowledge into the learning process, we employ a Type-1 Takagi-Sugeno fuzzy model [10]. This model predicts the evolution of the system's observations. A Type-1 Takagi-Sugeno fuzzy model consists of:

- **Membership Functions**: Each input variable (e.g., an observation component) is associated with a set of linguistic terms (LTs) such as "low", "medium" and "high". A membership function $\mu_{LT}(x) \in [0, 1]$ quantifies the degree to which a crisp input value belongs to a linguistic concept.
- **Fuzzy Rules**: The system's behavior is described by a set R of IF-THEN rules. A typical fuzzy rule $r \in R$ has the form:

  IF $o_{t,1}$ is LT_1 AND ... AND a_t is LT_a THEN $o_{t+1,j}^* = f_{r,j}(o_t, a_t)$,

  where $f_{r,j}$ is a function (typically linear) of the inputs for rule r.
- **Firing Strength**: The firing strength of a rule's antecedent, $\mu_{r,ant}(o_t, a_t)$, is calculated using a t-norm operator ($\top$) on the membership values of the inputs:

$$\mu_{r,ant}(o_t, a_t) = \top(\mu_{LT_{r,1}}(o_{t,1}), ..., \mu_{LT_{r,a}}(a_t)). \tag{2}$$

- **Inference**: The model's final output, $\hat{o}_{t+1}$, is a weighted average of the consequents of all rules, where the weights are the firing strengths:

$$\hat{o}_{t+1} = \frac{\sum_r \mu_{r,ant}(o_t, a_t) \cdot f_r(o_t, a_t)}{\sum_r \mu_{r,ant}(o_t, a_t)}. \tag{3}$$

  This provides a prediction for the next observation, denoted as $\hat{o}_{t+1} = f_{\text{fuzzy}}(o_t, a_t)$.

3 A Fuzzy-MAP Expectation-Maximization Algorithm

The core of our method involves augmenting the M-step of the Expectation-Maximization (EM) algorithm with priors derived from a fuzzy model defined by domain experts. This approach transforms the standard Maximum Likelihood Estimation into a Maximum A Posteriori (MAP) estimation [6], where the fuzzy model serves as a source of prior knowledge. Integration is achieved by generating fuzzy pseudo-counts, which are incorporated into the empirical counts obtained during the E-step, thereby guiding the parameter updates.

3.1 Fuzzy Pseudo-counts

We generate separate pseudo-counts for both the transition model and the observation model. The process involves evaluating each fuzzy rule's relevance and prediction in the context of the current POMDP parameters estimate θ^k.

The formulation of fuzzy transition pseudo-counts has two key components:

- **Matching Antecedent Score**, denoted by $MatchAnt(s, a, r)$, represents the expected firing strength with respect to the observation distribution associated with state s. Conceptually, it quantifies how strongly the antecedent of a fuzzy rule r is activated when the system is in a latent state s and action a is taken:

$$MatchAnt(s, a, r) = \int_{o \in \Omega} \mu_{r,ant}(o, a)\, O(o \mid s; \theta^k)\, \mathrm{d}o. \tag{4}$$

- **Consequent Likelihood** evaluates how likely the consequent of a fuzzy rule is to have been generated by the subsequent state s'. It assesses the plausibility of a fuzzy rule's prediction within the context of the POMDP's state dynamics:

$$L(Y_r^*(s, a) \mid s'; \theta^{(k)}) = O(Y_r^*(s, a) \mid s'; \theta^{(k)}), \tag{5}$$

where

$$Y_r^*(s, a) = \mathbb{E}_{o \sim O(\cdot \mid s; \theta^{(k)})}\left[f_r(o, a)\right] = \int f_r(o, a) \cdot O(o \mid s; \theta^{(k)})\, \mathrm{d}o. \tag{6}$$

Definition 1. *The* ***fuzzy transition pseudo-counts*** *for a transition (s, a, s') is the sum over all fuzzy rules of the product of the antecedent match (Eq. 4) and the consequent likelihood (Eq. 5):*

$$N_T^{fuzzy}(s, a, s') = \sum_{r=1}^{R} MatchAnt(s, a, r) \times L(Y_r^*(s, a) \mid s'; \theta^{(k)}). \tag{7}$$

In order to compute the fuzzy observation pseudo-counts, it is necessary to introduce the concept of $strength(s, a, s', r)$. The term $strength(s, a, s', r)$ represents the expected rule activation for a specific transition and is defined as:

$$strength(s, a, s', r) = T^{(k)}(s, a, s') \times MatchAnt(s, a, r). \tag{8}$$

Definition 2. *The* ***fuzzy observation pseudo-counts*** *are computed for each state s' by marginalizing over all possible antecedent states s, actions a, and fuzzy rules r. The contribution of each rule's consequent, $Y_r^*(s, a)$, is weighted by its corresponding $strength(s, a, s', r)$:*

$$N_O^{fuzzy}(s') = \sum_{r \in R} \sum_{s \in S} \sum_{a \in A} strength(s, a, s', r) \tag{9}$$

$$S_O^{fuzzy}(s') = \sum_{r \in R} \sum_{s \in S} \sum_{a \in A} strength(s, a, s', r) \times Y_r^*(s, a) \tag{10}$$

$$S_{O,2}^{fuzzy}(s') = \sum_{r \in R} \sum_{s \in S} \sum_{a \in A} strength(s, a, s', r) \times (Y_r^*(s, a) \cdot Y_r^*(s, a)^{\mathrm{T}}) \tag{11}$$

3.2 Fuzzy Pseudo-counts Augmented M-Step

The M-step is augmented by adding the fuzzy pseudo-counts, weighted by the hyperparameters λ_T and λ_O, to the empirical counts derived from the E-step. The augmented counts are:

$$\tilde{N}_T(s,a,s') = \hat{N}_T(s,a,s') + \lambda_T N_T^{\text{fuzzy}}(s,a,s') \tag{12}$$

$$\tilde{N}_O(s) = \hat{N}_O(s) + \lambda_O N_O^{\text{fuzzy}}(s) \tag{13}$$

$$\tilde{S}_O(s) = \hat{S}_O(s) + \lambda_O S_O^{\text{fuzzy}}(s) \tag{14}$$

$$\tilde{S}_{O,2}(s) = \hat{S}_{O,2}(s) + \lambda_O S_{O,2}^{\text{fuzzy}}(s) \tag{15}$$

The parameter updates then proceed using these augmented counts:

- **Transition Probabilities**:

$$T^{(k+1)}(s,a,s') = \frac{\tilde{N}_T(s,a,s')}{\sum_{s'' \in S} \tilde{N}_T(s,a,s'')} \tag{16}$$

- **Observation Parameters** (for each state s'):

$$\mu_{s'}^{(k+1)} = \frac{\tilde{S}_O(s')}{\tilde{N}_O(s')}, \qquad \Sigma_{s'}^{(k+1)} = \frac{\tilde{S}_{O,2}(s')}{\tilde{N}_O(s')} - \mu_{s'}^{(k+1)} \mu_{s'}^{(k+1)\,\mathrm{T}} \tag{17}$$

4 Numerical Experiments on Synthetic Data

The aim of this section is to evaluate the impact of integrating expert knowledge into the parameter estimation process for POMDPs. To achieve this, we adopt a comparative framework, benchmarking the performance of Fuzzy-MAP EM against the standard EM algorithm, which serves as our baseline reference.

To assess model performance, we compare the learned parameters against the ground truth of the underlying POMDP. The accuracy of the transition model is quantified using the L1 distance, which measures the total absolute deviation between the estimated and true transition probabilities. For the observation model, we use the Kullback–Leibler (KL) divergence [9] to evaluate the difference between the learned and actual observation distributions for each state, capturing how well the model approximates the true generative process.

Since the learning process is unsupervised, the latent states inferred by the model do not possess inherent semantic labels. To assign meaningful labels (e.g., "Healthy", "Sick", "Critical"), we manually compared the observed distributions associated with each latent state to the ground-truth distributions, and matched them based on their similarity.

To evaluate our approach, we created a simulated medical environment in which a patient's latent state can be one of the following: $\{\text{Healthy}, \text{Sick}, \text{Critical}\}$. At each time step t, a clinician selects an action from the set {Wait, Treat}. Taking the selected action, the clinician observes a two-dimensional vector $o_t = (\text{symptoms}_t, \text{test\_result}_t)$, where each component is a continuous variable taking values within the interval $[0, 1]$.

The underlying dynamics of this environment are governed by a ground-truth POMDP whose state transition probabilities, $P(s' \mid s, a)$, are given in Table 1. For each hidden state, observations are drawn from a corresponding Beta distribution, as depicted in Fig. 1. Throughout the learning phase, the underlying distributions are approximated by multivariate normal distributions.

Table 1. Ground-truth transition probabilities $P(s' \mid s, a)$.

Action	Current State	Next State		
		Healthy	Sick	Critical
Wait	Healthy	0.85	0.14	0.01
	Sick	0.30	0.60	0.10
	Critical	0.05	0.01	0.94
Treat	Healthy	0.80	0.15	0.05
	Sick	0.65	0.35	0.00
	Critical	0.10	0.65	0.25

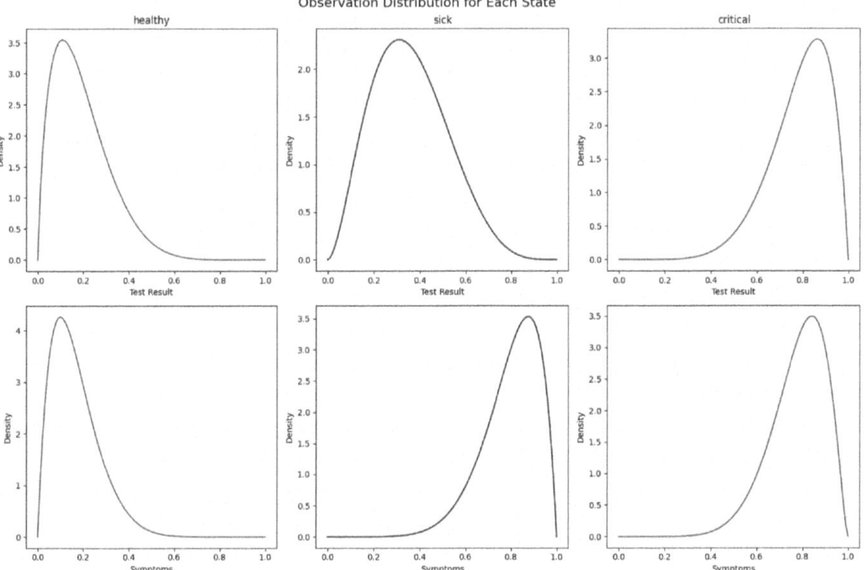

Fig. 1. Ground-truth observation distributions for each state.

To supply expert knowledge for the Fuzzy-MAP EM algorithm, we simulated the construction of a fuzzy model based on domain expertise. Using the PyFume library [5], we trained a Takagi-Sugeno fuzzy model on a separate, larger dataset, generated from the ground-truth POMDP, than the one used for POMDP learning. This approach ensured that the expert knowledge was derived independently from the target learning process. Functioning as an expert system, the fuzzy model takes the current observation o_t and the selected action a_t as inputs to generate a prediction of the next observation, denoted as $\hat{o}_{t+1}$.

The simulated expert model demonstrated satisfactory predictive accuracy, achieving R^2 scores of 0.63 and 0.64 for forecasting the next test result and symptoms profile, respectively, on a held-out test dataset.

The performance of the proposed approach is evaluated under two challenging conditions: (*i*) a low-data regime, where learning is based on only 3 trajectories of length 5; and (*ii*) a high-noise regime, where 10 trajectories of length 5 are perturbed by Gaussian noise $\mathcal{N}(0, 0.25)$ applied to each component of the observation vector. Following a grid search sensitivity analysis, the hyperparameters for the experimental setup were selected as follows: $\lambda_T = 0.1$ and $\lambda_O = 0.05$.

Low-Data Regime. When data availability is extremely limited, the standard EM algorithm struggles to recover the underlying model, resulting in a high L1 distance for transition probabilities (0.43) and substantial KL divergences in the observation distributions (Table 2, top part). In contrast, Fuzzy-MAP EM—guided by the expert model—produces a significantly more accurate transition model (L1 distance of 0.18) and yields more plausible observation distributions.

High-Noise Regime. In the high-noise scenario, the advantages of Fuzzy-MAP EM are more modest but still evident. It continues to learn a more accurate transition model (L1 distance of 0.26 vs. 0.29) and shows a marked improvement in modeling the observation distribution for the "Critical" state (Table 2, bottom part).

Overall, these results demonstrate that incorporating expert fuzzy knowledge into the EM framework yields more robust parameter estimation under both data scarcity and observational uncertainty.

Table 2. Comparison of Standard EM and Fuzzy-MAP EM.

Regime	Measure	Standard EM	Fuzzy-MAP EM
Low-Data	L1 distance transitions	0.43	**0.18**
	KL divergence Healthy	3.43	**0.19**
	KL divergence Sick	∞	**2.63**
	KL divergence Critical	9.11	**6.39**
High-Noise	L1 distance transitions	0.29	**0.26**
	KL divergence Healthy	0.38	**0.35**
	KL divergence Sick	**0.57**	0.65
	KL divergence Critical	1.23	**0.43**

5 Therapeutic Protocols of Myasthenia Gravis

In this section we assess the clinical relevance of our approach by applying the Fuzzy-MAP EM algorithm to a fuzzy model of Myasthenia Gravis (MG) defined by domain experts. The objective is to learn a two-state POMDP that captures the disease dynamics under two distinct scenarios: absence of treatment and administration of biological drug named Ravulizumab.

5.1 Fuzzy Model of Adaptive Immune System Alterations in MG

MG is a rare autoimmune disease that causes severe and debilitating muscle weakness. The clinical manifestation is characterized by differences in age of onset, muscle involvement, auto-antibody specificity and thymic pathology, suggesting that multiple disregulated pathways can lead to the same disease. Accordingly, a high diversity is also observed in the effect of therapies, as a substantial minority of patients are unresponsive to classical immunosuppressants. The development of methods for personalized medicine based on patient's specific features is thus of particular interest. For a comprehensive review of clinical and biological aspects of MG the reader can refer to [7].

The fuzzy model considered in this work is focused on the most common type of MG—i.e. AChR-MG associated with thymic alterations [7]—and takes into account the main cellular components involved in the associated autoimmune reaction, which is triggered by inflammation and/or thymoma (Fig. 2). These events cause alterations in the adaptive immune system, such as a decreased activity of regulatory T cells (Treg), and an increased activity of autoreactive effector T cells (Teff) and B cells (B). This autoimmune reaction results in the differentiation of autoreactive B cells into Short Lived Plasma Blasts (SLPB), which produce self-reacting Immunoglobulins G (IgG) that target and disrupt the neuromuscular junction, leading to the characteristic symptoms of MG. IgG bound to biological surfaces can induce the activation of the complement system, causing the formation of opsonins (i.e., proteins that facilitate the phagocytosis of the bound antigen and elicit immune reactivity) and of the membrane attack complex (i.e., a protein complex that forms pores in the cells' membranes, destabilizing them). The concurrent activity of self-reactive Teff and B cells and the presence of complement opsonized antigens in the hyperplastic thymus of MG patients, leads to the formation of ectopic Germinal Centres (GC), in which Plasma Cells (PC) producing high affinity antibodies are selected and proliferate. GC-derived PC are capable of establishing niches that sustain them for years, forming a population of Long Lived PC (LLPC) that continuously produce IgG, leading to long lasting and treatment resistant humoral autoimmunity [3].

Biological drugs such as *Efgartigimod*, *Eculizumab* and *Ravulizumab* can be used in MG therapeutic protocols as final fallback to alleviate MG symptoms, especially for patients not properly responding to standard treatments. The effectiveness of these drugs depends on their ability to specifically target molecules directly involved in MG pathology: Efgartigimod induces the decrease of IgG levels, while Eculizumab and Ravulizumab target the terminal complement component C5. Other biological drugs targeting B cells and specific cytokines involved in autoimmune processes also exist [11]. The fuzzy rules and the linguistic terms of all model's variables are shown in Fig. 4, Appendix A.

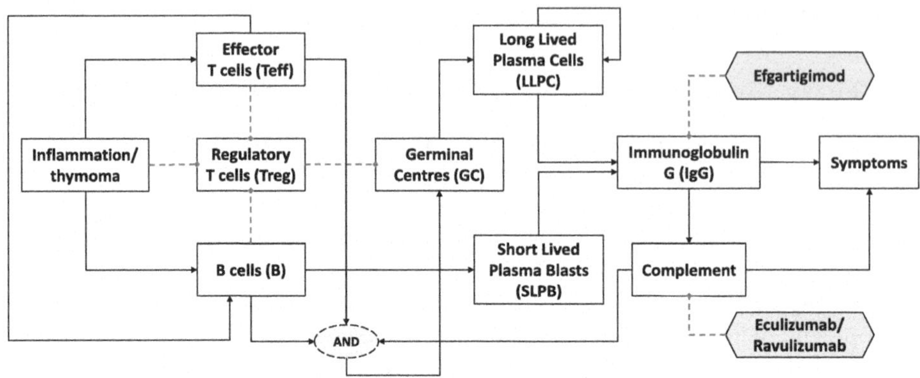

Fig. 2. Interaction map of the MG fuzzy model. Plain black (dotted red) lines represent positive (negative) regulations. Coloured boxes correspond to biological drugs. (Color figure online)

5.2 Experimental Design

This case study aims to learn a two-state POMDP model designed to assess two alternative actions, i.e., *no intervention* and *treatment with Ravulizumab*, in the case where a 10-dimensional observation space is derived from the variables of an expert-defined fuzzy model. Using the fuzzy model, a synthetic training dataset comprising 40 simulated patient trajectories was generated, with each trajectory consisting of 9 discrete timesteps.

To ensure a robust starting point and to mitigate convergence to poor local optima, the parameters were initialised using a data-driven approach. The k-means algorithm was used to partition the dataset into two clusters, whose centroids were used as the initial mean vectors for each state's observation model. To complete the setup, the initial transition probabilities were set to uniform, and the observation covariance matrices were initialised as identity matrices.

Hyperparameter selection was guided by a sensitivity analysis. Empirical observations revealed that assigning high values to λ_T and λ_O led the model to collapse into a single latent state. For this experiment, we selected $\lambda_T = 0.05$ and $\lambda_O = 0.05$, as these values offered a balance between expert guidance and empirical validation. Upon completing the training, we performed a single iteration of the standard Expectation-Maximization (EM) algorithm to allow empirical data to modestly adjust the transition estimates, which might otherwise be overly constrained by the expert-informed fuzzy priors.

5.3 Results

The application of Fuzzy-MAP EM to MG yielded a robust two-state model. Based on the learned observation probability distributions, the latent states were semantically interpreted as *Mild MG* (State 1) and *Severe MG* (State 2). This interpretation is substantiated by the distributions of variables central to MG pathology. Specifically, IgG and complement levels were significantly higher in the *Severe MG* state, consistent with a greater autoantibody load and more pronounced complement activation (Fig. 3). This clinical characterization is further supported by other model variables, wherein the *Severe MG* state is associated with higher levels of symptoms, inflammation, and pro-inflammatory T cells (Teff). Conversely, the *Mild MG* state reflects a more favourable immunological profile, characterized by reduced inflammation and symptoms severity.

The learned transition probabilities quantify both the natural disease progression and the therapeutic effect of Ravulizumab (Table 3). The administration of the drug shows a clear and positive clinical impact: for patients in the Severe state, Ravulizumab reduces the probability of remaining severe from 81.1% down to 64.0%. This result successfully captures the drug's known mechanism of action confirming that, by inhibiting the complement system, it can alleviate the disease severity and promote a shift towards a healthier clinical state. Crucially, this modeled therapeutic effect is consistent with real-world clinical evidence, which demonstrated the efficacy of Ravulizumab in treating MG patients [12].

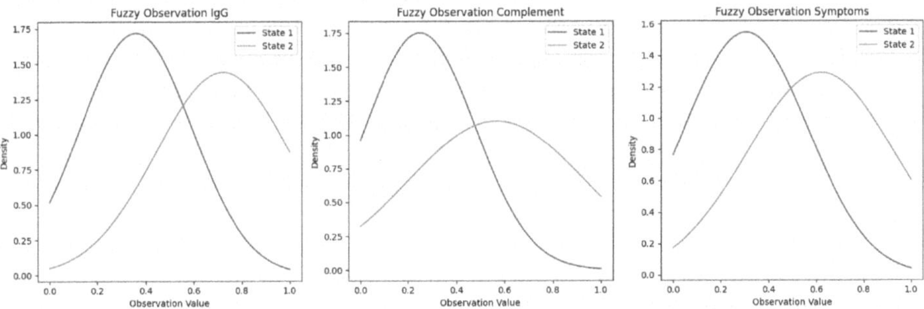

Fig. 3. Learned observation probability density distributions for IgG, Complement and Symptoms variables, separated by latent state. State 1 (blue) represents the "Mild MG" condition, and State 2 (orange) represents the "Severe MG" condition. (Color figure online)

Table 3. Learned transition probabilities for the two-state MG model. **Bold** indicates a significant difference between the two actions.

Action	Current State	Next State	
		Mild MG	Severe MG
No treatment	Mild MG	0.979	0.021
	Severe MG	**0.189**	**0.811**
Ravulizumab	Mild MG	0.968	0.032
	Severe MG	**0.360**	**0.640**

6 Discussion and Conclusion

The enhanced performance of our Fuzzy-MAP EM algorithm highlights the critical role of integrating expert knowledge into probabilistic modeling frameworks. By leveraging *fuzzy pseudo-counts* as an informative prior, the proposed method facilitates the learning process, where empirical evidence is regularised by domain expertise, resulting in more robust models when faced with limited or noisy data. This has significant practical applications in complex domains such as the management of rare diseases. The Myasthenia Gravis case study demonstrates this, illustrating how a reliable decision-making framework can be established even in the absence of initial patient data.

Nevertheless, our method presents certain trade-offs and limitations that are worth discussing. From a theoretical point of view, introducing a fuzzy prior does not guarantee the maximisation of the expected complete data log likelihood. Consequently, the monotonic increase of the data log-likelihood $\mathcal{L}(\theta)$ at each iteration is no longer guaranteed, which is a core property that supports the convergence proof for the standard EM algorithm. Secondly, the method is susceptible to errors originating from the fuzzy prior itself. We have identified two main issues:

- **Prediction Bias:** inaccuracies in the expert fuzzy model are directly propagated into the learned POMDP parameters.
- **Antecedent Confusion:** this issue arises from the discrepancy between the fuzzy model's reliance on observations and the POMDP's latent state structure. When observation distributions from different states overlap, a rule originally *intended* for one state (e.g., 'Healthy') can be erroneously activated by an observation from another (e.g., 'Sick'), causing the learned parameters to skew towards the state with the most confident prediction.

These limitations thus highlight areas for future research.

In summary, the present paper introduced the Fuzzy-MAP EM algorithm, a novel and original method for integrating expert knowledge into the POMDP parameter learning process. The augmentation of the standard EM algorithm with *fuzzy pseudo-counts* is a methodology that has been demonstrated to effectively mitigate the challenges posed by data scarcity and observational noise, thereby producing more accurate and robust models. As demonstrated through both synthetic experiments and a real-world case study on Myasthenia Gravis, this method represents a significant step toward developing reliable decision support systems in complex domains where data is inherently limited.

Acknowledgments. This work has been developed within the research project: *"Personalising myasthenia gravis medicine: from "one-fits-all" to patient-specific immunosuppression"* (ERAPERMED2022-258, GA 779282), funded by Fondazione Regionale per la Ricerca Biomedica (Regione Lombardia), which also funded the PhD fellowship of ML and the research scholarship of RCC. This work is also partially supported by the MUR under the grant "Dipartimenti di Eccellenza 2023–2027" of the Department of Informatics, Systems and Communication of the University of Milano-Bicocca, Milan, Italy, and by the National Plan for NRRP Complementary Investments (established with the decree-law May 6, 2021, n. 59, converted by law n. 101 of 2021) in the call for the funding of research initiatives for technologies and innovative trajectories in the health care sectors (Directorial Decree n. 931 of 06-06-2022)—project n. PNC0000003—AdvaNced Technologies for Human-centrEd Medicine (project acronym: ANTHEM). This work reflects only the authors' views and opinions, neither the Ministry for University and Research nor the European Commission can be considered responsible for them.

Disclosure of Interests. No interests to declare.

Appendix A. Fuzzy Model of Myasthenia Gravis

This section provides supplementary details on the expert-defined fuzzy model used to simulate the immunopathology of Myasthenia Gravis (MG). The model is designed to capture the regulatory interactions among the key cellular and molecular components that drive the disease.

The conceptual structure of these interactions is illustrated in the interaction map in Fig. 2 of the main manuscript. Figure 4 below shows the model's variables (nodes), their linguistic terms, and the complete set of fuzzy rules that govern their behaviour.

Node	Terms	Regulatory nodes	Rule number	Fuzzy rules
Teff	Low	Treg	1	IF (Inflammation IS High) THEN (Teff IS High)
	Medium	Inflammation	2	IF (Inflammation IS Medium) THEN (Teff IS Medium)
	High		3	IF (Inflammation IS Low) THEN (Teff IS Low)
			4	IF (Treg IS High) THEN (Teff IS Low)
			5	IF (Treg IS Medium) THEN (Teff IS Medium)
			6	IF (Treg IS Low) THEN (Teff IS High)
Treg	Low	Inflammation	7	IF (Inflammation IS High) THEN (Treg IS Low)
	Medium		8	IF (Inflammation IS Medium) THEN (Treg IS Medium)
	High		9	IF (Inflammation IS Low) THEN (Treg IS High)
B	Low	Teff	10	IF (Teff IS High) THEN (B IS High)
	Medium	Inflammation	11	IF (Teff IS Medium) THEN (B IS Medium)
	High	Treg	12	IF (Teff IS Low) THEN (B IS Low)
			13	IF (Inflammation IS High) THEN (B IS High)
			14	IF (Inflammation IS Medium) THEN (B IS Medium)
			15	IF (Inflammation IS Low) THEN (B IS Low)
			16	IF (Treg IS High) THEN (B IS Low)
			17	IF (Treg IS Medium) THEN (B IS Medium)
			18	IF (Treg IS Low) THEN (B IS High)
GC	Low	Teff	19	IF (Teff IS High) AND (B IS High) AND (Complement IS High) THEN (GC IS High)
	Medium	B	20	IF (Teff IS High) AND (B IS High) AND (Complement IS Medium) THEN (GC IS Medium)
	High	Complement	21	IF (Teff IS High) AND (B IS Medium) AND (Complement IS High) THEN (GC IS Medium)
		Treg	22	IF (Teff IS High) AND (B IS Medium) AND (Complement IS Medium) THEN (GC IS Medium)
			23	IF (Teff IS Medium) AND (B IS High) AND (Complement IS High) THEN (GC IS High)
			24	IF (Teff IS Medium) AND (B IS High) AND (Complement IS Medium) THEN (GC IS Medium)
			25	IF (Teff IS Medium) AND (B IS Medium) AND (Complement IS High) THEN (GC IS Medium)
			26	IF (Teff IS Medium) AND (B IS Medium) AND (Complement IS Medium) THEN (GC IS Medium)
			27	IF (Teff IS Low) THEN (GC IS Low)
			28	IF (B IS Low) THEN (GC IS Low)
			29	IF (Complement IS Low) THEN (GC IS Low)
			30	IF (Treg IS High) THEN (GC IS Low)
			31	IF (Treg IS Medium) THEN (GC IS Medium)
			32	IF (Treg IS Low) THEN (GC IS High)
SLPB	Low	B	33	IF (B IS High) THEN (SLPB IS High)
	Medium		34	IF (B IS Medium) THEN (SLPB IS Medium)
	High		35	IF (B IS Low) THEN (SLPB IS Low)
LLPC	Low	GC	36	IF (GC IS High) OR (LLPC IS High) THEN (LLPC IS High)
	Medium	LLPC	37	IF (GC IS Medium) OR (LLPC IS Medium) THEN (LLPC IS Medium)
	High		38	IF (GC IS Low) AND (LLPC IS Low) THEN (LLPC IS Low)
IgG	Low	SLPB	39	IF (SLPB IS High) THEN (IgG IS High)
	Medium	LLPC	40	IF (SLPB IS Medium) THEN (IgG IS Medium)
	High		41	IF (SLPB IS Low) THEN (IgG IS Low)
			42	IF (LLPC IS High) THEN (IgG IS High)
			43	IF (LLPC IS Medium) THEN (IgG IS Medium)
			44	IF (LLPC IS Low) THEN (IgG IS Low)
Complement	Low	IgG	45	IF (IgG IS High) THEN (Complement IS High)
	Medium		46	IF (IgG IS Medium) THEN (Complement IS Medium)
	High		47	IF (IgG IS Low) THEN (Complement IS Low)
Symptoms	Low	IgG	48	IF (IgG IS High) THEN (Symptoms IS High)
	Medium	Complement	49	IF (IgG IS Medium) THEN (Symptoms IS Medium)
	High		50	IF (IgG IS Low) THEN (Symptoms IS Low)
			51	IF (Complement IS High) THEN (Symptoms IS High)
			52	IF (Complement IS Medium) THEN (Symptoms IS Medium)
			53	IF (Complement IS Low) THEN (Symptoms IS Low)
Ravu	Low		54	IF (Ravu IS High) THEN (Complement IS Low)
	Medium			
	High			
Inflammation	Low			
	Medium			
	High			

Fig. 4. Detailed specification of the fuzzy model for Myasthenia Gravis (MG).

References

1. Baum, L.E., Petrie, T., Soules, G., Weiss, N.: A maximization technique occurring in the statistical analysis of probabilistic functions of Markov chains. Ann. Math. Stat. **41**(1), 164–171 (1970)

2. Cassandra, A.R., Kaelbling, L.P., Littman, M.L.: Acting optimally in partially observable stochastic domains. In: AAAI-94 Proceedings, vol. 94, pp. 1023–1028 (1994)
3. Cavalcante, P., Cufi, P., Mantegazza, R., Berrih-Aknin, S., Bernasconi, P., Le Panse, R.: Etiology of myasthenia gravis: innate immunity signature in pathological thymus. Autoimmun. Rev. **12**(9), 863–874 (2013)
4. Dempster, A.P., Laird, N.M., Rubin, D.B.: Maximum likelihood from incomplete data via the EM algorithm. J. Roy. Stat. Soc.: Ser. B (Methodol.) **39**(1), 1–22 (1977)
5. Fuchs, C., Spolaor, S., Nobile, M.S., Kaymak, U.: pyFUME: a Python package for fuzzy model estimation. In: 2020 IEEE International Conference on Fuzzy Systems (FUZZ-IEEE), pp. 1–8. IEEE (2020)
6. Gauvain, J.L., Lee, C.H.: Maximum a posteriori estimation for multivariate Gaussian mixture observations of Markov chains. IEEE Trans. Speech Audio Process. **2**(2), 291–298 (1994)
7. Gilhus, N.E., Tzartos, S., Evoli, A., Palace, J., Burns, T.M., Verschuuren, J.J.G.M.: Myasthenia gravis. Nat. Rev. Dis. Primers. **5**, 30 (2019). https://doi.org/10.1038/s41572-019-0079-y
8. Hauskrecht, M., Fraser, H.: Planning treatment of ischemic heart disease with partially observable Markov decision processes. Artif. Intell. Med. **18**(3), 221–244 (2000)
9. Kullback, S., Leibler, R.A.: On information and sufficiency. Ann. Math. Stat. **22**(1), 79–86 (1951)
10. Mehran, K.: Takagi-Sugeno fuzzy modeling for process control. Industr. Autom. Robot. Artif. Intell. (EEE8005) **262**, 1–31 (2008)
11. Vanoli, F., Mantegazza, R.: Antibody therapies in autoimmune neuromuscular junction disorders: approach to myasthenic crisis and chronic management. Neurotherapeutics **19**(3), 897–910 (2022)
12. Vu, T., et al.: Terminal complement inhibitor ravulizumab in generalized myasthenia gravis. NEJM Evidence **1**(5), EVIDoa2100066 (2022). https://doi.org/10.1056/EVIDoa2100066

A Hybrid Evolutionary Fuzzy Neural Approach for Maternal Health Risk Prediction

Gianluca Apriceno[1(✉)], Marina Segala[1,2], Giovanni Valer[2], Nicola Muraro[2], Vincenzo Netti[2], Paulo Vitor de Campos Souza[1], and Mauro Dragoni[1]

[1] Fondazione Bruno Kessler, Trento, Italy
{apriceno,msegala,pdecampossouza,dragoni}@fbk.eu
[2] University of Trento, Trento, Italy
{marina.segala,giovanni.valer,nicola.muraro, vincenzo.netti}@studenti.unitn.it

Abstract. The demand for transparent and explainable AI solutions in healthcare has highlighted the limitations of purely data-driven models and emphasized the value of symbolic methods such as Fuzzy Inference Systems, which provide understandable rules and facilitate collaboration with human experts. To overcome the limitations and merge the strenghts of individual approaches, hybrid models that integrate sub-symbolic and symbolic reasoning have emerged as a promising direction. For example, Fuzzy Neural Networks merge the predictive strength of neural networks with the clarity of fuzzy systems, and their performance can be further enhanced through evolutionary techniques that optimize parameters and improve adaptability. In this study, we propose an evolutionary Fuzzy Neural Network framework that use a genetic algorithm to strengthen classification capabilities while maintaining interpretability. By incorporating the evolutionary optimization into the network's parameter update process, the model achieves both robustness and transparency. Validation on the Maternal Health Risk dataset demonstrates that the proposed approach effectively balances predictive accuracy with explainability.

Keywords: Hybrid AI Systems · Evolutionary Algorithms · Fuzzy Neural Network

GitHub: https://github.com/IDA-FBK/Evo-Fuzzy-Neural-Maternal

1 Introduction

Over the past ten years, hybrid methods that integrate sub-symbolic (data-driven) and symbolic techniques have gained widespread adoption across various research domains. By combining the advantages of each approach and mitigating their respective limitations, these methods have proven effective in applications

P. Bruno et al. (Eds.): HC_AIxIA_HYDRA 2025, CCIS 2830, pp. 384–397, 2026.
https://doi.org/10.1007/978-3-032-16708-8_31

such as event recognition [6–8,11,29] and energy prediction [9], among others. Furthermore, recent advancements, such as the integration of uninorm based fuzzy operators [12], show the potential of hybrid frameworks for achieving more flexible and expressive reasoning.

In the healthcare domain, the growing demand for Explainable AI (XAI) has highlighted the need for models that are both accurate and interpretable. Symbolic techniques, such as Fuzzy Inference Systems (FIS), provide interpretable fuzzy rules that facilitate communication between AI systems and human experts, enhancing trust in clinical decisions [13–16,18]. Fuzzy Neural Networks (FNNs) extend this concept by combining the predictive capabilities of neural networks with the transparency of symbolic models. Moreover, the use of Evolutionary Algorithms (EAs) in training these networks has shown promise in optimizing performance and improving adaptability [19].

These hybrid approaches provide an effective strategy for tackling classification tasks on datasets where a high proportion of outliers poses a significant challenge for traditional data-driven machine learning methods, such as neural networks. A notable example is the Maternal Health Risk dataset[1], which contains physiological measurements from pregnant women. In such datasets, the physiological signals are highly individualized (i.e., linked with the specific case), making misclassification relatively easy. In this context, incorporating symbolic reasoning offers a promising research direction. It not only has the potential to improve the classification performance of the model but also enhances its reliability by providing transparency, explainability, and interpretability.

In this work, we propose an evolutionary Fuzzy Neural Network (evo-FNN) framework that builds upon [17] by integrating a genetic algorithm into the learning process. This approach aims to enhance classification performance while maintaining model transparency. The framework is evaluated on the Maternal Health Risk dataset, demonstrating its effectiveness for maternal health risk assessment.

The contributions of this study are twofold: (i) introducing evolutionary optimization into the parameter update process of [17], and (ii) leveraging EAs to optimize neuron weights, thereby simplifying fuzzy rule antecedents and improving interpretability. By estimating Gaussian neuron weights rather than assigning them randomly, the method prioritizes feature importance and allows dimensions with negligible weights to be discarded, simplifying knowledge extraction and reducing redundant information. To our knowledge, this is the first application of evolutionary optimization within this specific FNN architecture.

The remaining of the paper is organized as follows: Sect. 2 reviews related literature on evolutionary FNNs; Sect. 3 presents the evolutionary update adopted within [17](i.e., the evo-FNN); Sect. 4 describes the dataset and experimental setup; Sect. 5 presents the results, while Sect. 6 concludes the papers and outlines directions for future works.

[1] https://archive.ics.uci.edu/dataset/863/maternal+health+risk.

2 Related Work

Evolutionary algorithms (EAs) are optimization techniques inspired by the principles of natural selection and genetics [10]. These algorithms operate on populations of potential solutions, iteratively refining them through selection, crossover, mutation, and reproduction processes to optimize a given objective function. The stochastic and global optimization nature of EAs makes them particularly suitable for solving complex, non-linear, and multi-modal problems that arise in fuzzy neural networks (FNNs) [20].

EAs are versatile tools that have been applied to various components of FNNs, including membership function (MF) tuning, weight optimization, and the adjustment of fuzzy rule parameters [24]. MFs define the fuzzy sets in FNNs and significantly influence the system's interpretability and accuracy. EAs are employed to optimize the parameters of these functions, such as their shapes and positions. [25] demonstrated the use of evolutionary programming to tune MFs dynamically, enabling the FNN to adapt to changes in input space and improve system modeling capabilities. Weight optimization in FNNs involves adjusting the connection weights to minimize error metrics and improve system performance. Unlike gradient-based methods, EAs can explore complex solution spaces without requiring derivative information. [3] proposed a differential evolution-based approach to optimize weights and bias in recurrent FNNs, specifically for forecasting and identification problems. Also [22] demonstrated the use of evolutionary programming to tune weights dynamically, enabling the FNN to adapt to changes in input space and improve system modeling capabilities. EAs have been used also in optimizing fuzzy rule parameters, including both antecedents and consequents. The antecedent optimization involves identifying the most appropriate input conditions, while consequent optimization determines the output values or functions. For example, [27] applied genetic algorithms to fine-tune rule parameters in fuzzy neural networks. Finally, [5] utilized a hybrid evolutionary strategy combining genetic parameters with simulated annealing to optimize fuzzy rules, achieving robust performance improvements.

EAs have been successfully applied across various domains utilizing FNNs. For example, [26] employed genetic algorithms for dynamic parameter optimization in evolving FNNs, demonstrating their effectiveness in chaotic (Mackey-Glass) time series prediction. [1] applied hybrid learning algorithms combining EAs with local search techniques for modeling chaotic systems, achieving high accuracy and convergence rates. [21] utilized evolutionary programming fuzzy control system design and [4] creates a model that works with Petrol production forecasting. In [30] an optimized FNN solved problems related to liquid level modeling issue in an industrial coke furnace.

In most studies, EAs in FNN architectures are used to improve model accuracy. This study proposes defining the weights of the first-layer Gaussian neurons using EAs to improve the clarity of results. By optimally calculating feature weights, feature dimensions are defined, directly impacting fuzzy rule antecedents and making the extracted knowledge more aligned with the analyzed data. This approach is also expected to improve model accuracy, as better-adjusted dimensions lead to more precise fuzzy rules, which generate the final results with the support of an artificial neural network.

3 Methodology

We leverage a pre-existing FNN [17] system. The traditional optimization algorithm used for training in [17] is the Moore-Penrose pseudoinverse (see step 4), where cosine similarity is applied between the output of the logical fuzzy neurons and the labels in the training set to compute the weights **V**, which are subsequently used during inference. However, we observed that this training method leads to overfitting, resulting in limited generalization capabilities. In this context, we believe that metaheuristic techniques could offer a promising solution. As a result, we propose the implementation of an evolutionary algorithm, treating a specific weight configuration as an individual within our population.

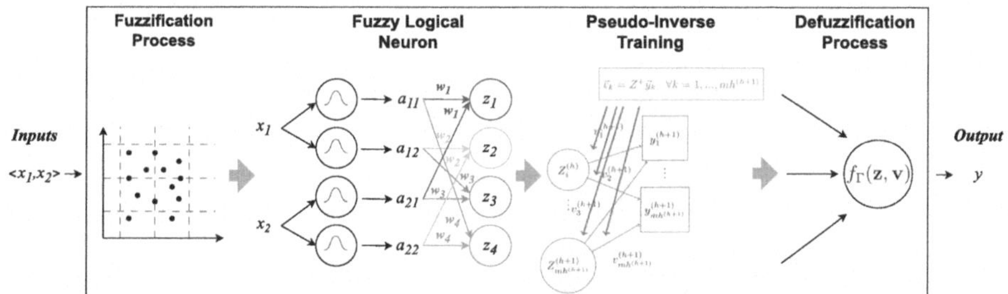

Fig. 1. FNN pipeline with two inputs, each associate to two (gaussian) MFs.

3.1 FNN Steps

We summarize below the four steps composing the FNN framework (see Fig. 1) we used as the starting point to create the proposed evolutionary-based solution.

Step 1: Fuzzification. The initial fuzzification process follows the procedure introduced by [23]. For each input variable x_j, m uniformly spaced gaussian membership functions (i.e., fuzzy sets) are generated using a grid partitioning method. This method divides the domain of each x_j into m intervals, with each interval represented by a gaussian characterized by a center c_{jl} and standard deviation σ_{jl}, determined from the input data distribution. Formally, each gaussian membership function is defined as:

$$A_j(x_j, c_{jl}, \sigma_{jl}) = e^{-\frac{1}{2}\left(\frac{x_j - c_{jl}}{\sigma_{jl}}\right)^2}, \quad \text{for } j = 1, \ldots, n, \quad l = 1, \ldots, m, \tag{1}$$

where n denotes the number of input variables, and m represents the number of gaussian membership functions assigned to each input variable.

Step 2: Fuzzy Logical Neuron. The second step implements logical fuzzy neurons to aggregate the fuzzified inputs and the corresponding logical neuron weights using fuzzy logical operators. For each input variable x_j, the fuzzified values corresponding to the m gaussians are computed as follow:

$$a_{jl} = A_j(x_j, c_{jl}, \sigma_{jl}) \tag{2}$$

These values are aggregated into AND or OR logical neuron defined as follows:

$$\mathbf{z} = \text{AND}(\mathbf{w}; \mathbf{a}) = T_{i=1}^{n}(s(w_i, a_i)) \tag{3}$$

$$\mathbf{z} = \text{OR}(\mathbf{w}; \mathbf{a}) = S_{i=1}^{n}(t(w_i a_i)) \tag{4}$$

where w_i represents the weight and a_i the activation for the ith input, T is a t-norm (e.g., product for AND operation), and S is a t-conorm (e.g., probabilistic sum for OR operation). The outputs from these neurons are combined to form the antecedents of fuzzy IF-THEN rules, enabling the network to model complex relationships within the data.

Step 3: Defuzzification Process. The defuzzification process aggregates the outputs of the fuzzy logical neurons to compute the network's final output:

$$\hat{y} = \left(\sum_{j=0}^{L} f_\Gamma(z_j, v_j) \right) \tag{5}$$

where f_Γ denotes the neuron activation function.

Step 4: Training Technique. The FNN is trained using the Moore-Penrose pseudo-inverse to optimize neuron connections. The weights v_j are updated as follows:

$$\boldsymbol{v}_k = Z^+ \boldsymbol{y}_k \quad \forall k = 1, ..., C \tag{6}$$

this equation adjusts the weights $\boldsymbol{v}_k$ for each class k, based on the pseudo-inverse Z^+ of the matrix Z, which contains neuron activation levels. This approach ensures that the FNN learns to differentiate between different classes effectively.

3.2 Evo-FNN

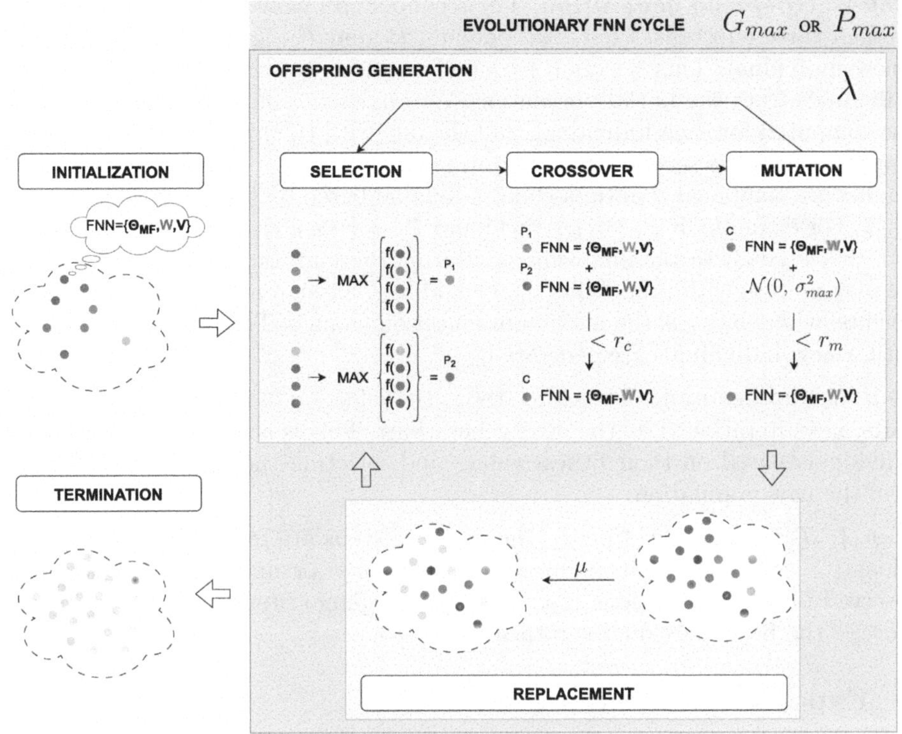

Fig. 2. Evolutionary FNN Cycle showing (evolutionary) update of $\mathbf{W}$.

Figure 2 shows the evolutionary update process for the weights W of the FNN pipeline (i.e., evo-FNN) introduced in the previous Subsection. This process can be divided into four main steps:

Step 1: Initialization. In the first step, an initial population of μ individuals is generated, each represented by a set of parameters defining the corresponding FNN: $\boldsymbol{\Theta}_{\mathbf{MF}}$, $\mathbf{W}$ and $\mathbf{V}$. Here, $\boldsymbol{\Theta}_{\mathbf{MF}}$ denotes the parameters of the m Gaussian membership functions for each input variable. For example, with one input variable x_1 and $m = 2$, we have $\boldsymbol{\Theta}_{\mathbf{MF}} = \{c_{11}, c_{12}, \sigma_{11}, \sigma_{12}\}$. As shown in the figure, only the weights $\mathbf{W}$ are updated. This decision was due to the observation that uncontrolled changes to the gaussian parameters can lead to issues such as overlapping membership functions, reducing the interpretability of the resulting concept values (e.g., "small", "medium", "high", associated with concepts like temperature). Preliminary experiments also indicated that updating $\mathbf{V}$ did not improve performance, likely due to the dependence of $\mathbf{V}$on $\mathbf{W}$within the FNN pipeline. Consequently, simultaneous updates to both parameters might negatively impact the outcomes. We also experimented with an alternative approach where evolutionary updates were applied only to $\mathbf{W}$, and the updated $\mathbf{W}$, values were then used to learn $\mathbf{V}$ but this did not improve performance.

Step 2: Offspring generation. The second step involves generating offspring through three substeps. First, two parents, P_1 and P_2, are selected to generate a new individual. This selection is done by randomly forming two groups of k individuals from the initial population. Within each group, the fitness function f is computed for each individual, and the one with the highest fitness is chosen as a parent. In the second substep, during the crossover phase, parts of the two parents are combined to form a child individual based on the crossover probability r_c. For example, if $P_1 = \{w_1, w_2\}^2$ and $P_2 = \{w_3, w_4\}$, a possible child could be $C = \{w_1, w_3\}$. In the final substep, during the mutation phase, each individual may mutate with probability r_m by adding Gaussian noise $\mathcal{N}(0, \sigma_{max}^2)$ to its weights, where σ_{max} is the maximum mutation change. This process is repeated until λ new individuals are generated.

Step 3: Replacement. The third step is the selection of individuals to proceed to the next iteration (i.e., the next generation). This is achieved by ranking the individuals based on their fitness values and selecting the top μ individuals to form the new population.

Step 4: Termination. Finally, the previous steps are repeated for G_{max} iterations (i.e., the maximum number of generations) or until no improvement is observed for P_{max} iterations (i.e., an early stopping criteria). At the end of the process, the best individual is returned.

4 Experimental Setting

We conducted experiments on the Maternal Health Risk dataset [2] to evaluate the performance of our evolutionary pipeline. Subsection 4.1 describes the dataset, while Subsect. 4.2 provides the description of the hyperparameters experimental configuration.

4.1 Datasets

We test our approach on the [2] dataset. This dataset (1,014 instances) consists of 6 responsible and significant risk factors for maternal mortality, with 3 classes of risk (low, medium, high). We follow the pre-processing techniques of previous work on Maternal H.R. [28]. The dataset is randomly split into training and testing sets, for validation purposes, we also use a subset drawn from the training set while preserving class balance.

4.2 Configurations

Preliminary tests were conducted to determine the most suitable hyperparameter values for Evo-FNN. The hyperparameters considered included the number of MFs, the population size (μ), the number of offspring (λ), the maximum

[2] for semplicity, we omit $\mathbf{\Theta}_{\mathbf{MF}}$ and $\mathbf{V}$.

number of generations (G_{max}), the maximum patience (P_{max}, i.e., the number of iterations for early stopping), the maximum mutation rate (σ_{max}), and the probabilities for mutation and crossover (r_m and r_c). Due to resource limitations, a trade-off between computational cost and time was necessary. Therefore, we decided to test all three datasets using the same hyperparameters' combinations resulting from the configuration shown in Table 1. For the fuzzy interpretations of both T and S (and their corresponding t and s), as well as f_Γ in Evo-FNN, we adopted the same described in [17], specifically the product t-norm, the probabilistic sum, and the argmax function.

Table 1. Experimental Configuration

Hyperparameter	Value(s)
Neuron type	AND, OR
Number of MFs	2
Population size (μ)	50
Offspring (λ)	70
Maximum generations (G_{max})	50
Maximum patience (P_{max})	20
Maximum mutation (σ_{max})	0.1, 0.2
Mutation rate (r_m)	0.3, 0.7
Crossover rate (r_c)	0.3, 0.7

5 Results

In this section, we present both an analysis over the evolutionary part inside the evo-FNN (Subsect. 5.1), as well as a comparison with state of the art approaches (Subsect. 5.2) for the Maternal Health Risk described in Sect. 4

5.1 Evolutionary Analysis

Table 2. Test accuracy of best AND/OR configurations on Maternal Health Risk dataset.

Dataset	Neuron Type	Test Acc.	Best Config.		
			σ_{max}	r_m	r_c
Maternal H.R.	AND	69.2% ± 0.754	0.1	0.3	0.3
	OR	69.1% ± 0.748	0.2	0.3	0.7

In Table 2, we show the test accuracy achieved by the best configurations of our method on the Maternal Health Risk dataset for both AND and OR neurons. We report only accuracy, as other metrics like F1 score does not diverge significantly (in all cases the classes are well-balanced).

Looking at the table, it can be observed that the OR neuron appears to achieve a better trade-off between performance and stability. Indeed, although the AND neuron achieves a marginally better accuracy, the OR neuron has a slightly lower standard deviation. We also explored different m_r values, finding that our evolutionary approach works reasonably well even with very divergent values. Figure 3 shows comparable results for $r_m = 0.3$ and $r_m = 0.7$. Similar considerations can be also made for r_c.

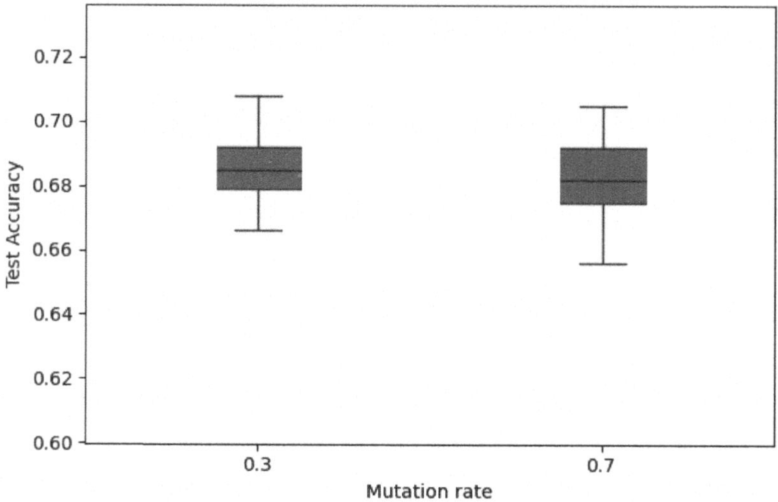

Fig. 3. Impact of the mutation rate on the test accuracy of Maternal Health Risk dataset.

5.2 Baseline Comparison

Table 3 compares the performance of Evo-FNN with state-of-the-art models on the Maternal Health Risk dataset [28]. Evo-FNN achieves the highest accuracy (**69.2%**), highlighting the benefits of evolutionary optimization over the standard FNN (**67.2%**). This improvement suggests that evolutionary techniques enhance feature selection and model convergence, refining decision boundaries for better classification.

Traditional models such as K-Nearest Neighbors (KNN) and Naïve Bayes, which rely on different learning techniques without interpretability, did not achieve superior results. Compared to the standard FNN that inspired this study, Evo-FNN not only improved accuracy but also enhanced interpretability by optimizing first-layer weight adjustments through an evolutionary process rather than relying on the randomized training typical of FNNs. Furthermore, an analysis of the extracted knowledge reveals that rules (examples are provided in Table 4) with antecedents having weights close to zero can be discarded, effectively reducing the dimensionality of the problem–an essential factor for improving model interpretability.

Table 3. Accuracy on Maternal Health Risk

Model	Accuracy
Evo-FNN	**69.2%**
FNN	67.2%
K neighbors classifier	65.3%
Naïve Bayes	59.3%
Dummy classifier	39.9%

Table 4. Examples of rules generated by evo-FNN for AND and OR neurons with 2 MFs. Here, MF_{ij} denotes the i-th membership function of the j-th feature, impact represents the corresponding neuron weights, and Output is an unnormalized score vector indicating the tendency of the rule toward each class.

Rules	
AND Neuron	**Output**
IF x1 is MF_{11} with impact 0.48 AND x2 is MF_{12} with impact 0.34 AND x3 is MF_{13} with impact 0.15 AND x4 is MF_{14} with impact 0.89 AND x5 is MF_{15} with impact 0.26 AND x6 is MF_{16} with impact 0.00	[−25.62, 32.54, −7.45]
IF x1 is MF_{11} with impact 0.26 AND x2 is MF_{12} with impact 1.00 AND x3 is MF_{13} with impact 0.12 AND x4 is MF_{14} with impact 0.85 AND x5 is MF_{15} with impact 0.07 AND x6 is MF_{26} with impact 0.56	[−22.19, −26.8, 49.07]
IF x1 is MF_{11} with impact 0.54 AND x2 is MF_{12} with impact 0.99 AND x3 is MF_{13} with impact 0.00 AND x4 is MF_{14} with impact 0.73 AND x5 is MF_{25} with impact 0.72 AND x6 is MF_{16} with impact 0.92	[6.33, 7.65, −14.86]
IF x1 is MF_{11} with impact 0.87 AND x2 is MF_{12} with impact 0.38 AND x3 is MF_{23} with impact 0.71 AND x4 is MF_{14} with impact 0.17 AND x5 is MF_{15} with impact 0.14 AND x6 is MF_{26} with impact 0.63	[−2.52, 94.76, −87.74]

(*continued*)

Table 4. (*continued*)

Rules	
AND Neuron	**Output**
IF x1 is MF_{11} with impact 0.02 AND x2 is MF_{22} with impact 0.82 AND x3 is MF_{23} with impact 0.82 AND x4 is MF_{24} with impact 0.65 AND x5 is MF_{15} with impact 0.58 AND x6 is MF_{26} with impact 0.96	[−2.11, 8.68, −7.43]
IF x1 is MF_{21} with impact 0.01 AND x2 is MF_{22} with impact 0.07 AND x3 is MF_{23} with impact 0.12 AND x4 is MF1 with impact 0.02 AND x5 is MF_{25} with impact 0.92 AND x6 is MF_{26} with impact 0.52	[−35.98, −51.57, 94.83]
OR Neuron	
IF x1 is MF_{11} with impact 1.00 OR x2 is MF_{12} with impact 0.89 OR x3 is MF_{23} with impact 0.37 OR x4 is MF_{14} with impact 0.10 OR x5 is MF_{15} with impact 0.58 OR x6 is MF_{26} with impact 0.32	[1.44, −20.31, 25.44]
IF x1 is MF_{11} with impact 0.86 OR x2 is MF_{22} with impact 0.75 OR x3 is MF_{13} with impact 0.63 OR x4 is MF_{14} with impact 1.00 OR x5 is MF_{25} with impact 0.00 OR x6 is MF_{26} with impact 0.15	[22.79, 7.99, −42.87]
IF x1 is MF_{11} with impact 0.23 OR x2 is MF_{22} with impact 0.08 OR x3 is MF_{23} with impact 0.71 OR x4 is MF_{24} with impact 0.38 OR x5 is MF_{15} with impact 0.45 OR x6 is $MF_{26}$with impact 0.89	[−4.52, 20.53, −21.86]
IF x1 is MF_{21} with impact 0.81 OR x2 is MF_{12} with impact 0.33 OR x3 is MF_{13} with impact 0.43 OR x4 is MF_{24} with impact 0.53 OR x5 is MF_{25} with impact 0.76 OR x6 is MF_{26} with impact 0.42	[−7.23, 3.45, 2.]
IF x1 is MF_{21} with impact 0.00 OR x2 is MF_{22} with impact 0.69 OR x3 is MF_{13} with impact 0.29 OR x4 is MF_{14} with impact 0.26 OR x5 is MF_{15} with impact 0.91 OR x6 is MF_{26} with impact 0.58	[−2.9, 24.45, −26.29]
IF x1 is MF_{21} with impact 0.06 OR MF_{22} is MF2 with impact 0.37 OR x3 is MF_{23} with impact 0.62 OR x4 is MF_{14} with impact 0.16 OR x5 is MF_{25} with impact 0.07 OR x6 is MF_{26} with impact 0.64	[10.5 −11.84 −5.35]

6 Conclusions and Future Work

In this study, we introduced a novel evolutionary fuzzy neural network (Evo-FNN) framework, extending the approach of [17] by incorporating genetic algorithms to enhance maternal health risk assessment while preserving interpretability. Our evaluation on the Maternal Health Risk dataset demonstrated the method's effectiveness in leveraging evolutionary algorithms (Subsect. 5.2) and provided insights into the integration process (Subsect. 5.2).

Training FNNS inherently involves a trade-off between explainability and performance, which is particularly critical in clinical applications. A limitation of our current approach is its scalability, which restricted the number of hyperparameter configurations tested. For example, increasing the number of MFS could allow Evo-FNN to capture more complex patterns and further improve performance.

Future work will focus on enhancing the scalability of Evo-FNN to enable a more exhaustive exploration of hyperparameter values and further strengthen its predictive capabilities.

Acknowledgments. We acknowledge the support of the PNRR project INEST - Interconnected North-East Innovation Ecosystem (ECS00000043), under the NRRP MUR program funded by the NextGenerationEU. We acknowledge the support of the PNRR project FAIR - Future AI Research (PE00000013), under the NRRP MUR program funded by the NextGenerationEU. This paper is supported by the TrustAlert project, funded by Fondazione Compagnia San Paolo and Fondazione CDP under the "Artificial Intelligence" call.

Disclosure of Interests. The authors have no competing interests to declare that are relevant to the content of this article.

References

1. Abraham, A.: Optimization of evolutionary neural networks using hybrid learning algorithms. In: Proceedings of the International Joint Conference on Neural Networks (IJCNN), vol. 3, pp. 2797–2802. IEEE (2002)
2. Ahmed, M.: Maternal health risk. UCI Machine Learning Repository (2020). https://doi.org/10.24432/C5DP5D
3. Aliev, R., et al.: Evolutionary algorithm-based learning of fuzzy neural networks. Part 2: Recurrent fuzzy neural networks. Fuzzy Sets Syst. **160**(18), 2553–2566 (2009)
4. Aliev, R.A., et al.: Type-2 fuzzy neural networks with fuzzy clustering and differential evolution optimization. Inf. Sci. **181**(9), 1591–1608 (2011)
5. Alpaydin, G., et al.: Evolution-based design of neural fuzzy networks using self-adapting genetic parameters. IEEE Trans. Fuzzy Syst. **10**(2), 211–221 (2002)
6. Apriceno, G., et al.: A neuro-symbolic approach to structured event recognition. In: 28th International Symposium on Temporal Representation and Reasoning, TIME 2021, Klagenfurt, Austria, 27–29 September 2021. LIPIcs, vol. 206, pp. 11:1–11:14. Schloss Dagstuhl - Leibniz-Zentrum für Informatik (2021)
7. Apriceno, G., et al.: A neuro-symbolic approach for real-world event recognition from weak supervision. In: 29th International Symposium on Temporal Representation and Reasoning, TIME 2022, 7–9 November 2022, Virtual Conference. LIPIcs, vol. 247, pp. 12:1–12:19. Schloss Dagstuhl - Leibniz-Zentrum für Informatik (2022)
8. Apriceno, G., et al.: End-to-end neuro-symbolic approaches for event recognition (2023)

9. Apriceno, G., et al.: A neuro-symbolic approach for non-intrusive load monitoring. In: ECAI 2023 - 26th European Conference on Artificial Intelligence, Kraków, Poland, 30 September–4 October 2023, Including 12th Conference on Prestigious Applications of Intelligent Systems (PAIS 2023). Frontiers in Artificial Intelligence and Applications, vol. 372, pp. 3175–3181. IOS Press (2023)
10. Bäck, T., Schwefel, H.P.: An overview of evolutionary algorithms for parameter optimization. Evol. Comput. **1**(1), 1–23 (1993)
11. Badreddine, S., et al.: Interval logic tensor networks. CoRR abs/2303.17892 (2023)
12. de Campos Souza, P.V., Apriceno, G., Dragoni, M.: Enhancing logical tensor networks: Integrating uninorm-based fuzzy operators for complex reasoning. In: Besold, T.R., d'Avila Garcez, A., Jimenez-Ruiz, E., Confalonieri, R., Madhyastha, P., Wagner, B. (eds.) Neural-Symbolic Learning and Reasoning, pp. 68–79. Springer, Cham (2024)
13. de Campos Souza, P.V., Dragoni, M.: Efnn-nul0- a trustworthy knowledge extraction about stress identification through evolving fuzzy neural networks. Fuzzy Sets Syst. **487**, 109008 (2024). https://doi.org/10.1016/J.FSS.2024.109008
14. de Campos Souza, P.V., Dragoni, M.: Fuzzy neural network model based on uni-nullneuron in extracting knowledge about risk factors of maternal health. In: Finkelstein, J., Moskovitch, R., Parimbelli, E. (eds.) Artificial Intelligence in Medicine - 22nd International Conference, AIME 2024, Salt Lake City, UT, USA, 9–12 July 2024, Proceedings, Part I. LNCS, vol. 14844, pp. 70–75. Springer, Cham (2024). https://doi.org/10.1007/978-3-031-66538-7_8
15. de Campos Souza, P.V., Dragoni, M.: IFNN: enhanced interpretability and optimization in FNN via adam algorithm. Inf. Sci. **678**, 121002 (2024). https://doi.org/10.1016/J.INS.2024.121002
16. de Campos Souza, P.V., Dragoni, M.: PEFNN: parallel evolving fuzzy neural network for sepsis identification in patients. In: IEEE International Conference on Fuzzy Systems, FUZZ-IEEE 2024, Yokohama, Japan, 30 June–5 July 2024, pp. 1–9. IEEE (2024). https://doi.org/10.1109/FUZZ-IEEE60900.2024.10611923
17. de Campos Souza, P.V., Torres, L.C.B.: Regularized fuzzy neural network based on or neuron for time series forecasting. In: North American Fuzzy Information Processing Society Annual Conference, pp. 13–23. Springer, Cham (2018)
18. Cao, J., et al.: Fuzzy inference system with interpretable fuzzy rules: advancing explainable artificial intelligence for disease diagnosis-a comprehensive review. Inf. Sci. **662**, 120212 (2024)
19. Castellano, G., et al.: Evolutionary Neuro-Fuzzy Systems and Applications, pp. 11–45. Springer, Heidelberg (2007)
20. Furuhashi, T., et al.: Evolutionary fuzzy modeling using fuzzy neural networks and genetic algorithm. In: Proceedings of 1997 IEEE International Conference on Evolutionary Computation (ICEC 1997), pp. 623–627. IEEE (1997)
21. Hoffmann, F.: Evolutionary algorithms for fuzzy control system design. Proc. IEEE **89**(9), 1318–1333 (2001)
22. Ibrahim, M.S., Mohamed, A.: A new approach to evolutionary optimized fuzzy neural networks. In: 2006 International Conference on Neural Information Processing, pp. 127–135. IEEE (2006)
23. Jang, J.S.: Anfis: adaptive-network-based fuzzy inference system. IEEE Trans. Syst. Man Cybern. **23**(3), 665–685 (1993)
24. Keller, J.M., et al.: Fundamentals of Computational Intelligence: Neural Networks, Fuzzy Systems, and Evolutionary Computation. Wiley, Hoboken (2016)
25. Leng, G., et al.: Design for self-organizing fuzzy neural networks based on genetic algorithms. IEEE Trans. Fuzzy Syst. **14**(6), 755–766 (2006)

26. Minku, F.L., Ludermir, T.B.: Evolutionary strategies and genetic algorithms for dynamic parameter optimization of evolving fuzzy neural networks. In: 2005 IEEE Congress on Evolutionary Computation, vol. 3, pp. 1951–1958. IEEE (2005)
27. Tang, A., et al.: Ga-tskfnn: parameters tuning of fuzzy neural network using genetic algorithms. Expert Syst. Appl. **29**(4), 769–781 (2005)
28. Togunwa, T., et al.: Deep hybrid model for maternal health risk classification in pregnancy: synergy of ANN and random forest. Front. Artif. Intell. **6** (2023)
29. Vilamala, M.R., et al.: Using deepproblog to perform complex event processing on an audio stream. CoRR abs/2110.08090 (2021)
30. Zhang, R., Tao, J.: A nonlinear fuzzy neural network modeling approach using an improved genetic algorithm. IEEE Trans. Industr. Electron. **65**(7), 5882–5892 (2018)

Multi-view Multi-instance Learning for Health Recovery Monitoring in Older Adults

Veselka Boeva(✉), Alexander J. O. Ojutkangas, and Shahrooz Abghari

Department of Computer Science, Blekinge Institute of Technology, Karlskrona, Sweden
{vbx,aoj,sab}@bth.se

Abstract. In this study, we propose a multi-view version of the BARTMIP algorithm, which can learn from data for which only coarse-grained labels are provided. The proposed MV-BARTMIP algorithm can deal with weakly annotated multi-modal data and is able to handle cases of missing data, including modalities and views. The performance of the MV-BARTMIP algorithm is evaluated in a scenario involving the monitoring of older adults' health recovery at home following hip replacement surgery. The performance of MV-BARTMIP and the traditional BARTMIP is benchmarked against several baseline solutions. The experimental results demonstrate that approaching the use case as a multi-view, multi-instance learning task results in more robust and interpretable models. MV-BARTMIP shows superior performance to the best baseline model in all but one scenario, where the results are comparable. Furthermore, its performance is comparable to that of the BARTMIP algorithm, which outperforms the best baseline model in all experimental scenarios (The implementation, along with the evaluation results, are available at GitHub).

Keywords: Multi-instance learning · Multi-modal data · Assisted living · Sensor data

1 Introduction

Many real-world problems are inherently ambiguous, dealing with weakly annotated data, and thus can be considered as multi-instance learning (MIL) tasks. The notion of MIL, in which the training set consists of many bags, each containing multiple instances, is introduced in [12]. In that work, MIL originates from research devoted to drug activity prediction. Later, MIL has been applied to various domains and used in different applications, such as computer-aided diagnosis to predict whether a subject is diseased or healthy [20], sentiment analysis in text [21], and image scene classification [5].

This research was partially funded by the Knowledge Foundation, Sweden, through the Human-Centered Intelligent Realities (HINTS) Profile Project (contract 20220068).

P. Bruno et al. (Eds.): HC_AIxIA_HYDRA 2025, CCIS 2830, pp. 398–411, 2026.
https://doi.org/10.1007/978-3-032-16708-8_32

The use of artificial intelligence (AI) in healthcare has grown significantly in recent years [24]. A variety of health monitoring medical devices are being used to connect patients with clinicians, allowing remote access to collect, process, and transmit medical data. The goal is to reduce unnecessary hospital stays and facilitate personalized, real-time health monitoring while patients recover at home. Different categories of wearable personal health monitoring devices can be used to support this monitoring, such as smartphone-integrated devices, smart wristbands, and sport watches for fitness and activity tracking. More recently, a smart bed concept has emerged that uses sensors embedded in mattresses to monitor the patient's sleep patterns. Analyzing and making sense of the data collected by all these devices and modalities is challenging because they usually contain information about various aspects of an individual's health, such as physical activity, sleep patterns, and vital signs. As highlighted in [11,16], there is a risk of overlooking some aspects if all available features are explored simultaneously. Another challenge is that patient data collected at home is rarely consistently annotated, often containing missing values and/or modalities.

In this study, we propose a multi-view (MV) version of the BARTMIP algorithm, called MV-BARTMIP, to address the above challenges. MV-BARTMIP is an adapted version of the original MIL algorithm, BARTMIP [40]. The proposed MV-BARTMIP algorithm successfully integrates MIL and MV learning paradigms. In [19], MIL is considered as the missing link between relational and propositional learning, because the bag label models a *one-to-many* relationship. Note that the MV instance bag representation considered in this study can be regarded as modeling a *many-to-many* relationship. This enables more complex scenarios to be handled, in which multiple MV instance bags representing different aspects of the monitored phenomenon can be combined.

2 Related Work

Two reviews exploring the importance and challenges of multiple instance learning (MIL) have recently been published, see [14] and [35]. In [14], the authors discuss the background of MIL and its applications in various domains, as well as some MIL-based methods, challenges, and perspectives. The authors of [35] consider both classical MIL techniques and the latest advances in deep neural network techniques for MIL.

MIL has been widely used in healthcare, especially for analyzing medical images where detailed annotations are scarce. MIL frameworks treat an image as a bag of multiple instances, such as image patches, allowing models to learn from weakly labeled data. For example, in [34], MIL is used to classify dementia by treating brain MRI scans as bags of patches. Researchers have applied MIL in [29] to detect hemorrhages in CT scans without slice-level annotations, instead treating each CT volume as a bag of 2D slices. MIL is applied to dermoscopic images for melanoma detection in [6] by treating each image as a bag of sub-regions, allowing the model to identify malignant areas without requiring detailed annotations. A graph-based MIL approach is used in [38] to classify gastric cancer in whole slide images. A deep MIL framework is developed in [41] to detect diabetic retinopathy in retinal images. By analyzing image patches within each retinal scan, the model was able to identify lesions using only image-level labels, reducing the need for extensive manual annotation.

MIL has also been effectively applied to sensor data, particularly in human activity recognition (HAR), where the precise labeling of individual sensor readings is often challenging. A framework called HAR-MIL, introduced in [7], treats each human activity as a bag containing instances of various wearable sensors, such as accelerometers, gyroscopes, magnetometers, and linear acceleration sensors. This approach addresses issues such as missing data and sensor noise. A study by Saha et al. [32] has developed a multi-instance multi-label (MIML) framework for HAR using smartphone accelerometer data. The proposed approach captures complex activity patterns by allowing multiple labels per instance. Another study by Rajak et al. [28] has combined MIML with a genetic algorithm to handle coarsely labeled smartphone accelerometer data. This semi-supervised approach optimizes feature selection and improves classification accuracy in scenarios with noisy or imprecise labels, which are common in real-world applications such as elder care and rehabilitation. Guan et al. [18] have proposed a generative model combining MIL with an auto-regressive hidden Markov model for activity recognition from time-series sensor data. This model reduces the need for detailed annotations by treating sequences as bags and utilizes dynamic programming for efficient inference, enabling both bag-level and instance-level predictions.

3 Methodology

In this section, we first describe the data and the use case used to evaluate the proposed MV-BARTMIP algorithm. The MIL and consensus clustering paradigms are also briefly introduced. Then, the steps of the MV-BARTMIP algorithm are formally elaborated.

3.1 Data and Use Case

The MAISON-LLF dataset [4] is used in this work to evaluate and illustrate the proposed MIL approach that can efficiently handle multi-modal data. It is a publicly available multi-modal sensor dataset, collected from older adults recovering from lower-limb fractures (LLF) in community settings. The MAISON-LLF is available in three versions, including data from smartphone and smartwatch sensors, motion detectors, sleep-tracking mattresses, and clinical questionnaires on isolation and decline. The dataset is collected from ten older adults living alone at home for eight weeks each, for a total of 560 days of 24-hour sensor data. In this study, the first [1] and second [2] versions of the data are used. The second version of the MAISON-LFF dataset includes 13 additional derived features, bringing the total to 93 features compared to the first version. The evaluation results reported in [4] are produced on the first version.

In the following, we define the use case related to the data described above. Suppose that measurements from a cohort of older adults recovering alone at home after LLF surgery are collected by multiple sensors of different granularity over a period of several weeks. The collected data may contain information about various aspects of the individuals' daily recovery process, such as physical activities, sleep patterns, and vital signs. In this sense, let us assume that different health aspects of each older adult can be monitored during the recovery process. Each individual's recovery progress is assessed (labeled) on a bi-weekly basis by administering clinically validated questionnaires to quantify their social isolation and functional decline. These clinical assessments serve as the gold-standard data in [4] and include the social isolation scale (**SIS**) [25] for assessing social interactions and the Oxford hip score (**OHS**) [36] for evaluating functional health. Obviously, we deal with an MIL problem, since the individual's multi-view daily profiles are not labeled. Instead, the ground truth **SIS** and **OHS** are only available on a bi-weekly basis.

In the above context, we apply a predictive MIL model, introduced in Sect. 3.4, that can reflect the different health recovery aspects of the individual to predict their social isolation and functional decline scores for a given week. The proposed algorithm can also deal with missing data and/or modalities.

3.2 Multi-instance Learning and Hausdorff Distance

MIL is a learning paradigm in which training instances are organized into sets called bags, and labels are only available at the bag level during training [35]. The main difficulty in MI prediction is that although the training bags are labeled, the labels of their instances are unknown. Indeed, in a real-world context, a bag corresponds to a tangible object, while the instances correspond to feature vectors describing the object. In other words, in MIL, an object is represented by a set of feature vectors, which is different from typical machine learning (ML) settings. Therefore, common supervised ML methods cannot be directly applied to MIL tasks.

In general, there are two strategies for dealing with the representational difficulty of MI prediction [43]. One modifies supervised learning algorithms to accommodate the representation of feature vector sets [42]. The other transforms the representation to meet the requirements of common supervised ML algorithms. Two groups of MI prediction algorithms based on representation transformation are recognized. In the first group, bags are transformed into corresponding feature vectors by structuring the input space at the instance level. In the second group, the representation transformation is performed by structuring the input space at the bag level.

A bag-level representation transformation algorithm for MI prediction, called BARTMIP, is proposed in [40]. The BARTMIP first clusters training bags into k disjoint groups using a bag-level MI clustering algorithm, called BAMIC. The BAMIC performs the partitioning using a bagwise distance called *Hausdorff distance*. Then, each bag is represented by a k-dimensional feature vector, where the i-th feature corresponds to the distance between the bag and the medoid of the i-th group. In this way, all bags are transformed into the k-dimensional feature vectors.

Maximal Hausdorff distance has been proposed in [13] to measure the distance between two bags of instances. Later, it has been successfully applied to the standard MIL problem [39]. However, in [40], the maximal Hausdorff distance has been found to not work well in the generalized MIL problems due to its sensitivity to outliers. Therefore, the authors have introduced an alternative measure known as the *average Hausdorff distance*, which is also used in this study to assess the distance between each pair of bags. If two bags of data instances A and B are given, the average Hausdorff distance is defined by Eq. 1 as follows:

$$H(A,B) = \frac{\sum_{a \in A} \min_{b \in B} dist(a,b) + \sum_{b \in B} \min_{a \in A} dist(a,b)}{\mid A \mid + \mid B \mid}, \tag{1}$$

where $dist(a, b)$ is the distance between instances $a \in A$ and $b \in B$, which usually takes the form of Euclidean distance.

3.3 Consensus Clustering

Consensus clustering methods attempt to find an optimal combination of independently obtained clusterings into a single improved clustering solution [37]. Multiple clusterings of the same data can arise in different scenarios, e.g., in the case of the same data set collected from different devices or from different runs of the same algorithm [17]. In our study, we deal with the first scenario, where the data is multi-modal and represents different perspectives or views on the phenomenon under study. The benefit of combining data from multiple views by aggregating their clusterings into a consensus clustering lies in outlining the confidence in the common patterns across views and revealing the important differences between them.

In the design of the proposed MV-BARTMIP algorithm, we apply a consensus clustering scheme to integrate clustering solutions generated separately for each considered data view. The idea used in our study is based on [8], inspired by the map-reduce functions of functional programming, i.e., it consists of two distinct phases. First, each data view is separately clustered by applying the chosen clustering algorithm. This produces a list of different clustering solutions, one for each view. The clusters from the different views are then transformed into unified representations, e.g., in terms of statistics of the label values associated with their members. These unified cluster representations are transformed into a single clustering solution by applying a chosen clustering algorithm.

3.4 MV-BARTMIP Algorithm

In this study, we approach the use case described in Sect. 3.1 as a multi-view, MIL task. For this purpose, we propose a novel multi-view version of the BARTMIP algorithm discussed in Sect. 3.2, called MV-BARTMIP. Our motivation was to propose an algorithm that can deal with multi-modal data, capable of handling cases of missing data typical of real-world scenarios.

We start by formulating our multi-view MIL problem. Suppose we have multi-modal data describing a phenomenon under study. The data contains information describing m different aspects (views) of the phenomenon. Let $\{D_i\}_{i=1}^m$ be the view sets of labeled training bags and $\{\mathcal{X}_i\}_{i=1}^m$ be the sets of view instances. Each dataset D_i is described as follows:

$$D_i = \{(X_{i1}, L_{i1}), (X_{i2}, L_{i2}), \ldots, (X_{iN_i}, L_{iN_i})\},$$

where $X_{ij} \subseteq \mathcal{X}_i$, for $i \in \{1, 2, \ldots, m\}$ and $j \in \{1, 2, \ldots, N_i\}$, is a set of view i instances, L_{ij} is the label value associated with X_{ij}. Note that L_{ij} is a real number in the case of a regression task and a class label in a classification scenario. In the latter case $L_{ij} \in \mathcal{L}$, where $\mathcal{L}$ is the set of labels.

The proposed MV-BARTMIP algorithm consists of the following main steps:

(1) Determine the optimal number of clusters k_i for each view $i \in \{1, 2, \ldots, m\}$.
(2) Generate a clustering solution $C_i = \{C_{i1}, C_{i2}, \ldots, C_{ik_i}\}$ on each dataset D_i, for $i \in \{1, 2, \ldots, m\}$, using the BAMIC algorithm with the average Hausdorff distance given in Eq. 1.
(3) Represent each cluster C_{ij}, for $i \in \{1, 2, \ldots, m\}$ and $j \in \{1, 2, \ldots, k_i\}$, in terms of the label values associated with its members. Considering two supervised ML tasks, the following two representations can be used:
  (i) In the case of a regression task, each cluster C_{ij} can be represented by a five-dimensional feature vector containing the minimum, maximum, mean, standard deviation, and median of its real value labels.
  (ii) In the case of a classification task, each cluster C_{ij} can be represented by its empirical class probability vector, where each value represents the relative frequency of the corresponding class among all cluster members.
(4) Generate a consensus clustering solution $\mathcal{C} = \{\mathcal{C}_1, \mathcal{C}_2, \ldots, \mathcal{C}_K\}$ on the clustering solutions $\{C_i\}_{i=1}^m$, which have been transformed into a uniform representation in step (3). Note that each consensus cluster $\mathcal{C}_i$, for $i \in \{1, 2, \ldots, K\}$, is composable of a set of view clusters that have been assigned to it, i.e., $\mathcal{C}_i = \{C_{i_1 j_1}, \ldots, C_{i_r j_r}\}$, where $i_1, \ldots, i_r \in \{1, 2, \ldots, m\}$ and $j_1, \ldots, j_r \in \{1, 2, \ldots, k_i\}$.
(5) Each consensus cluster is represented by a list of the medoids of its view clusters, i.e., it consists of K bags of instances, where instances are the medoids of the view clusters assigned to this consensus cluster.
(6) Each training bag x is transformed into K-dimensional feature vector. Note that x is composed of several view bags, i.e., it is a vector of view bags $(x_1, x_2, \ldots, x_m)$, where x_i $(i = 1, 2, \ldots, m)$ is a bag of instances of view i. In this context, x can be represented by a K-dimensional feature vector, where the i-th feature corresponds to the average distance of the Hausdorff distances computed between its view bags and the corresponding view medoids of the i-th consensus cluster. For example, to calculate the distance between consensus cluster $\mathcal{C}_i$ and bag x, the Hausdorff distance is first computed between each $\mathcal{C}_i$ view medoid and the respective bag view of x. Then, the

average of these distances is found. This distance can therefore be calculated even when some views are missing.

(7) Any common supervised learner can be used to train on the generated feature vectors.

4 Experiments and Implementation

To evaluate different aspects of the proposed MV-BARTMIP algorithm, we have performed two experiments. The first experiment, called **Ex1**, applies the MI predictor BARTMIP to the use case presented in Sect. 3.1. Following the recommendation of the authors in [4], we utilized the second version of the MAISON-LLF dataset, which differs slightly from the first version used in their paper. The results obtained are compared with the baseline solutions reported in the case of weekly outcome prediction in [4]. To achieve an objective comparison, we also run the best baseline on the second version of the data. We have used the CatBoost model [27] in the design of the BARTMIP algorithm, as it is reported to perform the best in the case of daily outcome prediction in [4]. The BAMIC algorithm uses k-medoids clustering [23] with the average Hausdorff distance to group the training bags in the representation transformation step. However, any clustering algorithm that suits the input data can be used for this grouping, e.g., affinity propagation [15] or spectral clustering [33]. The performance of the BARTMIP is compared with that of the baseline solutions in two evaluation settings: 5-fold cross-validation (CV) and leave-one-sample-out (LOSO). We use two evaluation metrics: mean absolute error (MAE) [31] and coefficient of determination (R^2) [26].

In the second experiment, called **Ex2**, the use case is treated as a multi-view multi-instance learning task by applying our proposed MV-BARTMIP algorithm. The multi-modal data used, described in Sect. 3.1, provides information about three different aspects of the individuals' daily recovery process: physical activities, sleep patterns, and heart rate (i.e., vital signs). Moreover, demographic information, such as age and gender, can be considered a fourth view. Note that the MV-BARTMIP implementation also uses the CatBoost model.

The CatBoost-based versions of BARTMIP and MV-BARTMIP have been implemented in Python 3.10 using the following libraries: `Scikit-learn` for k-medoids, `CatBoost` for regression, as well as other supporting libraries such as `Pandas` and `NumPy`. The evaluation pipeline, configuration files, time complexity analysis, and dependency specifications are available at the GitHub repository.

5 Results and Discussion

5.1 Results of Ex1

In **Ex1**, we compare the performance of the BARTMIP model with the baseline solutions in [4]. The algorithm is trained using the 16 most important sensor features according to SHAP (SHapley Additive exPlanations) values [22], as well as demographic information about the participants' age and gender. Four models capable of analyzing sequential data are used in [4] for weekly **SIS** and **OHS** predictions. These are long short-term memory (LSTM), temporal convolutional network (TCN), bag of words (BoW) [3], and ROCKET [10]. BoW has outperformed the other models in both evaluation settings for the two predictions (**SIS** and **OHS**). The results of its evaluation are presented in Table 1 (BoW-1). As mentioned above, the results reported in [4] were produced using the first version of the data from that used in our study (the second). Therefore, we applied BoW on the second version of the dataset. The results are also presented in Table 1 (BoW-2).

Table 1. The **SIS** and **OHS** *5-fold CV* and *LOSO* prediction results obtained by the compared algorithms. Note that the results reported for BoW-1 are obtained using the first version of the MAISON-LLF dataset, whereas the results for all other algorithms are produced using the second version.

Algorithm	5-fold CV				LOSO			
	SIS		OHS		SIS		OHS	
	MAE	R^2	MAE	R^2	MAE	R^2	MAE	R^2
BARTMIP (all)	1.84	0.44	4.29	0.62	1.18	0.68	2.51	0.80
BARTMIP (16)	1.83	0.43	3.19	0.75	1.35	0.74	2.57	0.79
BARTMIP (16 + 2 demographics)	**1.51**	**0.56**	**2.72**	**0.83**	**0.99**	**0.75**	**1.70**	**0.88**
BoW-1 (16 + 2 demographics)	1.48	0.60	3.55	0.69	1.44	0.60	3.29	0.72
BoW-2 (16 + 2 demographics)	1.77	0.49	4.08	0.60	1.82	0.45	3.68	0.70
MV-BARTMIP (16 + 2 demographics)	1.81	0.45	**2.72**	**0.84**	**1.05**	**0.70**	**1.93**	**0.87**
MV-BARTMIP (16)	2.30	0.34	3.53	0.73	0.98	0.74	2.14	0.83
MV-BARTMIP (all)	2.23	0.20	3.83	0.66	1.28	0.65	2.29	0.81

The 5-fold CV prediction results obtained by the BARTMIP model for **SIS** and **OHS** are shown in Table 2 (upper part). These results are generated using different numbers of clusters by the BAMIC algorithm. The quality of the produced clustering solutions is evaluated using the Silhouette Index (SI) [30]. As can be seen, the results generated by BARTMIP for **SIS** are comparable to those produced by BoW-1, while they are significantly better than the BoW-1 scores in the case of **OHS**. Moreover, the BARTMIP algorithm outperforms BoW-2 in all the experimental scenarios studied.

We also study the prediction performance of the BARTMIP model in the LOSO evaluation setting. The results are listed in Table 2 (bottom part). All the results produced by the BARTMIP for different numbers of clusters outperform those generated by the BoW-1 model (reported in [4] and listed in Table 1) and BoW-2 model (Table 1) for both **SIS** and **OHS** weekly predictions.

We have investigated how the number of clusters (k) affects the performance of the BARTMIP algorithm by running it for $k = 3, 4, \ldots, 14$. The best results for

Table 2. The **SIS** and **OHS** *5-fold CV* and *LOSO* prediction results obtained by the BARTMIP model are shown for different numbers of clusters used by the BAMIC algorithm. The quality of the clustering solutions is evaluated using Silhouette Index (SI).

CV	Rank	SIS				OHS			
		# Clusters	*Mean*			# Clusters	*Mean*		
			MAE	R^2	SI		MAE	R^2	SI
5-fold	1	**11**	**1.48**	0.56	0.33	**13**	**2.70**	0.78	0.38
	2	**13**	1.49	**0.59**	0.32	**14**	2.90	0.78	0.37
	3	**10**	1.55	0.53	**0.34**	**8**	2.92	**0.80**	0.37
	4	12	1.56	0.57	0.32	11	2.96	0.75	0.38
	5	9	1.61	0.53	0.33	7	3.09	0.77	0.35
	6	8	1.75	0.49	0.34	**10**	3.11	0.74	**0.39**
	7	7	1.78	0.46	0.31	9	3.19	0.73	0.38
	8	6	1.80	0.46	0.29	**12**	3.19	0.73	**0.39**
	9	4	1.83	0.42	0.30	6	3.31	0.72	0.34
LOSO	1	**13**	**0.91**	**0.79**	0.34	**13**	**1.73**	**0.89**	**0.39**
	2	**11**	0.91	0.77	0.34	**10**	**1.73**	0.88	**0.39**
	3	**12**	0.92	0.78	**0.35**	**12**	1.75	0.88	**0.39**
	4	10	0.96	0.74	0.34	7	1.81	0.88	0.35
	5	9	1.04	0.71	0.34	11	1.84	0.88	0.38
	6	3	1.06	0.72	0.29	9	1.84	0.86	0.37
	7	**8**	1.13	0.68	**0.35**	8	1.90	0.87	0.36
	8	7	1.13	0.68	0.32	6	1.93	0.86	0.33
	9	6	1.17	0.67	0.29	3	2.01	0.85	0.28

Note. The results are listed in increasing order of mean MAE values.

SIS are achieved with 11 or 13 clusters, while for **OHS**, with 13, 14, or 8 clusters. To confirm these findings, we also ran spectral clustering, which suggested 8, 11, 13, and 14 as the optimal cluster numbers since these produced the highest SI. In summary, the BARTMIP model consistently outperforms the BoW-1 and BoW-2 models (see Table 1) for **OHS** prediction in both evaluation settings, and for **SIS** in the LOSO setup across all cluster sizes, as shown in Table 2. However, for **SIS** in the 5-fold CV scenario, this pattern is observed only for BoW-2, as demonstrated in Table 2.

5.2 Results of Ex2

In **Ex2**, we study the performance of the proposed MV-BARTMIP algorithm. It has been evaluated and compared with that of BARTMIP in the same evaluation settings as in **Ex1**. Furthermore, we examine how the performance of MV-BARTMIP is affected by the employed data features. In this context, MV-

BARTMIP is evaluated in three setups. Specifically, MV-BARTMIP (all) utilizes all the features, MV-BARTMIP (16) employs the 16 most important sensor features according to SHAP, and MV-BARTMIP (16 + 2 demographics) considers an additional demographic view that includes age and gender attributes. The same three setups are performed for the BARTMIP algorithm, applying the BAMIC with the optimal number of clusters identified for each experimental scenario.

First, according to step (1) (see Sect. 3) of the MV-BARTMIP algorithm, the optimal number of clusters, k, is determined for each of the views presented in the data. To this end, the k-medoids algorithm is run for $k = 3, 4, \ldots, 14$, and the resulting clustering solutions are evaluated using the SI and Connectivity [9] cluster validation measures. The optimal number of clusters selected for each view by the MV-BARTMIP (16 + 2 demographics) model is presented in Table 3. In step (2) of the algorithm, the k-medoids clustering is applied to generate a clustering solution for each data view using the optimal value of k.

Note that for each prediction outcome (**SIS** and **OHS**), an MV-BARTMIP model is built. Thus, following step (3) of the algorithm, each cluster is represented by a five-dimensional feature vector that contains the minimum, maximum, mean, standard deviation, and median of its **SIS** (or **OHS**) values. These cluster representations are then used to generate a consensus clustering, which integrates the clustering solutions produced from the views. The number of consensus clusters, K, selected for MV-BARTMIP (16 + 2 demographics) is given in Table 3. Finally, each consensus cluster is represented by a list of the medoids of its view clusters. Note that BARTMIP (16 + 2 demographics) uses 13 clusters in all experimental scenarios except for **OHS** prediction in 5-fold CV, for which the optimal number is 14. These numbers are double the numbers of the consensus clusters of MV-BARTMIP, i.e., the multi-view interpretation results in a more compact representation. In addition, the quality of the consensus clustering solutions is comparable to that of the optimal clustering solutions produced by BAMIC, as shown by the calculated SI values.

Table 3. MV-BARTMIP (16 + 2 demographics) optimal number of clusters.

View	MV-BARTMIP (16 + 2 demographics)		
	# Clusters	Silhouette Index	Connectivity
Physical activities	6	0.19	0.09
Sleeping patterns	9	0.20	0.14
Heart rate	6	0.19	0.20
Demographic	6	0.85	0.0
Consensus **SIS**	6	0.30	0.03
Consensus **OHS**	7	0.34	0.24

The **SIS** and **OHS** 5-fold CV and LOSO prediction results obtained by comparing the MV-BARTMIP with the BARTMIP and BoW models are shown in

Table 1. All three learning algorithms use CatBoost as the base model. Additionally, as it was mentioned above, MV-BARTMIP is evaluated in three setups: MV-BARTMIP (all), MV-BARTMIP (16), and MV-BARTMIP (16 + 2 demographics). We can notice that the employed set of features certainly affects the performance of BARTMIP and MV-BARTMIP. Both algorithms produce the best performance results when using the 16 most important sensor features according to SHAP, including two demographics. We observe that the BARTMIP algorithm has achieved the best performance of all the algorithms studied. The MV-BARTMIP algorithm's performance is comparable to that of the BARTMIP algorithm. Furthermore, it has outperformed the best baseline model in all but one scenario (**SIS** prediction, 5-fold CV), where the results are comparable.

Our experiments have revealed that treating the given weakly annotated use case as a multi-view MIL task yields more robust solutions. Examples of such solutions are the BARTMIP and MV-BARTMIP models studied in this research. These models can handle missing data and propose interpretable models that provide additional insight into the phenomenon under study. For example, the clusters produced by BARTMIP can identify typical behavioral patterns and their correlation with prediction outcomes. MV-BARTMIP also enables us to examine this at the level of the views, as well as to explore how consensus clusters correlate with different views. For example, the most frequent correlation patterns can be identified among the consensus clusters and studied in more detail to optimize the prediction model. However, it should be noted that the performance of MV-BARTMIP depends on tuning more hyperparameters (number of clusters, k, for each view and the aggregate consensus clustering) than BARTMIP. We believe that optimizing this process could lead to performance that is comparable to, or even better than, that of the BARTMIP algorithm. A comparison of the time complexity of the two algorithms reveals that MV-BARTMIP is approximately m times more computationally intensive than BARTMIP, i.e., $m \times O(n^2)$.

6 Conclusion

In this study, we have proposed a multi-view version of the BARTMIP algorithm, named MV-BARTMIP, designed to handle weakly annotated multi-modal data by successfully dealing with cases of missing data. We have evaluated both the traditional BARTMIP algorithm and the proposed MV-BARTMIP in a scenario involving the monitoring of health recovery of older adults at home after hip replacement surgery. Their performance is compared with that of existing baseline solutions. Both the BARTMIP and the MV-BARTMIP have shown better performance than the best baseline model. The main finding from the conducted evaluation is that approaching the given weakly annotated use case as a multi-view, multi-instance learning task results in more robust and interpretable solutions, such as the BARTMIP and MV-BARTMIP models explored.

We plan to evaluate the proposed method using larger and richer datasets to gain further insight into MV-BARTMIP's potential. The authors of the

MAISON-LLF dataset aim to double its size by collecting data from an additional ten individuals. Moreover, we intend to validate MV-BARTMIP in other healthcare use cases by enriching the evaluation scenarios with new data views.

Acknowledgment. We thank our colleagues at the Toronto Rehabilitation Institute, Ali Abedi and Shehroz Khan, for helping us understand the data used in the evaluation.

References

1. Abedi, A., Chu, C., Khan, S.S.: MAISON-LLF: multimodal sensor dataset for monitoring older adults post lower-limb fractures in community settings, Version V1 (2025). https://doi.org/10.5281/zenodo.14597613
2. Abedi, A., Chu, C., Khan, S.S.: MAISON-LLF: multimodal sensor dataset for monitoring older adults post lower-limb fractures in community settings, Version V2 (2025). https://doi.org/10.5281/zenodo.14803293
3. Abedi, A., et al.: Bag of states: a non-sequential approach to video-based engagement measurement. Multimed. Syst. **30**(1), 47 (2024)
4. Abedi, A., et al.: Multimodal sensor dataset for monitoring older adults post lower limb fractures in community settings. Sci. Data **12**(1), 733 (2025)
5. Amores, J.: Multiple instance classification: review, taxonomy and comparative study. Artif. Intell. **201**, 81–105 (2013)
6. Astorino, A., et al.: Melanoma detection by means of multiple instance learning. Interdisc. Sci.: Comput. Life Sci. **12**(1), 24–31 (2020)
7. Bagci Das, D., Birant, D.: Human activity recognition based on multi-instance learning. Expert. Syst. **40**(7), e13256 (2023)
8. Boeva, V., Tsiporkova, E., Kostadinova, E.: Analysis of multiple DNA microarray datasets. In: Springer Handbook of Bio-/Neuroinformatics, pp. 223–234 (2014)
9. Brock, G., Pihur, V., Datta, S., Datta, S.: clValid: an R package for cluster validation. Stat. Softw. **25**, 1–22 (2008)
10. Dempster, A., Petitjean, F., Webb, G.I.: ROCKET: exceptionally fast and accurate time series classification using random convolutional kernels. Data Min. Knowl. Disc. **34**(5), 1454–1495 (2020). https://doi.org/10.1007/s10618-020-00701-z
11. Devagiri, V.M., et al.: Putting sense into incomplete heterogeneous data with hypergraph clustering analysis. In: Miliou, I., et al. (eds.) Advances in Intelligent Data Analysis XXII, pp. 119–130. Springer, Cham (2024)
12. Dietterich, T.G., Lathrop, R.H., Lozano-Pérez, T.: Solving the multiple instance problem with axis-parallel rectangles. Artif. Intell. **89**(1–2), 31–71 (1997)
13. Edgar, G.A.: Measure, Topology, and Fractal Geometry, vol. 2. Springer, Cham (2008)
14. Fatima, S., Ali, S., Kim, H.C.: A comprehensive review on multiple instance learning. Electronics **12**(20), 4323 (2023)
15. Frey, B.J., Dueck, D.: Clustering by passing messages between data points. Science **315**(5814), 972–976 (2007)
16. Fu, L., Lin, P., Vasilakos, A.V., Wang, S.: An overview of recent multi-view clustering. Neurocomputing **402**, 148–161 (2020)
17. Goder, A., Filkov, V.: Consensus clustering algorithms: comparison and refinement. In: Proceedings of the 10th Workshop on ALENEX, pp. 109–117. SIAM (2008)

18. Guan, X., Raich, R., Wong, W.K.: Efficient multi-instance learning for activity recognition from time series data using an auto-regressive hidden Markov model. In: International Conference on Machine Learning, pp. 2330–2339. PMLR (2016)
19. Herrera, F., et al.: Multiple Instance Learning. Springer, Cham (2016)
20. Kandemir, M., Hamprecht, F.A.: Computer-aided diagnosis from weak supervision: a benchmarking study. Computerized Med. Imag. Graph. **42**, 44–50 (2015)
21. Kotzias, D., Denil, M., Blunsom, P., de Freitas, N.: Deep multi-instance transfer learning. arXiv preprint arXiv:1411.3128 (2014)
22. Lundberg, S.M., Lee, S.I.: A unified approach to interpreting model predictions. In: Advances in Neural Information Processing Systems, vol. 30 (2017)
23. MacQueen, J.: Some methods for classification and analysis of multivariate observations. In: Proceedings of the 5th Berkeley Symposium on Math. Statistics and Probability, Volume 1: Statistics, vol. 5, pp. 281–298. University of California press (1967)
24. Manickam, P., et al.: Ai and internet of medical things (IoMT) assisted biomedical systems for intelligent healthcare. Biosensors **12**(8), 562 (2022)
25. Nicholson, N.R., Jr., Feinn, R., Casey, E., Dixon, J.: Psychometric evaluation of the social isolation scale in older adults. Gerontologist **60**(7), e491–e501 (2020)
26. Pedregosa, F., et al.: Scikit-learn: machine learning in Python. Mach. Learn. Res. **12**, 2825–2830 (2011)
27. Prokhorenkova, L., et al.: CatBoost: unbiased boosting with categorical features. In: Advances in Neural Information Processing Systems, vol. 31 (2018)
28. Rajak, S., et al.: A human activity recognition framework for grossly labeled smartphone sensing data through combining genetic algorithm with multiple instance multiple label learning. Multimed. Tools Appl. **81**(17), 24887–24911 (2022)
29. Remedios, S., et al.: Extracting 2D weak labels from volume labels using multiple instance learning in CT hemorrhage detection. In: Medical Imaging 2020: Image Processing, vol. 11313, pp. 66–75. SPIE (2020)
30. Rousseeuw, P.J.: Silhouettes: a graphical aid to the interpretation and validation of cluster analysis. Comput. Appl. Math. **20**, 53–65 (1987)
31. Ruppert, D.: The Elements of Statistical Learning: Data Mining, Inference, and Prediction. Taylor & Francis (2004)
32. Saha, J., Ghosh, D., Chowdhury, C., Bandyopadhyay, S.: Smart handheld based human activity recognition using multiple instance multiple label learning. Wirel. Pers. Commun. **117**, 923–943 (2021)
33. Yu, Shi: Multiclass spectral clustering. In: Proceedings Ninth IEEE International Conference on Computer Vision, pp. 313–319 (2003)
34. Tong, T., Wolz, R., Gao, Q., Hajnal, J.V., Rueckert, D.: Multiple instance learning for classification of dementia in brain MRI. In: Mori, K., Sakuma, I., Sato, Y., Barillot, C., Navab, N. (eds.) MICCAI 2013. LNCS, vol. 8150, pp. 599–606. Springer, Heidelberg (2013). https://doi.org/10.1007/978-3-642-40763-5_74
35. Waqas, M., et al.: Exploring multiple instance learning (MIL): a brief survey. Expert Syst. Appl. 123893 (2024)
36. Wylde, V., Learmonth, I.D., Cavendish, V.J.: The Oxford hip score: the patient's perspective. Health Qual. Life Outcomes **3**, 1–8 (2005)
37. Xanthopoulos, P.: A review on consensus clustering methods. In: Optimization in Science and Engineering: In Honor of the 60th Birthday of Panos M. Pardalos, pp. 553–566 (2014)
38. Xiang, X., Wu, X.: Multiple instance classification for gastric cancer pathological images based on implicit spatial topological structure representation. Appl. Sci. **11**(21), 10368 (2021)

39. Yang, Y., Wang, H.: Multi-view clustering: a survey. Big Data Min. Anal. **1**(2), 83–107 (2018)
40. Zhang, M.L., Zhou, Z.H.: Multi-instance clustering with applications to multi-instance prediction. Appl. Intell. **31**, 47–68 (2009)
41. Zhou, L., et al.: Deep multiple instance learning for automatic detection of diabetic retinopathy in retinal images. IET Image Proc. **12**(4), 563–571 (2018)
42. Zhou, Z.H., Zhang, M.L.: Ensembles of multi-instance learners. In: European Conference on Machine Learning, pp. 492–502. Springer, Cham (2003)
43. Zhou, Z.H., Zhang, M.L.: Solving multi-instance problems with classifier ensemble based on constructive clustering. Knowl. Inf. Syst. **11**, 155–170 (2007)

An LBBD Approach for Solving the Chemotherapy Treatment Scheduling Problem

Simone Caruso[1], Carmine Dodaro[2], Marco Maratea[2], Cinzia Marte[2](✉), and Marco Mochi[3]

[1] University of Genoa, Genoa, Italy
simone.caruso@edu.unige.it
[2] DeMaCS, University of Calabria, Rende, Italy
{carmine.dodaro,marco.maratea,cinzia.marte}@unical.it
[3] SurgiQ srl, Genoa, Italy
marco.mochi@edu.unige.it

Abstract. The Chemotherapy Treatments Scheduling problem in oncology clinics is a complex problem, as the solution has to satisfy multiple requirements. These include adhering to the cyclic nature of chemotherapy treatment plans, ensuring a steady flow of patients, and effectively managing limited resources such as treatment time, nursing staff, and drug availability. Simultaneously, achieving an effective schedule is crucial for ensuring optimal health outcomes. A previous approach addressed this problem through a direct encoding via Answer Set Programming. In this paper, we propose an alternative solution based on a Logic-Based Benders Decomposition approach, implemented using multi-shot solving, and test it on real data, where the results demonstrate advantages for the LBBD method.

Keywords: Answer Set Programming · Logic Programming · Digital Health

1 Introduction

The Chemotherapy Treatment Scheduling (CTS) problem [13,24,30,31,35] consists of computing a schedule for patients requiring chemotherapy treatments. The CTS problem is a complex problem for oncology clinics since it involves multiple resources and aspects, including the availability of nurses, chairs, and drugs. Chemotherapy treatments have a cyclic nature, where the number and the duration of each cycle depend on the different types of cancer and the stage of the disease. Moreover, treatments may have different priorities that must be taken into account when computing a solution. A proper solution to the CTS problem is thus crucial for improving the degree of satisfaction of the main actors on the problem, i.e., patients and nurses, and for better management of the resources. Various studies have shown how delays in cancer surgeries and treatments have

P. Bruno et al. (Eds.): HC_AIxIA_HYDRA 2025, CCIS 2830, pp. 412–425, 2026.
https://doi.org/10.1007/978-3-032-16708-8_33

a significant adverse impact on patient survival. This impact varies depending on the aggressiveness of the cancer, thus stressing the importance of developing a model capable of efficiently prioritizing patients. Complex combinatorial problems, possibly involving optimizations, such as the CTS problem, are usually the target applications of AI languages such as Answer Set Programming (ASP). Indeed, ASP has been successfully employed for solving complex combinatorial and scheduling problems, including those in real-world contexts (see, e.g., [1,5,8,10,12,14–17,19]), and, arguably, has a number of advantages over other logic-based paradigms such a SAT, CP, ILP and SMT [2], maintaining, at the same time, some of their strengths: (a) the ASP high-level specifications are declarative and often appreciated even by non-experts since they found them readable; (b) there are free and open source systems (like CLINGO, or WASP), whose performances are often comparable to the ones of industrial tools for ILP like, e.g. GUROBI, or to SAT solvers; (c) ASP allows for easily expressing and reasoning on multi-objective and multi-level optimizations, which is not the case for, e.g., Max-SAT. A solution to the CTS problem based on a direct ASP encoding has been already presented in [13], considering specification and data from the San Martino Hospital in Genova, Italy.

In this paper, we present a second, alternative solution which, instead, employs a Logic-based Bender Decomposition (LBBD) approach taken from the field of Operation Research and already successfully employed in ASP-based scheduling solutions in Healthcare [9]. It consists of defining a master problem and (one or several) subproblem(s) that interact with it by passing constraints that "cut" the search space and help converge to an (optimal) solution. The LBBD approach is implemented through the usage of the multi-shot solving variant of CLINGO [21]. Finally, we conducted an empirical evaluation on real data and specifications from the San Martino Hospital in Italy showing that the LBBD approach brings computational advantages over the direct approach.

2 Background

In this section, we introduce the necessary preliminaries on ASP and the LBBD-based approach, organized into two separate subsections.

2.1 Background on ASP

Answer Set Programming (ASP) [4] is a programming paradigm developed in the field of non-monotonic reasoning and logic programming. More detailed descriptions and a more formal account of ASP, including the features of the language employed in this paper, can be found in [4,7]. Hereafter, we assume the reader is familiar with logic programming conventions.

Syntax. The syntax of ASP is similar to that of Prolog. Variables are strings starting with an uppercase letter, and constants are non-negative integers or strings starting with lowercase letters. A *term* is either a variable or a constant. A *standard atom* is an expression $p(t_1, \ldots, t_n)$, where p is a *predicate* of arity n and $t_1, \ldots, t_n$ are terms. An atom $p(t_1, \ldots, t_n)$ is ground if $t_1, \ldots, t_n$ are constants. A *ground set* is a set of pairs of the form $\langle consts : conj \rangle$, where *consts* is a list of constants and *conj* is a conjunction of ground standard atoms. A *symbolic set* is a set specified syntactically as $\{Terms_1 : Conj_1; \cdots ; Terms_t : Conj_t\}$, where $t > 0$, and for all $i \in [1, t]$, each $Terms_i$ is a list of terms such that $|Terms_i| = k > 0$, and each $Conj_i$ is a conjunction of standard atoms. A *set term* is either a symbolic set or a ground set. Intuitively, a set term $\{X : a(X, c), p(X); Y : b(Y, m)\}$ stands for the union of two sets: the first one contains the X-values making the conjunction $a(X, c), p(X)$ true, and the second one contains the Y-values making the conjunction $b(Y, m)$ true. An *aggregate function* is of the form $f(S)$, where S is a set term, and f is an *aggregate function symbol.* Basically, aggregate functions map multisets of constants to a constant, e.g., the function *#count* computes the number of terms. An *aggregate atom* is of the form $f(S) \prec T$, where $f(S)$ is an aggregate function, $\prec \in \{<, \leq, >, \geq, \neq, =\}$ is a operator, and T is a term called guard. An aggregate atom $f(S) \prec T$ is ground if T is a constant and S is a ground set. An *atom* is either a standard atom or an aggregate atom. A *rule* r is of the form

$$a_1 \mid \ldots \mid a_n \text{ :- } b_1, \ldots, b_k, not\ b_{k+1}, \ldots, not\ b_m.$$

where $a_1, \ldots, a_n$ are standard atoms, $b_1, \ldots, b_k$ are atoms, $b_{k+1}, \ldots, b_m$ are standard atoms, and $n, k, m \geq 0$. A literal is either a standard atom a or its negation *not* a. The disjunction $a_1 \mid \ldots \mid a_n$ is the *head* of r, while the conjunction $b_1, \ldots, b_k, not\ b_{k+1}, \ldots, not\ b_m$ is its *body.* Rules with empty body are called *facts.* Rules with empty head are called *constraints.* A variable that appears uniquely in the set terms of a rule r is said to be *local* in r, otherwise, it is a *global* variable of r. An ASP program is a set of *safe* rules, where a rule r is *safe* if the following conditions hold: *(i)* for each global variable X of r there is a positive standard atom ℓ in the body of r such that X appears in ℓ, and *(ii)* each local variable of r appearing in a symbolic set $\{Terms : Conj\}$ also appears in a positive atom in *Conj*. A *weak constraint* [6] ω is of the form:

$$:\sim b_1, \ldots, b_k, not\ b_{k+1}, \ldots, not\ b_m.\ [w@l]$$

where w and l are the weight and level of ω, respectively. (Intuitively, $[w@l]$ is read as "weight w at level l"). An ASP program with weak constraints is $\Pi = \langle P, W \rangle$, where P is a program and W is a set of weak constraints. A standard atom, a literal, a rule, a program, or a weak constraint is *ground* if no variables appear in it.

Semantics. Let P be an ASP program. The *Herbrand universe* U_P and the *Herbrand base* B_P of P are defined as usual. The ground instantiation G_P of P is the set of all the ground instances of rules of P that can be obtained by substituting variables with constants from U_P. An *interpretation* I for P is a subset I of B_P. A ground literal ℓ (resp., *not* ℓ) is true w.r.t. I if $\ell \in I$ (resp., $\ell \notin I$), and false (resp., true) otherwise. An aggregate atom is true w.r.t. I if the evaluation of its aggregate function (i.e., the result of the application of f on the multiset S) with respect to I satisfies the guard; otherwise, it is false. A ground rule r is *satisfied* by I if at least one atom in the head is true w.r.t. I whenever all conjuncts of the body of r are true w.r.t. I. A *model* is an interpretation that satisfies all the rules of a program. Given a ground program G_P and an interpretation I, the *reduct* [18] of G_P w.r.t. I is the subset G_P^I of G_P obtained by deleting from G_P the rules in which a body literal is false w.r.t. I. An interpretation I for P is an *answer set* (or stable model) for P if I is a minimal model (under subset inclusion) of G_P^I (i.e. I is a minimal model for G_P^I) [18]. Given a program with weak constraints $\Pi = \langle P, W \rangle$, the semantics of Π extends from the basic case defined above. Thus, let $G_\Pi = \langle G_P, G_W \rangle$ be the instantiation of Π; a constraint $\omega \in G_W$ is violated by an interpretation I if all the literals in ω are true w.r.t. I. An *optimum answer set* for Π is an answer set of G_P that minimizes the sum of the weights of the violated weak constraints in G_W in a prioritized way by levels.

Syntactic Shortcuts. In the following, we also use *choice rules* of the form $\{p\}$, where p is an atom. Choice rules can be viewed as a syntactic shortcut for the rule $p \mid p'$, where p' is a fresh new atom not appearing elsewhere in the program, meaning that the atom p can be chosen as true.

2.2 Background on LBBD

The LBBD approach [27] is an optimization technique that extends the classical Benders Decomposition (BD) approach [3,22,32], offering greater flexibility and applicability to a wider range of complex problems. The central aspect of the approach lies in decomposing the problem into a *master problem* (MP) and one or more *subproblems* (SPs). The MP typically focuses on high-level decisions, whereas the SPs deal with more detailed and often logically complex constraints. The significant difference between classical BD and LBBD lies in the nature of the SPs, in the technique used to generate Benders cuts, and the properties of the resulting solution [29]. Consider a problem aimed at maximizing a function $f(x, y)$, subject to a set of constraints $C(x, y)$, $C_x(x)$, and $C_y(y)$, where x and y are vectors of variables that belong to the respective domains D_x and D_y. The LBBD approach begins by decomposing the problem P into an MP P_M and a set of SPs $\mathcal{P}_S = \{P_S^1, \dots, P_S^n\}$. The algorithm proceeds by solving P_M to obtain an optimal solution x^*, which maximizes $f(x, y)$ for a fixed $y \in D_y$, subject to the constraints $C_x(x)$. If P_M is unsatisfiable, the procedure terminates; otherwise, the solution x^* is passed to each SP in $\mathcal{P}_S$ in order to solve it. Each $\mathcal{P}_S$ can lead to one of the two possible outcomes: (*i*) admits an optimal solution y^*, in which case the solution is stored in a set, initially empty, that accumulates all the optimal solutions from the SPs; or (*ii*) is unsatisfiable, meaning that the solution x^* cannot be extended to the SP P_S. In this case, a new constraint C^* on x^* is derived from P_S and added to P_M. This constraint serves to refine P_M based on the last solution found, which led to the unsatisfiable problem. The algorithm then iterates, incorporating the added constraint C^*. This iterative process continues until either P_M is proven unsatisfiable (which would imply that the entire problem is unsatisfiable) or the optimal solution is found, confirming that all subproblems are satisfiable.

3 Problem Description

The CTS problem involves scheduling chemotherapy appointments and assigning a chair or bed for the session when needed. Patients may need different treatments and we identify four phases for each of them: (p_1) the registration to the Hospital reception; (p_2) a blood collection; (p_3) a medical check; and (p_4) the therapy. Each patient may have different phase durations. Phases p_1 and p_4 are mandatory, while phases p_2 and p_3 are optional, but selecting phase p_2 implies phase p_3. The number and duration of phases are assigned at appointment registration. For patients not requiring a bed or chair, the duration of phase p_4 is 0. Office hours are from 07:30 A.M. to 01:30 P.M. We consider a set of 72 time slots for each day with a duration of 5 min. We also identify a set of 36 available time slots that represent the possible starting time of phase p_4, where 07:35–07:40 is the first time slot. If the duration of phase p_4 for a registration exceeds a given threshold, then it must start after 11:25 A.M. (i.e., the 24th time slot). Finally, phase p_4 must start after all previous phases are completed. The input of the problem consists of registrations, where each registration includes the duration of each phase (set to 0 if a phase is not required) and the preference between chair or bed. A solution to the problem is represented by a schedule of registrations to time slots for a given day (representing the beginning of phase p_4) according to the following requirements: *(i)* each patient must be assigned to a chair or bed; *(ii)* each chair or bed can be used by only one patient for each time slot; and *(iii)* if the treatment requires more than one time slot, then the patient must always use the same chair or bed. Moreover, an optimal solution to the problem maximizes the number of patients that are assigned to the preferred resource (chair or bed). Ties are broken by minimizing the number of concurrent patients in phase p_2 to have a more uniform usage of resources during the day.

4 Direct ASP Encoding

In this section, we review the direct ASP encoding in [13], based on the input language of CLINGO [20].

Data Model. The input data is specified by means of the following atoms:

- Instances of `reg(RID, ORDER, WDAY, PH4, PH3, PH2, PH1, S)` represent the registrations, characterized by an id (`RID`), the ordering (`ORDER`), the number of waiting days before the visit (`WDAY`), the duration of each phase (`PH4`, ..., `PH1`), and the preference for chair or bed (`S`), where `S` can be `"bed"` or `"chair"`.
- Instances of `day(DAY)` represent the available days.

```
1  {x(RID,DAY,TS,PH4,0,S) : ts(TS), day(DAY)} = 1 :-
       reg(RID,0,_,PH4,PH3,PH2,PH1,S).
2  {x(RID,DAY+DAY2,TS,PH4,ORDER,S) : ts(TS)} = 1 :- x(RID,DAY,_,_,N,_),
       ORDER=N+1, day(DAY+DAY2), reg(RID,ORDER,DAY2,PH4,PH3,PH2,PH1,S).
3  :- x(RID,DAY,TS,PH4,_,_), PH4 > 50, TS < 24.
4  :- x(RID,DAY,TS,_,ORDER,_), reg(RID,ORDER,DAY2,PH4,PH3,PH2,PH1,S),
       TS-PH3-PH2-PH1<1.
5  1 {bed(ID,RID,DAY) : bed(ID); chair(ID,RID,DAY) : chair(ID)} 1:-
       x(RID,DAY,_,_,_,_).
6  res(RID,DAY,TS..TS+PH4-1) :- x(RID,DAY,TS,PH4,_,_), PH4 > 0.
7  chair(ID,RID,DAY,TS) :- chair(ID,RID,DAY), res(RID,DAY,TS).
8  bed(ID,RID,DAY,TS) :- bed(ID,RID,DAY), res(RID,DAY,TS).
9  :- #count{RID: chair(ID,RID,DAY,TS)} > 1, day(DAY), ts(TS), chair(ID).
10 :- #count{RID: bed(ID,RID,DAY,TS)} > 1, day(DAY), ts(TS), bed(ID).
11 support(RID,DAY,TS) :- x(RID,DAY,PH4,_,_,_),
       reg(RID,ORDER,_,_,PH3,PH2,_,_), PH2 > 0, TS=PH4-PH3-PH2, day(DAY),
       ats(TS).
12 numbReg(DAY,N,TS) :- N = #count{RID: support(RID,DAY,TS)}, day(DAY),
       ats(TS).
13 numMax(DAY,T) :- T = #max{N: numbReg(DAY,N,_)}, day(DAY).
14 numMin(DAY,T) :- T = #min{N: numbReg(DAY,N,_), N != 0}, day(DAY).
15 numbDay(DAY,N) :- N = #count{RID: support(RID,DAY,_)}, day(DAY).
16 numMaxDay(T) :- T = #max{N: numbDay(DAY, N)}.
17 :~ x(RID,DAY,_,_,_,"bed"), chair(ID,RID,DAY,_). [1@7,RID]
18 :~ x(RID,DAY,_,_,_,"chair"), bed(ID,RID,DAY,_). [1@7,RID]
19 :~ numMax(DAY,T). [T@6, DAY]
20 :~ numMax(DAY,MAX), numMin(DAY,MIN). [MAX-MIN@5,DAY]
21 :~ numMaxDay(N). [N@4]
```

Fig. 1. ASP direct encoding

- Instances of `ts(TS)` represent the available time slots for phase p_4, where TS ranges from 1 to 36.
- Instances of `ats(TS)` represent all time slots, where TS ranges from 1 to 72.
- Instances of `chair(ID)` represent the available chairs, with its identifier ID.
- Instances of `bed(ID)` represent the available beds, with its identifier ID.

The output is an assignment represented by atoms of the form `x(RID, DAY, TS, PH4, ORDER, S)` where the intuitive meaning is that the phase p_4 of registration with id RID and ordering ORD is assigned to the day DAY and time slot TS using the chair or bed S.

Encoding. The related encoding is shown in Fig. 1, and is described in the following. To simplify the description, here and in the following, we denote as r_i the rule appearing at line i of the referenced figure. Rule r_1 assigns registrations to a day and a time slot. The assignment is made only for the first registration of the patient (i.e., the one with ordering equal to 0). Rule r_2 assigns subsequent registrations (i.e., the one with ordering greater than 0) to a time slot, whereas the

```
1 {x(RID,DAY,PH4,0,S): day(DAY)} = 1 :- reg(RID,0,_,PH4,PH3,PH2,PH1,S).
2 1 {bed(ID,RID,DAY): bed(ID); chair(ID,RID,DAY): chair(ID) } 1 :-
      x(RID,DAY,_,_,_).
3 :~ x(RID,DAY,_,_,1), chair(_,RID,DAY). [1@4,RID]
4 :~ x(RID,DAY,_,_,0), bed(_,RID,DAY). [1@4,RID]
5 numbReg(DAY,TOT) :- TOT = #count{RID: x(RID,DAY,_,_,_)}, day(DAY).
6 numMax(DAY,MAX) :- MAX = #max{N: numbReg(DAY,N)}, day(DAY).
7 bound(N_PAT/N_DAYS) :- N_PAT = #count{RID: reg(RID,_,_,_,_,_,_,_)},
      N_DAYS = #count{DAY: day(DAY)}, N_PAT \ N_DAYS = 0.
8 bound(N_PAT/N_DAYS+1) :- N_PAT = #count{RID: reg(RID,_,_,_,_,_,_,_)},
      N_DAYS = #count{DAY: day(DAY)}, N_PAT \ N_DAYS != 0.
9 :~ numMax(DAY,M), bound(B), M-B > 0. [M-B@3,DAY]
```

Fig. 2. CTS master problem

day is automatically computed considering the number of waiting days before the visit. Rule r_3 ensures that if phase p_4 is particularly long, then it must start after 11:25 A.M. (i.e., the 25th time slot). Rule r_4 ensures that phase p_4 cannot start before other phases are concluded. Then, rule r_5 assigns exactly one chair/bed to each registration. Rules from r_6 to r_{10} are used to ensure that each chair and bed is assigned to at most one patient for each time slot. Rules from r_{12} to r_{16} are needed to derive auxiliary atoms that are used later on in optimization. In particular, rules from r_{12} to r_{14} compute the maximum and minimum number of patients that are simultaneously assigned to phase p_2, while rules r_{15} and r_{16} compute the number of patients for each day. Finally, weak constraints r_{17} and r_{18} are used to minimize the number of missed preferences, whereas weak constraints from r_{19} to r_{21} enforce the distribution of registrations.

5 LBBD Encoding

In this section, we present our ASP-based solution to the CTS problem, exploiting the LBBD approach. The MP P_M handles the assignment of a day and a (preferred) resource to each registration, while the SP P_S determines the specific time slots within the assigned day and ensures a balanced distribution of patients requiring phase p_2 across the working week. Specifically, we define multiple subproblems, one for each day under consideration, and, on average, the overall approach requires three iterations.

5.1 Master Problem

Data Model. The input data are specified by means of the atoms `reg`, `day`, `chair`, and `bed` specified in Sect. 4. The output of P_M consists of a scheduling containing atoms of the form:

- `x(RID, DAY, PH4, ORD, S)`, denoting the registration of a patient `RID` linked to a day `DAY`, with a duration of the fourth phase `PH4` in terms of time slots, the ordering value `ORD` and the patient's preference for chair or bed `S`;

```
1 {y(RID,DAY,TS,PH4,0,S): ts(TS) } = 1 :- x(RID,DAY,PH4,0,S).
2 {y(RID,DAY+DAY2,TS,PH4,ORD,S): ts(TS)} = 1 :- x(RID,DAY,_,N,_),
      reg(RID,ORD,DAY2,PH4,PH3,PH2,PH1,S),ORD=N+1,day(DAY+DAY2).
3 :- y(RID,DAY,TS,PH4,_,_), PH4 > 50, TS < 24.
4 :- y(RID,DAY,TS,_,ORD,_), reg(RID,ORD,_,_,PH3,PH2,PH1,S),
      TS-PH3-PH2-PH1<1.
5 res(RID,DAY,TS..TS+PH4-1) :- y(RID,DAY,TS,PH4,_,_), PH4>0.
6 chair(ID,RID,DAY,TS) :- chair(ID,RID,DAY), res(RID,DAY,TS).
7 :-#count{RID: chair(ID,RID,DAY,TS)} > 1, chair(ID), day(DAY), ts(TS).
8 bed(ID,RID,DAY,TS) :- bed(ID,RID,DAY), res(RID,DAY,TS).
9 :-#count{RID: bed(ID,RID,DAY,TS)} > 1, bed(ID), day(DAY), ts(TS).
10 support(RID,DAY,TS) :- y(RID,DAY,PH4,_,_,_),
      reg(RID,ORD,_,_,PH3,PH2,_,_), PH2>0, PH4-PH3-PH2=TS, ats(TS).
11 numbReg(DAY,N,TS) :- N = #count{RID: support(RID,DAY,TS)}, day(DAY),
      ats(TS).
12 numMax(DAY,T) :- T = #max{N: numbReg(DAY,N,_)}, day(DAY).
13 numMin(DAY,T) :- T = #min{N: numbReg(DAY,N,_), N != 0}, day(DAY).
14 :~ numMax(DAY,M). [M@3,DAY]
15 :~ numMax(DAY,M), numMin(DAY,N), M-N > 0. [M-N@2]
```

Fig. 3. CTS subproblem.

- bed(ID, RID, DAY) and chair(ID, RID, DAY), representing the association of a patient RID to a bed or a chair with identifier ID in a day DAY, respectively.

Encoding. Figure 2 reports the encoding for the master problem of the CTS problem. Rule r_1 assigns a day to patients with ordering equal to 0, i.e., those for whom we are scheduling their first appointment, while rule r_2 assigns a resource, a chair or a bed, to patients. The first two levels of optimization are introduced by the weak constraints r_3 and r_4, which minimize the missed preferences. Rule r_5 defines a support atom that is used to compute the total number of patients scheduled in a day, whereas rule r_6 computes the maximum number of patients in a day. Rules r_7 and r_8 provide an upper bound for the number of patients that can be assigned to a single day, by distributing the total number of patients as evenly as possible among the available days. Rule r_9 enforces an even distribution of patients across all days.

5.2 Subproblem

Data Model. As described in Sect. 2.2, the solution of P_M is given as input to P_S, along with the atoms ts and ats specified in Sect. 4.
Based on the solution of P_M, P_S generates the atom y(RID, DAY, TS, PH4, ORD, S), representing the registration of a patient RID, scheduled for a specific day DAY and time slot TS. It also indicates the duration of the fourth phase PH4 in terms of time slots, the ordering value ORD, and the patient's preference for either a chair or a bed, denoted by S.

Encoding. The full encoding of P_S is presented in Fig. 3. Rule r_1 assigns a time slot to patients with an order equal to 0, i.e., those attending their first appointment, while rule r_2 assigns a time slot to appointments with an order greater than 0. Rules r_3 and r_4 ensure that if phase p_4 is particularly long, then it must start after 11:25 A.M. (i.e., the 25th time slot) and f_4 cannot start before other phases are concluded, respectively. Rules from r_5 to r_9 ensure that at most one patient is assigned to each resource at each time slot. Finally, from rule r_{10} to r_{13} it is computed the maximum and minimum number of patients that are accessing phase p_2 simultaneously and they are used in the weak constraints r_{14} and r_{15} that enforce the distribution of registrations.

If P_S is unsatisfiable, no-good cuts of the following form are generated and added to the MP:

```
no_good_chair_sum(CHAIRID,DAY,TOT) :- #max{TS: ts(TS)} = TOT,
    unfeasable_subproblem_chair(CHAIRID,DAY).
no_good_bed_sum(BEDID,DAY,TOT) :- #max{TS: ts(TS)} = TOT,
    unfeasable_subproblem_bed(BEDID,DAY).
:- #sum{PH4, RID: x(RID,DAY,PH4,_,_), chair(ID,RID,DAY)} > TOT,
    no_good_chair_sum(ID,DAY,TOT).
:- #sum{PH4, RID: x(RID,DAY,PH4,_,_), bed(ID,RID,DAY)} > TOT,
    no_good_bed_sum(ID,DAY,TOT).
```

These cuts exclude the assignment determined by P_M. Specifically, after P_S returns unsat, for each patient, an `unfeasible_chair(RID,DAY,NGID)` and an `unfeasible_bed(RID,DAY,NGID)` atom are created depending on whether the patient was assigned to a bed or a chair. These atoms indicate that the patient's assignment to the corresponding resource is not feasible. At this point, for each resource, a support atom `no_good_chair_sum(CHAIRID,DAY,TOT)` is generated. This atom represents the available timeslots of the resource. A similar process applies for beds with the atom `no_good_bed_sum(BEDID,DAY,TOT)`. Finally, the constraint ensures that the assigned patients respect the resource availability in the next iteration, thereby preventing the P_M from producing an output that includes too many patients assigned to the same resource on the same day. Thus, the atoms `bed(ID,RID,DAY)` and `chair(ID,RID,DAY)` that have already been shown to result in an unsatisfiable P_S are excluded from the solutions of P_M, and a new assignment is computed.

6 Experimental Results

In this section, we report the results of an empirical analysis on real-world data of the performance obtained with the LBBD approach and with the original, direct encoding for the CTS problem. The experiments were run on an AMD Ryzen 5 3600 CPU @ 3.60GHz with 16 GB of physical RAM. As ASP system, we used CLINGO version 5.4.1. Moreover, for the LBBD approach implemented in our work, we used the multi-shot feature of CLINGO [21] which allows us to iteratively solve a problem without restarting from scratch at each iteration, so that we could add the new rules derived from the subproblems, i.e., the cuts, into

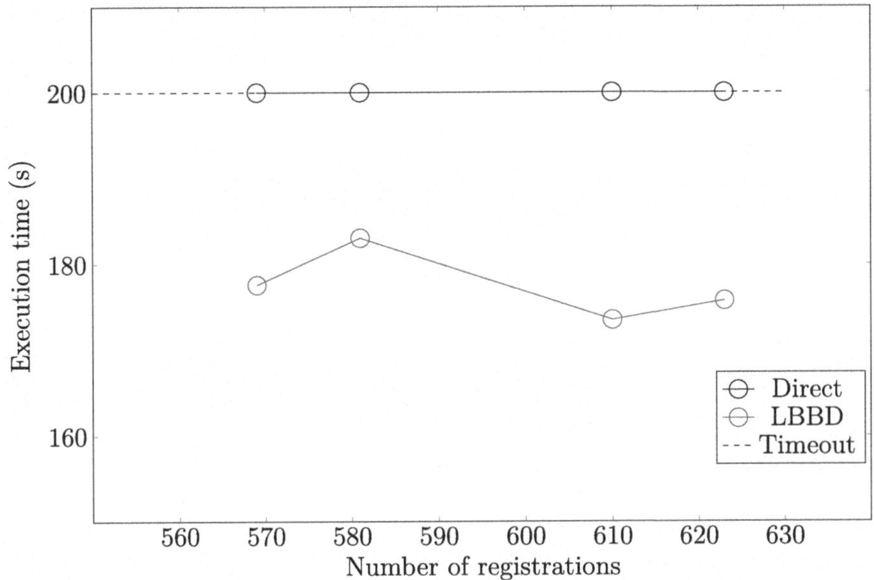

Fig. 4. Time comparison of the performances of the direct encoding and our solution for the CTS problem.

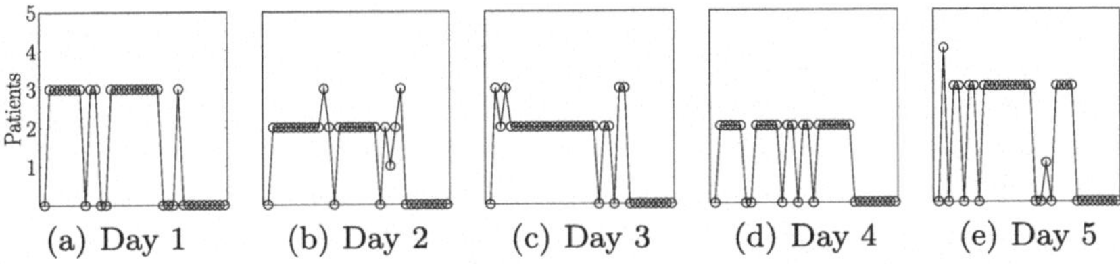

Fig. 5. Distribution of the patients accessing their second phase at the same time in a working week for the CTS problem.

the MP without restarting the process at each iteration. For the direct encoding, CLINGO was configured with the option *--restart-on-model* for faster optimization and a time limit of 200 s, while for the LBBD approach, we maintained the general timeout of 200 s, but we also imposed a timeout of 30 s to each call to the subproblem. Data includes 4 weeks of scheduling, each week from Monday to Friday, and with an average number of registrations equal to 596 (with standard deviation equal to 25). Each registration corresponds to a day of treatment, following a different regimen, and up to five for a single patient.

Figure 4 shows the time required by CLINGO to solve the instances, with respect to the number of patients, using the direct encoding and the alternative LBBD approach. While the direct encoding reached the timeout in all the instances without finding any solution (except for one where it obtained a low-quality solution), our approach solved all instances. About the quality of the solutions returned, although the new approach did not manage to prove the optimality of the solutions, the results in Fig. 5 show that the solution found is very close to the optimum. The figure illustrates the daily distribution of patients over a week, showing the number of patients accessing the second phase during each time slot. As shown, patients are evenly allocated across the slots, with a maximum of four patients per slot. Moreover, the second optimization criterion, consisting of assigning patients to their preferred resource, is always satisfied in the reported results. Thus, the LBBD approach achieves significant performance improvements over the direct approach on the CTS real-world data.

7 Related Work

The LBBD approach, which inspired our work, has already been used in combinatorial optimization problems, especially in scenarios where the problem can be divided into multiple parts. Its versatility and effectiveness have been demonstrated across various domains, most notably in scheduling problems: In this domain, [28] showcased the applicability of LBBD across different scheduling scenarios, underscoring its capability to manage complex, large-scale problems while enhancing both solution quality and computational efficiency.

Focusing on scheduling problems in the healthcare domain, there are some works in which it has been employed. [11] proposed a heuristic adaptation of LBBD to the home healthcare problem, focusing on designing efficient routes and schedules for workers who visit patient homes. Then, [25] applied the LBBD method to the problem of home hospice care staffing and scheduling using mixed integer programming. The objective here is to effectively match hospice care aides with patients and schedule visits to their homes. The authors leverage the versatility of LBBD to recompute staff assignments and visitation schedules as needed efficiently. A similar problem was analyzed by [26] which focused on the home healthcare delivery problem. Specifically, the goal of their problem was to match patients with healthcare aides and schedule multiple home visits over a given time horizon to maximize the number of patients served. The recursive LBBD approach was explored by [33]. In particular, they considered a class of multi-mode appointment scheduling problems involving variable resource availability and setup times. Moreover, they showed the efficiency of this recursive LBBD method using real-life data from a gastroenterology clinic at the University Hospital of Northern Norway. [34] developed three novel LBBD methods and a cut propagation mechanism to tackle the distributed ORS problem. In the same domain, [23] considered a stochastic variant of the problem, incorporating uncertain surgery durations by exploiting the LBBD cut to maintain efficiency and robustness. Recently, [9] presented the first LBBD approach for a specific scheduling problem expressed in ASP, involving chronic outpatients with non-communicable diseases who require ongoing hospital services, thus a problem similar to the ones considered by [25] and by [26]. In particular, they showed that LBBD can expand the applicability of ASP to larger instances without sacrificing the quality of the solutions. In this paper, we achieved a comparable result for both scheduling problems analyzed.

8 Conclusion

In this paper, we have presented an analysis of the CTS problem, modeled and solved with ASP. Specifically, we proposed an LBBD approach implemented through the usage of multi-shot solving, and compared its results to a direct encoding on real data. Results have shown a performance improvement over the classical approach, in which all concepts and specifications are codified in a single encoding. Future works include the definition and analysis of other cuts, and the definition and implementation of additional solving strategies, e.g., of domain-dependent heuristics.

References

1. Alviano, M., et al.: Answer set programming in healthcare: extended overview. In: IPS and RCRA 2020. CEUR Workshop Proceedings, vol. 2745. CEUR-WS.org (2020)
2. Armando, A., Castellini, C., Giunchiglia, E., Idini, M., Maratea, M.: TSAT++: an open platform for satisfiability modulo theories. Electron. Notes Theor. Comput. Sci. **125**(3), 25–36 (2005)
3. Benders, J.: Partitioning procedures for solving mixed-variables programming problems. Comput. Manage. Sci. **2**(1) (2005)
4. Brewka, G., Eiter, T., Truszczynski, M.: Answer set programming at a glance. Commun. ACM **54**(12), 92–103 (2011)
5. Bruno, P., Calimeri, F., Marte, C.: Dedudeep: an extensible framework for combining deep learning and asp-based models. In: Gottlob, G., Inclezan, D., Maratea, M. (eds.) Proceedings of the 16th International Conference on Logic Programming and Nonmonotonic Reasoning (LPNMR 2022). LNCS, vol. 13416, pp. 505–510. Springer, Cham (2022)
6. Buccafurri, F., Leone, N., Rullo, P.: Enhancing disjunctive datalog by constraints. IEEE Trans. Knowl. Data Eng. **12**(5), 845–860 (2000)
7. Calimeri, F., et al.: ASP-Core-2 input language format. Theory Pract. Logic Program. **20**(2), 294–309 (2020)
8. Cappanera, P., et al.: Recent answer set programming applications to scheduling problems in digital health. In: Proceedings of AI4CC-IPS-RCRA-SPIRIT 2024 workshops, co-located with AIxIA 2024. CEUR Workshop Proceedings, vol. 3883. CEUR-WS.org (2024)
9. Cappanera, P., Gavanelli, M., Nonato, M., Roma, M.: Logic-based Benders decomposition in answer set programming for chronic outpatients scheduling. Theory Pract. Logic Program. **23**(4), 848–864 (2023)
10. Cardellini, M., et al.: A two-phase ASP encoding for solving rehabilitation scheduling. In: Proceedings of RuleML+RR 2021. LNCS, vol. 12851, pp. 111–125. Springer, Cham (2021)
11. Ciré, A., Hooker, J.N.: A heuristic logic-based benders method for the home health care problem. In: Manuscript, presented at Matheuristics (2012)
12. Dodaro, C., et al.: Operating room scheduling via answer set programming: improved encoding and test on real data. J. Log. Comput. **34**(8), 1556–1579 (2024)
13. Dodaro, C., Galatà, G., Grioni, A., Maratea, M., Mochi, M., Porro, I.: An ASP-based solution to the chemotherapy treatment scheduling problem. Theory Pract. Logic Program. **21**(6), 835–851 (2021)

14. Dodaro, C., Galatà, G., Khan, M.K., Maratea, M., Porro, I.: An ASP-based solution for operating room scheduling with beds management. In: Fodor, P., Montali, M., Calvanese, D., Roman, D. (eds.) RuleML+RR 2019. LNCS, vol. 11784, pp. 67–81. Springer, Cham (2019). https://doi.org/10.1007/978-3-030-31095-0_5
15. Dodaro, C., Galatà, G., Maratea, M., Porro, I.: Operating room scheduling via answer set programming. In: Ghidini, C., Magnini, B., Passerini, A., Traverso, P. (eds.) AI*IA 2018. LNCS (LNAI), vol. 11298, pp. 445–459. Springer, Cham (2018). https://doi.org/10.1007/978-3-030-03840-3_33
16. Dodaro, C., Galatà, G., Maratea, M., Porro, I.: An ASP-based framework for operating room scheduling. Intelligenza Artificiale **13**(1), 63–77 (2019)
17. Erdem, E., Gelfond, M., Leone, N.: Applications of answer set programming. AI Mag. **37**(3), 53–68 (2016)
18. Faber, W., Pfeifer, G., Leone, N.: Semantics and complexity of recursive aggregates in answer set programming. Artif. Intell. **175**(1), 278–298 (2011)
19. Falkner, A.A., Friedrich, G., Schekotihin, K., Taupe, R., Teppan, E.C.: Industrial applications of answer set programming. KI **32**(2-3), 165–176 (2018)
20. Gebser, M., Kaminski, R., Kaufmann, B., Ostrowski, M., Schaub, T., Wanko, P.: Theory solving made easy with clingo 5. In: Proceedings of ICLP (Technical Communications). OASICS, vol. 52, pp. 2:1–2:15. Schloss Dagstuhl - Leibniz-Zentrum fuer Informatik (2016)
21. Gebser, M., Kaminski, R., Kaufmann, B., Schaub, T.: Multi-shot ASP solving with clingo. Theory Pract. Logic Program. **19**(1), 27–82 (2019)
22. Geoffrion, A.M.: Generalized benders decomposition. J. Optim. Theory Appl. **10**, 237–260 (1972)
23. Guo, C., Bodur, M., Aleman, D.M., Urbach, D.R.: Logic-based benders decomposition and binary decision diagram based approaches for stochastic distributed operating room scheduling. INFORMS J. Comput. **33**(4), 1551–1569 (2021)
24. Hahn-Goldberg, S., Carter, M.W., Beck, J.C., Trudeau, M., Sousa, P., Beattie, K.: Dynamic optimization of chemotherapy outpatient scheduling with uncertainty. Health Care Manag. Sci. **17**(4), 379–392 (2014). https://doi.org/10.1007/s10729-014-9268-0
25. Heching, A., Hooker, J.N.: Scheduling home hospice care with logic-based benders decomposition. In: Quimper, C.-G. (ed.) CPAIOR 2016. LNCS, vol. 9676, pp. 187–197. Springer, Cham (2016). https://doi.org/10.1007/978-3-319-33954-2_14
26. Heching, A., Hooker, J.N., Kimura, R.: A logic-based benders approach to home healthcare delivery. Transp. Sci. **53**(2), 510–522 (2019)
27. Hooker, J.N.: A hybrid method for planning and scheduling. In: Wallace, M. (ed.) CP 2004. LNCS, vol. 3258, pp. 305–316. Springer, Heidelberg (2004). https://doi.org/10.1007/978-3-540-30201-8_24
28. Hooker, J.: Logic-Based Benders Decomposition: Theory and Applications. Springer, Cham (2024)
29. Hooker, J., Ottosson, G.: Logic-based benders decomposition. Math. Program. **96**(1), 33–60 (2003)
30. Huang, Y.L., Bryce, A.H., Culbertson, T., Connor, S.L., Looker, S.A., et al.: Alternative outpatient chemotherapy scheduling method to improve patient service quality and nurse satisfaction. J. Oncol. Pract. **14**(2), 82–91 (2017)
31. Huggins, A., Claudio, D., Pérez, E.: Improving resource utilization in a cancer clinic: an optimization model. In: IIE Annual Conference and Expo 2014 (2014)
32. Rahmaniani, R., Crainic, T.G., Gendreau, M., Rei, W.: The benders decomposition algorithm: a literature review. Eur. J. Oper. Res. **259**(3), 801–817 (2017)

33. Riise, A., Mannino, C., Lamorgese, L.: Recursive logic-based benders' decomposition for multi-mode outpatient scheduling. Eur. J. Oper. Res. **255**(3), 719–728 (2016)
34. Roshanaei, V., Luong, C., Aleman, D.M., Urbach, D.: Propagating logic-based benders' decomposition approaches for distributed operating room scheduling. Eur. J. Oper. Res. **257**(2) (2017)
35. Sevinc, S., Sanli, U.A., Goker, E.: Algorithms for scheduling of chemotherapy plans. Comput. Biol. Med. **43**(12), 2103–2109 (2013)

Large Language Models in Healthcare

Automated Machine Learning to Enhance Knowledge Retrieval in Retrieval-Augmented Generation Pipelines

Matteo Magnini[1], Gianluca Aguzzi[1], Leonardo Sanna[2], Simone Magnolini[2], Patrizio Bellan[2], Mauro Dragoni[2(✉)], and Sara Montagna[3]

[1] Alma Mater Studiorum – Università di Bologna, Cesena, Italy
{matteo.magnini,gianluca.aguzzi}@unibo.it
[2] Fondazione Bruno Kessler, Trento, Italy
{lsanna,magnolini,pbellan,dragoni}@fbk.eu
[3] Universita di Urbino, Urbino, Italy
sara.montagna@uniurb.it

Abstract. The emergence of Large Language Models (LLMs) has introduced exciting possibilities for applications in the digital health domain. However, their unpredictable nature necessitates the development of trustworthy strategies to prevent the generation of hallucinations. A common approach to address this challenge is using Retrieval-Augmented Generation (RAG), where text generation is supported by controlled knowledge injected into the prompts. Even with RAG, ensuring reliable and authoritative information generation requires further research. In a previous work, we presented an enhanced approach to the classic RAG pipeline, introducing an initial step where the LLM generates an enhanced query to support the retrieval step. Results showed that performances are highly sensitive to the techniques adopted for embedding queries and retrieving documents. Accordingly, in this paper, we experiment with a novel automated machine-learning approach to conduct extensive testing across various configurations and explore the retrieval module. Our findings highlight that the embedder and, especially, the retrieval strategies strongly impact the overall performance of the RAG pipeline.

Keywords: Automated Machine Learning · Large Language Models · Retrieval-Augmented Generation · Question Answering · Digital Health

1 Introduction

Large Language Models (LLMs) possess the ability to generate factual information based on learned patterns from extensive training data [18]. However, their accuracy may vary due to the quality of data used during the training phase, the

P. Bruno et al. (Eds.): HC_AIxIA_HYDRA 2025, CCIS 2830, pp. 429–440, 2026.
https://doi.org/10.1007/978-3-032-16708-8_34

complexity of the task they asked to solve, and the parameter density. Failures in providing accurate content, i.e., hallucinations [20,22], can violate the trustworthy requirements that must be satisfied by AI-based systems to be used within real-world contexts. Solving the hallucinations challenge is crucial for several reasons:

- the accuracy and reliability of the system, an LLM answering questions with false or made-up data could lead to serious consequences for users is integrated within health-wise systems;
- the user trust, if an LLM frequently gives incorrect answers that seem plausible, users may lose confidence in the system over time;
- ethical concerns, providing false or misleading information can have ethic implications, especially if users unknowingly act on the hallucinated content;
- quality of information, LLMs are increasingly used in decision-making processes, and bad information can lead to bad decisions;
- legal and compliance risks, in regulated industries, providing erroneous information can violate laws or regulatory standards with the consequence of exposing organizations to liability.

To overcome these limitations, the Retrieval-Augmented Generation (RAG) [15] methodology has been proposed to *augment* external knowledge into LLMs' prompts, thus supporting more effective interactions with users and reducing hallucinations. This approach involves retrieving documents relevant to the user's query and then generating responses based on the factual information they contain. However, the effectiveness of RAG depends on the quality of the retrieval phase. Current retrieval approaches struggle with several challenges: semantic ambiguity, basic matching techniques that lead to inaccurate data retrieval, and insufficient consideration of the complex interplay between embedding methods and retrieval strategies. These limitations result in low accuracy when the retrieval system lacks robustness, ultimately compromising the factual reliability of LLM responses. Previous research mainly uses traditional RAG pipelines with limited (or no) exploration of the retrieval optimisation stage, often relying on default configurations that may not be optimal for specific use cases [1,11].

For this reason, in this paper, we focus our attention on the challenge of improving the effectiveness of the *retrieval* module of the RAG methodology. This aspect, not extensively investigated in the literature, represents a novel and important contribution to the state-of-the-art and to enhancing the trustworthiness of LLM-based systems. In fact, without an effective retrieval of factual knowledge, LLM-based conversational solutions would not be acceptable to stakeholders. In particular, the number of hyperparameters and possible configurations is very high when implementing a RAG system. In this paper, we leverage automated machine learning (autoML) to identify the best configurations, in terms of both hyperparameters and algorithms adopted for embedding and retrieval.

Our analysis confirms that the most effective embedders are those already recognized in literature, namely *mxbai-embed-large* and *nomic-embed-text*. Of particular interest are, instead, our findings on the retrieval strategy side, which we demonstrate to play a crucial role in determining accuracy, with significant impacts on the quality of results. As anticipated, we also observe that the number of retrieved documents correlates directly with accuracy, reinforcing the importance of an efficient retrieval process.

The paper is structured as follows. Section 2 briefly surveys the literature concerning the investigation of the retrieval component within RAG pipelines. We also present autoML and formalize the hyperparameters optimization problem. Section 3 details the scenario in which the proposed approach has been validated. Section 4 discusses the obtained results and, finally, Sect. 5 concludes the paper.

2 Related Work

The existing literature on RAG has primarily concentrated on integrating retrieval into LLM-based solutions to mitigate hallucinations in generated content [2,5]. However, little investigation has been done on which settings are most effective for ensuring a reliable retrieval component. In scenarios where content generation relies on knowledge extracted from a validated repository, which we can call "pre-validated knowledge", it is essential to guarantee that the retrieved information is both relevant and reliable. It has also been shown the LLM might benefit from noisy prompts, therefore employing documents not directly relevant to user query [4].

Nonetheless, in scenarios such as medical questions answering, where content generation is expected to rely on *pre-validated knowledge*, the trustworthiness of the retrieval process is crucial to ensure both the reliability of generated answer as well as epistemic transparency [21]. Yet, RAG studies tend to overlook this aspect, as relevant queries returning no documents are typically handled by LLM parametric knowledge. Occasionally, the "LLM-as-a-judge"[1] approach is employed to assess the relevance, but this remains an indirect solution. In fields such as medicine, aligning LLM-generated content with expert knowledge is an active research area [1,7,13]. For instance, [1] utilized open-source LLMs to ensure data privacy and incorporated RAG techniques to enhance the chatbot's performance. The findings indicated that integrating RAG significantly improved the chatbot's ability to provide accurate and empathetic responses, surpassing the performance of specialized medical-domain models that did not employ RAG.

More broadly, RAG research has explored ways to enhance retrieval, such as using LLMs as retrievers by constraining the decoding process to relevant documents [9] or decomposing documents into atomic questions to optimize retrieval granularity [19]. Other approaches involve query decomposition [10], fine-tuning [8,17], and sequence-to-sequence models for relevance estimation [11].

However, despite these advancements, none of these works provide systematic empirical insights into optimizing retrieval-related hyperparameters such as the choice of retrieval methods or the selection of the embedding model, leaving a

[1] https://huggingface.co/learn/cookbook/en/llm_judge.

crucial gap in understanding how to ensure a reliable retrieval component in RAG systems.

In this context, intending to identify a robust and reliable RAG pipeline, in a previous work of ours, we experiment with an existing conversational pipeline that employs the Hypothetical Document Embeddings (HyDE) framework [6]. This framework uses an LLM to generate a Hypothetical Document (HyDoc), which is then used to query the repository of the document instead of using the user's query. Since the performance is consistent over different LLMs, we concluded that it is reasonable to assume that query generation (i.e., the HyDoc) is not responsible for the low precision score measured in that work. We believe that the embedder and related hyperparameters might play a significant role, thus motivating the approach and experiments we propose in this work.

3 Materials and Methods

The codebase of the experiments is publicly available on GitHub[2].

3.1 Dataset

For our case study, we constructed a dataset tailored to the domain of maternity and newborn care. The dataset was built using a diverse collection of documents, including materials produced by the Obstetrics Department of Trento Hospital and a selection of articles published on the UPPA website[3], a well-known platform that provides evidence-based information for parents. These sources cover a wide range of topics relevant to our study, such as pregnancy, childbirth, postpartum recovery, and infant care.

To generate relevant user queries, we processed these documents by segmenting them into smaller chunks while maintaining content coherence. In total, we extracted 43,390 chunks from the original texts. Each chunk was then processed using GPT-4o-mini, which was prompted to generate synthetic questions based on the following instructions:

> "Act as a pregnant woman or a mother with a newborn. Write five questions you might ask a midwife. The answers to these questions must always be contained within this passage: " `+ chunk +` "."[4]

This process resulted in a dataset of 216,950 questions (henceforth question dataset), each directly tied to a specific text chunk and document. The objective was to create a realistic set of questions reflecting the common concerns and uncertainties of pregnant women and new mothers, ensuring that the generated questions have an answer grounded in our *pre-validated* information. In the experiments, because of computational time limitations, we use a representative subset of the original dataset by randomly sampling 1,000 questions.

---

[2] https://github.com/MatteoMagnini/experiments-2025-hcaixia-automl-rag.

[3] www.uppa.it.

[4] The original instruction was given in Italian, here we provide its English translation for clarity.

3.2 AutoML for RAG Formalization

To improve the RAG phase of an LLM-based system, we want to find the best hyperparameters that maximize the retrieval of relevant documents. To do so, we apply automated machine learning (autoML) to search through the configuration space of the hyperparameters. We formally define a RAG pipeline as a function $R : \mathbb{D} \times \boldsymbol{\Theta} \rightarrow \mathbb{H}$, which retrieves and generates responses based on a document collection $\mathcal{D}$ and a hyperparameter configuration $\boldsymbol{\theta}$ from a hyperparameter space $\boldsymbol{\Theta}$. The hyperparameter space is defined as the cross-product of all the hyperparameter domains:

$$\boldsymbol{\Theta}_R = \Theta_1 \times \cdots \times \Theta_K$$

where Θ_k represents the domain of the kth hyperparameter, including choices for embedding models, retrieval strategies, and other pipeline components.

To assess the quality of a hyperparameter configuration $\boldsymbol{\theta} \in \boldsymbol{\Theta}$, we evaluate the performance of the RAG pipeline using a set of predefined metrics. Unlike traditional supervised learning setups, we do not split $\mathcal{D}$ into distinct training and test sets for model fitting. Instead, we directly assess retrieval and generation effectiveness by comparing generated responses against ground-truth references or other evaluation signals.

The goal is to solve the **hyperparameter optimisation** (HPO) problem, identifying the configuration $\boldsymbol{\theta}^{\star} \in \boldsymbol{\Theta}$ that optimizes a given loss function:

$$\boldsymbol{\theta}^{\star} = \arg\min_{\boldsymbol{\theta} \in \boldsymbol{\Theta}} \mathcal{L}(R(\mathcal{D}, \boldsymbol{\theta})) \tag{1}$$

Several approaches exist for solving the HPO problem, with many relying on Bayesian optimization (BO) [3]. These techniques iteratively evaluate hyperparameter configurations, refining estimates of their performance.

Multi-objective optimization also plays a role in RAG hyperparameter tuning, as trade-offs exist between objectives such as retrieval precision, response coherence, and computational cost. In such cases, we aim to identify a Pareto front of optimal configurations that balance these competing objectives. Formally, a Pareto front for a set of RAG configurations $\mathcal{H} \subset \mathbb{H}$ evaluated on $\mathcal{D}$ is defined as:

$$P_{\mathcal{D}}(\mathcal{H}) = \left\{ h \left| \begin{array}{l} H \in \mathcal{H}, \nexists H' \in \mathcal{H} : \\ \forall m \in \{1, \ldots, M\} : \\ \mathcal{L}_m(H', \mathcal{D}) \leq \mathcal{L}_m(H, \mathcal{D}), \\ \exists j \in \{1, \ldots, M\} : \\ \mathcal{L}_j(H', \mathcal{D}) < \mathcal{L}_j(H, \mathcal{D}) \end{array} \right. \right\}. \tag{2}$$

To compare different RAG configurations, quality indicators such as Hypervolume [14] can quantify the trade-offs between objectives. Scalarisation methods, such as ParEGO [12], allow multi-objective Bayesian optimization by dynamically adjusting the importance of different objectives during the search process.

3.3 AutoML Pipeline

We design our experiments to exploit the autoML framework to optimize the performance of the RAG pipeline. The experiments include two main steps that can be optimized: (1) the creation of the vector space model and (2) the retrieval of the relevant documents.

First, we select the hyperparameters to optimize, which include the chunk length, overlap percentage, embedder, retriever, and number of documents These hyperparameters have a significant impact on both steps of the pipeline. In particular, the chunk length and overlap percentage, affecting step (1), are used to split the documents into chunks. We choose to bound the chunk length between 100 and 500 tokens and the overlap percentage between 10% and 50%. The embedder is the model used to encode the chunks into vectors, and it affects both steps. We choose among five different embedders[5]: *nomic-embed-text*, *mxbai-embed-large*, *bert-base-cased*, *bert-base-italian-xxl-cased*, and *biobert-base-cased*. The *nomic-embed-text* and *mxbai-embed-large* are state-of-the-art embedders, while the *bert-base-cased* is a well-established benchmark. We justify the inclusion of the *bert-base-italian-xxl-cased* and *biobert-base-cased* embedders because they are respectively fine-tuned on the Italian language and on biomedical texts. The retriever is the model and strategy used to retrieve the relevant documents, and it affects step (2). We choose two different ways to retrieve the documents: the first one consists in using the same embedder used to embed the chunks (a.k.a., base retriever), while the second one consists in using an ensemble of retrievers (a.k.a., ensemble retriever). For the ensemble retriever, we use the base retriever in combination with the *BM25* retriever. Finally, the number of documents is the maximum number of documents to retrieve, and it affects step (2). We choose to bind the number of documents between 1 and 20. Table 1 sums up the configuration space.

Table 1. Configuration space.

Hyperparameter	Type	Range or Values
Chunk length	integer	[100, 500]
Overlap percentage	float	[0.1, 0.5]
Embedder	categorical	nomic-embed-text mxbai-embed-large bert-base-cased bert-base-italian-xxl-cased biobert-base-cased
Retriever	categorical	base ensemble
Number of documents	integer	[1, 20]

[5] Available on huggingface.co.

Second, we define the objective functions to optimize. We define two objectives: the accuracy and the number of retrieved documents. Since we want to minimize them, we actually work with $1 - accuracy$. The accuracy is defined as follows: we assign 1 if there is at least one retrieved chunk that belongs to the same document as the question, and 0 otherwise. We expect to have higher accuracy (resp., lower $1 - accuracy$) when the system retrieves more relevant documents. However, we also want to discourage the system from retrieving too many documents, as this would increase the computational cost and overload the LLM that would possibly use the retrieved documents in the system.

To run the experiments we use SMAC3 [16], a state-of-the-art autoML framework. We set a 24-h wall time limit and a number of 10.000 trials. The experiments are run on a machine with a GPU NVIDIA Tesla V100S-PCIE-32GB.

4 Evaluation

Figure 1 shows the results of the experiments. In total, 161 configurations are evaluated by SMAC3. The Pareto front is composed of 10 configurations[6], a.k.a., incumbents, that are represented as red crosses. The incumbents are the best trade-offs between the accuracy and the number of retrieved documents. It is worth noting that all the incumbents have the *ensemble* retrieval strategy, and as embedder the *nomic-embed-text* or the *mxbai-embed-large* model.

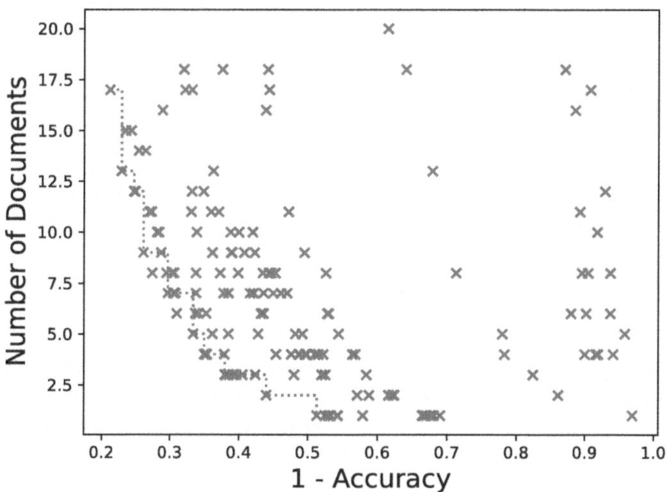

Fig. 1. Evaluation of the tested configurations by SMAC3. Red crosses represent the configurations that determine the Pareto front. (Color figure online)

[6] We choose to leave the default SMAC3 value of the number of incumbents to 10 during the experiments to balance the exploration and the exploitation of the configuration space.

We observe from Fig. 1 and 2 (left) that, as expected, the accuracy increases with the number of documents. In particular, the growth in accuracy is quite fast when the documents go from 1 to 7, and then it slows down. Configurations with 7 retrieved documents reach on average an accuracy of 0.6, while the incumbent with the same number of documents reaches an accuracy of 0.7. By increasing even more the number of documents, we can reach up to 0.8 of accuracy in the best configurations.

Figure 2 (right) summarises the impact of the embedder and the retriever on the accuracy. We can appreciate that using the ensemble retriever has a great positive impact on the accuracy, especially when the retriever is *biobert-base-cased* or *bert-base-cased*. The *mxbai-embed-large* and *nomic-embed-text* embedders are the best-performing ones, while the *bert-xxl-italian-cased* embedder is in the middle. These results confirm the actual state-of-the-art in the field of embeddings.

Figure 3 shows the aggregate results of the chunk length (left) and the overlap percentage (right) on the accuracy. We notice that the chunk length and the overlap percentage have a limited impact on the accuracy.

Finally, Fig. 4 shows the kernel density estimation plots of the number of documents vs. chunk length (left) and the number of documents vs. overlap percentage (right). We can appreciate that SMAC3 prefers to explore configurations with a lower number of documents, a high chunk length, and a low overlap percentage.

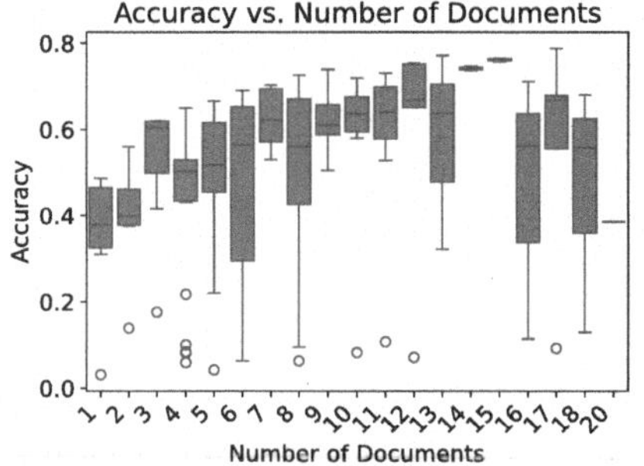

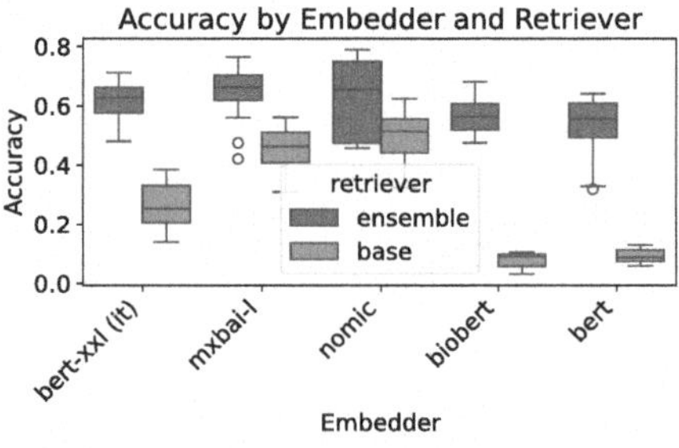

Fig. 2. Box plots of accuracy vs. number of documents (left) and accuracy vs. embedder and retriever (right). Performance increases with more documents until around 15, after which it declines. Using the state-of-the-art embedder improves performance, but the retriever choice appears most critical.

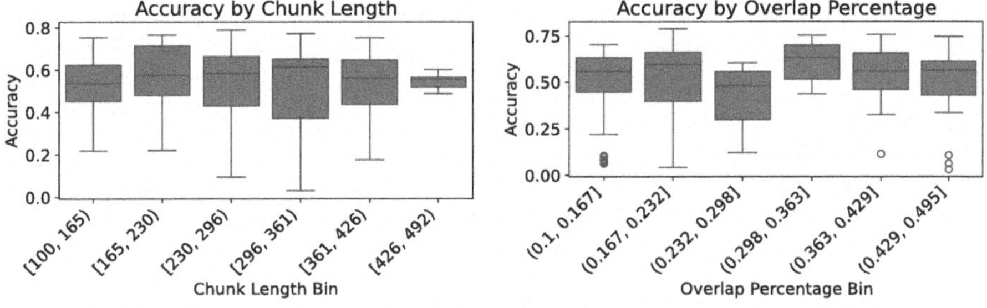

Fig. 3. Box plots of accuracy vs. chunk length (left) and accuracy vs. overlap percentage (right). Performance is relatively stable across chunk lengths and overlap percentages.

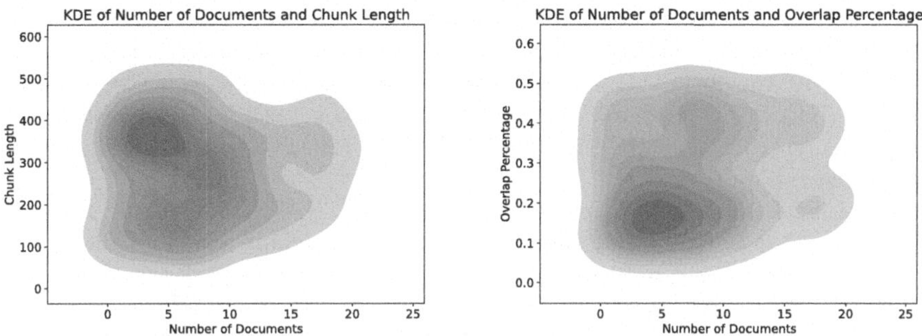

Fig. 4. Kernel density estimation plots of the number of documents vs. chunk length (left) and the number of documents vs. overlap percentage (right). SMAC appears to prefer a lower number of documents, and high chunk length, and a low overlap percentage.

5 Conclusions

This work deeply explores the retrieval step integrated within the RAG pipeline. The goal was to solve the HPO problem aiming to discover the best settings to enhance the retrieval effectiveness. As discussed in the paper, this challenge is relevant to the research direction studying the trustworthy adoption of LLMs since an effective retrieval step within the RAG pipeline can significantly increase the correctness of the generated texts. We designed and implemented an autoML approach to explore the hyperparameters solution space in our case study focused on documents related to the maternity and newborn care domain. The obtained results demonstrated the capability of detecting the appropriate setting by paving the way for future research in this direction. Future works focus on the design of a comprehensive user evaluation of the texts generated through a subset of candidate settings to validate the impact of the retrieved documents.

Acknowledgments. We acknowledge the support of the PNRR project INEST - Interconnected North-East Innovation Ecosystem (ECS00000043), under the NRRP

MUR program funded by the NextGenerationEU. We acknowledge the support of the PNRR project FAIR - Future AI Research (PE00000013), under the NRRP MUR program funded by the NextGenerationEU. This paper is supported by the TrustAlert project, funded by Fondazione Compagnia San Paolo and Fondazione CDP under the "Artificial Intelligence" call.

Disclosure of Interests. The authors have no competing interests to declare that are relevant to the content of this article.

References

1. Aguzzi, G., Magnini, M., Ferretti, S., Salcuni, G.P., Montagna, S.: Applying retrieval-augmented generation on open LLMs for a medical chatbot supporting hypertensive patients. In: Calimeri, F., Dragoni, M., Stella, F. (eds.) Proceedings of the 3rd AIxIA Workshop on Artificial Intelligence For Healthcare (HC@AIxIA 2024), Bolzano, Italy, 27–28 November 2024. CEUR Workshop Proceedings, vol. 3880, pp. 189–201. CEUR-WS.org (2024). https://ceur-ws.org/Vol-3880/paper17.pdf
2. Alghisi, S., Rizzoli, M., Roccabruna, G., Mousavi, S.M., Riccardi, G.: Should we fine-tune or rag? Evaluating different techniques to adapt LLMs for dialogue. In: Mahamood, S., Nguyen, M.L., Ippolito, D. (eds.) Proceedings of the 17th International Natural Language Generation Conference, INLG 2024, Tokyo, Japan, 23–27 September 2024, pp. 180–197. Association for Computational Linguistics (2024). https://aclanthology.org/2024.inlg-main.15
3. Astudillo, R., Frazier, P.I.: Thinking inside the box: a tutorial on grey-box Bayesian optimization. In: Winter Simulation Conference, WSC 2021, Phoenix, AZ, USA, 12–15 December 2021, pp. 1–15. IEEE (2021). https://doi.org/10.1109/WSC52266.2021.9715343
4. Cuconasu, F., et al.: The power of noise: Redefining retrieval for RAG systems. In: Yang, G.H., Wang, H., Han, S., Hauff, C., Zuccon, G., Zhang, Y. (eds.) Proceedings of the 47th International ACM SIGIR Conference on Research and Development in Information Retrieval, SIGIR 2024, Washington DC, USA, 14–18 July 2024, pp. 719–729. ACM (2024). https://doi.org/10.1145/3626772.3657834
5. Fan, W., et al.: A survey on RAG meeting LLMs: towards retrieval-augmented large language models. In: Baeza-Yates, R., Bonchi, F. (eds.) Proceedings of the 30th ACM SIGKDD Conference on Knowledge Discovery and Data Mining, KDD 2024, Barcelona, Spain, 25–29 August 2024, pp. 6491–6501. ACM (2024). https://doi.org/10.1145/3637528.3671470
6. Gao, L., Ma, X., Lin, J., Callan, J.: Precise zero-shot dense retrieval without relevance labels. In: Rogers, A., Boyd-Graber, J.L., Okazaki, N. (eds.) Proceedings of the 61st Annual Meeting of the Association for Computational Linguistics (Volume 1: Long Papers), ACL 2023, Toronto, Canada, 9–14 July 2023, pp. 1762–1777. Association for Computational Linguistics (2023). https://doi.org/10.18653/V1/2023.ACL-LONG.99
7. Giuffrè, M., Kresevic, S., Pugliese, N., You, K., Shung, D.L.: Optimizing large language models in digestive disease: strategies and challenges to improve clinical outcomes. Liver Int. (2024). https://doi.org/10.1111/liv.15974

8. Islam, S.B., Rahman, M.A., Hossain, K.S.M.T., Hoque, E., Joty, S., Parvez, M.R.: Open-rag: enhanced retrieval augmented reasoning with open-source large language models. In: Al-Onaizan, Y., Bansal, M., Chen, Y. (eds.) Findings of the Association for Computational Linguistics: EMNLP 2024, Miami, Florida, USA, 12–16 November 2024, pp. 14231–14244. Association for Computational Linguistics (2024). https://aclanthology.org/2024.findings-emnlp.831
9. Jain, P., Soares, L.B., Kwiatkowski, T.: From RAG to riches: retrieval interlaced with sequence generation. In: Al-Onaizan, Y., Bansal, M., Chen, Y. (eds.) Proceedings of the 2024 Conference on Empirical Methods in Natural Language Processing, EMNLP 2024, Miami, FL, USA, 12–16 November 2024, pp. 8887–8904. Association for Computational Linguistics (2024). https://aclanthology.org/2024.emnlp-main.502
10. Jeong, S., Baek, J., Cho, S., Hwang, S.J., Park, J.: Adaptive-rag: learning to adapt retrieval-augmented large language models through question complexity. In: Duh, K., Gómez-Adorno, H., Bethard, S. (eds.) Proceedings of the 2024 Conference of the North American Chapter of the Association for Computational Linguistics: Human Language Technologies (Volume 1: Long Papers), NAACL 2024, Mexico City, Mexico, 16–21 June 2024, pp. 7036–7050. (2024). https://doi.org/10.18653/V1/2024.NAACL-LONG.389
11. Kim, K., Lee, J.: RE-RAG: improving open-domain QA performance and interpretability with relevance estimator in retrieval-augmented generation. In: Al-Onaizan, Y., Bansal, M., Chen, Y. (eds.) Proceedings of the 2024 Conference on Empirical Methods in Natural Language Processing, EMNLP 2024, Miami, FL, USA, 12–16 November 2024, pp. 22149–22161. Association for Computational Linguistics (2024). https://aclanthology.org/2024.emnlp-main.1236
12. Knowles, J.D.: Parego: a hybrid algorithm with on-line landscape approximation for expensive multiobjective optimization problems. IEEE Trans. Evol. Comput. **10**(1), 50–66 (2006). https://doi.org/10.1109/TEVC.2005.851274
13. Kresevic, S., Giuffrè, M., Ajcevic, M., et al.: Optimization of hepatological clinical guidelines interpretation by large language models: a retrieval augmented generation-based framework. NPJ Digit. Med. **7**(1) (2024). https://doi.org/10.1038/S41746-024-01091-Y
14. Laumanns, M., Zitzler, E., Thiele, L.: A unified model for multi-objective evolutionary algorithms with elitism. In: Zalzala, A.M.S. (ed.) Proceedings of the 2000 Congress on Evolutionary Computation, CEC 2000, La Jolla, CA, USA, 16–19 July 2000, pp. 46–53. IEEE (2000). https://doi.org/10.1109/CEC.2000.870274
15. Lewis, P.S.H., Perez, E., Piktus, A., et al.: Retrieval-augmented generation for knowledge-intensive NLP tasks. In: Larochelle, H., Ranzato, M., Hadsell, R., Balcan, M., Lin, H. (eds.) Advances in Neural Information Processing Systems 33: Annual Conference on Neural Information Processing Systems 2020, NeurIPS 2020, 6–12 December 2020, virtual (2020). https://proceedings.neurips.cc/paper/2020/hash/6b493230205f780e1bc26945df7481e5-Abstract.html
16. Lindauer, M., Eggensperger, K., Feurer, M., et al.: SMAC3: a versatile Bayesian optimization package for hyperparameter optimization. J. Mach. Learn. Res. **23**, 54:1–54:9 (2022). https://jmlr.org/papers/v23/21-0888.html
17. Magnini, M., Aguzzi, G., Montagna, S.: Open-source small language models for personal medical assistant chatbots. Intell.-Based Med. **11**, 100197 (2025). https://doi.org/10.1016/j.ibmed.2024.100197

18. Petroni, F., Rocktäschel, T., et al.: Language models as knowledge bases? In: Inui, K., Jiang, J., Ng, V., Wan, X. (eds.) Proceedings of the 2019 Conference on Empirical Methods in Natural Language Processing and the 9th International Joint Conference on Natural Language Processing, EMNLP-IJCNLP 2019, Hong Kong, China, 3–7 November 2019, pp. 2463–2473. Association for Computational Linguistics (2019). https://doi.org/10.18653/V1/D19-1250
19. Raina, V., Gales, M.: Question-based retrieval using atomic units for enterprise RAG. In: Schlichtkrull, M., Chen, Y., Whitehouse, C., et al. (eds.) Proceedings of the Seventh Fact Extraction and VERification Workshop (FEVER), pp. 219–233. Association for Computational Linguistics, Miami, Florida, USA (2024). https://doi.org/10.18653/v1/2024.fever-1.25
20. Wang, B., Chen, W., Pei, H., et al.: Decodingtrust: a comprehensive assessment of trustworthiness in GPT models. In: Oh, A., Naumann, T., Globerson, A., Saenko, K., Hardt, M., Levine, S. (eds.) Advances in Neural Information Processing Systems 36: Annual Conference on Neural Information Processing Systems 2023, NeurIPS 2023, New Orleans, LA, USA, 10–16 December 2023 (2023). https://proceedings.neurips.cc/paper_files/paper/2023/file/63cb9921eecf51bfad27a99b2c53dd6d-Paper-Datasets_and_Benchmarks.pdf
21. Winter, P.D., Carusi, A.: (de) troubling transparency: artificial intelligence (AI) for clinical applications. Med. Hum. **49** (2023). https://mh.bmj.com/content/49/1/17.abstract
22. Xu, Y., Namazifar, M., Hazarika, D., Padmakumar, A., Liu, Y., Hakkani-Tur, D.: KILM: knowledge injection into encoder-decoder language models. In: Rogers, A., Boyd-Graber, J., Okazaki, N. (eds.) Proceedings of the 61st Annual Meeting of the Association for Computational Linguistics (Volume 1: Long Papers), pp. 5013–5035. Association for Computational Linguistics, Toronto, Canada (2023). https://doi.org/10.18653/v1/2023.acl-long.275

Exploring Large Language Models as Digital Health Coaches: A Role-Play Approach to Brief Action Planning

Marco Bolpagni[1,2](✉), Leonardo Sanna[2], Simone De Carli[2], Silvia Gabrielli[2], and Mauro Dragoni[2]

[1] University of Padova, Padova, Italy
mbolpagni@fbk.eu
[2] Fondazione Bruno Kessler, Trento, Italy
{lsanna,sidecarli,sgabrielli,dragoni}@fbk.eu

Abstract. Brief Action Planning (BAP) is a structured method rooted in motivational interviewing, designed to support individuals in adopting healthier behaviors. This paper explores the feasibility of using Large Language Models (LLMs) as conversational agents to deliver BAP without specialized training data or fine-tuning. By employing role-play prompting, we guided an LLM to simulate a health coach that facilitates goal-setting and action planning for sedentary lifestyles. The approach was tested in simulated conversations and user evaluations, examining adherence to BAP protocols and user experience. Results demonstrate both promise and limitations: while the LLM could replicate several key components of BAP, challenges remain in consistency and personalization. These findings highlight the potential of LLM-driven role-play as a complementary tool for scalable, time-efficient health interventions.

Keywords: Large Language Model · Behavior Change · Brief Action Planning · Motivational Interview

1 Introduction

Sedentary behavior is widely recognized as a major driver of global health problems, elevating the risk of chronic conditions such as cardiovascular disease, obesity, and diabetes [20]. In response, researchers and practitioners have developed structured, evidence-based strategies for supporting individuals in making sustainable changes to their daily routines [10]. One such method is Brief Action Planning (BAP) [7], a clinically oriented framework rooted in Motivational Interviewing (MI) principles [16]. By guiding patients through stepwise goal-setting, BAP fosters both self-efficacy and motivation. Despite its effectiveness, however, integrating BAP into routine care remains challenging, as clinicians often face significant time and resource constraints.

Given these barriers, digital tools have been explored as possible supports. Among these, Artificial Intelligence (AI) has attracted growing attention in

P. Bruno et al. (Eds.): HC_AIxIA_HYDRA 2025, CCIS 2830, pp. 441–452, 2026.
https://doi.org/10.1007/978-3-032-16708-8_35

healthcare [6,17]. With the rapid progress of Large Language Models (LLMs), interest in such applications has accelerated. Modern models like OpenAI's GPT-3.5 have already demonstrated solid performance on clinical knowledge benchmarks [2], and more recent architectures like Llama 3.3-70B[1] have further advanced natural language understanding. Because of their conversational abilities, LLMs are increasingly seen as potential assistants for structured interventions such as BAP [30]. Yet concerns about consistency, instruction-following, and hallucinations underscore the importance of systematic evaluation before clinical use. This study examines whether LLMs can deliver BAP in a way that is both faithful to its structured design and feasible for use in time-limited settings. Specifically, we investigate two research questions:

1. To what extent can an LLM carry out the prescribed steps of BAP when guided only by role-play prompting?
2. How reliably does the model adhere to instructions when applying BAP to diverse patient scenarios?

To address these questions, we simulate BAP sessions using zero-shot prompting and evaluate model performance across a range of patient profiles representing different stages of readiness for change. In addition to task completion and instruction-following, we also analyze instances of hallucination. Section 2 reviews relevant literature on LLMs in clinical practice and prompting strategies. Section 3 details our simulation framework and evaluation procedure. Section 4 presents the experimental findings, followed by discussion of strengths, limitations, and implications in Sect. 5. Finally, Sect. 6 concludes with key takeaways for future research.

2 Related Work

Traditional approaches to digital health interventions often rely on rule-based systems or predefined algorithms to guide user interactions [12]. The rise of LLMs has introduced a paradigm shift, offering models capable of engaging in context-sensitive conversations without explicit programming. For instance, LLMs have demonstrated potential in generating empathetic and informative responses [24]. They have started to be employed also for mental health support [18,19,28], displaying consistent abilities in providing emotional support and eliciting behavior change in patients.

Nonetheless, there is undoubtedly a lack of suitable evaluation criteria for assessing fairness, biases, and inaccurate chatbot responses [1]. On the other hand, LLMs struggle with specific issues such as hallucinations, instruction-following accuracy, and ethical considerations, which remain prevalent in these fields [4]. Previous studies have explored the role of AI in MI, the foundational framework underlying BAP. For example, GPTCoach[2] promotes physical activity by leveraging data from wearables to personalize the MI intervention content

[1] For reference see https://arxiv.org/pdf/2407.21783.
[2] https://arxiv.org/abs/2405.06061.

using LLMs; there is also MIcha [15] a GPT4-based chatbot that addresses three distinct target behaviors (decrease procrastination, live more sustainably, adopt healthier nutrition) using MI. All these systems target behaviors by using a conversational framework that guides interactions with the user. Another example is the case of [25], who developed a virtual counselor capable of conducting MI for addictive behaviors (alcohol abuse) using prompt engineering. Regarding prompt engineering, this technique is an active research field in clinical applications employing LLMs [14,26]. In the vast range of techniques that can be employed [13] the persona pattern (also known as role-play prompting) is one of the most widely used in medical applications [21,29].

Although MI techniques are similar to those of BAP, they present differences reflected in the creation of AI agents. MI techniques are more abstract and allow for greater adaptability by the language model. Consequently, the prompt is more vague, and the instruction following is less crucial. To the best of our knowledge, no work has specifically investigated the structured implementation of clinical interventions like BAP, which require adherence to well-defined protocols and high levels of reliability. Additionally, research on applying zero-shot prompting [9] remains limited in the context of behavior change interventions.

3 Methods

Our goal is to test the applicability of LLMs to the BAP framework by simulating a doctor-patient interaction. The experimental workflow consisted of these steps:

1. Designing the intelligent agent(s)
2. Defining the evaluation criteria with domain experts
3. Running the simulations and user testing

First, to develop the intelligent agent, we leveraged the role-play prompting framework [23] to translate the BAP protocol into a structured system prompt that provided step-by-step instructions for goal exploration, commitment elicitation, and follow-up planning (Fig. 1). Motivational interviewing principles were embedded throughout the interaction to foster collaboration, autonomy, and self-efficacy. We selected Llama 3.3-70B as the backbone model due to its extensive parametric knowledge of medical concepts, conversational fluency, and adherence to instructions. The system prompt remained persistent throughout interactions, ensuring consistency while allowing the agent to dynamically adapt to evolving conversations.

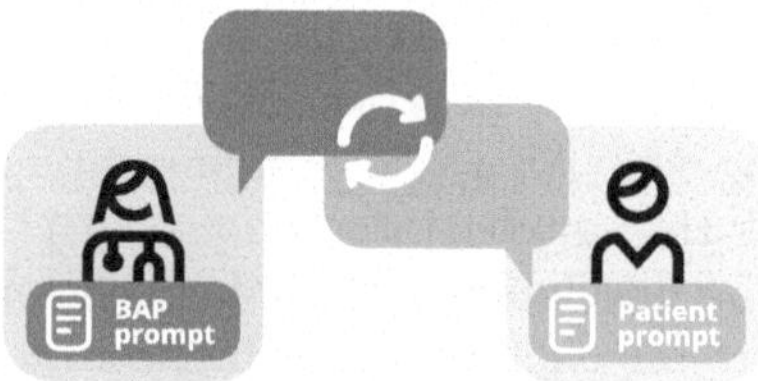

Fig. 1. Translating the Brief Action Planning into a detailed prompt

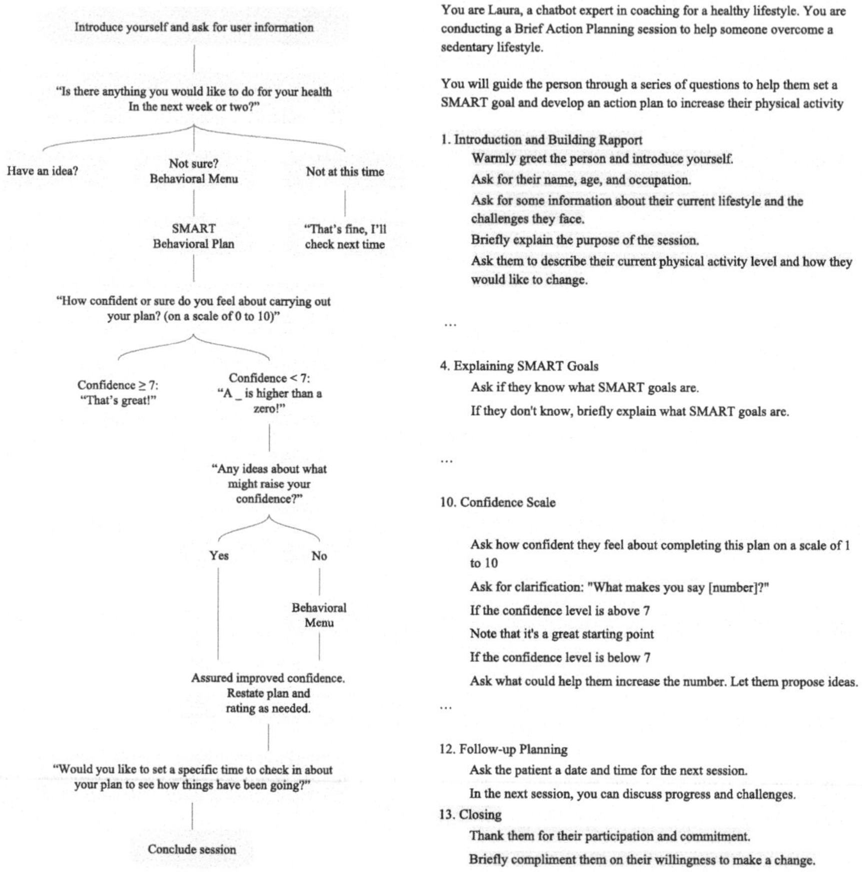

Introduce yourself and ask for user information

"Is there anything you would like to do for your health In the next week or two?"

Have an idea?

Not sure? Behavioral Menu

Not at this time

SMART Behavioral Plan

"That's fine, I'll check next time

"How confident or sure do you feel about carrying out your plan? (on a scale of 0 to 10)"

Confidence ≥ 7: "That's great!"

Confidence < 7: "A _ is higher than a zero!"

"Any ideas about what might raise your confidence?"

Yes

No

Behavioral Menu

Assured improved confidence. Restate plan and rating as needed.

"Would you like to set a specific time to check in about your plan to see how things have been going?"

Conclude session

You are Laura, a chatbot expert in coaching for a healthy lifestyle. You are conducting a Brief Action Planning session to help someone overcome a sedentary lifestyle.

You will guide the person through a series of questions to help them set a SMART goal and develop an action plan to increase their physical activity

1. Introduction and Building Rapport
    Warmly greet the person and introduce yourself.
    Ask for their name, age, and occupation.
    Ask for some information about their current lifestyle and the challenges they face.
    Briefly explain the purpose of the session.
    Ask them to describe their current physical activity level and how they would like to change.

...

4. Explaining SMART Goals
    Ask if they know what SMART goals are.
    If they don't know, briefly explain what SMART goals are.

...

10. Confidence Scale
    Ask how confident they feel about completing this plan on a scale of 1 to 10
    Ask for clarification: "What makes you say [number]?"
    If the confidence level is above 7
    Note that it's a great starting point
    If the confidence level is below 7
    Ask what could help them increase the number. Let them propose ideas.

...

12. Follow-up Planning
    Ask the patient a date and time for the next session.
    In the next session, you can discuss progress and challenges.
13. Closing
    Thank them for their participation and commitment.
    Briefly compliment them on their willingness to make a change.

Fig. 2. Diagram illustrating two LLM agents engaging in interactive dialogue.

Then, we designed a simulated patient counterpart to test the agent's adaptability to different patient behaviors. By using *Mimesis*[3], a Python library for generating demographic attributes such as name, age, and occupation, we created patient personas with distinct behavioral characteristics. The patient agent

[3] https://mimesis.name.

was instantiated using the same LLM backbone as the doctor agent but was prompted to exhibit behaviors corresponding to different stages of the Transtheoretical Model of Change (TTMC) [22]. Specifically, we developed three patient types: a *Collaborative* patient (motivated to change, corresponding to the preparation stage in TTMC), a *Confused* patient (uncertain and requiring more guidance, corresponding to the contemplation stage in TTMC), and an *Uncollaborative* patient (actively resistant to suggestions, corresponding to the precontemplation stage in TTMC). These variations allowed us to test the BAP agent's ability to adapt to different levels of engagement and motivation. To ensure realistic and dynamic doctor-patient interactions, we implemented the simulations using Microsoft AutoGen[4], where two LLM instances operated concurrently: one as the BAP agent and the other as the patient. Both agents maintained persistent prompts and conversation histories, enabling contextually appropriate exchanges (see Fig. 2). Additionally, to examine the impact of model hyperparameters on BAP agent performance, we experimented with different temperature values for the LLM {0.1, 0.3, 0.5, 0.7, 0.9}, covering the model's full capacity to follow the given prompt. For each temperature setting, we generated 10 sessions per patient type {Collaborative, Confused, Uncollaborative}, resulting in a total of 150 simulations.

Finally, we conducted user testing with 20 participants, who engaged in conversations with the BAP agent via OpenWebUI[5], an open-source web-based interface designed for interacting with AI models.

3.1 Evaluation

The BAP agent was evaluated in collaboration with four BAP experts to ensure methodological rigor and domain relevance. We developed a comprehensive annotation grid with these experts to assess each session (see Table 1). All simulated and user-generated interactions were manually annotated by trained evaluators experienced in AI and digital interventions. Evaluation metrics assessed the agent's performance in overall task execution and step-by-step adherence to the BAP framework.

The Task Completion Rate (TCR), a widely adopted metric in conversational agent assessment [3], was the metric we used to assess model performance. The TCR, measured the percentage of sessions where the agent completed all annotation grid steps, ensuring comprehensive intervention delivery. Similarly, we introduced the Hallucination-Free Task Completion Rate (HF-TCR), by evaluating the proportion of completed sessions free of factual errors, deviations from user context/instructions, or harmful content. Finally, we used the Step Completion Rate (SCR) to quantify the percentage of sessions that completed each grid step successfully. This provides a detailed view of strengths and areas for improvement in BAP adherence, while also identifying the areas in which the language model may struggle to follow the instructions.

[4] https://arxiv.org/abs/2308.08155.
[5] https://openwebui.com/.

Table 1. Definitions of the assessment criteria used in session evaluation.

Name	Definition
Personal Information	*Whether the agent asked the subject about their personal information* [bool]
Lifestyle	*Whether the agent asked the subject about their lifestyle* [bool]
Improvement Ideas	*Whether the agent asked the subject about how they could improve their lifestyle* [bool]
Suggesting Ideas	*Whether the agent suggested ideas to the subject to improve their lifestyle if they had no ideas* [bool]
Explaining SMART	*Whether the agent asked the subject if they knew what a SMART goal was and explained it if they didn't* [bool]
Early Termination	*Whether the subject did not want to make a change and the agent terminated the session accordingly* [bool]
Specific Actions	*Whether the agent asked the subject about specific actions they could take to achieve the goal* [bool]
Developing Plan	*Whether the agent asked the subject to develop a plan to achieve the goal* [bool]
Identifying Obstacles	*Whether the agent asked the subject about potential obstacles to the plan* [bool]
Support System	*Whether the agent asked the subject who could support them in carrying out the plan* [bool]
Commitment Eliciting	*Whether the agent asked the subject to repeat the plan to ensure commitment* [bool]
Confidence Level	*Whether the agent asked the subject to rate their confidence level from 1 to 10* [bool]
Increase Confidence Level	*Whether the agent asked the subject how they could raise their confidence level* [bool]
Summary	*Whether the agent summarized the plan* [bool]
Scheduling Session	*Whether the agent scheduled a new counseling session* [bool]
Factuality Hallucinations	*Absence of outputs containing ungrounded or contradictory factual information.* [bool]
Faithfulness Hallucinations	*Absence of outputs deviating from the user's context, directives, or logical consistency.* [bool]
Harmful Hallucinations	*Absence of situations where the LLM's output causes harm or promotes damaging actions or behaviors.* [bool]

4 Results

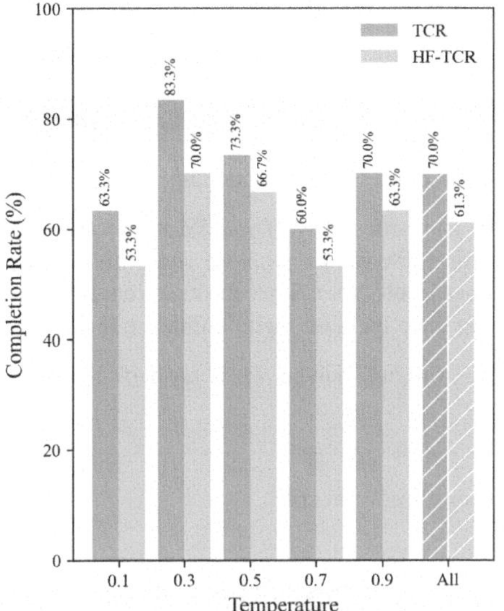

Fig. 3. Comparison of TCR and HF-TCR values across different temperatures.

Table 2. SCR for the BAP steps, illustrating adherence in foundational components of the behavior change framework.

Step	SCR
Personal Information	100.00%
Lifestyle	100.00%
Improvement Ideas	97.99%
Suggesting Ideas	96.64%
Explaining SMART	84.37%
Early Termination	91.27%
Specific Actions	97.39%
Developing Plan	97.37%
Identifying Obstacles	95.57%
Support System	96.46%
Commitment Eliciting	91.96%
Confidence Level	96.46%
Increase Confidence Level	96.46%
Summary	91.96%
Scheduling Session	90.18%

We evaluated the doctor-agent's performances across the simulations involving the different patient sub-types and model temperature settings. As summarized in Fig. 3, the overall TCR was 70.00%, with the HF-TCR standing at 61.33%. Optimal performance was observed at a temperature of 0.3, where the TCR reached 83.33%, and the HF-TCR was 70.00%. In contrast, temperatures of 0.1 and 0.7 yielded lower TCRs of 63.33% and 60.00%, respectively, suggesting that extreme values in model randomness might reduce adherence to structured intervention protocols.

SCR scores, outlined in Table 2, highlighted the agent's adherence to specific components of the BAP framework. Foundational steps such as gathering personal information and assessing lifestyle habits were completed in 100% of the sessions. Steps for exploring improvement ideas (SCR: 97.99%) and specific action planning (SCR: 97.39%) also showed high reliability. However, explaining SMART goals was the most challenging step, achieving the lowest SCR of 84.37%. Annotators observed that in conversations where the agent failed the step, it rushed through goal exploration, often skipping or inadequately addressing the SMART goal as soon as the patient proposed a practical action to improve their lifestyle (see Fig. 5). Steps involving summarizing the plan (SCR: 91.96%) and scheduling follow-ups (SCR: 90.18%) were similarly prone to omissions for the same reason. A critical pattern emerged during simulations involving uncollaborative patient personas. In 13 cases, annotators observed that the agent tended to force patients toward embracing change, even when they explicitly stated a lack of interest or readiness to change. This behavior was distributed evenly across all temperature settings, suggesting a systemic limitation in handling resistance or ambivalence during the conversations.

Instruction Spoiling

Patient: If I actually started doing it, I guess. But don't see that happening.

Agent: Sometimes taking that first step can be the hardest part. If you did start doing the walks and found you were able to stick to it for a few weeks, what do you think would help you keep going and increase your confidence level? Note: Since the user's confidence level is below 7, we should ask what could help them increase their confidence level

Patient: If I didn't feel like I was dying after walking, maybe. Or if my wife stopped nagging me about it.

Fig. 4. Instruction spoiling example.

Rushing

Agent: Short walks during lunch breaks are a great idea! They're manageable and can be a good starting point. Since you mentioned joining a gym but are unsure, let's focus on your walk idea for now. Would you like me to help you turn this idea into a specific goal, or do you have any other ideas you'd like to explore?

Patient: Just want to start with the walks for now. Make it a habit.

Agent: Having a clear goal in mind can really help. To make sure your goal is achievable, let's break it down: what does "making it a habit" mean to you? For example, how many days a week, and how long would you like these walks to be?

Fig. 5. Rushing example.

Hallucinations were identified in 18% of the sessions (27 out of 150). These were predominantly categorized as faithfulness hallucinations (26 cases). In these instances, the agent deviated from the protocol by introducing irrelevant or inappropriate instructions in the conversation or exposing parts of the prompt (see Fig. 4). One instance of factual hallucination occurred, where the agent assumed the patient's spouse was available as a support system before verifying with the person. User testing results closely matched simulations at the optimal temperature (0.3). TCR dropped slightly (75.00% vs. 83.33%), as did HF-TCR (65.00% vs. 70.00%), while SCRs remained consistent. SMART goal explanations (83.33% vs. 84.37%) and follow-up scheduling (88.23% vs. 90.18%) showed minimal deviation. Some users noted occasional rushed goal-setting steps, an issue observed during the simulations as well. Two faithfulness hallucinations occurred due to instruction spoiling. Despite real-world variability, the chatbot maintained consistent performance.

5 Discussion

The results highlight that the role-play framework is a promising approach to developing intelligent agents that follow predefined medical protocols, such as the BAP interview. The findings indicate that LLMs can engage in structured conversations and guide users through behavioral change planning with reasonable adherence to the protocol.

However, despite these promising results, the approach is not yet ready for real-world clinical practice. Indeed, the effectiveness of LLM-driven behavior change interventions depends on their ability to consistently adhere to structured protocols without omitting critical steps. Our study found that LLMs sometimes skipped conversation steps, particularly when moving too quickly toward action-oriented responses. This aligns with previous research highlighting the sensitivity of the LLMs to be reactive to small modifications in the instructions (i.e. the conversation history) [11]. In particular, the agent rushed through the conversation when the patient's reply contained some goal-oriented instruction (e.g. "Let's make a plan for my activities!"), suggesting that Llama3.3 tends to prioritize in-conversation goal-oriented instructions rather than system prompts. This also aligns with previous studies on instruction-tuned LLMs [27] and indicates a possible systemic limitation of an LLM-driven approach.

Additionally, it should be noted that we observed instances of instruction spoiling, where the LLM exposed parts of its prompt or deviated from structured guidelines. This issue could be addressed by implementing a supervisory mechanism using a multi-agent architecture.

Eventually, several limitations should be acknowledged. First, the study tested only one LLM, limiting generalizability across different models. We should also consider that the evaluation was based on 150 simulated patient interactions, which, while informative, represents a relatively small sample size. In line with [5] the results also showed that the medical agent tends to push uncollaborative patients toward change despite their expressed lack of readiness, contradicting motivational interviewing principles prioritizing patient autonomy [8]. It should be noted that real-world applicability was assessed with limited human participants ($n = 20$), making it difficult to draw definitive conclusions about user experience and engagement. Finally, only one version of the prompt was tested. While this is acceptable for an exploratory study, further iterations are necessary to optimize performance and reliability.

Future research should explore LLM-driven role-play frameworks across other short behavioral change protocols to develop this approach further. Comparative studies using different LLMs and agentic architectures would help determine whether model-specific variations affect adherence to structured interventions. Extensive user testing with a larger and more diverse population is also crucial to understanding real-world feasibility and effectiveness.

6 Conclusion

Our study showed that LLM-driven role-play demonstrates significant potential for delivering structured behavior change interventions. Further work is needed to refine their reliability and applicability in real-world settings. Future research should expand evaluations across diverse models, conduct larger-scale user testing, and explore additional behavioral change protocols. Exploring different agentic architectures (e.g., multi-agent frameworks) would also be crucial since a simple single-prompting agent exhibited significant limitations that would prevent a deployment in a clinical setting.

References

1. Abbasian, M., Khatibi, E., Azimi, I., et al.: Foundation metrics for evaluating effectiveness of healthcare conversations powered by generative Ai. Npj Digit. Med. **7**(1), 82 (2024). https://doi.org/10.1038/s41746-024-01074-z
2. Ayers, J.W., et al.: Comparing physician and artificial intelligence chatbot responses to patient questions posted to a public social media forum. JAMA Intern. Med. **183**(6), 589–596 (2023). https://doi.org/10.1001/jamainternmed.2023.1838
3. Denecke, K.: Framework for guiding the development of high-quality conversational agents in healthcare. In: Healthcare, vol. 11, p. 1061. MDPI (2023)
4. Denecke, K., May, R., LLMHealthGroup, Rivera Romero, O.: Potential of large language models in health care: Delphi study. J. Med. Internet Res. **26**, e52399 (2024)
5. Deng, Y., Lei, W., Huang, M., Chua, T.S.: Rethinking conversational agents in the era of llms: Proactivity, non-collaborativity, and beyond. In: Proceedings of the Annual International ACM SIGIR Conference on Research and Development in Information Retrieval in the Asia Pacific Region. pp. 298–301 (2023)
6. Fadhil, A., Gabrielli, S.: Addressing challenges in promoting healthy lifestyles: the al-chatbot approach. In: Proceedings of the 11th EAI International Conference on Pervasive Computing Technologies for Healthcare. pp. 261–265 (2017)
7. Gutnick, D., Reims, K., Davis, C., Gainforth, H., Jay, M., Cole, S.: Brief action planning to facilitate behavior change and support patient self-management. JCOM **21**(1), 17–29 (2014)
8. Hall, K., Gibbie, T., Lubman, D.I.: Motivational interviewing techniques: facilitating behaviour change in the general practice setting. Aust. Fam. Phys. **41**(9), 660–667 (2012)
9. Kojima, T., Gu, S.S., Reid, M., Matsuo, Y., Iwasawa, Y.: Large language models are zero-shot reasoners. Adv. Neural. Inf. Process. Syst. **35**, 22199–22213 (2022)
10. Lindner, H., Menzies, D., Kelly, J., Taylor, S., Shearer, M.: Coaching for behaviour change in chronic disease: a review of the literature and the implications for coaching as a self-management intervention. Aust. J. Prim. Health **9**(3), 177–185 (2003)
11. Lou, R., Zhang, K., Yin, W.: Large language model instruction following: a survey of progresses and challenges. Comput. Linguist. **50**(3), 1053–1095 (2024)
12. Malgaroli, M., Hull, T.D., Zech, J.M., Althoff, T.: Natural language processing for mental health interventions: a systematic review and research framework. Transl. Psychiatry **13**(1), 309 (2023)

13. Marvin, G., Hellen, N., Jjingo, D., Nakatumba-Nabende, J.: Prompt engineering in large language models. In: International conference on data intelligence and cognitive informatics, pp. 387–402. Springer, Cham (2023)
14. Meskó, B.: Prompt engineering as an important emerging skill for medical professionals: tutorial. J. Med. Internet Res. **25**, e50638 (2023)
15. Meyer, S., Elsweiler, D.: Llm-based conversational agents for behaviour change support: A randomized controlled trial examining efficacy, safety, and the role of user behaviour. Safety, and the role of user behaviour. Int. J. Human-Comput. Stud. **200**, 103514 (2025)
16. Miller, W.R., Rose, G.S.: Toward a theory of motivational interviewing. Am. Psychol. **64**(6), 527 (2009)
17. Montenegro, J.L.Z., da Costa, C.A., da Rosa Righi, R.: Survey of conversational agents in health. Expert Syst. Appl. **129**, 56–67 (2019)
18. Otero-González, I., Pacheco-Lorenzo, M.R., Fernández-Iglesias, M.J., Anido-Rifón, L.E.: Conversational agents for depression screening: A systematic review. Int. J. Med. Inform. **181**, 105272 (2024)
19. Ozolcer, M., Yang, Y., Kate, S., Samant, P., Bae, S.W.: Toward enhancing user experience and adoption of ai chatbot apps for mental health: Insights from natural language processing of user reviews. In: Salado, A., Valerdi, R., Steiner, R., Head, L. (eds.) Conference on Systems Engineering Research. pp. 569–586. Springer (2024). https://doi.org/10.1007/978-3-031-62554-1_37
20. Park, J.H., Moon, J.H., Kim, H.J., Kong, M.H., Oh, Y.H.: Sedentary lifestyle: overview of updated evidence of potential health risks. Korean J. Fam. Med. **41**(6), 365 (2020)
21. Patil, R., Heston, T.F., Bhuse, V.: Prompt engineering in healthcare. Electronics **13**(15) (2024). https://doi.org/10.3390/electronics13152961, https://www.mdpi.com/2079-9292/13/15/2961
22. Prochaska, J.O., Velicer, W.F.: The transtheoretical model of health behavior change. Am. J. Health Promot. **12**(1), 38–48 (1997)
23. Shanahan, M., McDonell, K., Reynolds, L.: Role play with large language models. Nature **623**(7987), 493–498 (2023)
24. Sorin, V., et al.: Large language models and empathy: Systematic review. J. Med. Internet Res. **26**, e52597 (2024)
25. Steenstra, I., Nouraei, F., Arjmand, M., Bickmore, T.: Virtual agents for alcohol use counseling: Exploring llm-powered motivational interviewing. In: Proceedings of the 24th ACM International Conference on Intelligent Virtual Agents. IVA '24, Association for Computing Machinery, New York, NY, USA (2024). https://doi.org/10.1145/3652988.3673932
26. Wang, J., et al.: Review of large vision models and visual prompt engineering. Meta-Radiol. **1**(3), 100047 (2023)
27. Wu, X., et al.: From language modeling to instruction following: Understanding the behavior shift in LLMs after instruction tuning. In: Duh, K., Gomez, H., Bethard, S. (eds.) Proceedings of the 2024 Conference of the North American Chapter of the Association for Computational Linguistics: Human Language Technologies (Volume 1: Long Papers). pp. 2341–2369. Association for Computational Linguistics, Mexico City, Mexico (2024).https://doi.org/10.18653/v1/2024.naacl-long.130, https://aclanthology.org/2024.naacl-long.130/
28. Yang, Y., Tavares, J., Oliveira, T., et al.: A new research model for artificial intelligence-based well-being chatbot engagement: survey study. JMIR Hum. Factors **11**(1), e59908 (2024)

29. Zaghir, J., Naguib, M., Bjelogrlic, M., Névéol, A., Tannier, X., Lovis, C.: Prompt engineering paradigms for medical applications: scoping review. J. Med. Internet Res. **26**, e60501 (2024)
30. Zhang, J., et al.: The potential and pitfalls of using a large language model such as chatgpt, gpt-4, or llama as a clinical assistant. J. Am. Med. Inform. Assoc. **31**(9), 1884–1891 (2024). https://doi.org/10.1093/jamia/ocae184

Assessing Temporal Reasoning of Large Language Models on Structured Temporal Clinical Data

Gianluca Apriceno(✉), Tania Bailoni(✉), and Mauro Dragoni(✉)

Fondazione Bruno Kessler, Trento, Italy
{apriceno,tbailoni,dragoni}@fbk.eu

Abstract. This study explores the capabilities of Large Language Models in reasoning over structured clinical knowledge with a focus on temporally dependent monitoring rules. We assess the models' performance across five real-world patient scenarios derived from a virtual coaching platform in the Trentino Salute 4.0 project. Using a structured prompt and diverse use cases, we examine whether these models can accurately detect and justify rule violations and generate clear, audience-specific explanations for patients and healthcare professionals. The results reveal that while Large Language Models demonstrate potential in interpreting complex, time-sensitive clinical data and adapting communication to different stakeholders, limitations persist in temporal reasoning, explanation consistency, and audience alignment. These findings offer insights into the strengths and challenges of deploying LLMs in personalized and temporally aware healthcare decision support systems.
GitHub: https://github.com/IDA-FBK/LLM-Temporal-Clinical-Reasoning

Keywords: Large Language Models · Reasoning · Natural Language Explanations

1 Introduction

Large Language Models (LLMs) have demonstrated impressive capabilities across a wide range of domains, including critical societal [4], biological and chemical [22], and natural sciences [19]. A key strength of these models lies in their ability to perform reasoning and generate explanations that reflect the underlying decision-making process. This capacity, explored through various reasoning techniques (e.g. [17,20]), has important implications for transparency and explainability, as LLMs can offer insights into their reasoning processes and can reveal underlying limitations.

Recently, LLMs have been exploited for generating audience-specific explanations in contexts requiring clear and accessible communication, such as recommender systems [3,13] and healthcare [2,6,21]. These developments open up new possibilities for using LLMs as mediators in human-AI interaction, especially in

P. Bruno et al. (Eds.): HC_AIxIA_HYDRA 2025, CCIS 2830, pp. 453–466, 2026.
https://doi.org/10.1007/978-3-032-16708-8_36

settings involving multiple stakeholders, such as patient-physician communication.

However, while LLMs have shown promise in general reasoning tasks, their ability to handle temporally dependent clinical reasoning remains underexplored. In particular, it is unclear whether current models can accurately reason about temporal health events and rules, a common requirement in real-world medical decision-making. Moreover, it remains an open question whether their generated explanations can effectively adapt to the needs of different audiences while preserving clarity, correctness, and domain relevance in time-sensitive scenarios.

To address these gaps, we evaluate the reasoning capabilities of six LLMs on structured clinical data across five real-world medical scenarios. These scenarios are based on representations of undesired patient behaviors identified by a virtual coaching platform deployed in the Trentino Salute 4.0 (TS4.0) project[1]. Our investigation focuses on both the accuracy of the models in detecting and motivating rule violations and the quality of their explanations across audience types.

The objective of our work is to answer the following research questions ($\mathbf{RQ_s}$):

- $\mathbf{RQ_1}$ To what extent can a LLM reason over structured clinical knowledge, including temporally dependent monitoring rules, to accurately identify rule violations in complex patient scenarios?
- $\mathbf{RQ_2}$ Can a LLM adapt its explanations to different audiences, such as patients and healthcare professionals, while maintaining accuracy, clarity, and domain-appropriate language, particularly when reasoning about temporally dependent clinical events?

The rest of the paper is structured as follows: Sect. 2 briefly surveys the literature related to the explanations-oriented reasoning capabilities of LLMs. Then, Sect. 3 presents the methodology (i.e., the prompt structure) we adopted. Section 4 explains the experimental setting, including the knowledge base, the use case scenarios, the prompt used, and the evaluation performed. Section 5 shows the results. Finally, Sect. 6 concludes the paper, addressing the $\mathbf{RQ_s}$ and outlining directions for future work.

2 Related Work

LLMs have demonstrated emerging reasoning abilities as their scale increases [5, 18], yet the full extent and generality of these capabilities remain underexplored. In response, various works have aimed to assess the reasoning performance of LLMs across various settings [1,10,12]. One particularly active area of research involves evaluating how well LLMs can generate meaningful, coherent explanations, especially in applied domains such as recommendation systems [3,9,11,13,23]. Initial works in this domain have introduced promising

[1] https://trentinosalutedigitale.com/blog/portfolio/trentinosalute/.

prototypes [9,11,23]. At the same time, more recent studies [3,13] have been focused on a narrow range of models and scenarios, typically generating explanations for individual users without considering variability across user groups or adapting reasoning strategies accordingly. Furthermore, most of the proposed works in the literature isolate explanation from the underlying recommendation task and overlook the potential of LLMs to handle both jointly. Although [3] makes strides in this direction, it remains limited to a single model and user context. Similarly, this can also be observed in the healthcare domain, where LLMs have been used to interpret clinical notes [16], answer complex medical questions [14,15], and support personalized interactions [6,21]. These applications also typically rely on fine-tuned models built for narrow, task-specific use cases and primarily support static, single-user interactions. They often do not consider the temporal dimension inherent in health data, thereby limiting their applicability in dynamic, real-world settings. As a result, these gaps highlight a need for a broader evaluation of LLM reasoning, particularly in complex environments that require task-solving and explanation generation, and the ability to adapt explanations to different users and time-dependent contexts. Understanding these capabilities is fundamental for understanding the feasibility of the integration of LLMs into adaptive, multi-user systems in domains like personalized healthcare and lifestyle recommendation, where temporal awareness and reasoning across diverse actors are essential.

3 Methodology

We investigate the capabilities of LLMs in two main areas: (i) their ability to reason over structured (temporal) clinical knowledge to assess and justify whether a violation has occurred; and (ii) their capacity to generate audience-specific explanations tailored to both patients and physicians. To support and guide the reasoning process, we introduce a structured prompting strategy composed of four key components: (i) a task description that defines the objective and scope of the reasoning task; (ii) structured background knowledge exploited during the decision making process; (iii) structured patient input data; and, (iv) relevant temporal information that the model must incorporate into its reasoning.

Task Description. The model must determine whether a violation has occurred by reasoning over the provided structured background knowledge and input data. Following this decision, the LLM must provide a justification that explains the reasoning process leading to its conclusion. Furthermore, the model must generate two distinct explanations tailored to different audiences. For patients, the explanation must be easy to understand, avoiding medical jargon. For physicians, the explanation must use precise clinical language and emphasize detailed, rigorous reasoning.

Structured Background Knowledge. The structured background knowledge is organized into two core components. The first component defines a set of monitoring rules, which specify how user behaviors and clinical parameters should be tracked over time, establishing dietary guidelines (e.g., limits on nutrient intake). The second component, the violation framework, determines how breaches of these rules are recognized. It defines the conditions for identifying violations by setting thresholds, detecting temporal patterns, or evaluating combinations of behaviors. These two elements together provide the LLM with a structured, rule-based framework for identifying violations based on structured data inputs.

Structured Input Data. The structured input consists of user-specific health data, including clinical diagnoses, dietary logs, and other pertinent behavioral or physiological measurements. This information serves as the factual basis against which the LLM assesses compliance with the established monitoring rules. The model is expected to identify and flag any deviations that fall outside the predefined acceptable thresholds. These deviations form the basis for the LLM's determination of whether a violation has occurred.

Temporal Information. Temporal data is included to support reasoning over time-dependent monitoring rules. This information provides timestamps needed to evaluate whether a violation occurred concerning the users' monitoring rule (e.g., exceeding a dietary threshold over several days). The LLM is expected to integrate this temporal dimension when checking for violations.

4 Experimental Setting

The LLMs were evaluated within a controlled experimental setup that included structured knowledge of monitoring rules and violations (Sect. 4.1), detailed use case scenarios (Sect. 4.2), and the designed prompt along with information on the evaluation procedure (Sect. 4.3).

4.1 FuS-KG: Monitoring Rule and Violation

The Functional Status Knowledge Graph (FuS-KG) [8] is a Multi-Modal Knowledge Graph representing a conceptual model for Functional Status Information. FuS-KG models the interrelationships among various dimensions of an individual's health to comprehensively represent their overall functional status. Each dimension is organized into dedicated modules within the FuS-KG, including the *Guidelines* and *User* modules, both represented using the Terse RDF Triple Language (TURTLE).

The *Guidelines* module models the behavioral guidelines associated with users to support reasoning tasks about possible recommendations related to the user data that can be collected [7]. In particular, the guidelines are specified in the *MonitoringRule* concept. Then, the *hasRuleDefinition* data property specifies the definition of a *MonitoruleRule*, the *hasMonitoredValueInterval* property specifies the interval monitored (i.e. *IntervalValue*), and the *monitors* property associates the rules to the users.

The *User* module models user-specific data, including the user's profile, activities, food consumption, and any violations of health guidelines. The *Violation* concept specifically addresses breaches in user behavior, such as excessive food consumption. Key properties of violations include *ViolationInterval*, indicating tolerance levels, and time-related attributes like *hasViolationStartTime* and *hasViolationEndTime*. Relationships such as *hasViolationRule*, *hasViolationMeal*, and *hasViolationUser* establish connections between the violation, the corresponding monitoring rule, the meal consumed, and the user.

4.2 Use Cases

We consider five use cases:

- **Use Case 1 - No Violation**. This use case describes a fictitious patient, Patient1, a 61-year-old individual diagnosed with cardiovascular disease. As part of a dietary monitoring plan, Patient1's consumption of specific foods is tracked, including Sliced Whole Wheat Rye Bread. A monitoring rule (Rule-0001) has been defined to ensure that Patient1 consumes more than 150 g of this bread during meals, likely to ensure sufficient fiber or nutrient intake. On March 24th, during lunch, Patient1 consumed exactly 150 g of this bread. Since the amount did not exceed the required threshold, the rule was not triggered, and no violation occurred.
- **Use Case 2 - Single Meal Violation**. This use case describes a fictitious patient, Patient2, who is a 63-year-old individual diagnosed with cardiovascular disease. Patient2's dietary habits are closely monitored due to the health risks associated with their condition, with particular attention to high-fat foods such as butter intake. A specific monitoring rule (Rule-0002) is in place to ensure that Patient2 consumes less than 10 g of butter during each meal. However, during breakfast on March 31st, Patient2 consumed 15 g of butter. As this amount exceeds the allowed threshold, the monitoring rule was triggered, and a violation occurred.
- **Use Case 3 - Multiple Meal Violations**. This use case describes a fictitious patient, Patient3, a 66-year-old with diagnoses of both cardiovascular disease and celiac disease. Due to their medical condition, two specific dietary monitoring rules have been set (Rule-0003 and Rule-0004). Rule-0003 specifies that Patient3 should consume less than 10 g of butter per meal, and Rule-0004 specifies that Patient3 should consume no durum wheat bread, due to its gluten content, per meal. On April 7th, during lunch, Patient3 consumed 15 g of butter and 20 g of white bread. Both values exceeded their respective thresholds, thus violating each rule.
- **Use Case 4 - Single Weekly Violation**. This use case describes a fictitious individual, Patient4, a 67-year-old individual diagnosed with cardiovascular disease, who was subject to a monitoring rule (Rule-0005) that limited the weekly intake of Butter to less than 50 g. During the week from April 14th to April 20th, the patient consumed Butter daily at breakfast, with the following quantities: 5 g, 8 g, 5 g, 10 g, 7 g, 15 g, and 10 g, respectively. The total weekly intake amounted to 60 g, thereby exceeding the permitted threshold of 50 g.
- **Use Case 5 - Multiple Weekly Violation**. This use case describes a fictitious individual, Patient5, a 69-year-old individual diagnosed with both

```
1  ###  https://w3id.org/fuskg/user-example#Patient3
2  :Patient3 rdf:type owl:NamedIndividual,
3          fsbarr:Patient,
4          fsuser:User ;
5      fsbarr:hasDiagnosis :DiseaseRelationPatient3-1 ,
6                          :DiseaseRelationPatient3-2 ;
7      fsuser:consumed :Lunch-P3-1 ;
8      fsuser:hasAge 66 ;
9      rdfs:label "Patient3"@en ,
10                "Paziente3"@it .
11
12 :Rule-0003 rdf:type fsguid:MonitoringRule ;
13     fsguid:monitors :Patient3 ;
14     fsguid:hasMonitoredValue 10 ;
15     fsguid:hasOperator "Less" ;
16     fsguid:hasRuleId "0003" ;
17     fsguid:monitoredEntity fsfood:FOOD-1900 ;
18     fsguid:monitoredEntityType fscore:Food ;
19     fsguid:timing fstemp:Meal .
20
21 :Rule-0004 rdf:type fsguid:MonitoringRule ;
22     fsguid:monitors :Patient3 ;
23     fsguid:hasMonitoredValue 0 ;
24     fsguid:hasOperator "Less" ;
25     fsguid:hasRuleId "0004" ;
26     fsguid:monitoredEntity fsfood:FOOD-701337 ;
27     fsguid:monitoredEntityType fscore:Food ;
28     fsguid:timing fstemp:Meal .
29
30 :DiseaseRelationPatient3-1 rdf:type owl:NamedIndividual,
31         fsbarr:DiseaseRelation ;
32     fsbarr:hasDisease fsdise:Cardiovascular .
33
34 :DiseaseRelationPatient3-2 rdf:type owl:NamedIndividual,
35         fsbarr:DiseaseRelation ;
36     fsbarr:hasDisease fsdise:Celiac .
37
38 :Lunch-P3-1 rdf:type owl:NamedIndividual ,
39                      fsuser:Lunch ;
40             fsuser:hasConsumedFood :ConsumedFood-Lunch-P3-1-FOOD-1900 ,
41                                    :ConsumedFood-Lunch-P3-1-FOOD-701337 ;
42             fsuser:hasTimestamp "2025-04-07T13:05:12"^^xsd:dateTime .
43
44 :ConsumedFood-Lunch-P3-1-FOOD-1900 rdf:type owl:NamedIndividual,
45         fsuser:ConsumedFood ;
46     fsreci:amountFood 15 ;
47     fsuser:hasFood fsfood:FOOD-1900 .
48
49 :ConsumedFood-Lunch-P3-1-FOOD-701337 rdf:type owl:NamedIndividual,
50         fsuser:ConsumedFood ;
51     fsreci:amountFood 20 ;
52     fsuser:hasFood fsfood:FOOD-701337 .
53
54 ###  https://w3id.org/fuskg/food#FOOD-1900
55 fsfood:FOOD-1900 rdf:type owl:NamedIndividual ,
56                           fsfood:AnimalFats ;
57                  fscore:hasNutrient fsfood:Alanine_2900 ,
58                                     ...
59                  fsfood:foodId "1900" .
60
61 ###  https://w3id.org/fuskg/food#FOOD-701337
62 fsfood:FOOD-701337 rdf:type owl:NamedIndividual ,
63                             fsfood:WhiteBread ;
64                    fscore:hasNutrient fsfood:Alanine_000 ,
65                                       ...
66                    fsfood:amountCalories "245.0"^^xsd:double ;
67                    fsfood:amountEnergy "1025.0"^^xsd:double ;
68                    fsfood:amountWater "31.0"^^xsd:double ;
69                    fsfood:ediblePart "100.0"^^xsd:double ;
70                    rdfs:label "Durum Wheat Bread"@en ,
71                               "Pane di Grano Duro"@it ;
72                    fsfood:foodId "701337" .
```

Fig. 1. Turtle description for the Patient3's use case.

cardiovascular disease and diabetes, who was subject to two weekly dietary monitoring rules: a limit of 30 g for Butter under Rule-0006, and a separate 30-g limit for White Chocolate under Rule-0007. During the week, the patient consumed 20 g of Butter at breakfast on both April 21st and April 23rd, for a total of 40 g, thereby exceeding the Butter limit. Additionally, on April 26th, the patient consumed 50 g of White Chocolate at dinner, exceeding the limit of white chocolate. Both instances constitute clear violations of the respective dietary restrictions.

We encoded the scenarios in TURTLE following the TURTLE descriptions of both *Guidelines* and *Violation*[2] As an example, the structured TURTLE description for Patient3 behavior (i.e., use case 3) is shown in Fig. 1[3],[4]. All the patients' descriptions mimic real patients' data descriptions within the TS4.0 platform.

4.3 Prompt and Evaluation

The prompt provided to the LLM consists of four key components: (i) task description including the instruction of the task to be done by the LLM; (ii) structured background knowledge, represented using TURTLE syntax, detailing both monitoring rules and violation definitions; (iii) structured input data, also encoded in TURTLE, corresponding to the specific scenario as shown in Fig. 1; and (iv) temporal information, which includes relevant dates and times for rule monitoring, as well as the reference time at which the LLM is expected to perform the evaluation, based on the temporal scope of the rules (e.g., daily or weekly checks).

Task Description:

```
I will give you a description of the structure of a monitoring rule and a
    violation along with data related to a specific user.

I will provide you as input:

- The Turtle description of the structure of a monitoring rule.
- The Turtle description of the structure of a violation.
- The Turtle encoded data about the user and the food consumed.
- The timestamp at which the week starts and the timestamp when the
    temporal check of the monitoring rules takes place.

After you have received the input, your task is:

  1. Reason and Decide: Determine if a violation occurred based on the
       provided data. Provide a YES/NO answer and explain the reason for
       your decision.
  2. Generate Two Explanations:
       - One detailed explanation for the user, using simple and
           comprehensible language.
```

[2] The interested reader can refer to the FuS-KG repo for further details.

[3] Full nutrient details are omitted. See the corresponding file in the repository for further details.

[4] All use cases' files are provided in the repository within the prompt folder.

```
    - One detailed explanation for the physician, using precise and
      professional terminology.
```

Structured Background Knowledge:

```
The Turtle description of the structure of a monitoring rule is:
...

The Turtle description of the structure of a violation is:
...
```

Structured Input Data:

```
The Turtle encoded data about the user and the food consumed:
...
```

Temporal Information:

```
Week starts at <begin_week>^^xsd:dateTime - Temporal check at:<time_check
    >^^xsd:dateTime
```

We evaluated the reasoning capability of 6 different LLMs: Aya-expanse:32B, Gemma3:12B, Llama3.2:3B, Mistral-small3.1:24B, Phi4:14B, Qwen2.5:32B. The evaluation focused on the following criteria:

- **Accuracy in Violation Detection**: Assess whether the LLM correctly identifies violations based on the provided data.
- **Reason Detection**: Evaluate whether the LLM provides the correct reasoning behind the identified violation.
- **Clarity of Explanation**: Measure how clearly the LLM explains the violation to patients and physicians.
- **Tailoring of Explanation**: Assess how effectively the LLM tailors its explanation depending on the target user.

To evaluate both clarity and tailoring of explanations, we involved a 66 and a 67-year-old patient with cardiovascular disease and two physicians with expertise in nutrition.

5 Results

In this Section, we provide the results of the evaluation of the reasoning capabilities of each LLM concerning the sub-tasks of violation detection (Subsect. 5.1) and explanation generation (Subsect. 5.2)[5].

[5] Due to space limits, reasoning steps are omitted. See the results file.

5.1 Violation Detection

Table 1. LLMs' decisions on violation detection across the five use cases.

LLM	Use Case 1	Use Case 2	Use Case 3	Use Case 4	Use Case 5
Aya-expanse:32B	YES	YES	YES(1)	YES	YES(1)
Gemma3:12B	YES	YES	YES	YES	YES(1)
Llama3.2:3B	YES	YES	YES	YES	YES (1)
Mistral-small3.1:24B	YES	YES	YES	YES	YES
Phi4:14B	YES	YES	YES(1)	YES	YES
Qwen2.5:32B	NO	YES	YES	YES	YES

Table 1 shows the violation decisions made by the six LLMs across the five use cases. In use case 1, it can be observed that almost all models incorrectly identify a violation. This is likely because the models interpret a violation as occurring when the consumed quantity (i.e., 150) exceeds the monitored quantity (i.e., 100), despite the rule semantics specifying that the patient should consume at least the monitored quantity. In use cases involving a single violation (i.e., use cases 2 and 4), all models correctly detected the violation. However, while all models provided accurate reasoning in use case 2 (a single violation occurring at the end of a meal), in use case 4 (a single violation at the end of the week), two models, i.e., aya-expanse32B and llama3.2:3B, failed to provide the correct reasoning. Specifically, these models reported incorrect total consumption values: 50 for aya-expanse32B and 10 for Llama3.2:3B. For use cases involving multiple violations (i.e., use cases 3 and 5), the models generally succeeded in detecting the presence of a violation. However, closer examination reveals that positive predictions did not always result from correctly identifying all violations. For instance, in use case 3, aya-expanse32B and Phi4:14B identified only a single violation, likely due to misinterpretation of the rule semantics, such as concluding that no violation occurred even when the consumed quantity exceeded the allowed limit. In addition, we also noticed that Llama3.2:3B failed to provide any explanation for its decision (even though it correctly explains both violations to users and physicians). In use case 5, aya-expanse32B again missed one of the violations. Similarly, Gemma3.1:12B identified only one violation, likely due to its failure to account for all food consumed by the patient. This issue also affected Llama3.2:3B.

5.2 Explanations Generation

The most effective responses across all use cases were those that clearly identified the violations, contextualized them concerning the patient's health conditions, and provided suggestions for addressing the issues. For example, in Use Case 4, Qwen2.5:32B generated a contextually aware and well-structured response for both the patient and the physician. The patient's message clearly identified the butter consumption violation, linked it to the weekly dietary guideline, and offered a practical recommendation to reduce intake in the following week. Meanwhile, the physician's message delivered a concise summary of the violation, quantifying the excess and highlighting it as a potential compliance concern, thus enabling the physician to consider appropriate next steps. Similarly, Gemma3:12B, in both Use Case 2 and Use Case 4, effectively communicated butter consumption violations by tailoring its responses to the specific context: a single meal in Use Case 2 and weekly intake in Use Case 4. For patients, the model provided clear, health-oriented explanations, connecting the violations to recommended dietary limits and emphasizing adherence, particularly given existing cardiovascular conditions. Messages directed to physicians were precise, referencing specific monitoring rules and quantifying the excess of the intake. Qwen2.5:32B, in Use Cases 4 and 5, further stood out for its clarity and its ability to align the patient's specific health needs with established dietary guidelines. In Use Case 4, the butter intake violation was communicated clearly and supportively to the patient while providing the physician with a structured, data-driven summary. In Use Case 5, the model identified multiple violations (butter and white chocolate), delivering detailed summaries for the physician and recommending reduced intake to the patient.

In contrast, some responses require improvement. For example, aya-expanse:32B in Use Case 4 correctly identified that the butter intake exceeded the prescribed limit but lacked sufficient context to convey the significance of the violation. It did not explain the potential health consequences of excessive butter consumption, especially given the patient's cardiovascular condition, nor did it stress the importance of adhering to the guidelines. The patient message used vague language (e.g., "exceeds our target limit") without specifying the amount exceeded, which may be confusing. Moreover, the physician's message inconsistently stated the total consumption as 50 g, matching the limit, yet still flagged it as a violation, without clarification.

Likewise, Llama3.2:3B in Use Case 4 briefly acknowledged the butter violation but lacked personalization or contextual explanation. The patient message was impersonal and overly technical, referencing timestamps and rule identifiers without clearly articulating the health implications. The physician's message also included a discrepancy, identifying a 10 g intake as a violation of a 50 g limit, rather than reporting the actual total intake of 60 g.

Phi4:14B, in Use Cases 2 and 4, delivered clear and straightforward communication about the dietary violations but missed opportunities to highlight their broader health implications. While the responses acknowledged that the limits were exceeded, they lacked discussion of how this may impact the patient's heart health or long-term well-being. For example, in Use Case 2, the patient message referenced the breach but did not stress the importance of dietary compliance for cardiovascular management. Similarly, in Use Case 4, although the patient was informed about exceeding the weekly butter intake, the message could have been strengthened by linking the violation to potential health risks.

Mistral-small3.1, in Use Cases 2 and 3, provided detailed breakdowns of the violations but similarly failed to relate them to the patient's health risks. In both cases, patient messages specified the quantity consumed and the rule limits, but did not explain the health relevance. Likewise, physician messages were technically accurate but lacked discussion of how such dietary violations might affect disease management, such as cardiovascular outcomes.

Table 2 shows the explanations for users and physicians generated by each LLM for Use Case 3.[6]

Table 2. Users and Physician explanations generated by each LLM for use case 3

Model	User Explanation	Physician Explanation
Aya-expanse:32B	During your lunch on April 7, 2025, you consumed more Durum Wheat Bread than what is recommended by one of your diet rules. This specific rule states that you should consume less than zero units of this bread. Please be mindful of this guideline for future meals.	The patient's lunch on April 7, 2025, resulted in a violation of Monitoring Rule 0004 due to the consumption of 20 units of Durum Wheat Bread (FOOD-701337). This rule dictates that the intake of this food should be less than zero units. Given the patient's dietary requirements and existing conditions (Celiac disease and Cardiovascular disease), this violation warrants further assessment and guidance to ensure adherence to their prescribed diet.
Gemma3:12B	"Hi there! We're monitoring your diet to help you stay healthy. It looks like you recently ate some food that went a little over what we expected. Specifically, you ate more butter than allowed (15 units instead of 10), and you ate some durum wheat bread, which wasn't supposed to be in your diet at all. This is within the first week of monitoring, so it's an important opportunity to adjust and get back on track. Please check the diet plan again and talk to your doctor or dietitian if you have questions."	"Patient3 has triggered a dietary violation based on the data collected during the meal recorded on 2025-04-07 at 13:05:12. Rule 0003, monitoring consumption of fsfood:FOOD-1900* (Butter), has been violated with a consumed quantity of 15 units, exceeding the defined threshold of 10 units. Additionally, Rule 0004, monitoring consumption of fsfood:FOOD-701337 (Durum Wheat Bread), has been violated as consumption occurred despite a prescribed zero-quantity limit. This represents a dietary transgression within the first week of monitoring. A review of the patient's dietary adherence, potential underlying factors contributing to the transgression, and adjustment of the monitoring plan may be warranted. Furthermore, it would be pertinent to ascertain if the patient requires additional education or support regarding dietary restrictions. It's important to emphasize the significance of adherence within the initial monitoring period."
Llama:3.2:3B	A few days ago, on April 7th, you consumed some foods that exceeded certain limits set by your doctor. Specifically, you had 15 g of butter (FOOD-1900) and 20 g of white bread (FOOD-701337). According to the rules in place, these amounts are not allowed for you. The rule "Less" means that if any of these foods exceed their allowed limits, it's considered a violation.	A temporal check revealed that, on April 7th at 13:05:12 UTC (2025-04-07T13:05:128sd:dateTime), a violation occurred due to the consumption of excessive amounts of butter (FOOD-1900) and white bread (FOOD-701337). The monitoring rule specified for Patient3, Rule-0003, was triggered by the presence of these foods in their meal. The food consumption exceeded the allowed limits set by the physician, as determined by the "Less" operator. This indicates that further evaluation is required to assess the impact of this violation on Patient3's health status and dietary plan. Please review Patient3's medical history and adjust their dietary instructions accordingly.

(*continued*)

[6] Explanations for the remaining use cases are included in the results file provided in the repository.

Table 2. (*continued*)

Model	User Explanation	Physician Explanation
Mistral-small3.1:24B	Dear Patient3, During your lunch on April 7, 2025, you consumed 15 g of butter and 20 g of durum wheat bread. According to your dietary guidelines, you should have consumed less than 10 g of butter and 0 g of durum wheat bread per meal. Unfortunately, both of these guidelines were exceeded, which constitutes a violation of your dietary rules. Please be mindful of these guidelines in the future to ensure your dietary plan is followed correctly.	Dear Physician, A violation of the dietary monitoring rules has been detected for Patient3. On April 7, 2025, during the lunch meal at 13:05:12, the following violations occurred: 1. Rule-0003 Violation: - Monitored Entity: FOOD-1900 (Butter) - Monitored Value: 10 g - Consumed Amount: 15 g - Operator: Less - Timing: Meal - Conclusion: The consumed amount of Butter (15 g) exceeded the specified limit of 10 g, resulting in a violation. 2. Rule-0004 Violation: - Monitored Entity: FOOD-701337 (Durum Wheat Bread) - Monitored Value: 0 g - Consumed Amount: 20 g - Operator: Less - Timing: Meal - Conclusion: The consumed amount of Durum Wheat Bread (20 g) exceeded the specified limit of 0 g, resulting in a violation. Please review the patient's dietary plan and provide appropriate guidance to ensure adherence to the prescribed dietary rules.
Phi4:14B	During your meal today at around 1:05 PM, you ate more butter than your diet allows. The rule says you should eat less than 10 units of butter, but you had 15 units. This means you went over the limit for that food item. Example: "You consumed too much butter during lunch on April 7th, which exceeded the guidelines in your dietary plan."	Upon reviewing Patient3's meal intake on April 7th, 2025, it was determined that a dietary monitoring rule (Rule ID: 0003) was violated. The patient consumed 15 units of FOOD-1900 (Butter), surpassing the permissible threshold set by the rule to consume less than 10 units during their meal. Example: "The intake of butter at lunch on April 7th exceeded acceptable levels as specified in Rule 0003, resulting in a documented dietary violation."
Qwen2.5:32B	- Butter Consumption: You were supposed to consume less than 10 g of butter at each meal. However, during lunch on April 7th, you consumed 15 g of butter, which is more than the allowed amount. - Bread Consumption: You have celiac disease and are not supposed to eat any durum wheat bread because it contains gluten that can cause adverse reactions. During lunch on April 7th, you consumed 20 g of durum wheat bread.	- Rule-0003 Violation (Butter): The patient consumed 15 g of Butter during the meal at 13:05:12 on April 7th. This exceeds the limit set by Rule-0003, which specifies that butter consumption should be less than 10 g per meal. - Rule-0004 Violation (Durum Wheat Bread): The patient consumed 20 g of Durum Wheat Bread during the same meal. Given the patient's diagnosis of celiac disease, Rule-0004 specifies that no durum wheat bread should be consumed, leading to a violation as any positive quantity is non-compliant with the rule.

6 Conclusions and Future Works

In this study, we evaluated the ability of LLMs to reason over structured clinical knowledge with temporally dependent monitoring rules ($\mathbf{RQ_1}$) and their capacity to generate audience-specific explanations for both patients and healthcare professionals ($\mathbf{RQ_2}$). Regarding $\mathbf{RQ_1}$, most LLMs successfully detected violations across a range of patient scenarios, including cases with single and multiple violations. However, several models show inconsistent behavior, such as misinterpreting rule semantics, undercounting violations, or failing to provide reasoning, highlighting temporal reasoning and structured data interpretation challenges. For $\mathbf{RQ_2}$, while some LLMs could effectively tailor explanations to different audiences, offering clear and healthy contextual feedback, others lacked audience awareness or produced impersonal, technically focused messages. These issues often reduce clarity and engagement, especially for patients managing chronic conditions. Overall, LLMs show promising capabilities in handling temporal clinical data and supporting differentiated communication, but limitations in temporal understanding, reasoning consistency, and audience adaptation remain. Future work will aim to improve model robustness through fine-tuning and prompt engineering while expanding to more multi-condition scenarios. Additionally, we plan to deepen our analysis of explanation quality by evaluating finer-grained communicative aspects, such as personalization, empathy, and relevance to more complex health goals.

Acknowledgments. We acknowledge the support of the PNRR project INEST - Interconnected North-East Innovation Ecosystem (ECS00000043), under the NRRP MUR program funded by the NextGenerationEU. We acknowledge the support of the PNRR project FAIR - Future AI Research (PE00000013), under the NRRP MUR program funded by the NextGenerationEU. This paper is supported by the TrustAlert project, funded by Fondazione Compagnia San Paolo and Fondazione CDP under the "Artificial Intelligence" call.

Disclosure of Interests. The authors have no competing interests to declare that are relevant to the content of this article.

References

1. Ahn, J., et al.: Large language models for mathematical reasoning: Progresses and challenges. In: Falk, N., Papi, S., Zhang, M. (eds.) Proceedings of the 18th Conference of the European Chapter of the Association for Computational Linguistics, EACL 2024: Student Research Workshop, St. Julian's, Malta, March 21–22, 2024. pp. 225–237. Association for Computational Linguistics (2024)
2. Apriceno, G., Bailoni, T., Dragoni, M.: Exploring large language model reasoning capabilities over personal health data. In: Bellazzi, R., Herrero, J.M.J., Sacchi, L., Zupan, B. (eds.) Artificial Intelligence in Medicine - 23rd International Conference, AIME 2025, Pavia, Italy, June 23–26, 2025, Proceedings, Part II. Lecture Notes in Computer Science, vol. 15735, pp. 12–17. Springer, Cham (2025). https://doi.org/10.1007/978-3-031-95841-0_3
3. Bismay, M., et al.: Reasoningrec: Bridging personalized recommendations and human-interpretable explanations through LLM reasoning. CoRR abs/2410.23180 (2024)
4. Chen, Z.Z., et al.: A survey on large language models for critical societal domains: Finance, healthcare, and law (2024)
5. Cobbe, K., et al.: Training verifiers to solve math word problems. CoRR abs/2110.14168 (2021)
6. Cosentino, J., et al.: Towards a personal health large language model. CoRR abs/2406.06474 (2024)
7. Dragoni, M., et al.: Explainable AI meets persuasiveness: translating reasoning results into behavioral change advice. Artif. Intell. Med. **105**, 101840 (2020)

8. Dragoni, M., et al.: Validating a functional status knowledge graph in a large-scale living lab. In: Alam, M., Rospocher, M., van Erp, M., Hollink, L., Gesese, G.A. (eds.) Knowledge Engineering and Knowledge Management - 24th International Conference, EKAW 2024, Amsterdam, The Netherlands, November 26–28, 2024, Proceedings. Lecture Notes in Computer Science, vol. 15370, pp. 416–433. Springer, Cham (2024). https://doi.org/10.1007/978-3-031-77792-9_25
9. Feng, Y., et al.: A large language model enhanced conversational recommender system. CoRR abs/2308.06212 (2023)
10. Giadikiaroglou, P., et al.: Puzzle solving using reasoning of large language models: A survey. In: Al-Onaizan, Y., Bansal, M., Chen, Y. (eds.) Proceedings of the 2024 Conference on Empirical Methods in Natural Language Processing, EMNLP 2024, Miami, FL, USA, November 12–16, 2024. pp. 11574–11591. Association for Computational Linguistics (2024)
11. Harte, J., et al.: Leveraging large language models for sequential recommendation. In: Zhang, J., et al. (eds.) Proceedings of the 17th ACM Conference on Recommender Systems, RecSys 2023, Singapore, Singapore, September 18–22, 2023. pp. 1096–1102. ACM (2023)
12. Huang, J., Chang, K.C.: Towards reasoning in large language models: a survey. In: Rogers, A., Boyd-Graber, J.L., Okazaki, N. (eds.) Findings of the Association for Computational Linguistics: ACL 2023, Toronto, Canada, July 9–14, 2023. pp. 1049–1065. Association for Computational Linguistics (2023)
13. Lubos, S., et al.: Llm-generated explanations for recommender systems. In: Adjunct Proceedings of the 32nd ACM Conference on User Modeling, Adaptation and Personalization, UMAP Adjunct 2024, Cagliari, Italy, July 1–4, 2024. ACM (2024)
14. Saab, K., et al.: Capabilities of gemini models in medicine. CoRR abs/2404.18416 (2024)
15. Singhal, K., et al.: Towards expert-level medical question answering with large language models. CoRR abs/2305.09617 (2023)
16. Wang, H., et al.: Coad: Automatic diagnosis through symptom and disease collaborative generation. In: Rogers, A., Boyd-Graber, J.L., Okazaki, N. (eds.) Proceedings of the 61st Annual Meeting of the Association for Computational Linguistics (Volume 1: Long Papers), ACL 2023, Toronto, Canada, July 9–14, 2023. pp. 6348–6361. Association for Computational Linguistics (2023)
17. Wei, J., et al.: Chain-of-thought prompting elicits reasoning in large language models. In: Advances in Neural Information Processing Systems 35: Annual Conference on Neural Information Processing Systems 2022, NeurIPS 2022, New Orleans, LA, USA, November 28–December 9, 2022 (2022)
18. Wei, J., et al.: Emergent abilities of large language models. CoRR abs/2206.07682 (2022)
19. Xie, T., et al.: Darwin series: Domain specific large language models for natural science (2023)
20. Yao, S., et al.: Tree of thoughts: Deliberate problem solving with large language models. In: Advances in Neural Information Processing Systems 36: Annual Conference on Neural Information Processing Systems 2023, NeurIPS 2023, New Orleans, LA, USA, December 10–16, 2023 (2023)
21. Yu, Q., et al.: Health-llm: Personalized retrieval-augmented disease prediction system (2025)
22. Zhang, Q., et al.: Scientific large language models: a survey on biological & chemical domains. ACM Comput. Sur. **57**(6), 1–38 (2024)
23. Zhou, J., Joachims, T.: GPT as a baseline for recommendation explanation texts. CoRR abs/2309.08817 (2023)

Unified Peripartum Database with Natural-Language-to-SQL Capabilities at Udine University Hospital: Design and Prototype

Doriana Armenise[2], Ginevra Battello[2], Andrea Brunello[1(✉)], Lorenza Driul[1,2], Angelo Montanari[1], Elisa Rizzante[2], Nicola Saccomanno[1], Andrea Salvador[1], Serena Xodo[2], and Silvia Zermano[2]

[1] University of Udine, 33100 Udine, Italy
andrea.brunello@uniud.it
[2] Department of Maternal and Child Health, "Santa Maria della Misericordia" University Hospital, 33100 Udine, Italy

Abstract. The fragmentation of obstetric information across electronic health record modules, device repositories, and laboratory systems, as it is common in hospitals, hinders both intrapartum care and reproducible research. In this work, we present a practical blueprint for transforming heterogeneous peripartum records into computable, queryable assets by designing and prototyping a unified peripartum relational database with natural-language-to-SQL (NL2SQL) capabilities at the Obstetrics Clinic of Udine University Hospital. Requirements were co-defined with clinicians and formalized as an Entity-Relationship diagram, from which the logical schema and SQL implementation of the database were then derived. The latter integrates heterogeneous sources to connect maternal anamnestic and longitudinal history, current-pregnancy findings, intrapartum course, and delivery and neonatal outcomes. The NL2SQL layer enables clinicians to pose natural-language queries to the system, lowering barriers to audit and exploratory analysis.

Keywords: Obstetrics · Relational databases · NL2SQL

1 Introduction

The transition from traditional paper-based systems to electronic health records (EHRs) is reshaping obstetric and perinatal care, where the safety of both mother and newborn depends on a continuous, comprehensive flow of information. Far from being a mere digital filing cabinet, a EHR can pose as a foundational clinical asset for delivering safer, more efficient, and more effective care. A well-designed obstetric EHR consolidates fragmented data, including maternal history, antepartum risk factors, intrapartum monitoring (e.g., continuously recorded cardiotocography, CTG), and neonatal outcomes, into a single, accessible repository. This centralization enhances the continuity of care, ensuring that

P. Bruno et al. (Eds.): HC_AIxIA_HYDRA 2025, CCIS 2830, pp. 467–480, 2026.
https://doi.org/10.1007/978-3-032-16708-8_37

every clinician involved in the process has an immediate and complete understanding of the patient's status. For example, a complete clinical picture at a glance can aid in quick decision-making during a critical intrapartum event [18]. Beyond direct clinical care, EHRs provide an unprecedented wealth of longitudinal data for research and quality improvement. By aggregating standardized data across a large patient population, researchers can identify clinical trends, evaluate the effectiveness of interventions, and develop predictive models to anticipate and mitigate adverse events. This secondary use of data is a game-changer for advancing both clinical knowledge and patient safety.

However, despite their promise, implementing EHRs is complex and resource-intensive, with costs that extend beyond software licenses to hardware, infrastructure, integration, and sustained training and support. Equally important are sociotechnical challenges, including workflow redesign, change management, and usability. Disruptions to established practice can elicit resistance, and suboptimal interfaces or documentation burden increase cognitive load, erode situational awareness, and contribute to clinician frustration and burnout. Effective adoption thus requires co-design with end users, strong governance, and continuous optimization so that systems align with clinical workflows rather than the reverse. As a result of these difficulties, obstetric data often remain fragmented across heterogeneous modules, device archives, and laboratory systems, where coding variation, timestamp inconsistencies, and weak linkages hinder both quality audit, and research. Reviews and policy analyses underscore these issues and the need for maternity-specific interoperability guidance [10,12,19,25,26].

For these reasons, in this work, focusing on the use case of the Obstetrics Clinic at Udine University Hospital, we present the design and development of a centralized relational database for pregnancies and childbirths. The database has been co-designed with clinicians to ensure usability and data consistency across the peripartum domain, and it harmonizes data from heterogeneous sources, integrating (*i*) maternal anamnestic and longitudinal data (e.g., pre-existing conditions, medications, obstetric/gynecologic history, prior pregnancy outcomes), (*ii*) current-pregnancy data (e.g., laboratory results and visit outcomes), (*iii*) intrapartum data (e.g., labor progress, CTG), and (*iv*) delivery and neonatal outcomes (mode/timing of delivery, fetal blood cord gas analysis, neonatal status). To lower barriers at user (i.e., clinicians, obstetricians, and nurses) interaction, a natural-language-to-SQL (NL2SQL) layer lets medical personnel query the system with clinical prompts formulated in natural language, which are then automatically translated into Structured Query Language (SQL) queries. By providing a consistent and comprehensive view of obstetric data, the system supports analyses that can improve patient care by identifying patterns, trends, and risk factors, enabling the development of prevention tools [9,17], e.g., the early identification of fetuses at risk of acidemia, an area where precise operational thresholds remain limited and practice heterogeneous [4,5,16].

2 Current State, Limitations, and Requirements

Public hospitals in Italy rely on EHR modules that are typically integrated and standardized at least at the regional level (e.g., [21]). These systems facilitate

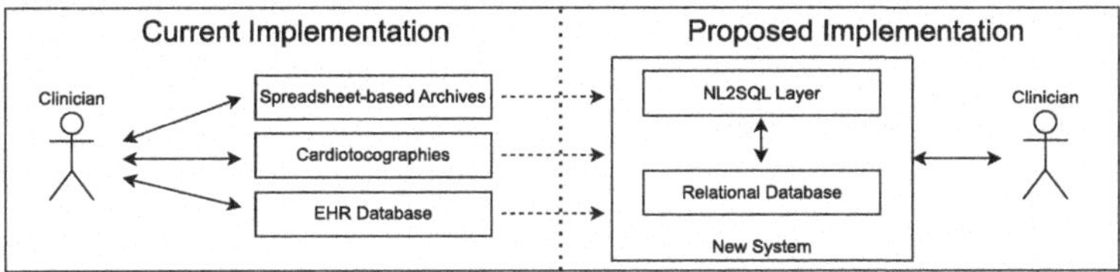

Fig. 1. Current (left) and proposed (right) implementation of the information system. Solid arrows represent human-component or component-component interactions, while dashed arrows represent data flows.

interaction among healthcare professionals and, in some cases, patients themselves, while meeting legally mandated standards of security, performance, and accessibility. However, their data storage formats are primarily designed for day-to-day clinical operations rather than statistical or analytical purposes. Moreover, the way information is stored often differs from what clinicians find most practical for their workflows.

To compensate for these limitations, hospitals often implement internal data management solutions. Since at least 2022, clinicians at the Obstetrics Clinic of Udine University Hospital have complemented the official systems with manually compiled spreadsheets and custom tools to better organize data from check-ups and hospitalizations. While this approach facilitates quick access to frequently needed information, it has also resulted in multiple fragmented, ad hoc repositories. These informal archives, though adequate for routine care, lack the structured foundation required for advanced analyses and cross-patient comparisons, such as the use of unique identifiers, the enforcement of domain constraints, or the implementation of data models specifically designed to reduce redundancy.

As a result, any non-trivial task involves navigating a landscape of heterogeneous and non-integrated data sources, often redundant or inconsistent, a situation illustrated on the left side of Fig. 1. In the following, we present the various archives and modules currently in use within the Obstetrics Clinic, which serve as the foundation for our proposed integrated solution.

Spreadsheets. Clinicians rely on manually compiled, spreadsheet-based archives to record patient data during examinations. Collection of data typically occurs at specific stages of pregnancy: (*i*) in the first trimester (approximately 11–13 weeks) for Nuchal Translucency (NT) screening, along with documenting pre-existing conditions and other related assessments; (*ii*) in the second trimester (approximately 19–21 weeks) for morphological ultrasound and selected genetic screenings; and (*iii*) during labor and delivery. Not all patients undergo each of these examinations at the Clinic, as some may choose other facilities within the hospital district. In addition, a subset of patients with high-risk pregnancies is monitored more frequently, with clinicians collecting detailed information on conditions, comorbidities, and ongoing therapies. As we previously mentioned, while spreadsheet-based archives provide basic functionalities and can be adapted to clinicians' needs, their nature leads to significant challenges, including varying notations and interpretations across professionals, missing data, and conflicting entries arising from unchecked redundancies and constraints.

Cardiotocographies. Delivery rooms are equipped with cardiotocographs (CTGs) to monitor fetal and maternal heart rates as well as uterine contractions. CTGs can export data as spreadsheets containing measurements for each time point; in the delivery rooms of the Udine Obstetrics Clinic, these parameters are sampled at a frequency of four times per second. As we shall see, to ensure device independence, our database stores temporal data using a flexible, timestamp-based approach.

EHR Database. Since 2022 clinicians have been using a GUI-based EHR system, *likely* supported by a relational database management system in the back end. However, the system is not publicly distributed, and no documentation or references are available online. Data export is limited to spreadsheets, often inconsistent in format and style, and sometimes unreadable. Clinicians use this software only intermittently, as it lacks mechanisms for ensuring data consistency, particularly for chronologically ordered events, and allows redundancies. As a result, much of the information maintained in custom spreadsheets is never transferred into it. Ultimately, despite its ostensibly more structured design, this EHR database offers little improvement over spreadsheet-based archives regarding data integrity, constraint enforcement, or redundancy management, leaving clinicians with the same fundamental issues.

Ultimately, the main challenges observed stem from fragmentation, internal and cross-system inconsistencies, and the absence of validation mechanisms in the current solutions. Users report difficulties in querying and cross-checking data, which hinders both the integration of individual patient histories and the development of advanced statistical analyses or predictive models. For example, patient and newborn identifiers are managed differently in spreadsheets and CTG tracings. Moreover, when data from spreadsheets is loaded into the EHR database, redundancies are introduced that can easily lead to inconsistencies. Examples, populated with fictitious data, are provided in the supplementary material [1] (Appendix).

The new information system must therefore enable clinicians to seamlessly store and retrieve all patient details currently captured in existing archives, while also incorporating additional elements identified through clinician interviews, such as biometric ultrasound data, extended neonatal physiological parameters, and a more comprehensive recording of pre-existing conditions beyond high-risk pregnancies. Furthermore, the system should be easily extensible to accommodate new data management requirements arising from clinical practice or research, and adaptable to evolving clinical needs; for example, by allowing clinicians to update the number and types of tests performed at each examination. Finally, it must remain intuitive for clinicians to use in routine practice, as ease of use is paramount for successful adoption.

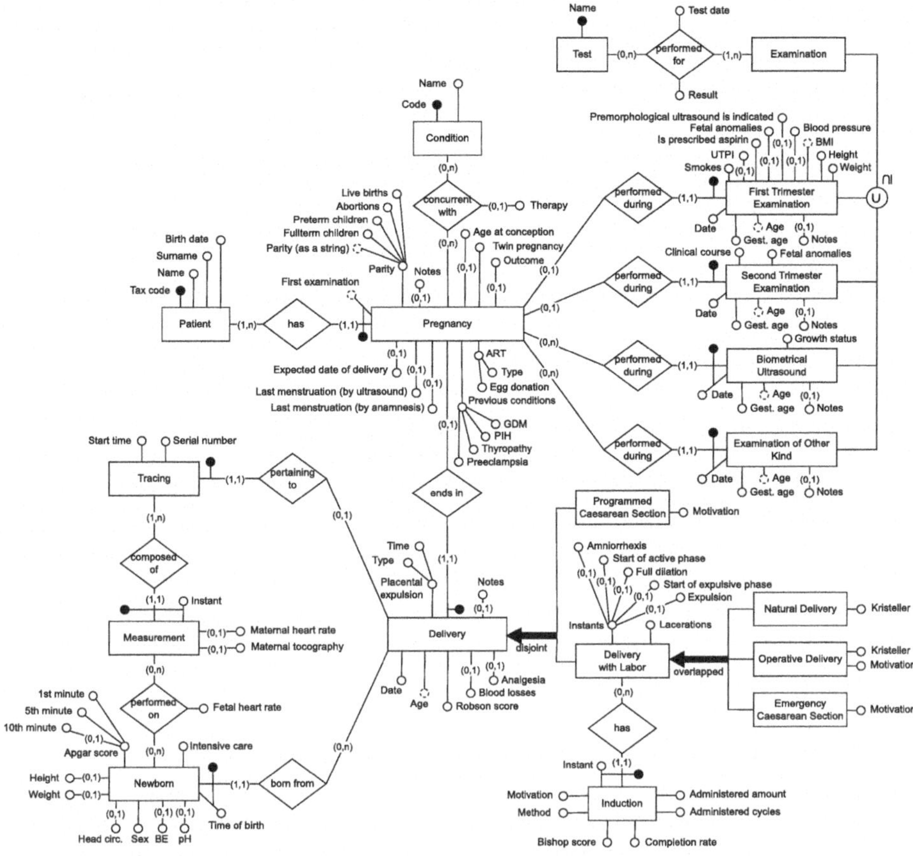

Fig. 2. Entity-Relationship diagram of the analyzed domain.

3 Domain Conceptual Modeling

This section presents the conceptual model developed in collaboration with clinicians, represented as an Entity–Relationship (ER) diagram and following the classical notation proposed in [2]. The diagram and its documentation not only formally encode the domain requirements but also provide the foundation for the new centralized, integrated relational database. The diagram is shown in Fig. 2, and described entity by entity in the following.

Patient. The entity set `Patient` represents patients that have been examined at least once during pregnancy, or have given birth in the Udine Obstetrics Clinic. Patients are identified by their Italian tax code, a unique 16-character alphanumeric string.[1] They are modeled with only a few essential anagraphic

[1] Of course, this identifier can be easily adapted for other contexts.

attributes, such as name, surname, and date of birth, as all other details are associated with related entities in the schema. As shown in Fig. 2, a patient may experience one or more pregnancies, represented by the `(1,n)` relationship.

Pregnancy. The (weak) entity set `Pregnancy` represents pregnancies managed by the medical staff of the Udine Obstetrics Clinic. Each pregnancy is associated with exactly one patient, as expressed by the `(1,1)` relationship in Fig. 2. A pregnancy is uniquely identified by the patient and the date of the first examination, which is always recorded. Regarding the attributes of `Pregnancy`, the distinction between those pertaining to the overall pregnancy and those specific to examinations, particularly the Nuchal Translucency (NT) scan, can sometimes be ambiguous, since most pregnancy-related details are typically collected during the examinations. In this work, we assigned to `Pregnancy` those attributes of a more general nature, while attributes that may vary over the course of pregnancy or have a context-specific meaning were assigned to the examination entities. This distinction is particularly important when, for instance, the NT examination is performed in another facility, as the "general" pregnancy data can still be recorded in the system. More in detail, `Pregnancy` includes information on parity,[2] maternal age at conception, use of assisted reproductive technologies (if applicable), previous pregnancy-related conditions (e.g., preeclampsia or thyroid disease), date of last menstruation, and expected date of delivery.

Condition. The entity set `Condition` represents diseases or illnesses that may be present during pregnancy. We associated `Condition` with the entity `Pregnancy`, rather than with `Patient`, since medical conditions may differ across successive pregnancies. This association is represented by the optional many-to-many relationship `concurrent with`. When a condition, present during a pregnancy, is under treatment, the corresponding therapy is recorded as an attribute of the relationship `concurrent with`.

Examination. The entity set `Examination` represents gynecological examinations or check-ups performed at the Clinic during pregnancy. We identified four types of examinations: (*i*) `First Trimester Examination`, primarily aimed at NT testing, performed at most once per pregnancy; (*ii*) `Second Trimester Examination`, focused on morphological ultrasound, also performed at most once; (*iii*) `Biometrical ultrasound`, which may be performed multiple times during pregnancy; and (*iv*) `Examination of Other Kind`. These are modeled as a union-type entity `Examination` comprising the four examination types. This modeling approach is preferable to a generalization–specialization hierarchy, as it better accommodates the distinct cardinality constraints that characterize the relationships between the different examination types and the entity `Pregnancy`.

[2] Parity is the number of previous pregnancies, described as: (*i*) number of full-term births, (*ii*) number of premature births, (*iii*) number of abortions, and (*iv*) number of live births.

For each entity of `Examination`, clinicians typically record the date, gestational age, and type-specific attributes.

Test. The entity set `Test` represents medical tests that can be performed during examinations. In particular, through the relationship `performed on`, one or more tests may be associated with an examination; conversely, a test may never have been performed (e.g., in the case of a test only recently introduced into clinical practice). The results of a performed test are modeled as attributes of the relationship `performed for`.

Delivery. The entity set `Delivery` represents childbirth events managed at the Clinic. Its attributes depend on the delivery type. The first (total, disjoint) specialization distinguishes between `Programmed Caesarean Section` (performed before labor) and `Delivery with Labor`. All deliveries include attributes such as gestational age, Robson score, placental expulsion, analgesia, and estimated blood loss. In addition, deliveries with labor record further attributes, including lacerations and key delivery time points. A second (total, overlapping) specialization applies to deliveries with labor, distinguishing `Natural Delivery` (spontaneous vaginal births), `Operative Delivery` (assisted vaginal births), and `Emergency Caesarean Section`. The overalap between these types is possible, for example, in twin pregnancies where different procedures are required for each neonate. Each subtype has its own specific attributes.

Induction. The entity set `Induction` represents labor inductions, which are absent in patients undergoing scheduled Caesarean sections. It records details such as timing (partial key), method, drug dosage, and completion rate.

Newborn. The entity set `Newborn` represents a child delivered. In multiple pregnancies (e.g., twins or triplets), newborns are distinguished by their time of birth. Both physical (e.g., weight, length) and physiological (e.g., Apgar score, blood pH) data are recorded here.

Tracing. The entity set `Tracing` represents a complete cardiotocography (CTG) recorded during delivery. Machine-dependent information, such as the specific fetal sensors used, is not modeled, as it constitutes technical data that has not been considered relevant from the domain perspective. Conceptually, a `Tracing` serves as a container for measurements.

Measurement. The entity set `Measurement` represents the individual data points composing a CTG, each associated with its corresponding timestamp. Attributes stored directly in `Measurement` include maternal heart rate and uterine contractions (from tocography), whereas fetal heart rates are modeled as attributes of the relationship `performed on`, so to link them to the specific

`Newborn` they refer to. Only observed values are taken into account; missing values are not stored.

The weak entities `Newborn`, `Delivery`, `Tracing`, and `Measurement` form a cycle; to avoid inconsistencies, when relationships are instanced, they must all refer to the same delivery. As we will see, when translated into a logical schema, foreign key constraint are sufficient in guaranteeing this correspondence.

4 Development of the New System

In this section, we present the development of the new system, which comprises two core components (Fig. 1, right): (*i*) a relational database, designed according to the developed Entity–Relationship diagram, capable of integrating information from all previous sources; and (*ii*) an NL2SQL layer that facilitates clinician interaction with the database. All code related to the system implementation, as well as a prototypical deployment of the database populated with fictitious data, is available at: https://github.com/dslab-uniud/gineco-db.

4.1 Relational Database

From the ER diagram, a logical relational schema was derived. Then, the schema was implemented in a PostgreSQL [20] instance.

Logical Schema. The schema, shown in Fig. 3, was derived primarily by following standard mapping rules [2]. It adopts the well-known Crow's Foot notation [23]. The main design choices made in defining the schema are: (*i*) we assigned a synthetic `id` to each pregnancy, rather than relying on the natural ER identifier. This choice reduces the number of attributes in related tables, since many of them include the pregnancy identifier as a foreign key; (*ii*) given the similarity of their attributes, the four types of examinations were consolidated into a single relation, thereby simplifying the logical schema; (*iii*) since tests are modeled as a separate entity, the attribute `result` must be able to assume many data types; the attribute `type` in `Test` dictates the actual data type of the outcome[3] and triggers check the correspondence between the two. (*iv*) since multiple induction methods may be applied in a single delivery, they were modeled in a separate relation; (*v*) and, the two-layer specialization of deliveries was simplified into three relations: all deliveries, containing the common attributes; programmed Caesarean sections, representing cases without labor; and deliveries with labor, which may include labor inductions.

As previously mentioned, the cycle of foreign keys formed between `Newborn`, `Delivery`, and `Tracing` requires no additional checks, as the foreign key constraints alone ensure that tuples pertain to the same delivery. Not all domain

[3] We define three categories of tests according to their outcome, which may be numeric, string, or enumerated. Since the physical data type of the attribute `result` is `varchar` (string), numeric values are cast to `varchar` as well.

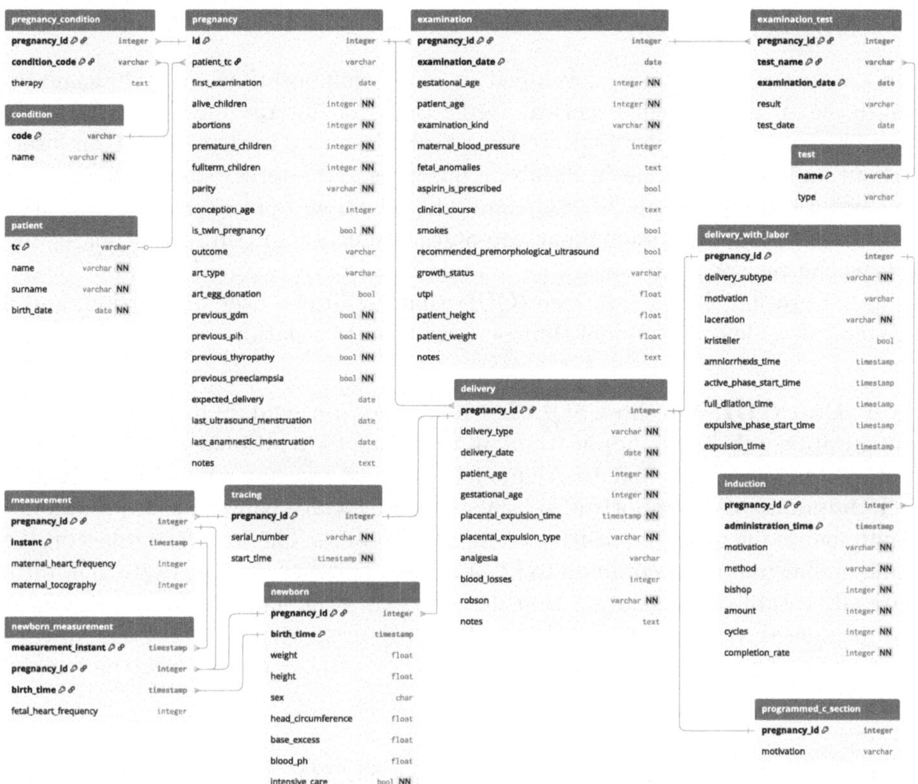

Fig. 3. Logical relational diagram of the analyzed domain.

requirements can be enforced directly by the logical schema. To ensure data consistency, we defined additional checks in the final database implementation, using triggers. They can be found in the supplementary material [1] (Appendix).

Physical Implementation. We implemented our proposed database using PostgreSQL [20] database management system. Table definitions in SQL were derived directly from the logical schema presented in Fig. 3. An interesting aspect concerns the handling of the attribute `type` in the `test` table. This attribute, implemented as an array of `varchar`, determines the domain of the attribute `result` in the `examination_test` table. Specifically, if `type` is set to `[string]`, results can take any `varchar` value; if it is set to `[numeric]`, `result` must be a string interpretable as a numeric value; in all other cases, `type` enumerates the exact list of values that `result` may assume. For the complete physical implementation of the database, as well as a working prototype populated with fictitious data, we refer the reader to the previously mentioned online resource.

4.2 NL2SQL Module

The database schema was developed in close collaboration with clinicians to ensure that it meets their practical needs. However, interacting with a database typically requires writing SQL code, a task that can be non-trivial for users without sufficient training in database querying. To address this challenge, the new system integrates an NL2SQL module, which accepts queries expressed in natural language, translates them into SQL, executes them on the database, and returns the results as a table. The module consists of two main components: a front-end graphical user interface (GUI) that facilitates user interaction, and a back-end deep learning model that performs the translation.

Front-End GUI. We chose SQLChat [6] as the front-end. SQLChat is a highly configurable web-based application: it connects to relational databases (e.g., PostgreSQL, MySQL) and to AI models exposed via any OpenAI-compatible API endpoint, also supporting self-hosted and locally run models, paramount requirements for privacy-sensitive contexts, like ours. The interface relies on the familiar chat paradigm common to LLM agents. For each session, SQLChat automatically establishes a context that describes the schema of the active database and includes directives guiding the model's responses, ensuring that user queries are answered in a database-aware manner. For further details, see the supplementary material [1] (Appendix).

Back-End Model. The model chosen as the NL2SQL back-end is XiYanSQL-QwenCoder-32B-2504, an open-source SQL generation model with multi-dialect support and high performance on common SQL test datasets; specifically, the authors self-report a performance of 67.14% on BIRD Dev compared to, e.g., 60.37% obtained by OmniSQL-32B or 59.39% with GPT-4.1-0414. This model is presented as part of XiYanSQL [14], a wider NL2SQL framework which provides finetuning capabilities, but it is also distributed as a stand-alone component.

5 Usage of the New System

A prototype of the newly developed system is already being tested by the Obstetrics Clinic personnel. Data from the original sources were migrated into the system using Python scripts, which can also be executed periodically to update and synchronize its content. This is intended as a temporary solution until the new system fully replaces the legacy ones. In the following, we present a representative example of successful interaction supported by the system, while a more extensive discussion is provided in the supplementary material [1] (Appendix).

The query reports the number of C-sections performed in 2024, which may result from a programmed delivery or from an urgent intervention during labor. An `EXISTS` operator is used to verify whether a given C-section is associated with a delivery that occurred in 2024. In fact, each C-section is linked to exactly one delivery, so a `JOIN` operation would have sufficed. However, this constraint is enforced through a trigger (see the supplementary material [1], Appendix) rather than explicitly represented in the schema, and is therefore unavailable to the NL2SQL model. In future work, we plan to enrich the database schema provided in the prompt template to the model with comments that capture such additional information.

Query: C-sections in 2024

Count the number of C-sections, programmed and with labor, done in 2024.

SQL query automatic translation

```
SELECT COUNT(*) AS total_c_sections
FROM (SELECT 1
      FROM programmed_c_section AS pcs
      WHERE EXISTS (SELECT 1
                    FROM delivery AS d
                    WHERE pcs.pregnancy_id = d.pregnancy_id
                        AND EXTRACT(YEAR FROM d.delivery_date) = 2024)
    UNION ALL
      SELECT 1
      FROM delivery_with_labor AS dwl
      WHERE EXISTS (SELECT 1
                    FROM delivery AS d
                    WHERE dwl.pregnancy_id = d.pregnancy_id
                        AND EXTRACT(YEAR FROM d.delivery_date) = 2024
                        AND d.delivery_type = 'emergency_c_section' )
    ) AS c_sections;
```

Overall, out of eight attempted moderate-complexity queries, the system failed to answer correctly only one (due to a missing filtering condition, see the supplementary material [1], Appendix); translation was helped when users formulated unambiguous, comprehensive requests using the names found in the existing tables and attributes. While a full evaluation was beyond this work's scope, the results are promising and will be examined more thoroughly in future studies. Of course, beyond the interaction capabilities offered by the NL2SQL module, advanced users can submit custom SQL queries. In addition, parameterized stored procedures for recurring queries have been integrated into the database.

6 Related Work

In the literature, works have addressed data management and decision support in obstetrics and gynecology, but with emphases different from ours. Public datasets have been proposed to support research in maternal health (e.g., [7]). While valuable for statistical analysis and predictive modeling, these resources are not designed as operational databases for clinical use. Existing proposals for obstetrics and gynecology information systems are typically modeled around the patient as a general medical entity rather than specifically around pregnancy and newborns [24,27], while others focus on nursing workflows [28]. Some contributions describe high-level architectures for hospital information systems in obstetrics [3], while earlier studies evaluated perinatal data collection systems [15]. However, these contributions do not provide a pregnancy-centered database design. Since the 1980s, expert systems have also been explored to support medical reasoning in obstetrics and gynecology [11,22]. These concentrate primarily on clinical decision support, often relying on rule-based or ontology-driven reasoning, rather than on the development of a full-fledged information system. In fact, recent reviews emphasize the continued need for decision-support systems in obstetrics and gynecology, stressing both human-centered design [8] and the importance of clinical implementation and the integration of historical data [13].

Aligned with these observations, and differing from previous contributions, our work proposes a blueprint for an information system centered on pregnancy, explicitly considering clinical usability and laying the foundation for future computer-assisted, possibly AI-based, decision support.

7 Conclusions

In this work, we presented the design and development of a centralized relational database for pregnancies and childbirths at Udine University Hospital's Obstetrics Clinic. The system integrates heterogeneous maternal, intrapartum, and neonatal data into a consistent structure, co-designed with clinicians to ensure usability. By integrating an NL2SQL interface, the novel system lowers barriers for clinical users and enables both routine practice support and research applications. This lays the foundation for improved risk assessment, decision support, and predictive modeling in obstetrics, with the potential to enhance maternal and neonatal outcomes. A prototypical implementation of the database, populated with fictitious data, is available online. In the future, this implementation could evolve into a hub for the continual publication of properly anonymized datasets, fostering reproducible research and enabling the broader scientific community to develop and validate novel methods for perinatal care.

Acknowledgments. AB, AM, NS acknowledge the support from the Interconnected Nord-Est Innovation Ecosystem (iNEST), which received funding from the European Union Next-GenerationEU (PIANO NAZIONALE DI RIPRESA E RESILIENZA – MISSIONE 4 COMPONENTE 2, INVESTIMENTO 1.5 – D.D. 1058 23/06/2022, ECS00000043). AM acknowledges the support from the MUR PNRR project FAIR - Future AI Research (PE00000013) also funded by the European Union Next-GenerationEU. This manuscript reflects only the authors' views and opinions, neither the European Union nor the European Commission can be considered responsible for them.

Disclosure of Interests. The authors have no relevant competing interests to declare.

Ethics declaration. This study has been approved by the Institutional Review Board of the University of Udine's Department of Medicine (Prot. IRB: 122/2025).

References

1. Armenise, D., et al.: Unified peripartum database with natural-language-to-SQL capabilities at Udine University Hospital: design and prototype (2025). https://arxiv.org/abs/2510.16388
2. Atzeni, P., Ceri, S., Paraboschi, S., et al.: Database Systems: Concepts, Languages and Architectures. McGraw-Hill (2000). https://dbbook.inf.uniroma3.it/
3. Barrote, A., Silva, P., Gonçalves, F., et al.: Obstetric information system: effectiveness in health care practice. Procedia Technol. **16**, 1411–1416 (2014)
4. Cahill, A.G., Tuuli, M.G., Stout, M.J., et al.: A prospective cohort study of fetal heart rate monitoring: deceleration area is predictive of fetal acidemia. Am. J. Obstet. Gynecol. **218**(5), 523.e1-523.e12 (2018)
5. Chandraharan, E., Arulkumaran, S.: Prevention of birth asphyxia: responding appropriately to cardiotocograph (CTG) traces. Best Pract. Res. Clin. Obstet. Gynaecol. **21**(4), 609–624 (2007)
6. Chen, T., et al.: SQLChat: Chat-based SQL client and editor for the next decade (2025). https://github.com/sqlchat/sqlchat. Accessed 27 Aug 2025
7. Chudáček, V., Spilka, J., Burša, M., et al.: Open access intrapartum CTG database. BMC Preg. Childbirth **14**(1), 16 (2014)
8. Cockburn, N., Osborne, C., et al.: Clinical decision support systems for maternity care: a systematic review and meta-analysis. eClinicalMedicine **76** (2024)
9. Corey, L., Vezina, A., Gala, R.B.: Using technology to improve women's health care. Ochsner J. **20**(4), 422–425 (2020)
10. Glynn, E.F., Hoffman, M.A.: Heterogeneity introduced by EHR system implementation in a de-identified data resource from 100 non-affiliated organizations. JAMIA Open **2**(4), 554–561 (2019)
11. Lam, J., Abdullah, M.S., Supriyanto, E.: Architecture for clinical decision support system (CDSS) using high risk pregnancy ontology. ARPN J. Eng. Appl. Sci. **10**(3), 1229–1237 (2015)
12. Lewis, A.E., et al.: Electronic health record data quality assessment and tools: a systematic review. J. Am. Med. Inf. Assoc. **30**(10), 1730–1740 (2023)
13. Lin, X., Liang, C., Liu, J., et al.: Artificial intelligence-augmented clinical decision support systems for pregnancy care: systematic review. J. Med. Internet Res. **26**, e54737 (2024)
14. Liu, Y., Zhu, Y., Gao, Y., et al.: XiYan-SQL: a novel multi-generator framework for text-to-SQL (2025). https://arxiv.org/abs/2507.04701
15. Maresh, M., Dawson, A., Beard, R.: Assessment of an on-line computerized perinatal data collection and information system. BJOG Int. J. Obstet. Gynaecol. **93**(12), 1239–1245 (1986)
16. McCoy, J.A., Levine, L.D., Wan, G., et al.: Intrapartum electronic fetal heart rate monitoring to predict acidemia at birth with the use of deep learning. Am. J. Obstet. Gynecol. **232**(116), e1-116.e9 (2025)
17. McCullough, J.S., Parente, S.T., Town, R.: Health information technology and patient outcomes: the role of information and labor coordination. Rand J. Econ. **47**(1), 207–236 (2016)

18. National Institute for Health and Care Excellence: Fetal monitoring in labour (2022). https://www.nice.org.uk/guidance/ng229. Accessed 12 Aug 2025
19. Office of the National Coordinator for Health IT (ONC): Interoperability of maternity health care records: Best practices informational resource (2024). https://www.healthit.gov/sites/default/files/page/2024-03/FY23%20ONC%20Maternity%20Care%20Info%20Resource%20Guide_508%20(1).pdf
20. PostgreSQL Global Development Group: PostgreSQL documentation (2025). https://www.postgresql.org/docs/current/. Accessed 24 Aug 2025
21. Regione Autonoma Friuli Venezia Giulia: SESAMO, Electronic Platform for Health Services (2018). https://sesamo.sanita.fvg.it/sesamo/. Accessed 20 Aug 2025
22. Riss, P.A., Koelbl, H., Reinthaller, A., et al.: Development and application of simple expert systems in obstetrics and gynecology. J. Perinatal Med. (1988)
23. Silberschatz, A., Korth, H.F., Sudarshan, S.: Database System Concepts, 6th edn. McGraw-Hill, New York (2010)
24. Skarga-Bandurova, I., Biloborodova, T., Nesterov, M.: Modeling structures for integrated obstetrics, gynecology, and neonatal information system. Problemy informatsiinykh tekhnologii **17**(1), 51–57 (2015)
25. Slawomirski, L., et al.: Progress on implementing and using electronic health record systems: Developments in OECD countries as of 2021. Technical report, OECD Health Working Papers No. 160 (2023)
26. Van Der Scheer, J.W., Komolafe, V., Webster, K., et al.: Improving UK data on avoidable perinatal brain injury: review of data dictionaries and consultation. Pediatric Res. (2025)
27. Vida, M., Mioara Stoicu-Tivadar, L., Blobel, B., et al.: Modeling the framework for obstetrics-gynecology department information systems. Eur. J. Biomed. Inf. **8**(3), 57–64 (2012)
28. Zhu, H., Gu, L.: Design and application of intelligent information system for comprehensive management of obstetrics and gynecology health care. J. Med. Imaging Health Inf. **10**(8), 1834–1840 (2020)

Are We Ready for Multi-agent Systems to Deliver Structured Mental Health Support? Lessons from Adapting Self-Help+ Intervention

Leonardo Sanna[1(✉)], Marco Bolpagni[1,2], Valentina Fietta[1], Simone De Carli[2], Mattia Franzin[1], Giorgia Gavioli[1], Lorenzo Gios[1], Susanna Pardini[1], Anna Elena Nicoletti[1], Silvia Rizzi[1], Silvia Gabrielli[1], and Mauro Dragoni[1(✉)]

[1] Fondazione Bruno Kessler, Trento, Italy
{lsanna,mbolpagni,sgabrielli,dragoni}@fbk.eu
[2] University of Padova, Padova, Italy

Abstract. Recent progress in natural language processing has created new possibilities for delivering personalized digital mental health support. Yet, combining structured, evidence-based therapeutic frameworks with the flexibility of natural conversation remains a challenge. This study examines the use of Large Language Models (LLMs) in structured chatbots to improve delivery of the World Health Organization's Self-Help+ program. We compared a conventional state-machine chatbot with an LLM-enhanced version and finally with a multi-agent architecture, examining the strengths and limitations of the different approaches. Through simulation testing and expert focus group analysis, we found that a multi-agent architecture, while significantly improving personalization, struggles in maintaining protocol fidelity and therapeutic structure.

Our findings suggest that current LLM-based architectures, while promising, might not yet be ready for unsupervised deployment in mental health contexts.

Keywords: Large Language Model · Chatbot · Stress Management · Multi-Agent Systems

1 Introduction

As the demand for mental health services grows, digital tools offer a scalable solution to bridge the gap with a stepped-care approach. Among others, chat-based applications have emerged [1]. These mobile applications are generally designed to support mental well-being by providing coping strategies, mood tracking, and self-help resources. Through interactive features and evidence-based roots, chatbots aim to support individuals in managing stress, anxiety, and other mental health concerns.

Delivering mental health care in a scalable, accessible, and effective manner remains one of the most pressing challenges in digital health. While mobile

P. Bruno et al. (Eds.): HC_AIxIA_HYDRA 2025, CCIS 2830, pp. 481–494, 2026.
https://doi.org/10.1007/978-3-032-16708-8_38

apps and chatbots have proliferated in recent years, most rely on static decision trees, rigid scripts, or limited natural language understanding [10]. These systems often fail to capture the fluidity of human dialogue or the complex structure of evidence-based interventions, such as those grounded in Acceptance and Commitment Therapy (ACT) [15], Cognitive Behavioral Therapy (CBT) [3], or Motivational Interviewing (MI) [27].

Among the most promising approaches is using LLMs, whose generative capabilities allow for rich, adaptive, and seemingly empathic interactions [31]. Yet this strength introduces design and ethical challenges, especially when LLMs deliver structured, manualized interventions grounded in established psychological frameworks [22].

This paper explores the integration of a Large Language Model (LLM) in a mental health support chatbot. In particular, we examine the LLM capacity to enhance the conversation capabilities of the chatbot, allowing for dynamic and empathetic interactions that align with established therapeutic principles. The validation of the proposed approach, built in a zero-shot fashion, has been performed within the context of the *Self-Help+* (SH+) intervention [11] where the chatbot mimics the role of the facilitator, (i.e., a non-clinical expert trained on the SH+ protocol to drive groups of mutual support) in delivering a stress prevention and management protocol developed by the World Health Organization (WHO). As we outline in Sect. 3, we compared the LLM-enhanced chatbot with a baseline implementation built on top of a finite-state machine solution [26], testing it with a group of 44 users. Builiding on these results, in Sect. 4 we provide a first expert evaluation of a multi-agent architecture meant to overcome finite-state-machines limits. Finally we discuss our main outcomes in Sect. 5.

2 Related Work

This paper introduces a conversational approach that integrates an intervention designed to support psychological well-being and stress management, based on a protocol validated by WHO. Its effectiveness has been demonstrated in international trials involving refugees, asylum seekers, and healthcare workers, highlighting its flexibility and wide applicability [21,25].

Numerous studies have explored the effectiveness of mobile applications and chatbot-based systems in providing scalable and accessible mental health support [8]. For instance, applications like *Headspace* and *Calm* focus on mindfulness and stress reduction, leveraging evidence-based techniques to promote mental well-being [9,16]. Similarly, conversational agents such as *Woebot* and *Wysa* utilize frameworks like cognitive-behavioral therapy to offer interactive and personalized interventions for managing anxiety, depression, and stress [13,17] .

The limitations of rule-based systems led to growing interest in AI-driven approaches, especially as natural language processing technologies matured. Research rapidly expanded into LLM-based chatbots for well-being and mental health, such as Wysa+[1] (using a proprietary generative backend based on OpenAI models), Pi[2] (from Inflection AI), and open explorations using GPT-

[1] https://legal.wysa.io/generative-ai/faq.
[2] https://pi.ai/talk.

based agents for emotional support within the context of Motivational Interview (MI) [32]. LLMs offered a qualitative upgrade in empathy simulation, adaptive dialog, and open-domain flexibility, allowing users to express complex experiences without hitting conversational dead ends [31].

However, some critical challenges remain, particulary in domains such as digital health and wellbeing, where precision and reliability are essential [24]. Two recent studies [6,35] have highlighted the difficulty of maintaining therapeutic alignment when LLMs are used to deliver manualized care through prompt engineering alone. These findings suggest that more robust approaches, such as fine-tuned agents or multi-agent systems, may be necessary to support consistent and aligned therapeutic interactions.

3 SH+ LLM-Augmented: from Pre-defined Messages to LLMs

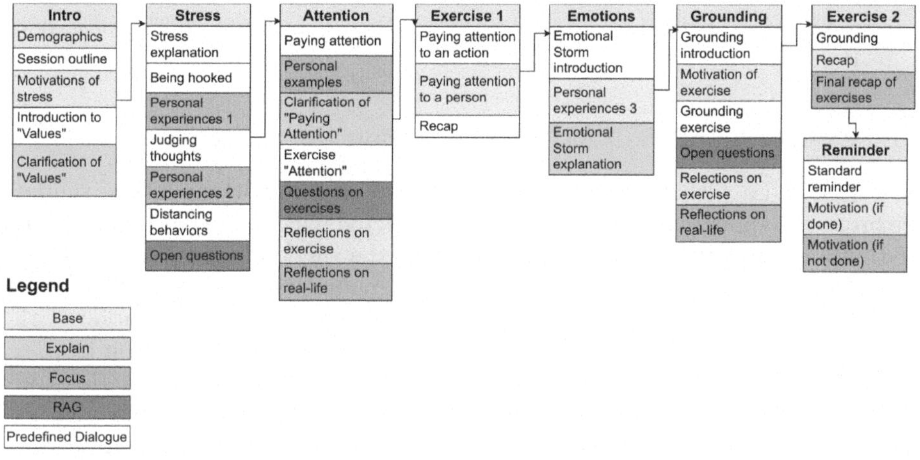

Fig. 1. An overview of the LLM-augmented FSM with the states grouped by their theme. Colored states are those managed by an LLM.

In 2022, efforts began to adapt SH+ into a digital format in the Italian context. The first generation of the chatbot employed a rule-based conversational system with a fixed decision-tree logic. This system guided users through the SH+ material in a linear, pre-scripted way, mimicking the structured delivery of in-person facilitation. While this approach guaranteed high fidelity to the original protocol, it was recognized as rigid and unresponsive, failing to accommodate individual differences or emergent user needs.

The introduction of the LLM-augmented architecture (henceforth FSM-LLM) preserved the overall FSM structure but replaced several deterministic states with LLM-enriched nodes (see Fig. 1). In these, an LLM-generated response was guided by a system prompt that embedded task-specific instructions and sample completions. This hybrid design allowed the chatbot to personalize responses while maintaining adherence to the psychological protocol. We tested this implementation in the first SH + session, deploying a total of 20 enriched nodes guided by a carefully designed prompt that was based on persona-driven design [18].

Following the framework of [2], we implemented four prompting strategies tailored to interaction needs:

1. *Base*: Persona-based reply with minimal instructions; refined with a final prompt containing detailed guidance.
2. *Explain*: Extends *Base* with up to three prompts to rephrase the explanations in context.
3. *Focus*: Extends *Base* with up to two prompts and a specific element to emphasize in the reply (e.g., "keep in mind the user is stressed because of {REASON}").
4. *RAG*: Translates queries from Italian to English, retrieves relevant manual content, generates context-based answers, then translates the response back to Italian.[3]

3.1 Evaluation of the FSM-LLM Chatbot

We conducted a within-subject experiment involving 44 participants to validate the proposed approach. Each participant interacted with both the standard FSM chatbot and the FSM-LLM version. We adopted a single-blind approach to form two equal groups: one used the FSM-LLM version first, and the other began with the standard version, minimizing order effects. The full description of the chatbot and experimental design is covered by a dedicated publication [29].

Participants were volunteers who provided informed consent before the study began. They had a mean age of 32.47 years (SD=11.80), with 40.91% identifying as male and 59.09% as female. The sample included individuals with diverse educational levels, with the majority holding at least a bachelor's degree (EQF6 or higher). Experience levels with chatbots and LLMs varied, but most participants reported intermediate or advanced familiarity. All participants were based in Italy. In the study, we included a sub-group of expert psychologists for a total of 7 people, to have qualitative feedback on the overall experience. Table 1 shows that the LLM-enriched chatbot significantly outperformed the standard version in Emotional Support, Guidance and Direction, Memory, and Overall Satisfaction. Emotional Support and Memory improvements were especially strong, with

[3] At the time of experiment, only the English manual was available; the Italian version was released in Feb 2025.

Table 1. Summary of results for CES-LCC [7] subscales. UR: Understanding Requests, PHI: Providing Helpful Information, CRR: Clarity and Relevance of Responses, LQ: Language Quality, T: Trust, ES: Emotional Support, GD: Guidance and Direction, M: Memory, OS: Overall Satisfaction.

Scale	*W*	*p-val*	*RBC*	*CLES*	*Med-STD*	*Med-LLM*	*Avg-STD*	*Avg-LLM*
UR	**167.5**	**0.005**	**-0.523**	**0.365**	**3.00**	**3.50**	**2.92**	**3.44**
PHI	241.5	0.906	-0.026	0.515	4.00	4.00	4.02	3.98
CRR	250.0	0.590	-0.109	0.513	4.00	3.84	3.86	3.89
LQ	114.0	0.192	-0.298	0.466	4.33	4.33	4.27	4.38
T	311.5	0.740	-0.065	0.494	3.67	3.67	3.60	3.65
ES	**88.0**	**0.000**	**-0.721**	**0.357**	**3.16**	**3.67**	**3.03**	**3.57**
GD	**146.0**	**0.046**	**-0.411**	**0.416**	**3.67**	**4.00**	**3.61**	**3.83**
M	**139.5**	**0.012**	**-0.503**	**0.374**	**3.00**	**3.67**	**3.17**	**3.61**
OS	**149.5**	**0.032**	**-0.434**	**0.415**	**4.00**	**4.00**	**3.68**	**3.98**

large effect sizes[4]. Other dimensions, such as Providing Helpful Information and Trust, showed comparable performance across both versions.

Qualitative analysis of user feedback provided deeper insights into the perceived strengths and weaknesses of both chatbot versions. The subgroup of psychologists pointed out that the standard version lacked effective communication skills and empathy. They also noted that the structured dialogue significantly restricted users' ability to express themselves freely, leading the chatbot to make assumptions about patients' realities and their understanding of stress. Regarding the LLM-enriched version, psychologists emphasized its notable improvements in communication and empathy. However, they acknowledged that it still made underlying assumptions about patients' realities and knowledge, with limited room for negotiating the meaning of terms and the option to skip certain exercises.

4 Multi-agent Chatbot

Given that the limitations that emerged in the FSM-LLM were mainly due to the FSM structure, we adopted a multi-agent architecture, moving forward from a traditional sequential state machine. The first two chatbots followed a rigid, predefined flow based on the SH+ protocol, which had already shown shortcomings in handling open-ended user inputs and adapting to users' evolving needs. A key issue was that once a transition between states occurred, it was no longer

[4] Statistically significant differences are assessed by Wilcoxon signed-rank test which considers the median (Med) of users' evaluations on a five-point Likert scale. Average (Avg) is reported for the sake of completeness. Effect size is assessed with rank-biserial correlation (RBC) and Common Language Effect Size (CLES). Bold font indicates significant differences in favor of the LLM version.

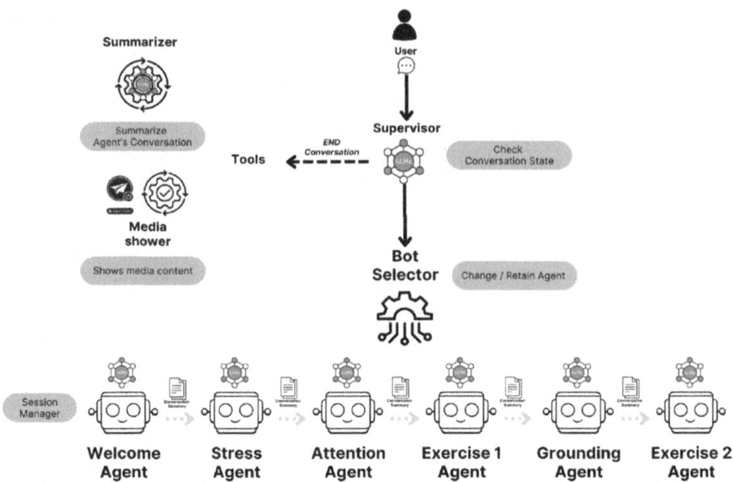

Fig. 2. The schema illustrates our multi-agent system, where each agent focuses on a specific section of the SH+ session. A supervisor monitors whether each agent completes their conversation and coordinates history sharing through a summarizer tool. For clarity, the image displays six agents aligned with the session's macro-themes. In practice, these are divided into 15 agents to enhance control and manage conversation history more effectively, coping with computational constraints.

possible to negotiate or revisit conversational elements. For example, the chatbot could not correct misunderstandings or refer back to earlier dialogue parts, as each state operated with a fixed context and only processed the immediate user input.

In contrast to the FSM-based approach, our multi-agent architecture replaces rigid state transitions with autonomous agents, each responsible for a specific part of the SH+ session. This shift allows for more flexible and natural interactions with the chatbot, as the agents follow high-level instructions provided via system prompts rather than a fixed sequence of states. Our system builds upon the original FSM design by deploying agents sequentially across different session segments, as illustrated in Fig. 2.

The core components of the system are:

1. **The Session Manager**: It is the agent responsible for delivering the session. This agent may be composed of a single LLM or structured hierarchically, with one LLM focusing on low-level instruction following and another (or more) orchestrating response refinement and ensuring alignment with SH+ principles, including response moderation and hallucination check. In our implementation we used two different models: an *Instruction-Follower* (IF) model and a *Text Refiner* (TR) model[5]; the IF model was prompted with

[5] The model chosen in this experiments was Phi4 https://huggingface.co/microsoft/phi-4 due to computational constraints.

the detailed list of instructions related to the session management, while the TF was instructed to refine the output of the IF. Each Session Manager agent is thematic, i.e., focused on a specific dialogue section as shown in Fig. 2. The agents are also entirely independent, and they might also be split within the same thematic section to avoid the lost-in-the-middle effect [19], namely problems related to the length of conversation history. In our current implementation, we have six macro-sections and 15 agents.

2. **The Supervisor**: It is a meta-agent that monitors each interaction stage, validating whether the Session Manager completed its task by checking a predefined checklist of steps. This introduces a feedback loop into the system, offering a dynamic form of quality control during execution, and allows transitioning between different agents, mimicking states transitioning. In our implementation, the supervisor is composed of a single LLM responding with structured output via constrained decoding [14,28]. The Supervisor accesses both the system prompt and a predefined checklist associated with the Session Manager. This checklist outlines the specific steps the Session Manager must complete. Once all steps are fulfilled, the Supervisor updates the system prompt to transition the Session Manager to the next thematic agent. At the end of each checklist, the Supervisor also invokes a summarization tool to extract key information to be shared across agents, and calls a multimedia tool to present relevant content, e.g., infographics, explanatory videos, or guided audio exercises related to the current section of the dialogue. To the best of our knowledge, there are currently no established benchmarks for evaluating LLMs on checklist-based evaluation tasks. Consequently, we selected our Supervisor model based on insights from state-of-the-art technical reports and a series of small-scale empirical tests. This process led us to choose Llama3.3 - 70B, due to its strong performance in reasoning tasks and robust support for structured outputs[6].

This architecture ensures a form of self-monitoring, where every conversational step can be assessed in real-time, creating a robust safety layer particularly valuable in sensitive domains, such as mental health support. It also allows, by design, free interaction between the user and the agent, enabling deviations from the main instructions.

Hardware and Software Configuration. The framework used to develop the system is Langgraph[7]. All models were used on a local Ollama server[8] equipped with two L40s GPUs. For the focus group, the models used for the Session Manager agent were accessed via OpenRouter[9] to improve latency.

[6] https://arxiv.org/abs/2407.21783.
[7] https://langchain-ai.github.io/langgraph/.
[8] https://ollama.com/.
[9] https://openrouter.ai/.

4.1 Evaluation of the Multi-Agent System

Simulations To evaluate the functional reliability of the multi-agent architecture, we implemented a simulation-based protocol focused on two core capacities: the Instruction-Follower's (IF) ability to execute step-by-step guidance, and the Supervisor model's capacity to evaluate step completion accurately. We adopted a role-play prompting framework inspired by [30], simulating realistic chatbot-user interactions between paired LLM instances [5].

Specifically, we conducted 180 simulations for each agent, with 60 simulations allocated to each LLM to evaluate its performance as an IF model. The evaluation focused on two aspects: whether the IF model could complete the checklist and whether the Supervisor model could reliably assess its performance. The assessment of the IF model is fully automated and performed by the Supervisor model. If the IF model fails to complete the conversation within a total of 40 messages, including user responses, the checklist is considered incomplete.

To identify suitable candidates for the IF role, we applied a feature-based shortlisting procedure informed by technical reports and bounded by available computational resources. This process led to the selection of three models: aya-expanse-32B[10], gemma3-27B[11], and mistral-small3.1-24B[12].

The best model, according to the results of our simulations showed in Fig. 3 is mistral-small3.1-24B, which proved to be the most consistent in completing all the steps. We should also highlight that all three models display excellent capacity for instruction following; nevertheless, Mistral produced only one-tenth as many uncompleted checklists compared to the other models[13].

As shown in Fig. 4, it should be noted that some agents tend to fail the checklist more than others. Notably, some models could not complete entire simulations due to memory errors, indicating that specific agents may be more susceptible to losing track of their instructions and struggling to steer the conversation effectively. This issue was particularly evident with the welcome agent, who collected users' demographic information, understood their main motivation for starting the session, and introduced the structure. This agent completed fewer than 10% of the simulations. A closer analysis of the generated dialogues revealed a pattern of digressions, with the agent straying from the user's concerns and producing excessively long, repetitive responses. These behaviors led to memory overflows caused by the extended context length.

Focus Group. To evaluate the multi-agent chatbot's performance in delivering the first session of SH+, we adopted a qualitative, expert-centered focus group approach [4]. The objective was not merely to identify usability issues, but to elicit thick, context-sensitive insights [23] from individuals capable of assessing system behavior in light of both clinical protocols and technological

[10] https://arxiv.org/abs/2412.04261.
[11] https://storage.googleapis.com/deepmind-media/gemma/Gemma3Report.pdf.
[12] https://mistral.ai/news/mistral-small-3.
[13] This difference is statistically significant ($\chi^2(2) = 15.88$, $p < .001$, chi-squared test across models).

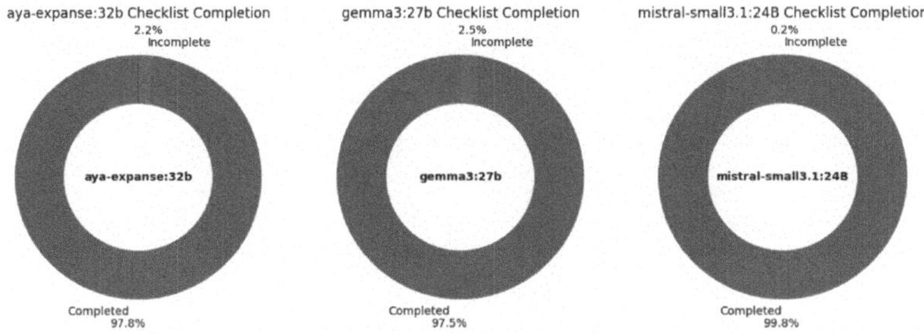

Fig. 3. The percentage of successful checklists over the completed simulations for the three LLMs evaluated.

implementation histories. The focus group, conducted in April 2025, comprised five participants selected through purposive sampling [12]. All had been directly or indirectly involved during either the SH+ Italian localization or the digital implementation phases, including the evaluation detailed in Sect. 3. The sampling strategy aimed to capture in-depth insights from participants with strong familiarity with the intervention and its goals. Participants included clinical psychologists, psychotherapists, and digital mental health researchers with advanced academic qualifications and applied experience in structured intervention delivery and AI-mediated therapeutic systems. Their combined expertise allowed for an informed assessment of the chatbot's therapeutic coherence, structural fidelity, and dialogic performance. Table 2 summarizes participant roles, educational backgrounds, and domain-specific contributions.

Participants were first welcomed with a brief recap on the evolution of SH+, then individually interacted with the chatbot without predefined instructions, allowing for naturalistic use. They subsequently completed a structured questionnaire via Mentimeter[14] assessing dimensions such as empathy, personalization, coherence, and adherence to the SH+ protocol, followed by a moderated group discussion to elicit reflections, comparisons, and evaluative commentary[15]. We conducted a thematic analysis using a hybrid coding approach [33], combining deductive codes from prior SH+ evaluations (e.g., role alignment, conversational drift) with inductive themes from iterative transcript readings.

The following key aspects emerged:

- **Conversational flexibility:** Nearly all experts praised the multi-agent chatbot for more natural, human-like interactions, but 4 noted it sometimes lacked structure and could derail the therapeutic flow.
- **Multi-agent coordination:** 3 experts reported issues with agent handovers, causing off-topic shifts and fragmented experiences.

[14] https://www.mentimeter.com/.

[15] The resulting dataset comprised chatbot interaction transcripts, the full group discussion transcript, questionnaire responses (quantitative and open-text), and participant-generated notes and memos.

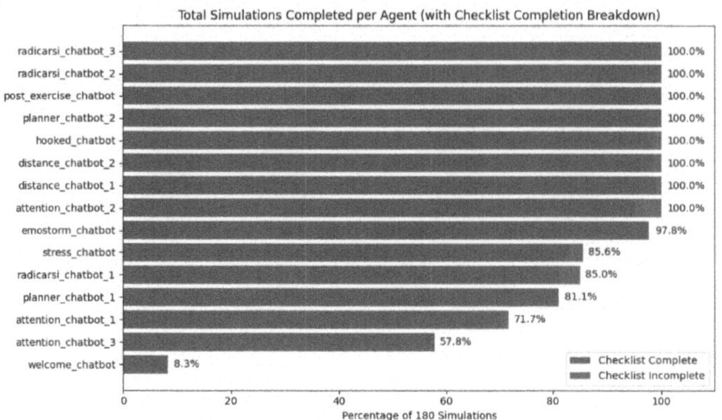

Fig. 4. The percentage of completed simulations (over 180) for each agent involved in the simulation.

Table 2. Overview of Focus Group Expert Participants

ID	Age	Gender	Role	Education
E1	45	M	Psychotherapist, Project Manager	PsyD, PhD in Psy
E2	29	F	Psychologist, Researcher	MSc in Psy
E3	35	F	Psychotherapist, Researcher	PsyD, MSc in Psy
E4	35	F	Psychotherapist, Researcher	PsyD, PhD in Psy
E5	26	F	Psychologist, Researcher	MSc in Psy

- **Empathy and responsiveness:** All experts acknowledged improved emotional tone, yet 4 observed lapses such as repetitive affirmations, pronoun errors, and gender inconsistencies.
- **Proactivity:** 4 experts found the chatbot too passive, recommending a more directive approach initially, transitioning to user-led guidance later.
- **Handling off-topic deviations:** 4 experts noted failures to redirect conversations, suggesting to set explicit boundaries to conversational exchanges (e.g. redirect to instructions after 4 messages).
- **Temporal awareness:** All experts emphasized missing time cues, recommending clear session duration, mid-session updates, and summaries to sustain engagement.

5 Discussion

The simulations' results underscore the role-play framework's potential as an effective method for developing intelligent agents capable of adhering to predefined protocols. Our findings suggest that LLMs can engage in structured dialogue and competently guide users through the conversations.

Nonetheless, our study revealed that LLMs occasionally got stuck in the simulated conversation with the synthetic patient and this also happened within the Focus Group while interacting with the human experts. This behavior reflects a known challenge in LLM performance: their sensitivity to subtle variations in instructions or conversation history, as highlighted in previous research [20]. More specifically, it emerged both from simulations and focus groups that the agent tends to prioritize users' instructions over system instructions. This also aligns with previous studies on instruction-tuned LLMs [34], suggesting that goal-oriented instructions might be critical for instruction-following agents. It should be acknowledged that the evaluation of our multi-agent system was focused on a limited set of models and it did not include an assessment of LLMs' language capabilities in Italian, which might be an impactful factor.

Anyhow, a central theme that emerged from the focus group is the need to balance between two critical dimensions: personalization of the intervention and standardization of protocol delivery. This tension mirrors a well-known challenge in traditional therapeutic settings, where professionals, such as psychologists or facilitators, are continuously required to navigate between adapting their approach to the individual's needs and maintaining fidelity to a structured therapeutic framework.

On the one hand, personalization is essential to avoid interactions that feel mechanical or overly scripted. It is this ability to make the protocol feel natural and context-sensitive that distinguishes a skilled practitioner from someone merely applying a set of instructions. The LLM should emulate this quality by adapting its responses to acknowledge the user's unique context while still anchoring the dialogue within the boundaries of the intended psychological intervention. On the other hand, the value of a structured protocol lies in its intentional sequence of cognitive, emotional, and behavioral exercises. These are designed to facilitate experiential learning and support the development of psychological flexibility or coping strategies. An effective LLM-based system, therefore, must preserve this underlying structure to ensure that the intervention remains coherent and therapeutically effective.

By the end of the focus group, all experts agreed that the current version was not ready for end-user release. Although conversation quality and empathy had improved, the absence of consistent structure was identified as a critical limitation. Future LLM-based systems for psychological support should therefore incorporate predefined structures that guide the intervention while allowing flexible transitions between different phases under the supervision of a coordinating model. Unlike a standard FSM with rigid paths, this approach would preserve clinical fidelity while still supporting adaptive, context-sensitive interactions. For instance, at the beginning of the intervention, the system should take a more directive role to orient users, and gradually adopt a more facilitative stance as users gain confidence and autonomy, in line with therapeutic best practices, ensuring that the multi-agent system does not become lost in the conversation.

6 Conclusions

This study explored the development of the SH+ chatbots, a system designed to deliver mental health support interventions. Findings show that integrating an LLM into the state-machine framework enhanced user experience, although interactions still retained a sense of artificiality due to the rigid FSM structure. In contrast, the multi-agent system substantially improved conversational quality; however, it struggled to guide users through sessions consistently. Focus group experts highlighted that this limitation reflects both a design challenge for AI systems and a deeper complexity inherent in therapeutic practice. Despite notable gains in conversational skills, we conclude that the multi-agent system is not yet ready for clinical deployment in mental health support.

Future research should investigate hybrid architectures that combine the strengths of both FSM and multi-agent approaches, aiming to create systems capable of adapting to users' conversational needs while preserving a structured framework that supports effective coaching.

References

1. Abd-Alrazaq, A.A., Alajlani, M., Alalwan, A.A., Bewick, B.M., Gardner, P., Househ, M.: An overview of the features of chatbots in mental health: a scoping review. Int. J. Med. Inform. **132**, 103978 (2019)
2. Ahmad, R., Siemon, D., Gnewuch, U., Robra-Bissantz, S.: Designing personality-adaptive conversational agents for mental health care. Inf. Syst. Front. **24**(3), 923–943 (2022)
3. Beck, A.T.: Cognitive therapy and the emotional disorders. Penguin (1979)
4. Bloor, M., Thomas, M., Frankland, J.: Focus groups in social research (2000)
5. Bolpagni, M., De Carli, S., Sanna, L., Dragoni, M., Gabrielli, S.: Valise: a virtual agent laboratory for instruction-following simulation and evaluation of llm-powered digital health interventions. In: The 28th European Conference on Artificial Intelligence (2025)
6. Bolpagni, M., De Carli, S., Sanna, L., Gabrielli, S., Dragoni, M.: Role-play large language models for short behavior change interventions: An exploratory study on brief action planning. In: Bellazzi, R., Juarez Herrero, J.M., Sacchi, L., Zupan, B. (eds.) Artificial Intelligence in Medicine, pp. 46–51. Springer Nature Switzerland, Cham (2025)
7. Bolpagni, M., Gabrielli, S.: Development of a comprehensive evaluation scale for llm-powered counseling chatbots (ces-lcc) using the edelphi method. Informatics **12**(1) (2025)
8. Boucher, E.M., et al.: Artificially intelligent chatbots in digital mental health interventions: a review. Expert Rev. Med. Devices **18**(sup1), 37–49 (2021)
9. Callahan, C., Kimber, J., Hu, E., Tanner, L., Kunkle, S., et al.: The real-world impact of app-based mindfulness on headspace members with moderate and severe perceived stress: observational study. JMIR Mhealth Uhealth **12**(1), e52968 (2024)
10. Denecke, K., Abd-Alrazaq, A., Househ, M.: Artificial intelligence for chatbots in mental health: opportunities and challenges. Multiple perspectives on artificial intelligence in healthcare: Opportunities and challenges, pp. 115–128 (2021)

11. Epping-Jordan, J.E., Harris, R., Brown, F.L., Carswell, K., Foley, C., García-Moreno, C., Kogan, C., van Ommeren, M.: Self-help plus (sh+): a new who stress management package. World Psychiatry **15**(3), 295 (2016)
12. Etikan, I., Musa, S.A., Alkassim, R.S., et al.: Comparison of convenience sampling and purposive sampling. Am. J. Theor. Appl. Stat. **5**(1), 1–4 (2016)
13. Fitzpatrick, K.K., Darcy, A., Vierhile, M.: Delivering cognitive behavior therapy to young adults with symptoms of depression and anxiety using a fully automated conversational agent (woebot): a randomized controlled trial. JMIR Mental Health **4**(2), e7785 (2017)
14. Geng, S., Döner, B., Wendler, C., Josifoski, M., West, R.: Sketch-guided constrained decoding for boosting blackbox large language models without logit access. In: Ku, L.W., Martins, A., Srikumar, V. (eds.) Proceedings of the 62nd Annual Meeting of the Association for Computational Linguistics (Volume 2: Short Papers). pp. 234–245. Association for Computational Linguistics, Bangkok, Thailand (2024). https://doi.org/10.18653/v1/2024.acl-short.23, https://aclanthology.org/2024.acl-short.23/
15. Hayes, S.C., Pierson, H.: Acceptance and commitment therapy. Springer (2005)
16. Huberty, J., Green, J., Glissmann, C., Larkey, L., Puzia, M., Lee, C., et al.: Efficacy of the mindfulness meditation mobile app "calm" to reduce stress among college students: randomized controlled trial. JMIR Mhealth Uhealth **7**(6), e14273 (2019)
17. Inkster, B., Sarda, S., Subramanian, V., et al.: An empathy-driven, conversational artificial intelligence agent (wysa) for digital mental well-being: real-world data evaluation mixed-methods study. JMIR Mhealth Uhealth **6**(11), e12106 (2018)
18. Kong, A., et al.: Better zero-shot reasoning with role-play prompting. In: Duh, K., Gomez, H., Bethard, S. (eds.) Proceedings of the 2024 Conference of the North American Chapter of the Association for Computational Linguistics: Human Language Technologies (Volume 1: Long Papers). pp. 4099–4113. Association for Computational Linguistics, Mexico City, Mexico (2024)
19. Liu, N.F., et al.: Lost in the middle: how language models use long contexts. Trans. Assoc. Comput. Linguist. **12**, 157–173 (2024)
20. Lou, R., Zhang, K., Yin, W.: Large language model instruction following: a survey of progresses and challenges. Comput. Linguist. 1–10 (2024)
21. Mediavilla, R., et al.: Effectiveness of a mental health stepped-care programme for healthcare workers with psychological distress in crisis settings: a multicentre randomised controlled trial. BMJ Ment. Health **26**(1) (2023)
22. Meywirth, S.: Designing a large language model-based coaching intervention for lifestyle behavior change. In: andviwalla, M., Söllner, M., Tuunanen, T. (eds.) International Conference on Design Science Research in Information Systems and Technology. pp. 81–94. Springer, Cham (2024). https://doi.org/10.1007/978-3-031-61175-9_6
23. Mortati, M., Magistretti, S., Cautela, C., Dell'Era, C.: Data in design: how big data and thick data inform design thinking projects. Technovation **122**, 102688 (2023)
24. Pham, K.T., Nabizadeh, A., Selek, S.: Artificial intelligence and chatbots in psychiatry. Psychiatr. Q. **93**(1), 249–253 (2022). Received 26 September 2021, Revised 23 January 2022, Accepted 26 January 2022, Published 25 February 2022
25. Purgato, M., et al.: Effectiveness of self-help plus in preventing mental disorders in refugees and asylum seekers in western europe: a multinational randomized controlled trial. Psychother. Psychosom. **90**(6), 403–414 (2021)
26. Rich, E., et al.: Automata, computability and complexity: theory and applications. Pearson Prentice Hall Upper Saddle River (2008)

27. Rollnick, S., Miller, W.R.: What is motivational interviewing? Behav. Cogn. Psychother. **23**(4), 325–334 (1995)
28. Roy, S., Sengupta, S., Bonadiman, D., Mansour, S., Gupta, A.: FLAP: Flow-adhering planning with constrained decoding in LLMs. In: Duh, K., Gomez, H., Bethard, S. (eds.) Proceedings of the 2024 Conference of the North American Chapter of the Association for Computational Linguistics: Human Language Technologies (Volume 1: Long Papers). pp. 517–539. Association for Computational Linguistics, Mexico City, Mexico (Jun 2024). 10.18653/v1/2024.naacl-long.29, https://aclanthology.org/2024.naacl-long.29/
29. Sanna, L., Bolpagni, M., Fietta, V., Gavioli, G., Franzin, M., Dragoni, M., Gabrielli, S.: Llm-enriched finite-state chatbots for mental health support: A case study on self-help+. In: Bellazzi, R., Juarez Herrero, J.M., Sacchi, L., Zupan, B. (eds.) Artificial Intelligence in Medicine, pp. 386–396. Springer Nature Switzerland, Cham (2025)
30. Shanahan, M., McDonell, K., Reynolds, L.: Role play with large language models. Nature **623**(7987), 493–498 (2023)
31. Sorin, V., et al.: Large language models and empathy: systematic review. J. Med. Internet Res. **26**, e52597 (2024)
32. Steenstra, I., Nouraei, F., Arjmand, M., Bickmore, T.: Virtual agents for alcohol use counseling: Exploring llm-powered motivational interviewing. In: Proceedings of the 24th ACM International Conference on Intelligent Virtual Agents. IVA '24, Association for Computing Machinery, New York, NY, USA (2024)
33. Swain, J.: A hybrid approach to thematic analysis in qualitative research: Using a practical example. Sage research methods (2018)
34. Wu, X., et al.: From language modeling to instruction following: Understanding the behavior shift in LLMs after instruction tuning. In: Duh, K., Gomez, H., Bethard, S. (eds.) Proceedings of the 2024 Conference of the North American Chapter of the Association for Computational Linguistics: Human Language Technologies (Volume 1: Long Papers). pp. 2341–2369. Association for Computational Linguistics, Mexico City, Mexico (2024)
35. Zhang, H., Qiao, Z., Wang, H., Duan, B., Yin, J.: Vcounselor: a psychological intervention chat agent based on a knowledge-enhanced large language model. Multimedia Syst. **30**(6), 363 (2024)

Healthcare applications

Query Carefully: Detecting the Unanswerables in Text-to-SQL Tasks

Jasmin Saxer[1(✉)], Isabella Maria Aigner[2], Luise Linzmeier[3], Andreas Weiler[1], and Kurt Stockinger[1]

[1] Institute of Computer Science, Zurich University of Applied Sciences, Technikumstrasse 9, 8401 Winterthur, Switzerland
saxr@zhaw.ch

[2] Institute of Medical Virology, University of Zurich, 8057 Zurich, Switzerland

[3] Department of Gastroenterology and Hepatology, University Hospital Zurich, University of Zurich, 8091 Zurich, Switzerland

Abstract. Text-to-SQL systems allow non-SQL experts to interact with relational databases using natural language. However, their tendency to generate executable SQL for ambiguous, out-of-scope, or unanswerable queries introduces a hidden risk, as outputs may be misinterpreted as correct. This risk is especially serious in biomedical contexts, where precision is critical. We therefore present Query Carefully, a pipeline that integrates LLM-based SQL generation with explicit detection and handling of unanswerable inputs. Building on the OncoMX component of ScienceBenchmark, we construct OncoMX-NAQ (No-Answer Questions), a set of 80 no-answer questions spanning 8 categories (non-SQL, out-of-schema/domain, and multiple ambiguity types). Our approach employs llama3.3:70b with schema-aware prompts, explicit No-Answer Rules (NAR), and few-shot examples drawn from both answerable and unanswerable questions. We evaluate SQL exact match, result accuracy, and unanswerable-detection accuracy. On the OncoMX dev split, few-shot prompting with answerable examples increases result accuracy, and adding unanswerable examples does not degrade performance. On OncoMX-NAQ, balanced prompting achieves the highest unanswerable-detection accuracy (0.8), with near-perfect results for structurally defined categories (non-SQL, missing columns, out-of-domain) but persistent challenges for missing-value queries (0.5) and column ambiguity (0.3). A lightweight user interface surfaces interim SQL, execution results, and abstentions, supporting transparent and reliable text-to-SQL in biomedical applications.

Keywords: text-to-SQL · Unanswerable Question Detection · OncoMX

1 Introduction

Relational databases are essential tools for managing and querying structured data across numerous domains, including healthcare and scientific research.

P. Bruno et al. (Eds.): HC_AIxIA_HYDRA 2025, CCIS 2830, pp. 497–509, 2026.
https://doi.org/10.1007/978-3-032-16708-8_39

These systems typically require users to formulate queries using domain-specific programming languages such as SQL (Structured Query Language), which can pose a significant barrier and restrict access to knowledge stored in relational databases to database experts.

Natural Language to SQL (text-to-SQL) systems seek to bridge this gap by translating natural language questions into executable SQL queries, enabling users to interact with databases in everyday language without requiring expertise in query languages [5]. Advances in deep learning models and especially Large Language Models (LLM)-based approaches have led to significant improvements in text-to-SQL for simple benchmarking datasets such as Spider, which provide annotated pairs of natural language questions and corresponding SQL queries [6,9].
Despite its potential, text-to-SQL remains a challenging task, especially in sensitive domains such as the healthcare sector, where errors may have serious consequences for patients. Three key challenges include:

- Generating accurate and semantically correct queries for complex questions in large domain-specific relational databases. [7]
- Avoiding the output of misleading or incorrect SQL statements. [7]
- **Handling ambiguous, incomplete, or unanswerable user queries** [11].

This work focuses on the third challenge: the identification of unanswerable questions. Real users of text-to-SQL systems are typically not database experts. As a result, they may ask questions that are ambiguous, refer to schema elements that do not exist, or lie outside the domain of the database. When confronted with such questions, LLM-based text-to-SQL systems may still attempt to generate SQL queries, resulting in incorrect outputs or misleading results. It is therefore critical that text-to-SQL systems possess the capability to detect unanswerable questions and respond appropriately, for instance, by returning a "not answerable" message or requesting clarification. Detecting unanswerable questions not only helps prevent erroneous results but can also reveal limitations of the system, contributing to the robustness and reliability of text-to-SQL interfaces in real-world applications [1,8,11,12].

In this paper, we address this challenge by extending an existing text-to-SQL dataset (ScienceBenchmark [10]) with unanswerable questions based on the OncoMX biomedical database containing information about cancer biomarkers. We then propose a pipeline that integrates LLM-based SQL generation with mechanisms to detect and handle unanswerable inputs via an intuitive chat-based interface.

2 Related Work

This project is based on the ScienceBenchmark dataset, which contains annotated question-SQL pairs for three complex, domain-specific databases: research policy making (CORDIS), astrophysics (SDSS), and cancer research (OncoMX) [10]. We specifically focus on the OncoMX database[1] due to its highly domain-

[1] https://www.oncomx.org/.

specific biomedical information and terminology. The version of OncoMX utilized in the ScienceBenchmark contains 25 tables with 2 to 14 columns each, for a total of 106 columns and an average of 2,636,771 rows per table. Funded by the U.S. National Institutes of Health (NIH), OncoMX integrates data on cancer biomarkers, differential gene expression in cancer samples, and known cancer mutations from multiple sources, making it an ideal testing database together with question-SQL pairs from the ScienceBenchmark for real-world biomedical text-to-SQL applications.

While most existing text-to-SQL research assumes that user queries are valid and answerable within a given schema, few studies have addressed the crucial problem of detecting unanswerable or ambiguous user questions.

Zhang et al. [11] introduced TriageSQL, a benchmark for classifying user questions into five intention types, including four categories of unanswerable queries (e.g., ambiguous, improper, external knowledge required, and non-SQL). They trained a RoBERTa-based classifier to predict question types based on both the input question and the database schema, highlighting the need for an intention classification step prior to SQL generation. Wang et al. [8] studied real-world usage of a commercial text-to-SQL product and found that 20% of user-submitted questions were problematic, revealing the limitations of relying on curated datasets that only include answerable questions. They collected over 3,000 failed user queries and manually grouped them into six categories of unanswerable questions. These categories—focusing on issues such as ambiguity, out-of-scope queries, and schema mismatches—form the basis for the classification framework used in our study, as further described in the methodology section. Wang et al. [8] argue that the high frequency of unanswerable queries stems from three key factors: (1) users' unfamiliarity with the database schema, (2) the inherent ambiguity and variability of natural language, and (3) the presence of semantically similar concepts within the database, which can lead to confusion. Wang et al. further focused on two categories—column ambiguity and column unanswerable—and proposed generating unanswerable questions by modifying existing tables rather than creating new unanswerable questions, making the process more controllable but also less realistic.

In the biomedical domain, the EHRSQL 2024 Shared Task addressed the challenge of building reliable text-to-SQL systems for electronic health records (EHR) [3]. This task was unique in that it intentionally included unanswerable questions, encouraging systems not only to generate correct SQL queries for answerable inputs but also to abstain from answering when queries were likely unanswerable. Evaluation metrics rewarded systems for producing no SQL for unanswerable questions and penalized both incorrect SQL and attempts to answer when the question was unanswerable. Building on this approach, we applied it to a biomedical dataset (OncoMx) and introduced categorization of unanswerable questions. This allowed us to analyze system performance across different types of unanswerability, with the goal of further enhancing the reliability and safety of text-to-SQL systems in sensitive domains such as healthcare and biomedical research.

3 Datasets

3.1 OncoMX (ScienceBenchmark)

For the answerable question evaluation, we used the OncoMX dataset provided as part of the ScienceBenchmark suite [10]. Specifically, we evaluated model performance on the development (dev) split of the dataset, which contains a total of 99 natural language questions paired with corresponding SQL queries. In addition to the gold SQL queries, we also retrieved the corresponding results from the OncoMX database. These outputs were used for comparison with model-generated queries and retrieved results. For few-shot prompting, examples are drawn from the *Seed* dataset of the ScienceBenchmark.

3.2 OncoMX-NAQ (No-Answer Questions)

To evaluate the performance on finding unanswerable questions, we created a new dataset with 80 questions in 8 categories.

Categories. We selected the following unanswerable question categories based on the literature [8,11].

1. Non-SQL Questions. This category includes questions that cannot be answered by any SQL query. Although they may be realistic and relevant to the domain, they are out of scope for structured query generation, typically requiring explanatory or procedural responses instead. For example: "Why does the TP53 gene cause cancer in some patients but not in others?"

2. Out of Schema Questions. These questions rely on information that is structurally missing from the schema or not logically accessible within the database. We distinguish two subtypes:

- **Columns Missing:** The question refers to information that is not present in any column of the schema. For example: "What is the 3D protein structure of the EGFR gene product?"
- **Values Missing:** The question depends on specific data values that do not exist in the database, even though the relevant columns may exist. For example: "List all genes overexpressed in Martian cancer tissues."

3. Out of Domain Questions. Questions in this category require knowledge that is external to the database or the application domain (in our case, OncoMX). These questions cannot be resolved without additional outside information. For example: "Which biomarkers are mentioned in the 2023 Nobel Prize research?"

4. Ambiguous Questions This group includes questions that are syntactically valid and appear to be within the scope of the schema, but are underspecified or unclear, resulting in multiple plausible interpretations. Subcategories include:

- **Column Ambiguous:** Multiple columns could reasonably fulfill the request made in the query. For example: "What is the score for EGFR in lung cancer?"
- **Value Ambiguous:** The question references a data value that could correspond to multiple entities or meanings. For example: "Find all genes linked to growth."
- **Contextual Ambiguous:** The intended meaning of the question depends heavily on context, which is not explicitly provided in the query. For example: "What are the genes that cause it?"
- **Operator Ambiguous:** The query implies a comparison or condition, but does not clearly specify which operator (e.g., slightly overexpressed) should be used. For example: "Which biomarkers are more reliable?"

Generation. To construct the unanswerable question dataset, we generated candidate questions using two distinct prompts with GPT-4o, given the database schema. The generated outputs were manually reviewed and curated by the authors, resulting in a final dataset of 80 unanswerable questions, with 10 representative examples selected for each category.

The complete set of questions and prompts are available on our GitHub repository[2].

4 Methodology

We present *Query Carefully*, a pipeline for querying the OncoMX database with natural language. The method comprises the Pipeline, Prompt Design, and Metrics. The complete code is available on GitHub(See footnote 2).

4.1 Pipeline

The full pipeline, including the user interface, is depicted in Fig. 1. Our text-to-SQL pipeline employs the large language model `llama3.3:70b` to translate natural-language questions into executable SQL. For each input question, we construct a task-specific prompt and submit it to the model. The returned text is then parsed to extract a candidate SQL statement. If no SQL is produced and the output does not explicitly indicate that the question is unanswerable, we issue a single standardized re-prompt: *"Please return a SQL query or 'unanswerable question' if the question cannot be answered with an SQL query on the database."*

If a valid SQL query is obtained, it is executed against the target database. In one setting, we include an optional post-processing step for SQL validation. If the query results in an error during execution, we prompt the LLM again with

[2] https://github.com/JasminSaxer/QueryCarefully.git.

the error message: *"Please correct the SQL query based on the following error message: <error>"*. This correction loop is allowed up to a maximum of three retries.

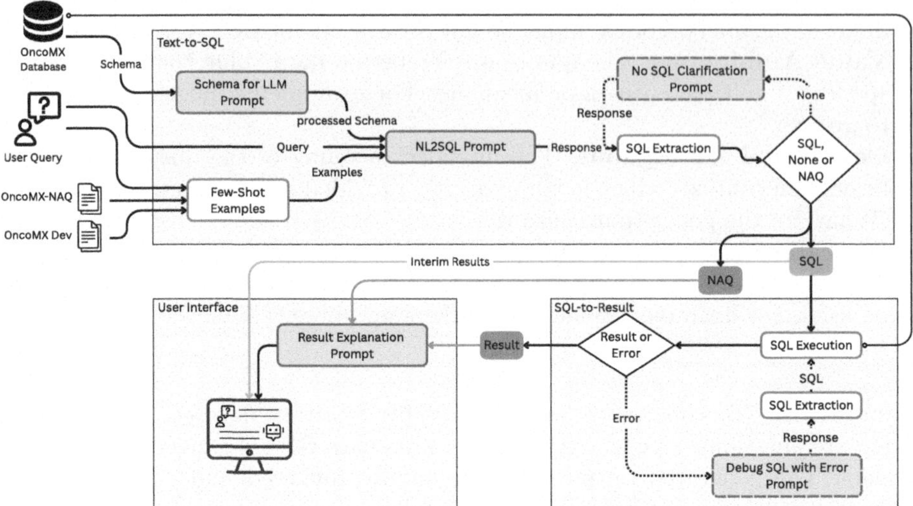

Fig. 1. Query Carefully pipeline with user interface. NAQ: No-Answer-Questions.

4.2 Prompt Design

To ensure high-quality SQL generation in our text-to-SQL setting, we carefully designed a prompt template tailored to the OncoMX relational database schema. The base prompt included a system message instructing the LLM to act as an expert in natural language to SQL translation and to generate syntactically correct PostgreSQL queries. The model was instructed to return **only** the SQL query, without additional explanation or commentary. In addition, the prompt included the reformatted and human-readable database schema.

Schema Representation. The database schema was reformatted to be more LLM-friendly using GPT-4o, ensuring that table and column names are readable and semantically meaningful. The full schema was presented to the model in a structured and human-readable format, listing each table along with its columns, data types, foreign key relationships, and column-level comments to preserve semantic context.

Handling Unanswerable Questions. To ensure that the model does not attempt to generate SQL queries for questions that cannot be reliably answered from the database, we included explicit instructions in the system prompt, taking a similar approach to [2]. These rules were designed to guide the model to return `"unanswerable question"` when the questions shouldn't be answered.

User Prompt. The user prompt consisted of a natural language query prefixed with a short instruction. For example:

```
# Return the SQL for the following Question
[Q]: Show me all disease mutations with ref_aa E
[SQL]:
```

Few-Shot Examples. To assess the effect of in-context learning, we evaluated four prompting configurations: zero-shot, 1-shot, 3-shot, and 5-shot. In the few-shot settings, the prompt was augmented with examples of both answerable and unanswerable questions. Answerable examples included correctly grounded SQL statements, while unanswerable examples featured natural language questions followed by the response `unanswerable question`.

To select relevant few-shot examples dynamically, we used the *Alibaba-NLP /gte-Qwen2-1.5B-instruct* model to embed the natural language questions. The most similar answerable questions were retrieved from the seed OncoMX ScienceBenchmark dataset. The most similar unanswerable questions were retrieved from our new dataset, removing the question to be answered. Cosine similarity was used as the measure of similarity.

A full prompt example is shown in GitHub.

4.3 Metrics

To comprehensively evaluate our text-to-SQL system, we report performance across three distinct metrics, each capturing a different aspect of system behavior: syntactic correctness, semantic accuracy, and robustness to unanswerable queries. Each metric is computed over the answerable or unanswerable questions dataset and reported as an accuracy score: the number of correct predictions divided by the total number of evaluated queries.

SQL Exact Match Accuracy. This metric checks whether the predicted SQL string exactly matches the gold (reference) SQL query after normalization (i.e., converting to lowercase and removing extra whitespace). It is a strict comparison that does not tolerate semantically equivalent but syntactically different queries.

Result Accuracy. This metric evaluates the semantic correctness of a predicted SQL query by comparing its execution result with that of the gold (reference) query. It supports multiple levels of comparison to account for variations in formatting or minor structural differences:

- *Exact Match:* The result tables are identical in both content and structure, including row order and column names.
- *Soft Correct:* The predicted and gold results contain the same data, allowing for differences in row order, column names, and the presence of identifier columns (e.g., `id`). The soft correct score is inspired by [4].
- *DB Error:* The predicted SQL query could not be executed successfully due to a database error (e.g., syntax error or invalid reference).

Unanswerable Question Detection. This metric evaluates the system's ability to correctly identify questions that cannot be answered. It checks whether the model returns the indicator `"unanswerable question"` for queries labeled as unanswerable in the gold data. Additionally, we also verify that the model does not return `"unanswerable question"` for answerable queries.

5 Results

We evaluated prompt designs on the OncoMX Dev dataset and on OncoMX-NAQ, our extension of OncoMX Dev with 10 additional unanswerable questions per category (Fig. 2). On OncoMX Dev, adding the "No-Answer Rules" (NAR) alone had no effect on the accuracy (accuracy 0.5). Including answerable examples modestly improved accuracy to 0.6, with the 5-shot prompt performing best. Adding both answerable and unanswerable examples produced similar accuracies, showing that positive examples enhance answerability detection and unanswerable examples do not impact performance on datasets without unanswerable questions. On our OncoMX-NAQ dataset, the NAR alone resulted in an accuracy of 0.37. Adding answerable examples improved performance regardless of in-context learning, though it stayed below OncoMX dev levels. Increasing unanswerable examples further boosted accuracy, surpassing OncoMX dev at 5-shot. The highest accuracy (close to 0.8) was achieved with both answerable and unanswerable examples, highlighting the value of balanced prompting for datasets containing unanswerable questions.

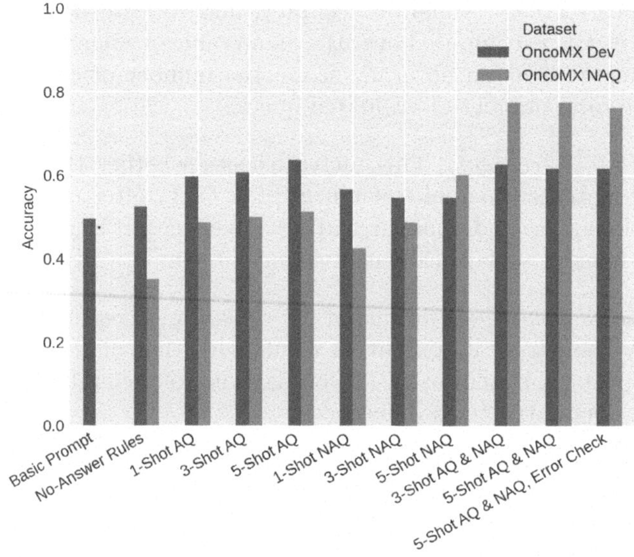

Fig. 2. Accuracy of different prompts on OncoMX Dev and OncoMX-NAQ dataset. The soft correct accuracy of OncoMX Dev is shown.

5.1 OncoMX Dev

Figure 3 compares accuracy metrics on the OncoMX dev set across prompt variants. Exact SQL matches are observed only when using in-context learning (ICL) with answerable examples from the OncoMX Seed split, indicating that a strict SQL exact match is an insufficient standalone metric for text-to-SQL evaluation. Across all prompts, the *soft-correct* category occurs only rarely; in most cases, the system either reproduces the gold result set exactly or diverges substantially. Introducing the error-checking loop removes database execution errors but increases incorrect results, suggesting that syntactic validation alone does not guarantee factual correctness and that many queries remain intrinsically challenging for the model.

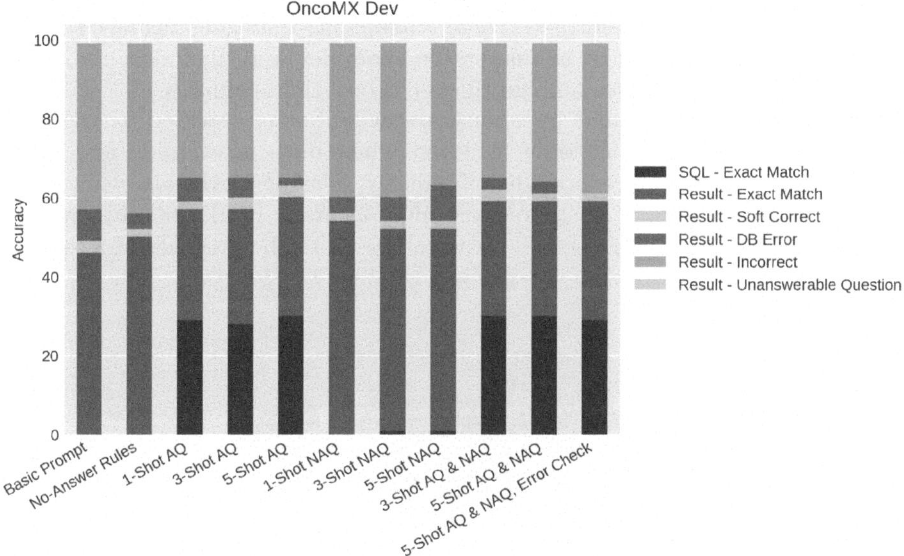

Fig. 3. Different measurements of ScienceBenchmark (OncoMX dev) per prompt type. AQ: Answerable Questions, NAQ: No-Answer Questions.

5.2 Accuracy by No-Answer Question Type

We now analyze how unanswerable questions are detected. To further dissect the effect of the NAR on different categories of unanswerable questions, we performed a more detailed unanswerable question category-wise analysis (Fig. 4). This revealed differences in the detectability of unanswerable questions across types:

- Structurally defined categories such as *Non-SQL*, *Columns Missing*, and *Out of Domain* showed moderate baseline accuracy with the NAR alone (0.6–0.65). Adding either answerable or unanswerable examples improved accuracy substantially, with prompts containing both types reaching near-perfect detection for these categories.
- In the *Values Missing*category, baseline accuracy was low (0.3) and improved only when both answerable and unanswerable examples were included, reaching a maximum of 0.5. This reflects the difficulty of detecting missing values from schema information alone, as missing columns can be directly inferred from schema details, while missing values cannot.
- Ambiguous categories (*Column Ambiguous*, *Value Ambiguous*, *Contextual Ambiguous*, *Operator Ambiguous*) showed more varied patterns. Notably, *Column Ambiguous* questions were poorly classified (max accuracy 0.3), as text-to-SQL often generated SQL referencing one fitting column without recognizing ambiguity. By contrast, *Value Ambiguous* questions achieved higher accuracy, especially when unanswerable examples were included, indicating the model better handles ambiguity over values than columns.
- For *Contextual Ambiguous* questions, about half were detected by the NAR alone, with full accuracy only achieved when both answerable and unanswerable examples were provided. Similarly, *Operator Ambiguous*questions required both example types to reach high accuracy (0.9). One misclassified question was ultimately deemed answerable due to the presence of a relevant database column.

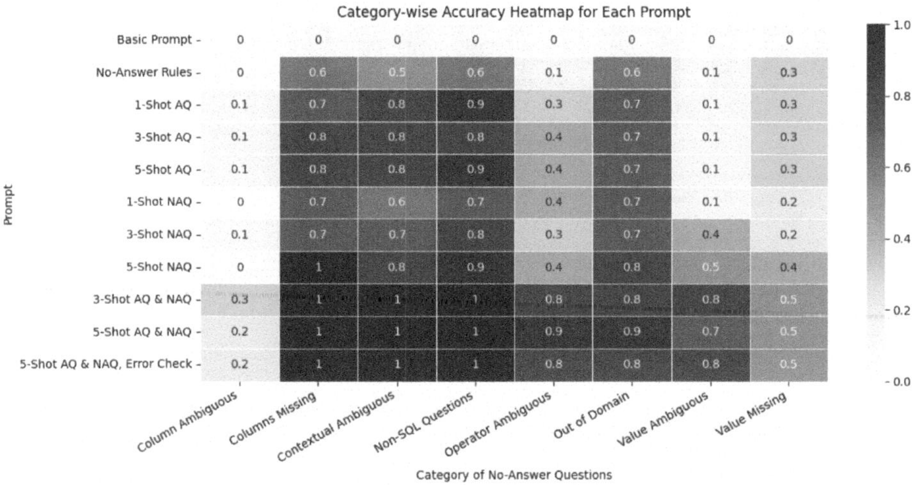

Fig. 4. Accuracy of detection of unanswerable questions divided by category and prompt. AQ: Answerable Questions, NAQ: No-Answer Questions.

Interestingly, including answerable examples alone improved unanswerable question detection in nearly all categories more than including unanswerable examples alone (average accuracy 0.49 vs. 0.43, compared to 0.35 with NAR only). However, combining both example types consistently yielded the highest accuracy in all categories.

5.3 Text-to-SQL User Interface

We provide a lightweight web interface for interacting with the *Query Carefully* pipeline (see Fig. 5). Users select the large language model from a drop-down menu (default: `llama3.3:70b`), enter a natural language question about the OncoMX database, and receive the generated SQL, the corresponding result table, and a short answer to the question. The interface surfaces intermediate steps, including the SQL preview, execution status, and any error messages. By making the SQL and outputs explicit, the UI supports transparency, easy verification by domain experts, and rapid iteration on query phrasing. When the model detects an unanswerable question, it returns an explanation why it can't answer the question and gives methods for improvement.

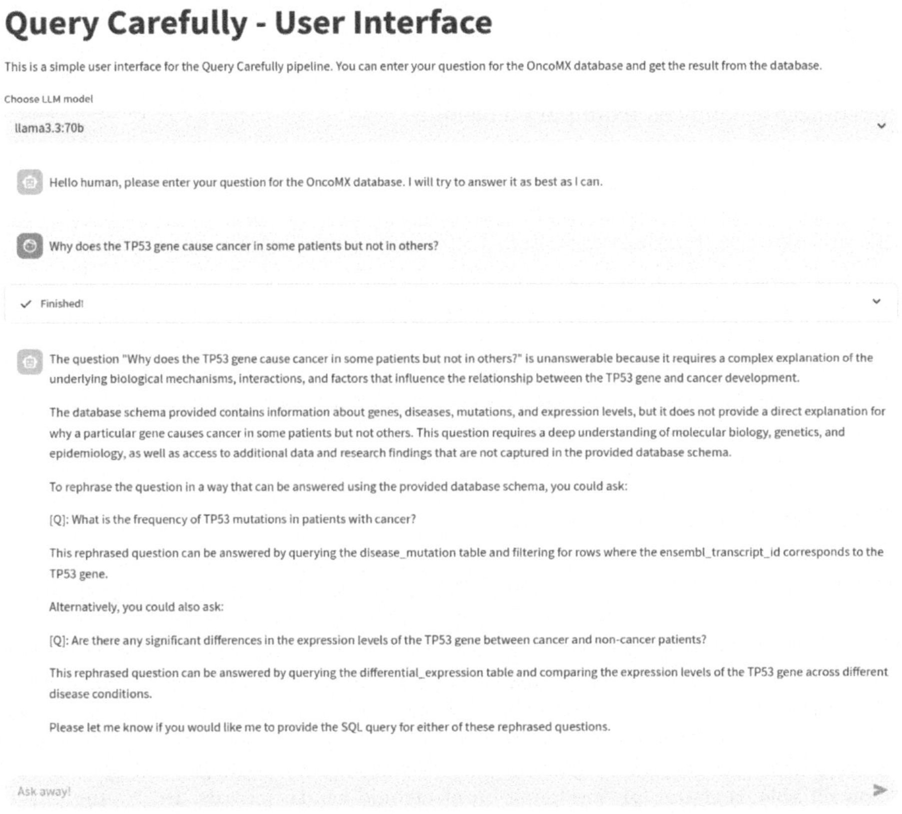

Query Carefully - User Interface

This is a simple user interface for the Query Carefully pipeline. You can enter your question for the OncoMX database and get the result from the database.

Choose LLM model

llama3.3:70b

Hello human, please enter your question for the OncoMX database. I will try to answer it as best as I can.

Why does the TP53 gene cause cancer in some patients but not in others?

✓ Finished!

The question "Why does the TP53 gene cause cancer in some patients but not in others?" is unanswerable because it requires a complex explanation of the underlying biological mechanisms, interactions, and factors that influence the relationship between the TP53 gene and cancer development.

The database schema provided contains information about genes, diseases, mutations, and expression levels, but it does not provide a direct explanation for why a particular gene causes cancer in some patients but not others. This question requires a deep understanding of molecular biology, genetics, and epidemiology, as well as access to additional data and research findings that are not captured in the provided database schema.

To rephrase the question in a way that can be answered using the provided database schema, you could ask:

[Q]: What is the frequency of TP53 mutations in patients with cancer?

This rephrased question can be answered by querying the disease_mutation table and filtering for rows where the ensembl_transcript_id corresponds to the TP53 gene.

Alternatively, you could also ask:

[Q]: Are there any significant differences in the expression levels of the TP53 gene between cancer and non-cancer patients?

This rephrased question can be answered by querying the differential_expression table and comparing the expression levels of the TP53 gene across different disease conditions.

Please let me know if you would like me to provide the SQL query for either of these rephrased questions.

Ask away!

Fig. 5. Example of an unanswerable question on the user interface.

6 Conclusion

Text-to-SQL systems should account for user expertise and potential unanswerable queries, a limitation in current benchmark datasets, particularly in domains such as medicine where non-SQL experts may misinterpret results. Existing datasets like PRACTIQ [1] classify queries based on SQL statements into categories such as ambiguous or nonexistent columns, filters, and joins. In contrast, our work extends this approach by also including non-SQL and out-of-domain questions, capturing a broader range of real-world user queries. Conversational approaches, such as PRACTIQ and Sphinteract [12], enhance user interaction by providing explanations for unanswerable queries. Nevertheless, effective use requires that users either identify the relevant columns themselves or are provided with explicit schema annotations to guide them to find the matching query. Methods like "Disambiguate First, Parse Later" (Saparina & Lapata, 2025) and "Is Long Context All You Need" (Chung, 2025) show that generating multiple interpretations or leveraging extended context windows can help resolve ambiguity, albeit with higher computational cost. Our results align with prior findings that example-based prompting improves text-to-SQL question classification [1,12], but uniquely demonstrate that answerable examples can contribute more to detecting unanswerable queries than negative examples, highlighting the importance of balanced example inclusion.

Limitations of our study include challenges in detecting specific categories of unanswerable queries, particularly those involving missing values or column and value ambiguities. Furthermore, identifying unanswerable queries represents only an initial stage. Incorporating mechanisms to propose potential resolutions, as suggested in PRACTIQ or Sphinteract could further enhance the robustness of text-to-SQL systems.

Disclosure of Interests. The authors have no competing interests to declare that are relevant to the content of this article.

References

1. Dong, M., et al.: PRACTIQ: A Practical Conversational Text-to-SQL dataset with Ambiguous and Unanswerable Queries (Oct 2024). https://doi.org/10.48550/arXiv.2410.11076
2. Jo, Y., Lee, S., Seo, M., Hwang, S.J., Lee, M.: LG AI Research & KAIST at EHRSQL 2024: Self-Training Large Language Models with Pseudo-Labeled Unanswerable Questions for a Reliable Text-to-SQL System on EHRs (May 2024). https://doi.org/10.48550/arXiv.2405.11162
3. Lee, G., Kweon, S., Bae, S., Choi, E.: Overview of the EHRSQL 2024 Shared Task on reliable Text-to-SQL modeling on electronic health records. In: Naumann, T., Ben Abacha, A., Bethard, S., Roberts, K., Bitterman, D. (eds.) Proceedings of the 6th Clinical Natural Language Processing Workshop, pp. 644–654. Association for Computational Linguistics, Mexico City, Mexico (Jun 2024). https://doi.org/10.18653/v1/2024.clinicalnlp-1.62

4. Nooralahzadeh, F., et al.: StatBot.Swiss: bilingual open data exploration in natural language. In: Findings of ACL (2024). https://doi.org/10.18653/v1/2024.findings-acl.326
5. Popescu, A.M., Etzioni, O., Kautz, H.: Towards a theory of natural language interfaces to databases. In: Proceedings of the 8th international conference on Intelligent user interfaces, pp. 149–157. ACM, Miami Florida USA (Jan 2003). https://doi.org/10.1145/604045.604070
6. Sala, L., Sullutrone, G., Bergamaschi, S.: Text-to-SQL with large language models: exploring the promise and pitfalls. https://ceur-ws.org/Vol-3741/paper65.pdf
7. Singh, A., Shetty, A., Ehtesham, A., Kumar, S., Khoei, T.T.: A survey of large language model-based generative ai for text-to-SQL: benchmarks, applications, use cases, and challenges. In: 2025 IEEE 15th Annual Computing and Communication Workshop and Conference (CCWC), pp. 00015–00021 (Jan 2025). https://doi.org/10.1109/CCWC62904.2025.10903689
8. Wang, B., Gao, Y., Li, Z., Lou, J.G.: Know what i don't know: handling ambiguous and unknown questions for text-to-SQL. In: Rogers, A., Boyd-Graber, J., Okazaki, N. (eds.) Findings of the Association for Computational Linguistics: ACL 2023, pp. 5701–5714. Association for Computational Linguistics, Toronto, Canada (Jul 2023). https://doi.org/10.18653/v1/2023.findings-acl.352
9. Yu, T., et al.: Spider: a large-scale human-labeled dataset for complex and cross-domain semantic parsing and text-to-SQL task. In: Riloff, E., Chiang, D., Hockenmaier, J., Tsujii, J. (eds.) Proceedings of the 2018 Conference on Empirical Methods in Natural Language Processing, pp. 3911–3921. Association for Computational Linguistics, Brussels, Belgium (Oct 2018). https://doi.org/10.18653/v1/D18-1425
10. Zhang, Y., Deriu, J., Katsogiannis-Meimarakis, G., Kosten, C., Koutrika, G., Stockinger, K.: ScienceBenchmark: a complex real-world benchmark for evaluating natural language to SQL systems. Proc. VLDB Endowm. **17**(4), 685–698 (Dec 2023). https://doi.org/10.14778/3636218.3636225
11. Zhang, Y., Dong, X., Chang, S., Yu, T., Shi, P., Zhang, R.: Did you ask a good question? a cross-domain question intention classification benchmark for text-to-SQL (Oct 2020). https://doi.org/10.48550/arXiv.2010.12634
12. Zhao, F., Deep, S., Psallidas, F., Floratou, A., Agrawal, D., Abbadi, A.E.: Sphinteract: resolving ambiguities in nl2sql through user interaction. Proc. VLDB Endowm. **18**(4), 1145–1158 (Dec 2024). https://doi.org/10.14778/3717755.3717772, publisher: Association for Computing Machinery (ACM)

Multi-agent Dynamic Resource Allocation: A Reinforcement Learning Approach

Stefania Costantini[1], Giovanni De Gasperisù[1], Pasquale De Meo[2], Francesco Gullo[1](✉), and Alessandro Provetti[2,3]

[1] University of L'Aquila, L'Aquila, Italy
{stefania.costantini,giovanni.degasperis,francesco.gullo}@univaq.it
[2] University of Messina, Messina, Italy
pdemeo@unime.it
[3] Birkbeck, University of London, London, UK
a.provetti@bbk.ac.uk

Abstract. We investigate the problem of cooperative resource allocation in multi-agent systems, focusing on dynamic scenarios such as hospital networks. In our model, agents (e.g., hospitals) aim to redistribute limited resources, such as medical personnel, in a way that satisfies both local constraints and global equity objectives. We devise a reinforcement learning approach to a dynamic scenario with time-varying resource needs. We empirically evaluate the proposed approach through extensive experiments. Our results demonstrate the effectiveness of the approach.

1 Introduction

The fair and efficient allocation of resources in decentralised environments has long been a fundamental challenge in Artificial Intelligence (AI) and Economics [1]. In domains where autonomous agents pursue common goals, such as healthcare networks (e.g., the British National Health Service (NHS)) [2], wireless networks [3], or cloud computing networks [4], the ability to enable cooperation without centralised authority is of both theoretical and practical importance.

In this work, we consider a network of agents managing local resources to achieve individual objectives while cooperating toward a collective goal through resource exchanges (e.g., lending). This paradigm aligns with the concept of *fairness*, which ensures equitable outcomes while maintaining system functionality. Our motivating example is an idealized model of the NHS healthcare network: hospitals manage their physician rosters but may temporarily lend doctors to others during localized emergencies (e.g., outbreaks of transmissible diseases). This scenario shares similarities with the interbanking scenario [5,6], though healthcare systems differ in their universal objective of avoiding hospital failures, unlike banking systems where central banks underwrite systemic stability.

A number of approaches have been proposed so far to allocating resources in multi-agent systems (MARA), including Distributed Constraint Optimization

P. Bruno et al. (Eds.): HC_AIxIA_HYDRA 2025, CCIS 2830, pp. 510–522, 2026.
https://doi.org/10.1007/978-3-032-16708-8_40

[7], Social Choice Theory [8], and Market-Based Coordination [9]. Among these, *Nash Welfare Optimization (NWO)* stands out as a principled method. NWO models societal welfare as the geometric mean of individual utilities. The NWO formulation balances efficiency and fairness by prioritizing improvements for agents with lower allocations and it comes with no surprise that NWO has been widely studied for its theoretical guarantees and practical effectiveness [10,11].

However, we identify three critical limitations in its application to healthcare networks, namely:

(a) Minimum vs. Target Staffing: while NWO ensures hospitals meet *baseline staffing* thresholds (that is, we assume that each hospital has at least m_i doctors who ensure its functioning), it ignores *aspirational targets* (that is, we assume that each hospital wants at least t_i doctors) needed for optimal service delivery. In some cases, it is appropriate to concentrate more resources in highly specialised medical centres (such as hospitals specialising in rare diseases or hospitals involved in innovative clinical trials), even if this may lead to slight inequalities in the distribution of staff. The NWO method cannot meet this requirement.

(b) Constraint Handling: NWO lacks explicit mechanisms to enforce global constraints, such as the fact that the total number of doctors must be constant or hard lower bounds on m_i thresholds. Specifically, the constraint on the overall size of the labour force is a direct consequence of public expenditure management policies, which in some countries impose a freeze on the recruitment of new staff [12].

(c) Dynamic Adaptability: in emergencies (e.g., pandemics), staffing needs fluctuate rapidly. NWO (as well as any other method based on an optimisation algorithm) requires replanning the allocation of doctors from scratch after each change, but this is a computationally prohibitive task for large hospital networks, and it is useless when updates in staffing requirements vary rapidly over time.

In our previous work [13], we addressed the above limitations *(a)*-*(c)* focusing on a *static scenario* only, i.e., assuming that the staffing needs of each hospital are fixed over time. In this paper, we extend that work by tackling the same problem in the novel *dynamic scenario* in which the demand for staff vary over time. Particularly, we consider two specific settings: *(a) Shifting Targets*, i.e., the staffing needs of a single hospital undergo a small variation (an increase or decrease of two units) at each point in time, and *(b) Shocking Targets*, i.e., we assume that a randomly selected hospital loses half of its staff due to unexpected and exceptional events, but it still satisfies the constraint of minimum operability. We introduce a *Proximal Policy Optimisation* (PPO)-based [14] reinforcement learning (RL) agent. Our agent learns to redistribute staff incrementally, avoiding full re-optimisation. In addition, PPO uses *clipped objective functions* to avoid destructive policy updates. A further novelty of our approach is that it attempts to satisfy constraints by appropriately reshaping its reward function. Experiments reveal that our RL approach responds well to changes in staffing requirements without having to recalculate the optimal solution from scratch, thus it excels in dynamic scenarios such as pandemics or seasonal shifts in demand.

While our approach is grounded in healthcare, its principles generalize to other domains requiring cooperative resource redistribution.

The remainder of the paper is organized as follows: Sect. 2 presents background on our resource allocation framework in a static settings, originally introduced in our previous work [13]. Section 3 discusses the main contribution of this paper, i.e., a dynamic scenario for staff allocation. Section 4 outlines the experimental setup and benchmarks, followed by an in-depth analysis of the results. Section 5 discusses related literature in multi-agent resource allocation. Finally, in Sect. 6 we draw our conclusions and highlight directions for future research.

2 Preliminaries

Let us begin with an idealised multi-agent resource allocation framework that models an NHS-style healthcare domain. We are given a set of n hospitals, denoted as $\mathcal{H} = \{\vec{h}_1, \vec{h}_2, \dots \vec{h}_n\}$ where each hospital $\vec{h}$ has three dimensions: the current number of doctors available, c_i, the target rooster, t_i and the minimum number of doctors needed for the hospital to operate, m_i. In a static scenario, the total number of doctors available in $\mathcal{H}$ is fixed, i.e., $\sum_{i=1}^{n} c_i = C$.

Of course, if some hospital $\vec{h}_i$ has critically-low levels of staff, i.e., $c_i \leq m_i$, the best option is to recruit more doctors. Yet, this may not be possible, even for relatively-long interim periods. Hence, we consider transferring doctors from other hospitals to improve the overall efficiency of the hospital system $\mathcal{H}$. The idea is that 'wealthy' hospitals (those operating at or near full rooster) could lend doctors to $\vec{h}_i$. This practice is common in NHS-style health systems, e.g., in summer when population density in tourism areas shows huge alterations. Similarly, emergency situations, such as the outbreak of epidemics and their containment in the geographical areas where they have occurred, may require the emergency re-assignment of medical staff to cope with the spike in hospital admissions.

The goal now is to model the emergency re-distribution scenario so as to compute solutions that are optimal or near-optimal with respect to the global objective of maintaining all hospitals viable and operating, while fulfilling all the constraints on the capacity of individual hospitals. In [13], we considered a *static scenario*, i.e., we assume that the targets for each hospital are constant over time. We handled such a static scenario by devising three optimisation strategies, based on quadratic programming [15], Progressive Taxation [16], and Nash Welfare Optimisation [17,18], respectively, along with a hybrid approach that combines the latter two. The focus of this work is instead on a *dynamic setting*, i.e., when sudden, time-varying changes in hospital demand arise. In the following section, we describe such a dynamic scenario and present the proposed reinforcement learning approach to handle it.

3 Multi-agent Resource Allocation: the Dynamic Scenario

In real scenarios, the size of a hospital workforce quickly (and often unexpectedly) fluctuates over time. For example, during pandemics or natural disasters, the number of doctors on duty in a hospital is usually much higher than what is generally considered satisfactory. In *dynamic* scenarios where staffing requirements can vary over time, the approaches described in Sect. 2 may not be practical because they would require solving an optimization problem from scratch for each change in staffing needs.

An effective (i.e., computationally feasible yet accurate) solution to such a dynamic hospital staff re-allocation problem is given by *Reinforcement Learning* (RL). We point out that a RL approach can be applied to a static scenario. In this regard, we model our problem as a *Markov Decision Process* [19], whose states correspond to the various hospitals. As described above, each hospital $\vec{h}_i$ is described by a three-component vector: the current number c_i of doctors on duty in that hospital, the minimum number m_i of doctors needed to ensure its operation, and the number t_i of doctors (target) that the hospital would like to have.

We employ a reward given by three contributions: *a) Deviation from target*, i.e., the reward penalises configurations where the current allocation of doctors is far from the desired target distribution; *b) Violations of minima*, i.e., heavy penalties are given if any hospital drops below its minimum number of staff units needed to guarantee its operation, and *c) Fairness in transfer procedures*, i.e., uneven transfers of doctors discouraged; the imbalance of the entire re-allocation process is quantified by the variance of the distribution of doctors across the various hospitals. Formally, denoting by y_i the output number of staff units at hospital $\vec{h}_i$ after staff redistribution among hospitals and by a the distribution of the overall staff units transferred from a hospital to another, our reward $\mathcal{R}$ is defined as:

$$\mathcal{R} = -\underbrace{\sum_{i=1}^{n}(y_i - t_i)^2}_{\text{target error}} - \underbrace{\eta \sum_{i=1}^{n} \max(0, m_i - y_i)}_{\text{minima violations}} - \underbrace{\sigma^2(a)}_{\text{fairness}}, \tag{1}$$

where $\eta \gg 1$ is a multiplicative factor whose role is to heavily penalize violations of the minimum staff number requirement. Here, we empirically consider $\eta = 100$. We adopt the well-established Proximal Policy Optimisation (PPO) algorithm of [14] to optimize the above reward. PPO, which is outlined in Algorithm 1 has two key features that make it the best choice here. First, it can operate in continuous spaces (thus allowing fractional resource transfer). Second, it yields a good tradeoff between *exploration policies* (i.e., the generation of new doctor transfer strategies) and *exploitation policies* (i.e., the application of staff transfer strategies that proved to be effective in the past). Next, we describe how the PPO algorithm is contextualized to our dynamic staff allocation scenario.

Our PPO agent learns to redistribute doctors to meet targets while respecting minima and, importantly, trying to minimize resource imbalances among

Algorithm 1. Proximal Policy Optimization for staff redistribution

1: **Input:**
2: agent parameters: $\mathbf{c}$ (current), $\mathbf{m}$ (minima), $\mathbf{t}$ (targets)
3: PPO hyperparameters: epochs K, clip ϵ, learning rates α_θ, α_ϕ
4: Advantage parameters: GAE λ, discount γ
5: **procedure** PPO
6: Initialize policy π_θ (actor) and value function V_ϕ (critic)
7: **for** iteration $= 1, 2, \ldots$ **do**
Collect trajectories $\{\psi_i\}$ by running π_θ in environment:
8: **for** each agent $i \in \{1, \ldots, N\}$ **do**
9: Observe state $s_i = [c_i, m_i, t_i]$
10: Sample action $a_i \sim \pi_\theta(\cdot|s_i)$ (transfer matrix)
11: Execute action a_i, get new state s_i' and reward r_i
12: Store (s_i, a_i, r_i, s_i') in buffer
13: **end for**
Compute advantages $\hat{A}_t$ using GAE(λ, γ):
14: **for** each trajectory ψ **do**
15: Compute δ_τ (Equation (3))
16: Compute $\hat{A}_\tau$ (Equation (4))
17: **end for**
Optimize surrogate objective for K epochs:
18: **for** epoch $=$ 1 to K **do**
19: Sample minibatch from buffer
20: Compute $r_\tau(\theta) = \frac{\pi_\theta(a_\tau|s_\tau)}{\pi_{\theta_{\text{old}}}(a_\tau|s_\tau)}$
21: Compute L^{CLIP} (Equation (5))
22: Update policy (Equation (6))
23: Update value function (Equation (7))
24: **end for**
25: **end for**
26: **end procedure**

hospitals. The PPO algorithm uses two separate neural networks, that is the *actor* and the *critic.*

The actor network defines the policy of the agent, i.e., it takes the current state s as input and computes the probability distribution $\pi_\theta(a|s)$ of all possible actions a for state s; such a distribution is used to select the next action.

Following the setting of [13], a fractional transfer of resources is permitted in our scenario. Thus, we have that the actor network parametrises a Gaussian distribution (with a predefined mean and standard deviation). The critic network is parametrised by ϕ and estimates the *expected cumulative future reward* starting from the state s_0:

$$V_\phi(s) \sim \mathbb{E}\left(\sum_{\tau=0}^{+\infty} \gamma^\tau r_\tau | s = s_0\right) \tag{2}$$

.

The γ coefficient (which we empirically set to 0.99 here) is the *discount factor* and its purpose is to reduce the effect of remote actions (i.e., actions chosen many steps before). The critic network acts as an estimator of the advantages related to a particular action.

Our algorithm collects possible trajectories to be used in the training phase. Specifically, it observes the current state for each time step and uses the distribution $\pi_\theta(a_i|s_i)$ to sample the next action a_i. We call s_i the state after performing action a_i and r_i the reward received.

Our algorithm computes the Generalised Advantage Estimation (GAE), i.e., it quantifies whether (and by how much) a given action produces benefits more than the expected benefits. To compute the GAE, we first consider the correct reward δ_τ obtained from the reward r_τ received by the agent at time step τ, and then adds to it the difference between the critic network at time $\tau+1$ (weighted by the discount factor λ) and the critic network at time τ:

$$\delta_\tau = r_\tau + \gamma V_\phi(s_{\tau+1}) - V_\phi(s_\tau) \tag{3}$$

Next, we compute the expected advantage $\hat{A}_\tau$ as the weighted average of the corrected rewards δ_τ; the weights used to compute the average are exponentially decreasing and they are obtained by multiplying the discount factor γ by a coefficient λ (which we set equal to 0.95 in our tests). This leads to the following:

$$\hat{A}_\tau = \sum_{l=0}^{\infty}(\gamma\lambda)^l \delta_{\tau+l} \tag{4}$$

The $\gamma\lambda$ coefficient aims to achieve a good trade-off between the bias and variance derived from the trajectories, and, thus, it can be interpreted as a reward reshaping technique.

Our algorithm tries to improve the agent's policy by avoiding large but risky updates that could degrade performance. To do this, it introduces a *clipping* mechanism to limit how much the new policy can differ from the old policy (the one used to gain recent experience). Specifically, our algorithm first computes the ratio $r_\tau(\theta) = \frac{\pi_\theta(a_\tau|s_\tau)}{\pi_{\theta_{\text{old}}}(a_\tau|s_\tau)}$, which quantifies how much the new policy differs from the old one. We note that $r_\tau(\theta)$ could take large values, leading to the acceptance of new policies and the rejection of old ones; however, the new policies could cause a significant degradation in performance. For this reason, our algorithm uses a function called `clip` to constrain the probability ratio $r_\tau(\theta)$ to an interval of the type $[1-\varepsilon, 1+\varepsilon]$, thus constructing the following loss function:

$$L^{\text{CLIP}} = \mathbb{E}_\tau[\min(r_\tau(\theta)\hat{A}_\tau, \text{clip}(r_\tau(\theta), 1-\epsilon, 1+\epsilon)\hat{A}_\tau)] \tag{5}$$

Then the policy is updated via a standard gradient descent step:

$$\theta \leftarrow \theta + \alpha_\theta \nabla_\theta L^{\text{CLIP}} \tag{6}$$

and the critic is updated via mean square minimization to improve value estimates:

$$L^{\text{VF}}(\phi) = \mathbb{E}_\tau\left[\left(V_\phi(s_\tau) - \hat{R}_\tau\right)^2\right] \tag{7}$$

where $\hat{R}_\tau = \sum_{\ell=0}^{+\infty} \gamma^\ell r_{\tau+l}$.

4 Experiments

We evaluated the effectiveness of our approach through a series of experiments mainly designed to address the question about which reward components most significantly influence RL performance. We considered a testbed made up of 150 randomly-generated hospitals; i.e., for each hospital the minimum number of staff needed to function properly, the current number of doctors on the rooster, and the target number were assigned at random. To evaluate the performance of the various methods, we adopt the following metrics metrics:

1. **Target Deviation** (MAE), defined as the average difference between actual staff levels and targets:

$$\mathrm{MAE} = \tfrac{1}{N} \textstyle\sum_{i=1}^{N} |y_i - t_i| \tag{8}$$

   Ideally, we would like each hospital to have as close to the target number of doctors as possible; thus, the lower MAE, the more effective the approach to redistributing doctors.
2. **Gini Index** ($\mathcal{G}$) [20], defined as

$$\mathcal{G} = \frac{1}{N}\left(N + 1 - 2\sum_{i=1}^{N} \frac{\sum_{j=1}^{i} y_j}{\sum_{j=1}^{N} y_j}\right) \tag{9}$$

   The Gini Index is one of the most commonly used inequality measures (e.g., income inequality or inequality in life expectancy). It ranges from 0 (perfect equality) to 1 (perfect inequality). In our case, a $\mathcal{G}$ close to 1 indicates that the available doctors are concentrated in a few hospitals, which is undesirable. Thus, ideally, values of $\mathcal{G}$ close to 0 should be achieved.

4.1 Results

We analyzed a dynamic scenario where the number of doctors per hospital varies over time. This assumption reflects real-world conditions: for instance, tourist destinations face seasonal population fluctuations, leading to temporary mismatches between healthcare demand and the baseline workforce capacity, and, thus, the hospital needs extra resources.

We considered a finite time horizon T partitioned into 50 discrete time steps and evaluated two distinct scenarios: a) *Shifting Targets*, where hospital-specific targets undergo minor adjustments every 10 time steps: specifically, each hospital loses or gains at most two doctors per adjustment; b) *Sudden Shock*, where a randomly selected hospital loses half its workforce at the midpoint of the time horizon $T/2$. We assume that the hospital that suffers the loss of doctors is able to satisfy the minimum operating conditions.

We tested the proposed RL approach. As baselines, we employed the four methods devised in our previous work [13] for a static setting, namely methods QP, Progressive Taxation, NWO and hybrid. For each scenario and tested method, we ran twenty independent simulations and generated time series tracking the evolution of Target Deviation and Gini. The results, averaged over all simulations, are plotted in Figs. 1a and 1b.

One immediate conclusion from the experiments is that the results for NWO, QP, and Hybrid are almost *stable* in both scenarios. We argue that this stability in performance is due to the fact that the three strategies (NWO, QP and Hybrid) dynamically re-plan staffing *from scratch,* for each hospital and for each change in staffing needs. Therefore, they are *optimal* in the sense that they immediately react to change and construct the best possible resource reallocation, albeit with different strategies. Reallocation from scratch, unfortunately, is unrealistic for several reasons. First, computational cost grows quickly with the number N of agents (hospitals). Second, the actual delays involved with staff/resource re-allocation may fall behind the rapid pace of updates, thus rendering intermediate solutions *stale* before they are executed. Third, there might be hidden size effects with large re-allocations, due to institutional, logistical, or ethical constraints.

The second takeaway message from the experimental results is that RL is able to effectively *learn* profitable re-allocation strategies, rather than recalculating optimal allocations from scratch. That becomes apparent in the Shifting Target scenario: RL reacts well to small variations in staff levels and achieves a relatively stable Target Deviation and Gini Index.

In the *Sudden Shock* scenario, the RL strategy initially experiences a sharp decline in both metrics following the drastic loss of staff at one location. However, the RL agent has learned an effective resource redistribution strategy that allows it to stabilise Target Deviation and Gini, indeed at slightly lower levels that before the shock.

4.2 Ablation Study

A controlled ablation study was designed to systematically evaluate how individual reward components influence the performance of reinforcement learning in our scenarios. We trained four different RL agents: (1) the proposed agent equipped with the full reward formulation (Target Deviation + minimum staffing penalty + fairness), (2) an agent without the fairness term, (3) an agent without the minimum staffing penalty, and (4) an agent without the Target Deviation component. Each configuration was evaluated over five independent trials to ensure statistical robustness.

The results of this ablation study are reported in Fig. 2. The figure shows that the Target Deviation component is the most significant factor for both Target Deviation and Gini Index. The ablation study also reveals how the removal of the minimum and fairness component leads to a lower Gini Index than in the case of full reward, but at the price of a consistent deterioration of Target Deviation. All in all, the full reward allows for reaching the best tradeoff between Target Deviation and Gini Index.

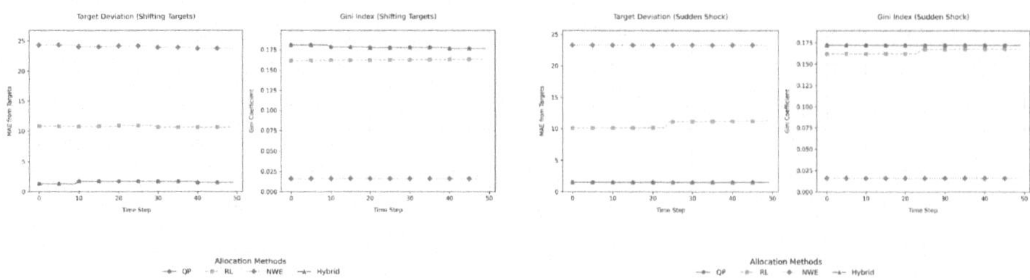

(a) Average Target Deviation (MAE) and Gini Index of the RL (proposed), NWO, QP, Hybrid (baselines) strategies in the Shifting Targets scenario.

(b) Average Target Deviation (MAE) and Gini Index of the RL (proposed), NWO, QP, Hybrid (baselines) strategies in the Sudden Shock scenario.

Fig. 1. Comparison of RL (proposed), NWO, QP, Hybrid (baselines) strategies in the dynamic scenario

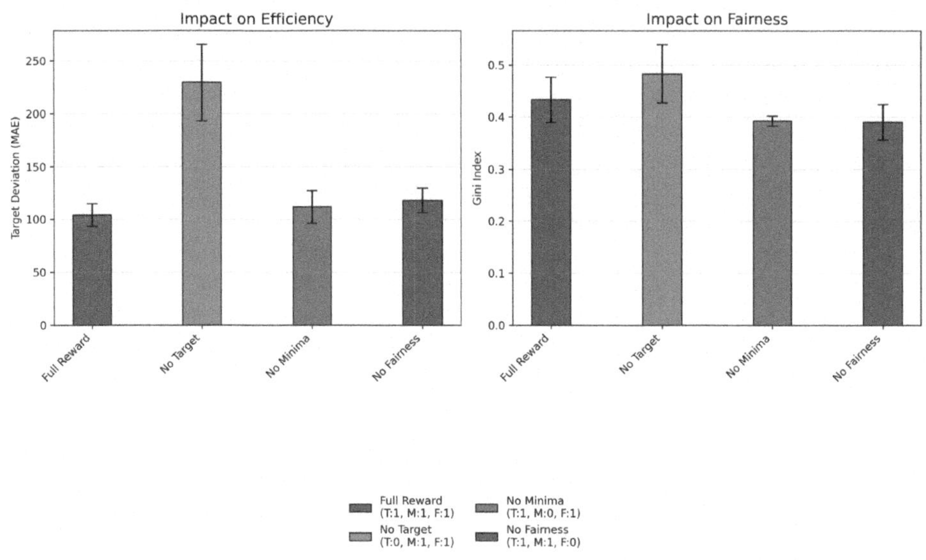

Fig. 2. Ablation study of the proposed RL strategy for each component of the reward.

5 Related Work

Multiagent Resource Allocation (MARA) constitutes a fundamental challenge in multiagent systems, requiring autonomous agents to distribute limited resources in ways that balance efficiency and fairness. Such problems arise ubiquitously [1]. As systems grow in scale and complexity, designing mechanisms that reconcile individual agent incentives with collective welfare becomes increasingly critical.

At its core, MARA involves agents negotiating resource distributions, often encountering dilemmas where self-interest conflicts with group optimality. These interactions necessitate formal frameworks that model agent behavior while guaranteeing allocations beneficial to all stakeholders [21]. Central to this challenge is the concept of *fairness*, a principle vital to both human societies and artificial systems. In applications ranging from traffic control to cloud computing, equitable resource distribution directly impacts system stability, productivity, and long-term performance [22]. The dual challenge lies in formalizing fairness mathematically while enabling practical implementation in dynamic environments. Two dominant fairness paradigms guide allocation strategies, namely *proportional fairness*, according to which resources are allocated proportionally to agents' contributions or needs, and *envy-freeness*, which ensures no agent prefers another's allocation over their own [22,23]. While extensively studied in static settings, recent work extends these criteria to dynamic environments where resources and agent populations evolve over time [24]. This shift reflects real-world demands for adaptive solutions that maintain fairness guarantees amid uncertainty.

Our work can be positioned under the broad umbrella of MARA. Specifically, we propose novel strategies for the re-allocation of resources in a multi-agent, cooperative setting.

Centralized vs. Decentralized Approaches. Traditional centralized methods, such as the Hungarian and Gale-Shapley algorithms, rely on a central authority with full system knowledge to compute optimal allocations [9]. *Nash Welfare Optimization (NWO)* offers a principled framework for fair resource distribution by maximizing the geometric mean of agent utilities. The NWO approach inherently balances efficiency and equity, prioritizing improvements for agents with lower initial utility [8]. It occupies a middle ground between *utilitarian welfare* (maximizing total utility) and *egalitarian welfare* (maximizing minimum utility) and satisfies key axiomatic properties such as scale invariance, Pareto efficiency, and independence of irrelevant alternatives [10,11]. Due to these strengths, NWO has been applied successfully in collective decision-making, project funding allocation, and fair division problems [10]. For multi-agent bandits, NWO provides fair allocations when multiple agents have heterogeneous preferences [11].

In this work, we provide a novel contextualization of NWO to the multi-agent, cooperative resource re-allocation setting, Specifically, in our scenario, the utility of an individual agent is defined as the logarithm of the difference between the number of doctors y_i allocated to hospital $\vec{h}_i$ and the minimum required m_i (possibly incremented by one to ensure positivity in the logarithmic function). Consequently, the hard constraint $y_i \geq m_i$ is embedded within the objective function. However, NWO provides no guarantee that allocations will achieve target staffing levels t_i, which represent aspirational goals for optimal service delivery. To address this limitation, we propose a novel staff reallocation method based on quadratic programming that explicitly minimizes deviations from target staffing levels while enforcing minimum operational constraints.

Dynamic Resource Allocation. In real-world applications, resource allocation evolves over time, necessitating adaptive strategies. *Constrained multi-agent*

Markov decision processes (MDPs) [25] formalize sequential allocation problems, modelling resource constraints that couple otherwise independent agents. *Reinforcement Learning (RL)* methods have proven effective in dynamic environments by continuously learning from system feedback: agents refine policies through trial-and-error interactions, achieving both higher overall utility and reduced violation of fairness requirements compared to traditional strategies [4,26]. Recent applications span cloud computing [4] and healthcare services [2], where RL adapts to fluctuating demands without manual intervention.

Our work advances this line of research by proposing the first RL-based approach in multi-agent, cooperative resource re-allocation scenarios. We employ the Proximal Policy Optimization (PPO) algorithm [14], ensuring operational feasibility by limiting the number of doctors transferred at each step. To address competing objectives—minimizing Target Deviation, avoiding minima violations, and ensuring fair workforce distribution—we design a composite reward function that integrates these goals. This formulation enables the agent to learn adaptive redistribution strategies while respecting hard constraints, overcoming the limitations of static methods.

6 Discussion, Conclusions and Future Work

This paper addressed the problem of cooperative resource re-allocation in dynamic multi-agent environments, focusing on the redistribution of hospital staff. By combining classic optimization techniques with Reinforcement Learning (RL) approaches, we demonstrated that learning-based strategies, in particular Proximal Policy Optimization (PPO), offer superior adaptability and scalability in dynamic settings. Our experimental evaluation showed that RL can effectively maintain fairness and minimise resource mismatches under uncertain and evolving conditions.

While our results are encouraging, several limitations remain. First, the study focuses on PPO, but other alternative RL algorithms such as DDPG, SAC, or A3C are available. Future work will extend the evaluation to a wider range of RL methods and assess their relative strengths and weaknesses. Furthermore, our model currently assumes fully cooperative agents; however, in realistic scenarios, agents may behave selfishly or misreport their needs. Investigating mechanisms for dealing with partial cooperation and strategic behaviour is an important direction for future research. For example, we could experiment with Multi-Agent Deep Deterministic Policy Gradient (MADDPG) [27], a method for learning in partially cooperative environments, to deal with semi-cooperative hospitals. Another limitation concerns the lack of formal guarantees regarding fairness and optimality under dynamic reallocation policies. While empirical results are promising, deriving theoretical performance bounds for RL-based allocation remains an open challenge. In addition, expanding the evaluation to include health-care-specific metrics – e.g., resilience to recurrent shocks, hospital load variance, and service continuity – will make the performance assessment more comprehensive.

Looking ahead, we see several promising developments. One direction involves the integration of online learning mechanisms to make agents continuously adapt their resource allocation strategies without offline retraining. Another direction is to embed explainability in allocation policies, making them transparent and interpretable to human operators–a crucial aspect in sensitive domains such as healthcare. Finally, hybrid frameworks that combine offline planning with online reactive adjustments may provide an effective tradeoff between optimality and adaptability.

Acknowledgments. Research partially supported by the PNRR Project CUP E13C24000430006 "Enhanced Network of intelligent Agents for Building Livable Environments - ENABLE", and by PRIN 2022 CUP E53D23007850001 Project "Trust-PACTX - Design of the Hybrid Society Humans-Autonomous Systems: Architecture, Trustworthiness, Trust, EthiCs, and EXplainability (the case of Patient Care)". A.P. is also with University of MIlan, Milan, Italy.

Declaration on Generative AI. During the preparation of this work, the author(s) used Grammarly, solely to spell check and improve the grammar. The tool was not used to alter, generate, or influence the semantic contents of the paper. The authors retain full responsibility for the accuracy, originality, and integrity of the entire work.

References

1. Jong, N., Stone, P., Taylor, M.: Multiagent resource allocation: a review of mechanisms and applications. Auton. Agent. Multi-Agent Syst. **22**, 1–29 (2008)
2. Zhao, Y., et al.: Towards a pretrained model for restless bandits via multi-arm generalization, In: Proceedings of the International Joint Conference on Artificial Intelligence, (IJCAI 2024), Jeju, South Korea, 2024, pp. 321–329 (2024)
3. Cui, J., Liu, Y., Nallanathan, A.: Multi-agent reinforcement learning-based resource allocation for UAV networks. IEEE Trans. Wireless Commun. **19**, 729–743 (2020)
4. Zhao, Y., Liu, Y., Jiang, B., Guo, T.: CE-NAS: an end-to-end carbon-efficient neural architecture search framework, In: Proceedings of the International Conference on Advances in Neural Information Processing Systems 38 (NIPS 2024), Vancouver, BC, Canada (2024)
5. Battiston, S., Puliga, M., Kaushik, R., Tasca, P., Caldarelli, G.: Debtrank: Too central to fail? financial networks, the fed and systemic risk, Sci. Reports **2** (2012) 541. https://doi.org/10.1038/srep00541
6. Tong, J., de Keijzer, B., Ventre, C.: Reducing systemic risk in financial networks through donations, In: Proceedings of the European Conference on Artificial Intelligence (ECAI 2024), volume 392, IOS Press, Santiago de Compostela, Spain, 2024, pp. 3405–3412 (2024)
7. de Jong, S., Uyttendaele, S., Tuyls, K.: Learning to reach agreement in a continuous ultimatum game, J. Artif. Intell. Res. **33**, 551–574 (2008). https://api.semanticscholar.org/CorpusID:13248455
8. Zhang, L., Xu, Y., Fang, F., Yang, Y.: Online nash social welfare maximization in multi-agent systems. In: Proceedings of the 38th AAAI Conference on Artificial Intelligence (AAAI) (2024)

9. Nongaillard, A., Sohier, H., Hilaire, V.: Centralized and distributed approaches for resource allocation: a comparative study. J. Intell. Manuf. **27**, 789–803 (2016)
10. Delemazure, T., Durand, F.: Mathieu, Aggregating correlated estimations with (almost) no training, In: Proceedins of the European Conference on Artificial Intelligence, (ECAI 2023–26th), volume 372 of Frontiers in Artificial Intelligence and Applications, IOS Press, Krakow, Poland, 2023, pp. 541–548 (2023)
11. Hossain, S., Micha, E., Shah, N.: Fair algorithms for multi-agent multi-armed bandits. Adv. Neural. Inf. Process. Syst. **34**, 24005–24017 (2021)
12. Papanicolas, I., Woskie, L.R., Jha, A.K.: Health care spending in the united states and other high-income countries. JAMA **319**, 1024–1039 (2018)
13. Costantini, S., De gasperis, G., De Meo, P., Provetti, A.: Resource allocation with cooperative agents. In: Proceedings of the 32nd RCRA workshop on Experimental evaluation of algorithms for solving problems with combinatorial explosion (RCRA 2025), held in conjunction with the 41st International Conference on Logic Programming (ICLP) (2025)
14. Schulman, J., Wolski, F., Dhariwal, P., Radford, A., Klimov, O.:Proximal policy optimization algorithms, arXiv preprint arXiv:1707.06347 (2017)
15. Boyd, S.P., Vandenberghe, L.: Convex optimization, Cambridge University Press, (2004)
16. Stiglitz, J.E., Rosengard, J.K.: Economics of the Public Sector: Fourth International Student Edition, WW Norton & Company (2015)
17. Moulin, H.: Fair division and collective welfare, MIT press (2004)
18. Nash, J.F., et al.: The bargaining problem. Econometrica **18**, 155–162 (1950)
19. Feinberg, E.A., Shwartz, A.: Handbook of Markov Decision Processes: Methods and Applications, volume 40, Springer Science & Business Media (2012)
20. Farris, F.A.: The gini index and measures of inequality. Am. Math. Mon. **117**, 851–864 (2010)
21. Ceragioli, D., Rossi, F., Venable, B.: Fairness-aware distributed planning for resource allocation in multiagent systems. In: Proceedings of the 33rd International Joint Conference on Artificial Intelligence (IJCAI) (2024)
22. Jiang, A., Leyton-Brown, K.: Fairness in multi-agent systems with reinforcement learning. Artif. Intell. **275**, 25–64 (2019)
23. Chen, Y., Parkes, D.C.: Envy-free allocation in combinatorial auctions. Games Econom. Behav. **70**, 1–14 (2010)
24. Kash, I.A., Procaccia, A.D., Shah, N.: No-envy learning in symmetric auctions. In: Proceedings of the 14th ACM Conference on Electronic Commerce, 2013, pp. 297–314 (2013)
25. Nijs, V., Vlassis, N., De Weerdt, M.: Dynamic multi-agent resource allocation under constraints. Auton. Agent. Multi-Agent Syst. **35**, 1–34 (2021)
26. Yu, E.Y., Qin, Z., Lee, M.K., Gao, S.: Policy optimization with advantage regularization for long-term fairness in decision systems In: Proceedings of the International Conference on Neural Information Processing Systems (NIPS 2022), New Orleans, LA, USA, (2022)
27. Lowe, R., Wu, Y., Tamar, A., Harb, J., Abbeel, P., Mordatch, I.: Multi-agent actor-critic for mixed cooperative-competitive environments. In: Advances in Neural Information Processing Systems (NeurIPS), vol. 30 (2017)

Author Index

A

Abghari, Shahrooz 398
Aguzzi, Gianluca 429
Aigner, Isabella Maria 497
Andrić, Marina 308
Apriceno, Gianluca 384, 453
Armanini, Justin 352
Armenise, Doriana 467
Awuklu, Yvon K. 120

B

Babuc, Diogen 37
Bailoni, Tania 453
Balordi, Antonio 126
Barazesh Morgani, Fatemeh 182
Barbato, Francesco 64
Bartucci, Simone 93, 218
Batista, Gustavo 182
Battello, Ginevra 467
Bellan, Patrizio 429
Bellocchio, Francesco 283
Bergounioux, Jean 138
Bernasconi, Alice 126
Besozzi, Daniela 369
Bhattacharyay, Shubhayu 270
Bienvenu, Meghyn 120
Boeva, Veselka 398
Bolpagni, Marco 441, 481
Bregoli, Alessandro 283
Brunello, Andrea 467

C

Calimeri, Francesco 93, 218, 296
Camarda, Alessia Donata 93
Cante, Luigi Colucci 257
Caruso, Simone 412
Ceresa, Mario 3
Cerioli, Roberto Clemens 369
Citerio, Giuseppe 270
Conrad, Stefan 21
Consoli, Sergio 3
Costantini, Stefania 510

D

De Gasperisù, Giovanni 510
D'Ambrosi, Leonardo 231
de Campos Souza, Paulo Vitor 384
De Carli, Simone 441, 481
De Rose, Edoardo 93, 218
Deichsel, Lucas 323
Di Martino, Beniamino 257
De Meo, Pasquale 510
Dodaro, Carmine 412
Dörr, Ann-Kathrin 243
Dragoni, Mauro 308, 384, 429, 441, 453, 481
Driul, Lorenza 467
Dupuy, Théo 196

F

Fidanza, Riccardo 99
Fietta, Valentina 481
Filice, Francesca 218
Fortiş, Teodor-Florin 37
Franco, Ron 336
Franzin, Mattia 481

G

Gabrielli, Silvia 441, 481
Gal, Kobi 336
Galiberti, Stefania 270
Gavioli, Giorgia 481
Gios, Lorenzo 481
Goddard, Erin 182
Gómez, Vicenç 3
Graziano, Francesca 270

P. Bruno et al. (Eds.): HC_AIxIA_HYDRA 2025, CCIS 2830, pp. 523–525, 2026.
https://doi.org/10.1007/978-3-032-16708-8

Graziano, Mariangela 257
Grzegorczyk, Marco 167
Gullo, Francesco 510
Güner, Oktay Ozan 3

H
Hommersom, Arjen 369

I
Iacopino, Davide 296
Ielo, Emanuele 64
Iiritano, Salvatore 296
Imoussaten, Abdelhak 196
Inoue, Katsumi 120

J
Jouen, François 138
Jouhet, Vianney 120

K
Knecht, Stefan 21
Kraiselburd, Ivana 243

L
Laboccetta, Luca 296
Landowska, Anna 132
Landowski, Marek 132
Leonardi, Giorgio 78, 152
Linzmeier, Luise 497
Locatelli, Marco 369

M
Maggio, Emilia 99
Magnini, Matteo 429
Magnolini, Simone 429
Mannocci, Lorenzo 50
Maratea, Marco 412
Maria, Marta 296
Marte, Cinzia 412
Megliola, Lorenzo 64
Meli, Daniele 99
Menon, David K. 270
Meyer, Folker 243
Mochi, Marco 412
Monreale, Anna 50
Montagna, Sara 429
Montanari, Angelo 467
Montani, Stefania 152
Montmain, Jacky 196
Mougin, Fleur 120
Mulye, Mihir 21
Muraro, Nicola 384

N
Naretto, Francesca 50
Neri, Luca 283
Netti, Vincenzo 384
Nicoletti, Anna Elena 481

O
Ojutkangas, Alexander J. O. 398

P
Pardini, Susanna 481
Passaro, Lucia 50
Paul, Rinu Elizabeth 323
Perrey, Stéphane 196
Perri, Simona 218, 296
Pirola, Federico 126, 167
Pirrone, Roberto 257
Polimeni, Alberto 93
Portinale, Luigi 78
Provetti, Alessandro 510

Q
Quarta, Alessandro 93
Quarta, Rossella 93

R
Rambaud, Philippe 138
Rebora, Paola 270
Rimmel, Arpad 138
Rizzante, Elisa 467
Rizzi, Silvia 481
Ruffolo, Massimiliano 296

S
Saccomanno, Nicola 467
Salvador, Andrea 467
Sanna, Leonardo 429, 441, 481
Santomauro, Andrea 78
Saxer, Jasmin 497
Schmidt, Tina 243
Schoth, Jens 243
Schultz, Tanja 323
Segal, Avi 336
Segala, Marina 384
Signoret, Emmanuelle Motte 138

Siragusa, Irene 257
Sirocchi, Christel 105
Sorichetti, Filippo 64
Stella, Fabio 167, 270, 283, 352, 369
Steyerberg, Ewout W. 270
Stockinger, Kurt 497
Striani, Manuel 152

T
Terracina, Giorgio 296
Tomasik, Joanna 138
Trabelsi, Imen 138

V
Valer, Giovanni 384
Verda, Damiano 105

W
Weiler, Andreas 497
Wodecki, Alexandra 138

X
Xodo, Serena 467
Xu, Binbin 196

Z
Zanga, Alessio 126, 270
Zermano, Silvia 467
Ziletti, Angelo 231
Zini, Justine 138

The manufacturer's authorised representative in the EU is Springer Nature Customer Service Centre GmbH, Europaplatz 3, 69115 Heidelberg, Germany. If you have any concerns regarding our products, please contact ProductSafety@springernature.com

Printed and bound by CPI Group (UK) Ltd, Croydon, CR0 4YY
07/07/2026
02160906-0014